Saunders

Review of Practical Nursing for NCLEX-PN

Saunders

Review of Practical Nursing for NCLEX-PN

2nd Edition

Esther Matassarin-Jacobs, Ph.D., R.N., O.C.N.
Associate Professor
Loyola University of Chicago
Chicago, Illinois

Consulting Editor
Diana I. Bubb, M.S.N., R.N.

W.B. SAUNDERS COMPANY
A Division of Harcourt Brace & Company
Philadelphia • London • Toronto • Montreal • Sydney • Tokyo

W.B. SAUNDERS COMPANY
A Division of
Harcourt Brace & Company

The Curtis Center
Independence Square West
Philadelphia, PA 19106

Library of Congress Cataloging-in-Publication Data

Matassarin-Jacobs, Esther.
    Saunders review of practical nursing for NCLEX-PN / Esther
Matassarin-Jacobs; consulting editor, Diana Bubb. — 2nd ed.
        p.   cm.
    Includes bibliographical references and index.
    ISBN 0-7216-3694-2
    1. Practical nursing—Examinations, questions, etc.   2. Practical
nursing—Outlines, syllabi, etc.   I. Bubb, Diana I.   II. Title.
[DNLM: 1. Licensure, Nursing—United States—examination
questions.   2. Nursing, Practical—examination questions.   WY   18
M4245s]
RT62.M38   1992
610.73'069'3076—dc20
DNLM/DLC   91-25279

Editor: Ilze Rader
Designer: Terri Siegel
Cover Designer: Charles Smith
Production Manager: Ken Neimeister
Manuscript Editor: Judith Redding
Illustration Specialist: Lisa Lambert
Indexer: Mary Chris Lindsay

SAUNDERS REVIEW OF PRACTICAL NURSING FOR NCLEX-PN
Second Edition   ISBN   0–7216–3694–2

This is dedicated to my husband, Philip B. Jacobs, who helps me in so many ways. I know I would never have been able to do any of this without you.

This is also dedicated to my parents, F.W. Matassarin, MD, and Grace Matassarin, RN. You two got me started. Thank you.

Contributors

Sandra Benson, R.N.
Instructor, Blount County LPN Program, Maryville, TN

Beulah Bloodworth, R.N.
Chairman, Practical Nursing Department, Foothills Vocational-Technical School, Searcy, Arkansas

Diane M. Chudomelka, B.S.N., M.S.Ed., R.N.
Instructor, Maternity Nursing, Waynesville School of Practical Nursing, Waynesville, Missouri

Jody A. Eckler, B.S.N., R.N.
Instructor, Sandusky School of Practical Nursing, Sandusky, Ohio

Judy M. Fair, M.Ed., R.N.
Instructor, Sandusky School of Practical Nursing, Sandusky, Ohio

Sally Winckler Flesch, M.A., R.N.
Chairperson, Practical Nursing Program, Black Hawk College, Moline, Illinois

T. Jan Woods, M.S.N., R.N.
Instructor, Aiken Technical College, Aiken, South Carolina

Reviewers

Susan Dickey, M.S.N., R.N.C.
Temple University, Philadelphia, Pennsylvania

Ruth Hall, M.A., R.N.
Augusta Technical Institute, Augusta, Georgia

Marjorie T. Livengood, M.Ed., R.N.
Athens Area Technical Institute, Athens, Georgia

Ruth Nicholson, B.S., R.N.
Iona College, Seton School, Yonkers, New York

Mary Patricia Norrell, B.S.N., R.N.C.
Indiana Vocational Technical College, Columbus, Indiana

Sandra Scherb, R.N.
Dakota County Technical College, Rosemount, Minnesota

Ruth A. Stagg, B.S.N., R.N.
T.H. Harris Technical Institute, Opelousas, Louisiana

Sandra D. Thompson, B.A., R.N.
Mercer County Technical Education Center, Princeton, West Virginia

Judith G. Winterhalter, D.N.Sc., R.N.
North Penn Counseling Center, Lansdale, Pennsylvania

Marietta G. Wood, R.N.
Mercer County Technical Education Center, Princeton, West Virginia

Frances Yankowski, R.N.
Albany-Schoharie-Schenectady BOCES, Albany, New York

Judith M. Young, M.S.N., R.N.
Upper Bucks County Area Vocational-Technical School, Perkasie, Pennsylvania

Preface

This is the second edition of a review book that has helped many PN graduates pass the NCLEX-PN and become licensed.

In 1990, the examination format was changed to a totally integrated approach based on the four-part nursing process and the four-part area of patient needs classification. This seemed confusing to students used to the old model, which was divided into categories such as medical nursing and surgical nursing. I have designed this text to help the PN candidate cope with these changes. Also, the expanded review content and questions sections in this edition will help you evaluate your learning needs. Although no book can replace your education, this text can help you tie it all together so that you can be successful in taking the NCLEX-PN.

As with the first edition, I have drawn considerably from practical nursing faculties throughout the country. They have helped me identify the needs of the PN graduates and determine how a review text could help them.

The National Council of State Boards of Nursing sets the standards, puts the examination together after it is written by PN faculty and supervisors, and validates the examination. The Council is actively involved in researching and constantly updating the examination. Since nursing and health care is in a state of constant flux, so is the examination. In the near future, the examination may be computerized, though this will not change the content or what you need to do to pass. You must demonstrate that you have the minimal competency to practice practical nursing.

I wish you well in your goal, licensure as a practical nurse. With hard work and proper preparation, you will be successful.

ESTHER MATASSARIN-JACOBS
Chicago, Illinois

Contents

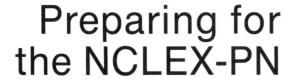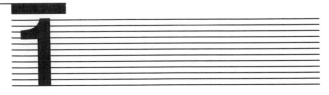

Preparing for the NCLEX-PN

Part 1
Preparing for the Test

The NCLEX-PN is a two-part examination of approximately 240 questions total. You will be given 2 hours in the morning to complete the first half of the examination, and 2 hours in the afternoon to complete the second half. You will have only about 1 minute to answer each question. Time constraint can be one of the most difficult things for you to handle in the testing situation. Suggestions are given in Chapter 2 on how to handle this potential problem.

The examination is composed of 240 single, multiple-choice items. "Single" means that for each question, there are only four single choices. This type of question tests your knowledge without unnecessarily confusing you, as the older multiple-multiple choice questions often did. You answer these questions directly on the test booklet by marking the circle next to the correct answer. You can get practice reading this type of question and marking the answer in the practice tests at the beginning and end of this review text.

There is no penalty for guessing on this examination, but be careful not to start "wild guessing." If you guess, make it an educated guess by eliminating one or two of the possible responses. This can double your chances of being correct.

The passing score for this test is set at the level of minimal competency for a safe, effective practical nurse. The score is referred to as criterion-referenced. The National Council of State Boards of Nursing sets this passing score, and each state is given the option of either accepting this score or choosing one of its own. At the present time, all states have chosen to use the National Council score. After you have taken the examination and it has been scored, you will receive a letter stating either PASS or FAIL. If you do not pass, you will receive feedback on your areas of weakness. This will help you to prepare if you have to retake the examination. Hints for retaking the examination are included in Part 2 of Chapter 2.

You should begin to prepare for the examination well in advance of the test date (listed in the Appendix). The best preparation is the course of study you have taken to prepare you as a practical nurse; nothing can replace that. If you were successful in your course of study, with proper and adequate preparation you should be able to successfully complete the NCLEX-PN. Your notes and your textbook can provide you with a great deal of material for your preparation. This review text can help you to organize and focus your study.

Part 2
Using This Text

This text is designed to help you approach your preparation in a systematic and logical manner. By carefully identifying the specific areas you know less about, you can target them for more review and improve your chances for success on the NCLEX-PN.

How should you use this text to help you prepare for the NCLEX-PN? One of the first steps you should take is to read the next section of this chapter. Part 3 tells you about the NCLEX-PN itself, how it is organized, the number of questions it contains, and the type of material included in this examination. This knowledge should improve your self-confidence when you finally see the examination of the test.

Of course, a simple list of the material to be covered is not the only thing you will need. Chapter 2 is directed at helping you improve your test-taking skills. By learning better ways of taking multiple-choice tests, you can improve your testing ability. Many people needlessly lose points because they are not "test-wise." Application of the information in Chapter 2 can help you avoid such pitfalls.

This review text, with proper use, can help you prepare for the examination. There are at least two ways to use the review material. First, you can simply review the sections containing material that you feel uncomfortable with. In this way, if you have already identified your own learning deficits, you can progress quickly through the material. The problem with this method is that most people either try to go through everything or spend unnecessary time reviewing material they have already mastered. Sometimes, it is hard to identify what you do not know.

In the other way to use this text, start by taking one of the practice examinations at the beginning of the text. You don't even have to take the whole test at once. Start with about 10 questions or two situations. Look up the answers and rationales, and identify the content included in any of the questions you missed and those that you got correct. Write this down and do another 10 or so questions, following the same pattern. By the time you have taken the practice test of about 120 to 125 questions, you will have a good list of the areas that you know and those that require more study. You should then spend your time on the areas

that you do not know, saving the areas you are familiar with until the end for a quick review. There are four practice tests included in this book, so you can use the two at the beginning of the book in this way and still have two to practice with, simulating an actual test situation.

Each section of content also has questions following it. You can use these as either pretests or post-tests. When you answer these questions, go back and review the material covered in the questions you missed. Always focus on the areas you do not know, and briefly review the areas of content you are most familiar with.

When you feel that you are prepared, you can take one of the practice tests as though it was the actual test. Set an alarm clock for 2 hours and try to take the test within the time limit. When you are finished, check your answers carefully, reading all the rationales, and write down those areas that are still giving you trouble. Go back and study those areas. You have four practice tests with questions similar to the actual test, and you have practice questions at the end of each chapter to help you study. Success in the practice tests can also be a great confidence builder. When you see how much you know, you will feel better able to handle the material that you do not know as well.

No review text can teach you everything you should have learned in your practical nursing program. If you find an area that you really do not understand and if the review book does not provide enough information, go back to your textbooks or class notes to cover that area in greater detail. Remember, this is just a review text; if used as such, it can help you be successful on the NCLEX-PN.

Part 3
Format of the NCLEX-PN

GENERAL DESCRIPTION

The NCLEX-PN is a 1-day examination designed by the National Council of State Boards of Nursing (NCSBN) to test the graduate's ability to practice practical nursing in a safe and effective manner. The graduate's knowledge of practical nursing is tested through the application of that knowledge to health care situations requiring practical nursing interventions. The contents of the examination were based on a study that analyzed the activities performed by practical nurses. This study produced a competency

model of entry-level practical nursing. The test plan was then derived from this competency model. Your course in practical nursing should have adequately prepared you to succeed in the examination and in the role of the practical nurse.

The examination consists of two separate examinations, with a total of 240 questions divided into the two books. These examinations are given during 1 day, with one book, or approximately half of the examination, in the morning 2-hour session, and one equal book in an afternoon 2-hour session. The questions are written by both faculty members who teach practical nursing and clinical practitioners from a wide variety of practice settings who supervise new graduates in practical nursing. The examination is given twice yearly, in April and October. The dates for the next few years can be found in the Appendix. The examination is graded on a PASS–FAIL basis. A PASS level is set by the NCSBN using criteria of minimal competence. Your goal will be to do as well as possible to demonstrate your mastery of the required knowledge.

TEST PLAN

The test plan is composed of two main areas: (1) phases of the nursing process, and (2) categories of client needs. Different percentages of the questions apply to these areas. In order to help you prepare for these questions, knowledge of what is included in these areas is useful.

Phases of the Nursing Process

The practical nurse assists in patient assessments, contributes to the planning of care, performs basic and therapeutic nursing interventions, and helps evaluate the outcomes of this nursing care. The beginning practitioner may assume a more dependent role in the planning and evaluation phases but should be fairly independent in assessing patients and implementing care.

Assessment (Collecting Data—30% of the Questions)—Code I

The practical nurse contributes to the devlopment of a database about clients by (1) observing physiologic, psychosocial, health, and safety needs of clients; (2) collecting information from the client, significant others, health team members, and records; (3) determining the need for more information; and (4) communicating findings of the data collected. The practical nurse also participates in the formulation of nursing diagnoses.

Planning (20% of the Questions)—Code II

The practical nurse contributes to the development of nursing care plans by (1) assisting in formulation of goals; (2) participating in identification of clients' needs and nursing measures required to achieve goals; (3) communicating needs that may require alteration of the care plan; and (4) communicating with the client, significant others, or health team members in planning nursing care.

Implementation (30% of the Questions)—Code III

The practical nurse implements care by (1) performing basic therapeutic and preventive nursing measures by following prescribed plan of care to achieve established client goals; (2) providing a safe and effective environment; (3) assisting the client, significant others, and health team members to understand client's plan of care; and (4) recording client information and reporting it to other health team members.

Evaluation (20% of the Questions)—Code IV

The practical nurse evaluates care by (1) participating in evaluating the effectiveness of the client's nursing care; (2) assisting in evaluating the client's response to nursing care and in making appropriate alterations; (3) evaluating the extent to which identified outcomes of the care plan are achieved; and (4) recording and describing the client's response to therapy or care.

Categories of Client Needs

In order to structure the health needs of individuals, the NCSBN, based on the results of its job analysis survey, identified four categories of client needs that the practical nurse addresses. These categories, rather than traditional subject matter areas, are the means by which the test is divided. Under each of these areas, specific nursing content is identified (NCSBN, 1989).

Safe, Effective Care Environment (24%–30% of the Questions)—Code 1

A safe, effective care environment includes the *basic* knowledge, skills, and abilities that include, but are not limited to, data-gathering techniques; interpersonal communication skills; alternative methods of communication for clients with special needs; preparation for prescribed treatments and procedures; providing safe and effective treatments and procedures for the patient; environmental and client safety; infection control, including signs and symptoms of infection; client rights, both legal and ethical; confidentiality; individualization of care, including religious, cultural, and developmental influences; team participation in care planning and evaluation; and general knowledge of community planning.

Physiologic Integrity (42%–48% of the Questions)—Code 2

Physiologic integrity includes the *basic* knowledge, skills, and abilities that include, but are not limited to, providing for physiologic adaptation of the patient; therapeutic and life-saving procedures; specialized equipment; principles of administering medications, including both expected and unexpected effects of medication; maintenance of optimal body functioning and prevention of complications; principles of body mechanics and assistive devices; comfort measures; reduction of risk potential; basic physical assessment skills; side effects of chemotherapy and radiation therapy; maintaining intact skin; providing for mobility and preventing its hazards; performing basic nursing measures; and reporting changes in a client's condition.

Psychosocial Integrity (7%–13% of the Questions)—Code 3

Psychosocial integrity includes the *basic* knowledge, skills, and abilities that include, but are not limited to, obvious signs of emotional and mental health problems; self-concept; life crises; chemical dependency; coping and adaptation; self-destructive behavior; sensory deprivation and overload; adaptive and maladaptive behavior; therapeutic communication; common therapies; and general knowledge of community resources.

Health Promotion and Maintenance (15%–21% of the Questions)—Code 4

Health promotion and maintenance includes the *basic* knowledge, skills, and abilities that include, but are not limited to, family interactions; concepts of wellness; adaptations to altered health states; reproduction and human sexuality; birthing and parenting; continued growth and development, including normal maternity nursing care; encouraging self-care; diet modification; death and dying; integrity of support systems; prevention and early treatment of disease; immunization; health teaching that is appropriate to the scope of practice; and general knowledge of community resources.

Although this test plan may seem somewhat complicated, it is important for the practical nurse candidate to be familiar with it so that preparation for the examination can be systematic and complete. By becoming familiar with the areas tested, the graduate can be ready for the examination.

Categories of Human Functioning

These content divisions are not imposed by the NCSBN but are given so that you can group the content into functional areas. This is how the content is divided within most chapters of this text, and the test items will be labeled this way so that you can find the content areas of your weakness more easily.

Growth and Development—Code A

This includes content on normal growth and development of children and adults, sexuality, reproductive disorders in both men and women, maturation throughout the life span, child bearing, and child rearing.

Oxygenation—Code B

This includes the body's ability to maintain fluid balance and to transport oxygen and other gases; fluid and electrolyte balance; acid–base balance; cardiopulmonary disorders; cardiopulmonary resuscitation (CPR); anemias; hemorrhagic disorders; and leukemia and lymphomas.

Sensory/Perceptual Alterations—Code C

This includes the ability to perceive, interpret, and respond to sensory and cognitive data; hearing, vision, and speech disorders; sensory deprivation or overload; cerebral and central nervous system (CNS) disorders; brain tumors; seizures; laryngectomy; organic brain syndrome; degenerative neurologic disorders; and learning disabilities.

Protective Functions—Code D

This includes physiologic defenses; prevention of trauma, infection, and threats to health; communicable diseases; sexually transmitted diseases; immunity; basic cancer and therapies; trauma; physical abuse; skin disorders; asepsis; safety hazards; poisoning; and surgical intervention.

Mobility/Activity/Comfort—Code E

This includes hazards of immobility, musculoskeletal disorders, fractures, and degenerative disorders.

Metabolism/Elimination—Code F

This includes the intake and utilization of essential nutrients, normal and therapeutic nutrition, diet in pregnancy and lactation, obesity, diabetes, gastric and metabolic disorders, the body's ability to remove waste products, endocrine disorders, gastrointestinal disorders, ulcers, hernias, neoplasms, liver disease, renal disorders, and prostatic disorders.

Psycho-Social-Cultural Functions—Code G

This includes the ability to function in intrapersonal, interpersonal, group and social–cultural relationships; loss and grieving; psychotic and neurotic behaviors; therapeutic communication; group dynamics; ethical–legal aspects; community resources; spiritual needs; situational crises; and substance abuse.

BIBLIOGRAPHY

National Council of State Boards of Nursing. (1989). *NCLEX-PN: Test Plan for the National Council Licensure Examination for Practical Nurses*. Chicago.

Improving Your Ability to Pass the Examination

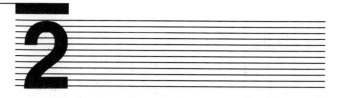

Part 1
Test-Taking Strategies

How do you successfully take a multiple-choice examination? The answer to this question is fairly long, but as your understanding of multiple-choice test items increases, so do your chances for successfully answering them. Hints and strategies can be learned to improve your ability to answer multiple-choice questions.

First, the most important point is to focus on *reading* and understanding the question. Reading may seem like a simple matter, but most mistakes are made because the test taker does not read the question carefully and completely. Along with reading the question, it is vital that you carefully read each response that follows the "stem" of the question. Test takers often read quickly and chose the first response that looks good; sometimes they do not even read all the possible responses.

When you read the question, pay close attention to any specific information within the question that can direct you to the correct answer. Sometimes the stem will contain statements such as "your first action," "which would be appropriate," "an inappropriate intervention for this patient," "all except," "an important assessment," "the best goal," and "the most appropriate response." Phrases such as these can focus the area of your response. If the question asks for a priority action, it means that all the responses might be correct, but you have to chose the first priority.

For example:

Unsuccessful adaptation to the middle years would be characterized by:
1. *Reassessment of role within the home*
2. *Achievement of career goals*
3. *Increased involvement in community activities*
4. *Acceptance of retirement*

A question such as this, which looks for the one thing that does not fit, can be easy to answer. The best way to approach it is to treat each response as a "true-false" question. In this question, look at each response. #1 is true: middle years is a time to reassess the roles within the family. #2 is true: it is a time when most adults achieve their career goals. #3 is also true: it is a time when adults focus more on their role in the community. #4 in this case is false and the correct answer for this question. The middle years is not a time of accepting retirement, only the beginning preparation for it. By focusing on the important part of the question—"unsuccessful"—and treating each response as a separate question, you should be able to find the one false response. This method is appropriate when the question contains a negative such as "least" or "inappropriate." Even if you can narrow down the possibilities to two responses, you have doubled your chances of guessing correctly.

Time control is another important factor. You will have only about 1 minute per question. Answering in this time is another skill that can be learned. Take one of the practice tests and block out 10 items. Set an alarm clock for 10 minutes and begin. Doing this several times will help to improve your speed. During the actual test situation, you can do two important things to help improve your speed. First, take a watch and set limits and checks for yourself, such as deciding that by $\frac{1}{2}$ hour you should be on at least question #30. If you are not, then you must speed up. Do not wait until the end to notice that you are behind. The other thing to do is to omit the very difficult items and come back to them at the end, or simply guess at the answer. If an item is taking you more than 1 minute, go on.

Understanding the focus of the question can also help direct your response to it. The focus of the question can be the phases of the nursing process. For instance, a question that asks for an assessment requires an answer that provides more data. One that asks for a plan requires you to focus on the specific problem addressed and find a measurable, realistic goal. Another major area of focus is the categories of client functioning. To give you some ideas on questions from both these categories, an example of each, along with an analysis, follows.

To assist with your understanding of the your learning needs, a code is included after each answer. The code is as follows:

I, II, III, or IV for the phase of the nursing process
1, 2, 3, or 4 for the category of client needs
A, B, C, D, E, F, or G for the category of human functioning
Specific content category by name; ie, cholecystectomy

PHASES OF THE NURSING PROCESS

Assessment (Collecting Data) (I)

Which of the following observations should the practical nurse make when the client returns from having a long leg cast applied to a newly broken tibia?
  1. Circulation and sensation proximal to the cast
  2. Temperature of the cast
  3. Capillary refill of the toes
  4. Presence of Homans' sign in the opposite leg

This item focuses on assessment. The correct answer is #3; the most important assessment for the nurse to make is the circulation and sensation distal to the cast. #1 is incorrect because it states "proximal." #2 is not important on a fresh cast, because "hot" spots of infection would not appear this soon and because casts become warm with drying. #4 is an important assessment at any time, but a fresh-fracture client would probably not have developed a thrombophlebitis yet. At the end of the rationales in this text you will see the following code: I, 2, E. Fractures/ Casts. This tells you exactly what was tested, so you can refer to those areas when studying.

Planning (II)

Which of the following is an appropriate goal for a primipara on her first postpartum day? Mother will be able to:
  1. Bathe infant without help
  2. Provide complete care of newborn
  3. Hold and interact with newborn
  4. Feed newborn without assistance

This question asks the nurse to set an achievable goal for a new mother with her first baby. #1, #2, and #4 are probably unrealistic goals for a new mother on the first day after birth. #3 is not only realistic, it is the most desirable goal, because mother–infant bonding is one of the most important goals to achieve. II, 4, A. Postpartal Care.

Implementation (III)

You have difficulty inserting the rectal catheter for an enema. Your best action is to:
  1. Wait a few minutes for the lubricant to take effect
  2. Tell the client to calm down
  3. Wait a few seconds until the sphincter relaxes, then proceed
  4. Chart that you were unable to give the enema

The best answer for this is #3. The nurse knows that temporarily waiting often allows the sphincter to relax. The other answers are not appropriate actions. III, 2, F. Lower GI.

Evaluation (IV)

Which of the following would indicate successful learning by your client, who you have been teaching an 1800 calorie diabetic diet?
  1. Patient eats all food on tray
  2. Patient states understanding of diet
  3. Patient's wife understands dietary restrictions
  4. Patient correctly marks menu for 1800 calorie ADA diet

In order to evaluate learning, the practical nurse must have measurable data. The only answer that provides this is #4. #1 does not reflect learning. #2 is not measurable; how do you know the patient understands? #3 is also not measurable and does not address the client directly. IV, 4, F. Diabetes Mellitus.

CATEGORIES OF CLIENT NEEDS

Safe, Effective Care Environment (1)

The patient at greatest risk for postoperative bleeding would be an arthritic who has been taking:
  1. Aspirin
  2. Maalox
  3. Prednisone
  4. Acetaminophen

This item focuses on patient safety and expected outcomes of treatment. In order to answer it, you need some knowledge of drug side effects. #1 is the answer, because aspirin has an anticoagulant effect on the blood and could predispose postoperative bleeding. A question like this could be followed with one or two related questions, such as "Precautions to take to decrease the risk of bleeding include," or "In order to prevent the bleeding risk in the above question, the nurse should." Questions often come in a series, so it important to be sure of your first answer and then follow along that same line to answer them all correctly. I, 1, D. Surgery.

Physiologic Integrity (2)

Mr. Wilson is admitted with COPD. He tells you that his breathing treatments leave him unable to eat because of all the mucus he brings up. To decrease his anorexia and improve his nutritional intake, the practical nurse should:
  1. *Suggest he have the treatments right after meals*
  2. *Administer frequent mouth care, especially before meals*
  3. *Request a change to a liquid diet*
  4. *Ask the physician about starting hyperalimentation*

This item focuses on a physiologic need for adequate nutrition and an expected result of treatment. #1 makes no sense, because it is likely to increase vomiting. #3 and #4 take away the normal diet, an important part of preventing debilitation in the chronically ill patient. Only #2 would be appropriate for this client. This question offers an example of a situation in which the test taker often wants another answer:

  5. *Schedule the treatments between meals*

This can be frustrating, because the answer you want isn't there. Forget it and go with the best answer there. You are not allowed to write in your choice! IV, 2, B. COPD.

Psychosocial Integrity (3)

Mary had a very bad day at work and is very angry with her supervisor. When she comes home from work, she punishes her daughter by grounding her for a week for not taking out the trash. This is an example of what defense mechanism?
  1. *Projection*
  2. *Denial*
  3. *Displacement*
  4. *Sublimation*

This is a fairly simple, comprehension level question. You should be able to recognize the description of #3, displacement. The items from this section test your knowledge of the mental health concepts, which make up the smallest percentage of questions on the test. The other responses are other defense mechanisms. I, 3, G. Defense Mechanisms.

Health Promotion and Maintenance (4)

Discharge instructions for Mr. Wilson, who has COPD, should not *include which of the following?*
  1. *Smoking cessation*
  2. *Avoidance of temperature extremes*
  3. *Avoidance of industrial air pollution*
  4. *Avoidance of humidified air*

This item asks for the one thing you would *not* teach Mr. Wilson about health promotion. Using the true-false approach, #1 and #3 are easily apparent as being true. Again, if you do not know at this point, guess. Looking at the other two, we know that the COPD client has thick tenacious sputum, so humidity should help, making #4 the false answer that is the correct answer in this case. Do not make the mistake of reading too fast and missing "avoidance." III, 4, D. COPD.

Another common mistake that test takers often make is changing their first answer. Many people continue to mentally rehash a question and convince themselves that there is a hidden meaning or some trick. There are no "trick" questions on this examination, and the items have been examined closely to make sure that there are no hidden meanings. It is rarely correct to change an answer. The odds of changing it to a correct response are very low, your first instinct usually being correct. Change an answer *only* if you have truly seen some missed information or suddenly remembered an important fact. Otherwise, leave that eraser alone. Also, changing answers undermines your confidence, and you start to change more and more as you panic. You should stop, take a deep breath, and go on without changing answers.

Your state of mind is another important factor. Many people have "test anxiety." This means that the simple thought of the test makes you tense and you are liable to freeze up or become very nervous during a test. If you have test anxiety, there are a number of things you can do ahead of time to prepare. First, practice some sort of relaxation exercises, such as those you teach mothers during childbirth. Practice those slow deep breaths and imagine yourself blowing away all your tension. If you become comfortable with this before the test, it can be very useful during the test. Practice this technique when you take the practice tests in this book.

People also tend to experience anger and frustration over certain test items, a feeling guaranteed to break their concentration. If you find this happening because you think an item is dumb or the situation unlikely to happen in nursing, laugh, do not get angry. Put the emotion away until after the test. Anger and frustration occur when the response you want is not listed. Don't let them. Your only choices are those listed, so chose the best one.

Another tension breaker is *not* studying the night before the examination or between your morning and afternoon sessions. It is a terrible temptation to do so, but it will not help. It will only increase your anxiety. Also, avoid talking about the questions with other test takers between tests. This also increases your tension and fears. Put the first test out of your mind and focus

your thoughts on doing well on the second test. Keep imagining yourself as having successfully completed the test and as a successful practical nurse.

Should you guess at answers? Yes, but make educated guesses. It means first try to decrease the number of possible responses. With four responses, you have a 1 in 4, or 25% chance at a correct answer. With three responses, you have a 1 in 3, or 33% chance; reducing the possible responses to two gives you a 50% chance of guessing correctly. Even on very difficult items, taking a little time to eliminate even one answer improves your odds. Do not just wild guess recklessly. This can decrease your confidence. When you reach a dilemma—is it #1 or #3—guess and go on. Do not spend time going back and forth between the two. Simply chose one, go on, and forget it!

These tips should improve your test-taking skills; combined with a proper planned review, they should help you do better on the licensure examination and achieve your goal.

Part 2
Hints for Retaking the Examination

What if you are not taking the test for the first time? The advice in this text applies to you especially. You must first decide why you did not pass the first time. Some of the suggestions above may help you if it was anxiety or lack of time that contributed to your failure. You need to look at your performance as honestly as you can. You must identify your areas of weakness so that you can change them and be successful at the next testing.

When you fail the examination, the National Council will send you a diagnostic profile showing you what your weaknesses were. This profile will first tell you approximately how close to passing you were. The ranges given are 12 or fewer items; 13–24 items; 25–36 items; or 37 or more items. If you were close, then a little more effort should lead to success. The other information given is the proximity you were to the reference point in the "Phases of the Nursing Process" and the "Categories of Client Needs." If you do well in all but one area, then focus on that area for your next attempt. An index in the front of each practice test divides the questions by categories to help you practice to retake the examination.

You need to be very honest with yourself about your reasons for not passing. Ask yourself if you truly studied for the examination. If you did not have a

regular program of preparation, that is exactly what you need to establish now. Prepare, and you will stand a much better chance of passing.

If you had a weakness in school, such as maternity nursing, and your lowest performance seemed to be in the area of "Health Promotion/Maintenance," then focus heavily on maternity nursing for the next examination. If you are a poor test taker, then use the suggestions in this book and practice your test-taking skills.

If you are lost as to what your weaknesses were, take the first two practice tests in this text. When you have finished, look up the answers and write down exactly what you were missing. This will then be the focus of your study.

You can also use some of the questions at the end of each chapter as pretests. That means that you answer these questions before studying the chapter to see if you already know the material. If you do well on this test, that content is less important to study; focus first on the areas you cannot answer questions on.

Will these suggestions help you pass next time? If you follow the guidelines in this text and study hard for the examination, you should be successful. Do not give up on yourself. With hard work and preparation, you can achieve your goal, becoming a licensed practical nurse.

Practice Test

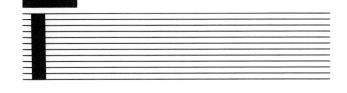

Questions

John, age 63 years, is married and has two children, ages 16 and 19 years. He is a Type I diabetic but has not followed the diabetic regimen prescribed by his physician: that is, diet, weight control, and insulin. On admission to the hospital, he is somewhat lethargic, and the physician believes he may be in early diabetic ketoacidosis. Because he is also incontinent, an indwelling catheter is inserted.

1. The nurse assesses for signs and symptoms of ketoacidosis, which include:

    ① Odor of acetone on breath
    ② Oliguria
    ③ Hypoglycemia
    ④ Absence of acetone in the urine

2. The nurse knows that initial treatment of diabetic ketosis usually includes administration of:

    ① Regular insulin.
    ② Intravenous glucose
    ③ Long-acting insulin
    ④ Intravenous diuretics

3. John is able to give himself insulin, but because he has not been compliant in the past, it might be of value if:

    ① He is given the phone numbers of the health department and nearest hospital
    ② Someone checked his urine daily to be sure he is taking his insulin
    ③ Someone else in his family also learned to give insulin
    ④ The doctor changed him to oral medications

Elaine, age 30 years, has had symptoms of Graves' disease for 4 years. She is admitted to the hospital for surgery.

4. Symptoms of Graves' disease may include:

    ① Weight loss
    ② Decreased energy
    ③ Bradycardia
    ④ Intolerance to cold

5. When admitting Elaine, the nurse's assessment would be most likely reveal:

    ① Swollen ankles
    ② A fine tremor of the hands
    ③ Ascites
    ④ Low blood pressure

6. Elaine's previous medical treatment for Graves' disease may have included:

    ① A low sodium diet
    ② A high sodium diet
    ③ Drugs that block production of thyroid hormones
    ④ Administration of synthetic thyroid hormones

7. Preoperatively, Elaine is given drugs in an attempt to establish a euthyroid state to decrease the risk of postoperative:

    ① Hypothyroidism
    ② Iodine intoxication
    ③ Loss of pituitary activity
    ④ Thyroid crisis

8. Elaine returns from the operating room. Once she is fully awake, the nurse should position the patient:

    ① With head of the bed elevated
    ② Flat in bed
    ③ Turned on her side
    ④ In any position she desires

9. Following surgery, Elaine is observed for symptoms of respiratory obstruction, which would most likely be due to:

    ① Bronchoconstriction owing to decrease in thyroid hormones
    ② Constriction of the airway by the surgical dressing
    ③ Enlargement of the remaining part of the thyroid gland
    ④ Edema in or near the operative area

10. A sudden temperature elevation to 106°F accompanied by restlessness, tachycardia, and delirium, would lead you to suspect:

① Pneumonitis
② Thyroid crisis
③ Atelectasis
④ Hemorrhage

11. Elaine complains of a feeling of fullness in her throat. On inspection, the dressing is dry and intact. Your *next* step is to:

① Check her chart and administer oxygen, if ordered
② Check for drainage on the bedding or pillow behind her neck
③ Call her physician
④ Turn her on her side and slightly hyperextend her head.

Mr. Ford, age 67 years, is admitted to the hospital for surgical treatment of benign prostatic hypertrophy.

12. Typical early symptoms of benign prostatic hypertrophy include:

① Burning and pain on urination
② Narrowing of the urinary stream and urinary frequency
③ Fever and chills
④ Hematuria

13. The type of prostatic surgery that poses the lowest risk for Mr. Ford is:

① Suprapubic
② Retropubic
③ Perineal
④ Transurethral (TUR)

14. If a TUR is done, Mr. Ford has a three-way Foley catheter inserted for continuous irrigation in order to:

① Prevent clots from obstructing the catheter
② Reduce the possibility of postoperative bladder infection
③ Control his pain
④ Monitor his intake

15. The nurse assesses that Mr. Ford's Foley catheter is not draining urine. Which of the following nursing actions is appropriate?

① Increase the rate of the irrigation
② Irrigate the catheter with 30 mL sterile saline solution

③ Notify the physician
④ Increase oral intake

Mrs. Martin, a 32-year-old homemaker with a 3-year-old child, had been trying to get pregnant for several months. She has been troubled with spotting between periods and excessive bleeding at menstruation. She consulted her physician, who performed a pelvic examination and a Pap smear. The result of her Pap smear was Class V. Mrs. Martin was admitted to the hospital and scheduled for insertion of a radioactive vaginal implant of cesium, to be followed in 1 week with a total abdominal hysterectomy and bilateral salpingo-oophorectomy.

16. A soapsuds enema was ordered prior to the procedure. The most important reason for this procedure is to:

① Prevent the patient from contaminating the operative field
② Provide comfort
③ Prevent constipation and straining to defecate
④ Prevent the rectum from becoming distended with feces and shifting into the path of radioactive rays

17. A Foley catheter was inserted. The chief reason for using an indwelling catheter in this patient is to:

① Prevent the patient from contaminating the packing in her vagina
② Prevent the bladder from becoming distended with urine and shifting into the path of the radioactive rays
③ Keep the bladder collapsed for the comfort of the patient
④ Prevent cystitis from frequent catheterizations

18. While the implant is in place, Mrs. Martin's nursing care will likely include:

① Maintaining a fully liquid diet
② Frequent perineal care
③ A cleansing enema prn to prevent constipation
④ Maintaining the head of the bed at 0 to 30 degrees

19. The following nursing interventions should be included on Mrs. Martin's nursing care plan *except*:

① Limit visitors to those over 18 years of age
② No pregnant visitors

③   Visits limited to the amount of time determined by the radiologist

④   No visitors allowed at this time

The implant is removed by the doctor, and Mrs. Martin is being prepared for surgery. When passing her room, the nurse hears her crying, enters the room, and sits beside her bed. Mrs. Martin says, "I wanted another baby so badly, and now I will never have another child."

20.   Which of the following statements by the nurse would be most helpful to Mrs. Martin?

①   "It is all right to cry. I understand it must be difficult to know you will never be able to have another child. I'll sit here with you for awhile, if you wish."

②   "No, you won't be able to have another child, but you can always adopt a child."

③   "Maybe you should talk to your doctor about postponing surgery until you have another child."

④   "At least you were lucky enough to have one child before the surgery."

21.   On her fifth postoperative day, Mrs. Martin complains of burning and itching of her perineal area and notices white, lumpy vaginal discharge. The nurse realizes that this is probably due to:

①   Delayed response to irritation from the vaginal implant

②   Associated infection from the Foley catheter

③   Suppression of normal vaginal flora by the postoperative prophylactic antibiotic therapy.

④   Irritation from wearing a perineal pad against the shaved area

Lee Anne had been noting progressive loss of ability to hear. After testing, she was informed that she had conduction deafness caused by otosclerosis. During the patient information session that followed, Lee Anne's disability and her options for treatment were discussed.

22.   The transmission of sound from the outer to the middle ear occurs in the following sequence:

①   Tympanic membrane, malleus, incus, stapes, oval window

②   Tympanic membrane, incus, malleus, stapes, oval window

③   Tympanic membrane, incus, stapes, malleus, oval window

④   Oval window, stapes, malleus, incus, tympanic membrane

23.   Otosclerosis produces loss of hearing because the:

①   Auditory nerve is permanently damaged

②   External canal of the ear is obstructed

③   Small bones of the middle ear cannot vibrate

④   Auditory nerve is inflamed

24.   Following surgery to correct the otosclerosis, the nurse should caution Lee Anne against blowing her nose suddenly or violently because this could:

①   Rupture the tympanic membrane–malleus junction

②   Decrease pressure in the middle ear and thus interfere with the healing process

③   Increase drainage from the external canal

④   Dislodge the prosthesis

Adam (age 30 years) was admitted to the hospital with a diagnosis of detached retina.

25.   During the assessment, which of the following symptoms would the nurse expect to find:

①   Feeling that a curtain is being drawn over the field of vision

②   Burning and itching of the eyes

③   Sharp, stabbing pain in the affected eye

④   Twitching and feelings of tiredness after doing close work such as reading

26.   Shortly after the admission procedure, Adam asks for assistance to walk to the bathroom. An appropriate response from the nurse would be to:

①   Orient him to his surroundings, lower the bottom side-rails, and give him permission to ambulate to the bathroom whenever necessary

②   Lower the side-rails, dangle the patient, then assist him to the bathroom by walking at his side with his arm through hers

③   Get an assistant and ambulate him with one nurse on each side, supporting him with an arm around his waist

④   Direct him to remain quietly in bed, obtain a bedpan or urinal, and assist him with a minimum of movement to his head

27. Adam becomes restless and is frequently moving his extremities around the bed and turning from side to side. Observing this behavior, which of the following statements by the nurse is most appropriate?

    ① "You should try to lie still for awhile."
    ② "I see that you are getting restless. How can I help you be more comfortable?"
    ③ "Please try to lie still so you don't damage your eye further."
    ④ "Don't move around so much, because if you increase the damage to your eye, you may become completely blind in that eye."

A nurse is working in a well-baby clinic and is responsible for normal growth and development assessments. In order to correctly report abnormalities to the physician, the nurse must have a good knowledge base of normal growth and development milestones.

28. Most infants are able to lift their heads by the age of:

    ① 2 weeks
    ② 2 months
    ③ 3 months
    ④ 1 month

29. At which age does the anterior fontanel close?

    ① 2 weeks of age
    ② 2 to 3 months of age
    ③ 6 months of age
    ④ 15 to 18 months of age

30. At birth, James weighed 7 lb. At his 12-month check-up, the nurse would expect his weight to be approximately:

    ① 14 lb
    ② 21 lb
    ③ 28 lb
    ④ Cannot be determined; weight gain varies widely

31. The child has a complete set of deciduous teeth at the age of:

    ① $1\frac{1}{2}$ years
    ② 2 years
    ③ $2\frac{1}{2}$ to 3 years
    ④ $3\frac{1}{2}$ to 4 years

32. The first permanent teeth appear approximately at age:

    ① $2\frac{1}{2}$ to 3 years
    ② 4 to 5 years
    ③ 6 to 7 years
    ④ 8 to 9 years

Mr. Antonio Rodriguez is to have abdominal surgery and is admitted the day before surgery.

33. The nurse should begin to prepare Mr. Rodriguez for discharge:

    ① When he is admitted
    ② The evening of surgery
    ③ After signs of improvement appear
    ④ During the last 2 days of hospital stay

34. Mr. Rodriguez is to receive the following preoperative medications: Demerol 100 mg at 8 AM IM and atropine g 1/150 at 8 AM IM. You have vials marked Demerol 50 mg/mL and atropine g 1/100 per mL. How much of each drug would you give?

    ① 0.5 mL Demerol and 0.67 mL atropine
    ② 0.5 mL Demerol and 1.5 mL atropine
    ③ 2.0 mL Demerol and 1.5 mL atropine
    ④ 2.0 mL Demerol and 0.67 mL atropine

35. After giving the preoperative medication, the nurse discovers that the operative permit had not been signed. The nurse should:

    ① Have the patient sign the permit before the medication begins to work
    ② Ask a family member to sign the permit
    ③ Sign the permit for the patient because she knows he gave his verbal permission
    ④ Notify the surgeon because surgery cannot now be performed

Mr. Rodriguez eventually goes to surgery, where he receives spinal anesthesia.

36. Mr. Rodriguez returns to his room. Which of the following written orders should the nurse question before carrying out?

    ① Regular diet
    ② Fluids as desired
    ③ Bathroom privileges beginning tomorrow at 8 AM
    ④ Fowler's position for 12 hours

37. Which of the following signs should alert the nurse to the possibility that Mr. Rodriguez may be hemorrhaging?

① Rapid pulse rate
② Labored respirations
③ Below-normal body temperature
④ Increasing blood pressure

38. Mr. Rodriguez demonstrates signs of shock. Which of the following positions is appropriate?

① Face-lying position
② Side-lying position
③ Low-Fowler's position
④ Modified Trendelenburg position

Mr. Rodriguez is to have the surgical dressings changed every 4 hours. In order to perform this procedure, the nurse must understand both medical and surgical asepsis.

39. Medical asepsis is a technique used to:

① Prevent the spread of infection during a surgical procedure
② Eliminate all organisms from any objects coming in contact with a patient
③ Prevent the spread of disease from one person to another
④ Remove bacteria from all objects that come in contact with an open wound

40. Surgical asepsis is based on the principle of:

① Destroying bacteria as they leave the body
② Destroying organisms before they enter the body
③ Isolating all patients who have infectious diseases
④ Basic cleanliness and sanitation

41. The best method of preventing the spread of infection is:

① Isolating all patients suspected of having an infection
② Wearing rubber gloves when performing all nursing procedures for surgical patients
③ Washing the hands thoroughly before and after each contact with a patient
④ Sterilizing the hands with a strong germicide at least once a day

42. Mr. Rodriguez's dressing is least likely to be used to:

① Restrict movement
② Cover a disfigurement
③ Keep microorganisms out of the wound
④ Prevent drainage from leaving the wound

43. When changing a patient's dressing, it is *best* when ventilation in a room can be provided *without*:

① Decreasing humidity
② Creating drafts
③ Using air conditioning
④ Dropping the room temperature

44. Mr. Rodriguez's dressing sticks to the wound when the nurse tries to change it. Which of the following actions is most appropriate?

① Apply petroleum jelly to the wound to prevent further problems
② Moisten the dressing with sterile normal saline
③ Pick up the dressing very slowly with sterile forceps
④ Cut the dressing off in small pieces with a sterile scissors

45. Mr. Rodriguez is to receive dressing changes frequently. His wound is to be cleansed with an antiseptic solution prior to application of the new dressing. Antiseptic solutions are generally used to:

① Stop the growth of bacteria on the skin or mucous membranes
② Destroy bacteria in the air around a wound
③ Disinfect the dressing materials
④ Kill all bacteria in open wounds or sores

46. A nurse is applying an elastic bandage to Mr. Rodriguez's foot, ankle, lower leg, and knee. The nurse should begin bandaging the extremity at the:

① Knee
② Middle of the lower leg
③ Ankle
④ Foot

47. Mr. Rodriguez has an order for a K-pad (thermal or heating pad) to be applied over his dressing. He says that his K-pad is too cool. Which of the following nursing actions is appropriate?

① Call the doctor to have the order changed
② Apply a warmer hot water bottle
③ Return the K-pad and get another one
④ Continue to apply heat with this K-pad

48. Mr. Rodriguez is at risk of infection. Which of the following do all pathogenic microbes need to grow?

   ① Oxygen
   ② Light
   ③ Moisture
   ④ Host

49. Mr. Rodriguez would be at increased risk for infection if he were incontinent of the bowel. The normal flora of the colon include which of the following?

   ① Rickettsiae
   ② *Escherichia coli*
   ③ *Pseudomonas aeruginosa*
   ④ *Streptococcus aureus*

After Mr. Rodriguez's dressing is changed, the equipment used must be once again rendered sterile.

50. When an object is being sterilized by chemical means, it is very important to:

   ① Avoid soaking the object too long
   ② Wash the article thoroughly to remove any blood or mucus before placing it in the chemical
   ③ Use a solution that will not damage living tissue
   ④ Rinse the article under running water before it is placed in the solution

51. Spore-forming bacteria are:

   ① Easily destroyed
   ② Destroyed only by boiling
   ③ Resistant to many methods of sterilization
   ④ Much less dangerous than other types of bacteria

52. The most reliable method used for sterilizing hospital equipment so that it is free of spores and active bacteria is:

   ① Soaking in a strong chemical
   ② Washing and drying it thoroughly after use
   ③ Applying steam under pressure in an autoclave
   ④ Boiling the equipment

53. The nurse changes Mr. Rodriguez's dressing as scheduled on the third postoperative day. She notes signs of inflammation. These may include:

   ① Redness, warmth, swelling

   ② Hemorrhage, pain
   ③ Formation of pus, tissue necrosis
   ④ Bruising, petechiae, ecchymosis

Mr. Rodriguez is diagnosed with a postoperative infection. He has an IV and antibiotic ordered.

54. The physician orders D5W 1000 mL IV to run at 125 mL/h. The IV tubing delivers 12 gtt/mL. What should the drip rate be?

   ① 12 gtt/min
   ② 20.5 gtt/min
   ③ 25 gtt/min
   ④ 200 gtt/min

55. The physician orders ampicillin 250 mg IV every 4 h. Your vial reads "ampicillin 100 mg." The directions on the vial read "Inject 1.2 mL of sterile water to yield 1.5 mL of solution." How much solution will you give Mr. Rodriguez?

   ① 1.5 mL
   ② 1.67 mL
   ③ 3.0 mL
   ④ 3.75 mL

56. Mr. Rodriguez is placed on drainage and secretion precautions. Which of the following actions by the nurse is appropriate?

   ① Using a mask when changing dressings
   ② Entering the room only when giving care
   ③ Placing soiled dressings in a waterproof bag
   ④ Wearing a gown whenever giving care

57. The nurse notes in the doctor's progress notes that there is now an area of necrosis in Mr. Rodriguez's wound. The term necrosis means that:

   ① The tissues have become hardened and useless
   ② The cells of the tissue are dead and in a state of decay
   ③ The tissues are inflamed
   ④ There is a new growth of abnormal cells in the tissue

58. As the nurse changes Mr. Rodriguez's dressing, she notes the surgical wound has separated and internal structures are partially exposed. The nurse should care for the area by:

   ① Exposing the area by leaving it uncovered
   ② Securing a dry dressing over the area

③ Covering the area with sterile gauze moistened with sterile normal saline
④ Placing the exposed organs gently into their original positions with a gloved hand

59. Evisceration is *best* described as:

① Turning a part of a body organ inside out
② Wound infection with involvement of underlying tissues
③ Separation of a wound with the exposure of a body organ
④ Slipping of one part of a body organ into another part of the organ

60. Mr. Rodriguez asks the nurse, "How do you think I am getting along now?" A question such as this should alert the nurse to think that *very likely* the patient is:

① Experiencing anxiety
② Developing a postoperative complication
③ Feeling better than his condition warrants
④ Having fears about the prospects of his recovery

61. One of the *best* measures to help prevent the postoperative complications of thrombi and emboli formation is:

① Ambulating the patient
② Massaging the patient's legs
③ Properly aligning the patient's legs in bed
④ Putting pillows under the patient's knees

62. Mr. Rodriguez's dressing changes are extremely painful for him. Which of the following actions would be *best* for the nurse to use in this situation?

① Have the patient take a nap immediately before and after the procedure
② Have the patient use relaxation exercises immediately before the procedures
③ Arrange to have a favorite television or radio program on during the procedure
④ Give the patient a prescribed pain medication an hour before the procedure

63. During the dressing change, Mr. Rodriguez demonstrates common signs of acute pain. Which of the following is *least* often associated with acute pain?

① An elevated temperature
② A higher blood pressure
③ A rapid pulse rate
④ Excessive perspiration

64. The nurse assesses Mr. Rodriguez's pain. Which of the following questions is most likely to provide information about the patient's discomfort?

① "Are you upset about something?"
② "Please describe the pain for me."
③ "Are you sure your pain comes and goes as you described?"
④ "Your pain started after you ate, didn't it?"

65. Which of the following statements *most accurately* describes a characteristic of pain?

① Pain is objective in nature
② Responses to pain vary widely
③ Consciousness is unnecessary for pain to be felt
④ Pain of anticipation is usually mild in nature

66. Which of the following nursing measures has been found *most helpful* when caring for a patient in pain?

① Leaving him to rest in a quiet room
② Asking the patient to describe his pain
③ Asking the family to remain with the patient
④ Turning the patient

67. The nurse palpates around Mr. Rodriguez's wound. If Mr. Rodriguez is in pain, the nurse would expect to find that his muscles are:

① Relaxed
② Twitching
③ Contracted
④ Become weakened

Mrs. James is a 22-year-old gravida 2, para 1 who is 39 weeks pregnant. When she arrives at the labor and delivery unit, she states that she has been having contractions every 5 to 6 minutes for the past hour. She also has a slight bloody show and tells you that she is becoming very uncomfortable.

68. The PN's first action should be to:

① Have Mrs. James get undressed and take her vital signs
② Tell Mrs. James not to worry about anything
③ Assist Mrs. James into a comfortable position and notify the charge nurse of her arrival
④ Tell Mrs. James that she is in early labor and that she will deliver soon

69. Labor that begins at 39 weeks is considered to be:

   ① Premature
   ② Full term
   ③ Postmature
   ④ Precipitate

Sterile vaginal examination (SVE) reveals that the cervix is 3 to 4 cm dilated, 50% effaced. The membranes are bulging, and the presenting part is at 0 station.

70. Complete dilatation of the cervix is:

   ① 6 cm
   ② 8 cm
   ③ 10 cm
   ④ 12 cm

71. Effacement refers to the:

   ① Amount of bloody show
   ② Thinning and shortening of the cervix
   ③ Position of the fetus
   ④ Amount of amniotic fluid present

72. Presenting part refers to:

   ① The part of the fetus coming through the pelvis first
   ② The relationship of the long axis of the fetus to the long axis of the mother
   ③ The part of the fetus most easily palpated
   ④ The degree of descent occurring in the maternal pelvis

73. After Mrs. James is admitted to the unit and the external fetal and maternal monitors are applied, the PN explains that the purpose of the monitors is to record:

   ① Fetal movement and maternal contractions
   ② Fetal activity and maternal heart rate
   ③ Fetal heart rate and maternal heart rate
   ④ Fetal heart rate and maternal contractions

74. Mr. James expresses concern about his wife's progress. Your best response would be:

   ① "Don't worry, she's doing fine."
   ② "I know you are concerned. I'll see if she can have some medication."
   ③ "Everything will be okay. Just tell her to relax."
   ④ "Her labor is progressing. Your support with the relaxation exercises is very helpful."

75. Which of the following observations indicates that Mrs. James is in the transition phase of active labor?

   ① Restlessness, nausea, doubts about ability to cope, cervix 8 to 9 cm dilated, and contractions 2 to 3 minutes apart
   ② Panicky, feels need to "bear down," vague communication, cervical dilitation complete
   ③ Somewhat apprehensive, wants someone with her, contractions moderately strong, and cervix 5 to 6 cm dilated
   ④ Fairly comfortable, relaxing well, contractions mild to moderate, and cervix 3 to 4 cm dilated

76. The physician performs an amniotomy. It is important for the nurse to assess and document the time and the:

   ① Duration and intensity of the following contractions
   ② Maternal vital signs and the fetal heart rate
   ③ Increase in bloody show and the amount of amniotic fluid
   ④ Color, character, and amount of amniotic fluid and the fetal heart rate

77. After delivery, the nurse may best facilitate bonding by:

   ① Taking the baby to the nursery and obtaining the weight and length so the parents can tell their family and friends
   ② Having the father carry the baby to the nursery and let the mother rest for a couple of hours
   ③ Keeping the baby in the delivery area with a warmer and encourage the parents to unwrap, hold, and touch the baby
   ④ Keeping the baby in the delivery area but wrap the baby warmly and allow the father to hold the baby and show it to the mother

78. Mr. and Mrs. James would like to carefully plan their next pregnancy. Mrs. James is breast-feeding and does not want to take birth control pills. The nurse teaches the couple that:

   ① Breast-feeding women do not ovulate, so no contraception is necessary
   ② A condom and vaginal foam used together are very effective
   ③ A tubal ligation is the most effective method and can be reversed at a later date

④ Periodic abstinence is best because it is the only "natural" method

Gene Ray, 76 years old, has experienced leg cramps for several years. He recently began to have severe headaches, syncope, and short memory lapses. He is admitted to the hospital with a diagnosis of atherosclerosis/arteriosclerosis.

79. Atherosclerosis is best described as:

① Hardening and widening of the arteries
② Loss of elasticity of blood vessels
③ Blood clots in the major arteries
④ Fatty deposits on the lining of blood vessels

80. The most accurate study used to diagnose atherosclerosis is a:

① Serum cholesterol level
② Prothrombin time
③ Arteriogram
④ Doppler study

81. Mr. Ray's current symptoms may indicate that the condition now includes:

① Pulmonary dysfunction
② Coronary occlusion
③ Cerebral involvement
④ Impending renal failure

82. The physician orders a low fat diet. Mr. Ray says that he always has bacon, scrambled eggs, and toast for breakfast. The nurse suggests that a better breakfast would be:

① Poached egg and fresh fruit
② Cooked cereal and orange juice
③ Pancakes and 2% milk
④ French toast and coffee

83. During the initial assessment of Mr. Ray's lower extremities, the nurse might expect to find:

① Moist, warm skin and regular pulses
② Edema, pain when touched, and bounding pulses
③ Tingling, numbness, and slowed pulses
④ Pale, cool skin and diminished pulses

84. The physician orders Cyclospasmol, a peripheral vasodilator. The nurse would observe Mr. Ray for symptoms of:

① Orthostatic hypotension
② Bradycardia

③ Nervousness
④ Lethargy

85. Mr. Ray was found to have a gangrenous ulcer in his right little toe. Which of the following would the nurse include in his care plan?

① Maintain strict bed rest until ulcer heals
② Apply hot compresses to increase blood flow
③ Keep a bed cradle in place to keep the covers off
④ Elevate the legs whenever sitting

Amy Marsh, a 42-year-old homemaker, comes to a medical clinic for a physical examination. Mrs. Marsh is a gravida 2, para 2, 5 feet 2 inches tall, and weighs 192 lb. Her blood pressure is 180/100. She has had no serious illnesses, nor any family history of hypertension.

86. Mrs. Marsh's type of hypertension will probably be classified as:

① Secondary
② Malignant
③ Essential
④ Latent

87. Which of the following is *not* considered to be a predisposing factor to hypertension?

① Smoking
② Aerobic exercises
③ Family history
④ Obesity

88. Mrs. Marsh denies having headaches. The nurse instructs her that other signs/symptoms of hypertension include:

① Blurred vision and ringing in the ears
② A slow pulse rate and anorexia
③ Increased energy and dry skin
④ Pallor and double vision

89. Mrs. Marsh is to begin antihypertension therapy and is to be taught to monitor her blood pressure. She is instructed that it is important to take her blood pressure:

① Using brachial and popliteal arteries
② Only in the early morning hours
③ About four times a day for the first month and then daily
④ Lying, sitting, and standing until she adjusts to medication

90. A 1000-calorie, low sodium diet is ordered for Mrs. Marsh. A food that is naturally high in sodium and should be avoided is:

① Fresh corn
② Orange juice
③ Cream of Wheat
④ Milk

91. An exercise program is important to the management of hypertension. An appropriate beginning exercise for Mrs. Marsh would be:

① Playing tennis
② Walking
③ Bicycling
④ Aerobics

92. In order to complete a teaching plan for Mrs. Marsh's medication regimen, the nurse must know:

① How quickly it causes the blood pressure to drop
② All the trade names of the drug
③ How it affects the serum potassium
④ If it causes hypernatremia

93. A complication common to hypertension is:

① Congestive heart failure
② Cataracts
③ Cirrhosis of the liver
④ Ulcerative colitis

94. A food that contains no cholesterol is:

① Broiled chicken
② Dinner rolls
③ Fresh asparagus
④ Tuna salad

Arnold Zimmer is admitted to the hospital with a diagnosis of congestive heart failure (CHF). Mr. Zimmer's vital signs are blood pressure, 160/110; temperature, 98°F; pulse, 130; and respiration, 30.

95. The objective symptom that is often present in left-sided CHF is:

① Nausea
② Insomnia
③ Orthopnea
④ Weight loss

96. Which of the following would be an early symptom of CHF?

① Fatigue

② Chest pain
③ Ringing in the ears
④ Insomnia

97. The physician orders furosemide (Lasix) 80 mg IV to be given stat. The nurse would expect a result to be:

① Increased serum magnesium
② Increased serum chloride
③ Decreased serum calcium
④ Decreased serum potassium

98. The therapeutic effect of furosemide is to:

① Slow the heart rate
② Increase urine output
③ Dilate the bronchi
④ Reduce anxiety

99. Mr. Zimmer also has an order for digoxin 0.25 mg to be administered IV. Before administering this medication, the nurse will:

① Check his apical pulse
② Take his temperature
③ Recount his respirations
④ Take his blood pressure

100. Mr. Zimmer asks what effect digoxin has on his body. He is instructed that it will:

① Slow and strengthen the action of his heart muscle
② Dilate the blood vessels of his heart
③ Cause fluid to drain out of his lungs by dilating the alveoli
④ Improve the function of the heart valves

101. Until Mr. Zimmer's heart is compensated, he will probably be more comfortable in which of the following positions?

① Supine position
② Prone position
③ Sims' position
④ Fowler's position

102. An intervention on the nursing care plan is to check the pulse pressure every 8 hours. This is done by:

① Checking the blood pressure lying and standing
② Assessing the amplitude of the pulse
③ Subtracting the diastolic blood pressure from the systolic
④ Describing the character and rate of the pulse

103. Fluid intake is to be restricted until the edema has subsided. This restriction usually involves:

① Cooperation between dietary and nursing personnel when planning all fluids
② Limiting intake of between-meal beverages only
③ Limiting all fluids except those needed for oral medications
④ Limiting the intake of water only

104. Mr. Zimmer is instructed that in following his low sodium diet, he can season his food with:

① Lemon juice
② Steak sauce
③ Catsup
④ Prepared mustard

105. Mr. Zimmer asks how long he will need to continue his digoxin. He is instructed that it will probably be necessary to continue this drug:

① Until his pulse rate returns to normal
② Until all the edema is gone
③ Until after the physician does a stress test to prove his heart is compensated
④ For the rest of his life

106. Kim Gray, a patient with leukemia, is admitted to the oncology unit. Early symptoms of leukemia include:

① Fatigue and generalized malaise
② Bone pain and epistaxis
③ Tachycardia and weight loss
④ Enlarged lymph nodes and heat intolerance

107. The test that is *most* accurate in diagnosing leukemia is a:

① Skeletal radiograph
② Erythrocyte sedimentation rate (ESR)
③ White blood cell count
④ Bone marrow biopsy

108. An expected side effect of chemotherapy for leukemia is:

① Bone marrow suppression
② Splenomegaly
③ Generalized edema
④ Cardiac toxicity

109. A major factor in the nursing care of Ms. Gray includes observation for and prevention of:

① Thrombus formation

② Urinary retention
③ Infections
④ Pedal edema

110. Radiation therapy may be included in the treatment of the leukemic patient to:

① Reduce white blood count
② Increase effectiveness of corticosteroids
③ Reduce side effects of chemotherapy
④ Reduce symptoms of splenomegaly

111. Ms. Gray is instructed to:

① Maintain a low fiber diet
② Avoid forceful nose blowing
③ Avoid using mouthwash
④ Come to clinic daily for Hickman catheter care

Mrs. Carson has been admitted to the medical floor with a diagnosis of bilateral pneumonia. She complains of chest pain, dyspnea, and a persistent productive cough.

112. Mrs. Carson's physician orders a sputum culture and sensitivity. This specimen should be obtained:

① Before starting an antibiotic
② After oral hygiene, by clearing the throat and expectorating into a container
③ Only after postural drainage
④ After she has eaten

113. The color of Mrs. Carson's sputum will probably be:

① Bright red
② White or grayish
③ Clear and frothy
④ Rust

114. Mrs. Carson is experiencing a chill. Her temperature will be highest:

① Just after the chill is over
② Just before the chill
③ About midway through the chill
④ About 30 minutes after the chill

115. Mrs. Carson's temperature is 104°F and she has joint aching. An antipyretic that also relieves joint pain is:

① Acetaminophen (Tylenol)
② Phenacetin
③ Aspirin
④ Codeine

116. The physician has ordered penicillin. Before starting the medicine, the nurse will:

① Instruct the patient that she might experience a skin rash
② Wait until the chest radiograph has been done
③ Check for a history of allergies
④ Hold until the C&S report is on the chart

117. A nursing measure that could assist Mrs. Carson in coughing up tenacious secretions would be to:

① Have her sit on the side of the bed to cough
② Increase oxygen flow rate
③ Provide frequent oral hygiene
④ Increase fluid intake

Martha Stuart is a patient on your unit. She is experiencing high blood pressure and fainting spells. While talking to her, you discover that her husband died suddenly 6 months ago.

118. Which of the following would be an important concept related to successful grieving?

① Resolution should occur within 6 months
② Shock and disbelief may last for months
③ Preoccupation with the image of the loss is abnormal
④ Awareness of the loss develops within weeks or months

119. Which of the following would indicate that Mrs. Stuart is having difficulty in grieving?

① Avoiding contact with others
② Expressing feelings of guilt
③ Showing feelings of hostility
④ Exhibiting symptoms of somatic distress

120. An appropriate intervention for any patient who is grieving would include:

① Sedating the patient to avoid a focus on the grief
② Allowing the patient to retreat from reality
③ Allowing the patient to talk about feelings, even if negative
④ Allowing the patient to avoid usual roles/responsibilities as long as possible

Answers & Rationales

Guide to item identification (see pp. 3–5 for further details about each category)

I, II, III, or IV for the phase of the nursing process
1, 2, 3, or 4 for the category of client needs
A, B, C, D, E, F, or G for the category of human functioning
Specific content category by name; ie, cholecystectomy

1. ① Symptoms of ketoacidosis include acetone on breath and in urine, polyuria, hyperglycemia. Other choices are incorrect, theoretical concepts.
I, 2, F. Endocrine/Diabetes.

2. ① Initial treatment is usually regular insulin, because it has a rapid action and will improve symptoms quickly. IV glucose and increased carbohydrate diet will worsen the symptoms.
III, 2, F. Endocrine/Diabetes.

3. ③ Others in the family may be able to assist John, or administer his insulin to him if he neglects to do so. Phone numbers would be valuable in an emergency, but will not prevent one; checking urine will not assure that he is taking his insulin, because diet and exercise also influence his metabolism. Oral medications are effective only if the patient has some functional pancreatic tissue and do not necessarily increase compliance.
III, 4, F. Endocrine/Diabetes.

4. ① Increased metabolism causes weight loss in spite of normal or increased intake. Patients have high levels of energy, rapid pulse, increased appetite, and increased heat production owing to the increased metabolic rate.
I, 2, F. Endocrine/Thyroid.

5. ② The increased metabolism increases muscle stimulation and interferes with fine muscle coordination. #1, #3, & #4 do not occur.
I, 2, F. Endocrine/Thyroid.

6. ③ If the production of thyroid hormones is blocked, the symptoms of Graves' disease will decrease or be eliminated. Sodium levels are not relevant to this disease. Thyroid hormones will increase symptoms.
I, 2 & 4, F. Endocrine/Thyroid.

7. ④ Handling of the thyroid gland in surgery may cause release of more hormones, causing extreme life-threatening hyperthyroid symptoms known as thyroid crisis. Decreasing production of hormones preoperatively is usually an effective preventive measure. Other choices represent incorrect theoretical concepts.
III, 2, H. Endocrine/Thyroid.

8. ① Elevation of the head decreases pressure to head and neck, which prevents edema and hemorrhage. Other choices may promote edema or hemorrhage.
III, 2, B, D, & F. Endocrine/Thyroid.

9. ④ Some edema is normal owing to the trauma of surgery. Due to the small size of the neck area, this edema can compress the trachea and is the most likely cause of respiratory obstruction. The other choices are incorrect theoretical concepts.
I, 2, B & F. Endocrine/Thyroid.

10. ② Increased and exaggerated postoperative symptoms of Graves' disease is the complication known as thyroid crisis. The other choices represent incorrect theoretical concepts.
I, 2, F. Endocrine/Thyroid.

11. ② The drainage will follow body contours and gravity so will be more likely to be in dependent areas. This assessment is imperative to gather adequate information to relay to the physician. #1 & #3 may possibly be done later, depending on the results of the first assessment, and #4 is an incorrect theoretical concept.
III, 2, B & F. Endocrine/Thyroid.

12. ② Narrow stream and frequency are early symptoms. The other choices represent symptoms of cystitis, which sometimes occurs later, owing to the incomplete emptying of the bladder, allowing urine to remain in the bladder for long periods of time.
I, 2, F. BPH.

13. ④ A transurethral resection presents the lowest risk for the patient because there is no abdominal or perineal incision and, therefore, fewer postoperative complications and shorter hospitalization. It can also be done easily under spinal anesthesia.
II, 1 & 2, F. BPH.

14. The prostate is very vascular, and some bleed-
① ing is expected postoperatively. The continuous flow of irrigating solution prevents clots
from obstructing the catheter.
II, 1 & 2, F. BPH.

15. The Foley catheter may be blocked with clots.
③ This is an abnormal finding that should be
reported immediately.
I & III, 1 & 2, D and F. BPH.

16. As stool fills the rectum, the area is distended
④ and moves pressure toward the vaginal area,
allowing the radioactive rays from the implant
to radiate and possibly damage rectal tissue.
Although the other answers are true to some
degree, they are not the most important rationale in this situation.
III, 1 & 2, A & D. Reproductive/Cancer.

17. If the bladder would fill, it would lie back
② toward the vagina and more directly into the
path of the radiation, which could damage the
bladder tissue. The other answers are true to
some degree, but are not the most important
rationale in this situation.
III, 1 & 2, A & D. Reproductive/Cancer.

18. Elevating the head may cause displacement of
④ the implant and radiation damage to other
organs. A 0- to 30-degree elevation is usually
allowed for comfort, because this does not
significantly alter the angle of the pelvis. #2
and #3 are contraindicated until the implant
is removed, to avoid disturbance of the implant. The patient need not be on a full liquid
diet.
III, 1 & 2, A & D. Reproductive/Cancer.

19. Visits are allowed but visitors must adhere to
④ imposed restrictions.
III, 1 & 3, A & D. Reproductive/Cancer.

20. This response uses a therapeutic technique of
① communication because it acknowledges the
patient's thoughts and feelings and gives permission to express emotion. The nurse is also
offering her presence if the patient wishes to
talk. The other responses block communication by expressing the nurse's opinion
and belittling the patient's feelings.
III, 3, A & G. Reproductive/Cancer.

21. It is common practice to order antibiotics for
③ postoperative patients, and this is a common
complication of antibiotic therapy. Vaginal
implant does not cause skin irritation; and

while the superimposed infection is possible
after the implant, it is more likely due to the
antibiotic. The Foley catheter does not cause
vaginal infection, and a perineal pad should
not irritate enough to cause vaginal infection.
IV, 2, D. Reproductive/Medication administration.

22. Tympanic membrane, malleus, incus, stapes,
① oval window is the correct anatomic sequence.
I, 2, C. Otosclerosis.

23. The ossicles or bones of the middle ear are
③ fused together and unable to vibrate to transmit the sound waves to the inner ear. This
disease does not involve obstruction or nerve
damage.
I, 2 & 4, C. Otosclerosis.

24. Sudden or violent blowing of the nose causes
④ increased pressure in the middle ear and may
dislodge the prosthesis that replaces the
stapes. #1, #2, & #3 represent incorrect theoretical concepts.
III, 2 & 4, C. Otosclerosis.

25. As the retina detaches, rods and cones are
① unable to receive images, which results in
gaps or black areas in the visual field. There
are no complaints of pain, burning, etc, with
detached retina; therefore, #2, #3, and #4
are not pertinent to this diagnosis.
I, 2, C. Detached Retina.

26. Increased head movement can increase the
④ pressure of the vitreous humor and allow
more of it to seep under the retina and further
the detachment. The patient should be kept as
quiet as possible; all answers indicating activity are incorrect.
III, 1 & 2, C. Detached Retina.

27. This statement reflects the nurse's observa-
② tion of behavior to the patient. The question is
open ended and thus encourages the patient
to discuss how his needs can be met. #1, #3,
& #4 block communication.
III, 3. Detached Retina.

28. Normally, at 3 months most infants can lift
③ their heads. Some infants may perform this
earlier. Premature babies may do so later.
I, 4, A. Peds Growth and Development.

29. The anterior fontanel closes and becomes use-
④ less as an assessment tool after age 15 to 18

months. The posterior fontanel closes much earlier.

I, 4, A. Peds Growth and Development.

30. ② By 12 months, the child usually triples the birthweight.

I, 4, A. Peds Growth and Development.

31. ③ All 20 deciduous teeth are in by 30 to 36 months of age.

I, 4, A. Peds Growth and Development.

32. ③ Although the child will lose the first tooth just prior to this age, the first permanent tooth, normally a bottom incisor, will present itself at about 6 to 7 years of age. #1 is the age when all deciduous teeth are in. #2 and #4 are incorrect.

I, 4, A. Peds Growth and Development.

33. ① When he is admitted, giving the patient time to learn. #2, #3, and #4 are all too late to begin discharge planning.

II, 1 & 2, D. Perioperitive Care.

34. ④ 2.0 mL Demerol and 0.67 mL atropine.

$$\frac{100\ mg}{x\ mL} = \frac{50\ mg}{1\ mL} \qquad 50x = 100$$
$$x = 2\ mL$$

$$\frac{g\frac{1}{150}}{x\ 2\ mL} = \frac{g\frac{1}{100}}{1\ mL} \qquad \frac{1}{100}x = \frac{1}{150}$$
$$x = \frac{\frac{1}{150}}{\frac{1}{100}}$$

$$\frac{1}{150} \div \frac{1}{100} = \frac{1}{150} \times \frac{100}{1} = \frac{100}{150} = 0.67\ mL$$

III, 1 & 2, D. Medication Administration.

35. ④ The permit must be signed by the patient, with a witness, before sedation and after thorough explanation of the surgical procedure.

IV, 1, D & G. Perioperiative Care.

36. ④ After spinal anesthesia, the patient is often ordered to lie flat for a period of time. In #1 and #2, the GI system is generally affected very little by spinal anesthesia. #3 is a common postoperative order.

III, 1 & 2, A. Perioperative Care.

37. ① The pulse increases with blood loss. Respirations may become rapid, temperature is often unaffected, and blood pressure decreases with blood loss.

I, 2, B. Shock.

38. ④ The head should be lower than the feet to assure blood flow to vital centers. #1, #2, and #3 do not demonstrate the head-lower-than-feet position.

III, 2, B. Shock.

39. ③ Medical asepsis is aimed at decreasing the number and growth of microbes to decrease the risk of spread of infection. The other options all describe surgical asepsis.

III, 1 & 2, D. Perioperative Care.

40. ② Surgical asepsis is aimed at the destruction of microbes before they enter the body. We do not destroy microbes as they leave the body, but aim to divert them away from others. #3 and #4 describe medical asepsis.

III, 1 & 2, D. Perioperative Care.

41. ③ Washing hands is still considered the most important infection prevention. Gloves are worn only during certain procedures, when the care giver is likely to come in contact with a moist body surface or substance. The hands cannot be sterilized.

III, 1 & 2, D. Perioperative Care/Isolation Precautions.

42. ④ Drainage is encouraged to leave the wound and is soaked up by the absorbent layer of the dressing. Movement of the incision line may cause disruption of sutures. The patient may not be tolerant of his wound yet, and dressings are sterile and changed often to decrease microbe invasion.

III, 2, A. Perioperative Care/Wound Care.

43. ② Microbes travel on air currents. #1, #3, and #4 do not relate to spread of microbes.

II, 1 & 2, A. Perioperative Care/Wound Care.

44. ② Moistening the dressing loosens it and using sterile saline assures the integrity of aseptic technique. #1, #3, and #4 are not recommended.

III, 1 & 2, D. Perioperative Care/Wound Care.

45. ① Antiseptics stop the growth and reproduction of microbes. #2, #3, and #4 all relate to a disinfectant solution that is not safe for application to the skin.

III, 1 & 2, D. Perioperative Care/Wound Care.

46. ④ Wrapping an extremity should begin at the lowest point to prevent pooling of venous blood below the wrap. #1, #2, and #3 are not the lowest point.

III, 2, B. Basic Skills.

47. Nerves that act as heat receptors adjust very
④ quickly to warmth, making the pad feel cool again. If the K-pad is properly functioning it should be used. #1, #2, and #3 are not appropriate actions.
III, 2, B. Perioperative Care/Wound Care.

48. All pathogens require moisture, food,
③ warmth, and darkness. Some need oxygen, but others do not.
II, 1 & 2, D. Perioperative Care.

49. This is the only example of a normal flora of
② the bowel.
II, 1 & 2, D. Perioperative Care.

50. The article must have all protein residue re-
② moved before the chemical used can reach its surface. Care must be taken to soak the object long enough, not too long. The solution will not be applied to tissue, and simply rinsing does not assure complete removal of protein residue.
III, 1, D. Perioperative Care.

51. Spores can be destroyed only by certain
③ methods. They are very resistant and hence dangerous.
III, 1, D. Perioperative Care.

52. This is the most reliable method of destroying
③ spores, the most resistant form of microbe. #1, #2, and #4 will not kill spores.
III, 1, D. Perioperative Care.

53. The five classic signs are redness, warmth,
① swelling, pain, and decreased mobility. #2, #3, and #4 do not indicate signs of inflammation.
I, 2, D. Perioperative Care.

54. $\dfrac{125 \text{ mL}}{60 \text{ mins}} \times 12 = 25 \text{ gtt/min}$
③

III, 2, D. Medication Administration.

55. $\dfrac{100 \text{ mg}}{1.5 \text{ mL}} = \dfrac{250 \text{ mg}}{\text{x mL}}$
④

$250 \times 1.5 = 100\text{x}$

$375 = 100\text{x}$

$3.75 = \text{x}$

III, 2, D. Medication Administration/Perioperative Care.

56. Infected dressings should be properly dis-
③ carded. The other actions are not necessary with this type of isolation.
II, 3, D & G. Perioperative Care/Isolation Precautions.

57. This is the correct definition.
② I, 2, D. Perioperative Care.

58. The internal structures must be kept moist
③ until the physician arrives. #1 and #2 do not keep it moist and #4 is not a nursing function.
III, 2, D. Perioperative Care.

59. This is the correct definition.
③ I, 2, A. Perioperative Care.

60. The patient is looking for confirmation, indi-
④ cating he is fearful about his condition. Most patients are able to have confidence in their own judgment if they are not fearful. There is no indication that #2 is correct, and his question denotes doubt rather than confidence.
I, 3, G. Psycho-socio-cultural Functions.

61. Ambulating encourages circulation and de-
① creases venous pooling, while massaging legs could dislodge a developing emboli. Alignment does not assure good circulation, and pillows under the knees can cause pressure and decrease circulation.
II, 2, B & D. Postoperative Complications.

62. This gives sufficient time for the medication to
④ be in effect when the dressing is changed. #1, #2, and #3 may help decrease anxiety associated with the pain, but #4 works directly on the pain.
II, 2, C. Perioperative Care.

63. Body temperature does not increase as a re-
① sult of pain. All others are common signs of pain.
I, 2, C. Perioperative Care.

64. This is an open-ended question that will allow
② the patient to describe the pain. #1, #3, and #4 are all answerable by one or two words and thus do not facilitate communication.
I, 3, G. Perioperative Care/Communication.

65. Pain is a subjective experience and people ex-
② perience pain differently.
I, 2, C. Perioperative Care.

66. The patient may be experiencing pain unasso-
② ciated with the incision.
I, 2, C, D, & G. Perioperative Care.

67. ③ Muscles around a painful area will be tense in an attempt to hold the area still.
I, 2, C & D. Perioperative Care.

68. ③ It is important to establish a sense of trust and security at admission. Although the nurse would certainly have her get undressed and take her vital signs, it is important to first talk to her and make her comfortable.
III, 3 & 4, A & G. Labor and Delivery/Interpersonal Relationships.

69. ② Full-term pregnancy is defined as one lasting 38 to 42 weeks. Premature delivery is define as delivery occurring before 37 weeks.
I, 4, A. Labor and Delivery.

70. ③ The cervix is fully dilated when it reaches 10 cm.
IV, 4, A. Labor and Delivery.

71. ② Effacement is defined as the thinning and shortening of the cervix in preparation for birth.
I, 4, A. Labor and Delivery.

72. ① The presenting part is defined as the part of the fetus attempting to come through the maternal pelvis first. It is usually the head, or possibly the feet or buttocks.
IV, 4, A. Labor and Delivery.

73. ④ The tocotransducer and the phonotransducer monitor uterine contractions and fetal heart rate, respectively.
III, 4, A. Labor and Delivery.

74. ④ Support for the father during labor includes helping him feel that he is a contributor to the birthing process. Medication at this time would be inappropriate, and the other answers are nonsupportive.
III, 1 & 4, E & G. Labor and Delivery/Interpersonal Relationships.

75. ① These are the signs of transition in the labor process. #2 occurs during the second stage of labor, and #3 and #4 indicate early phases of the first stage of labor.
I, 4, A. Labor and Delivery.

76. ④ An amniotomy may be referred to as an artificial rupture of the membranes. When the membranes rupture, the fetal heart rate should be assessed to determine any distress to the fetus. Color, character, and amount of fluid should be documented.
I, 4, A. Labor and Delivery.

77. ③ If there are no complications, the infant should spend as much time as possible with the parents to facilitate bonding. Care must be taken to provide a warm environment, and skin-to-skin contact should be encouraged.
III, 4, A & G. Labor and Delivery/Interpersonal Relationships.

78. ② This method, when used properly, is extremely effective. #1 is incorrect; it does not protect against pregnancy. #3 is considered permanent, and #4 is a personal response.
III, 4, A. Labor and Delivery.

79. ④ Atherosclerosis is characterized by a build up of fatty plaques within arteries. It does produce some hardening and loss of elasticity, but the cause is the plaque.
I, 2, B. Atherosclerosis.

80. ③ An arteriogram allows the visualization of the inside of an artery. Serum cholesterol suggests that plaque may be present, but the only way it can be seen is through an arteriogram.
I, 2, B. Atherosclerosis.

81. ③ The symptoms he is exhibiting are of decreased cerebral blood flow owing to narrowing of the cerebral vessels.
I, 2, B & C. Atherosclerosis.

82. ② The diet he usually follows is very high in fat and cholesterol. Eggs are high in cholesterol. Cereal and juice would provide the lowest amounts of fat and cholesterol for his breakfast.
III, 4, B & F. Atherosclerosis/Nutrition.

83. ④ The signs/symptoms the nurse is observing are typical signs of peripheral vascular disease. When a patient has atherosclerosis in one area of the body, it is likely to be present in other parts of the body also.
I, 2, B. Peripheral Arterial Disease.

84. ① When a patient is given a vasodilator, it causes dilation of all vessels, not just those affected by disease. When generalized vasodilation occurs, the patient's blood pressure can drop and cause lightheadedness and faintness.
I, 1 & 2, B. Peripheral Vascular Disease.

85. Peripheral venous disease can result in venous stasis with ulcer formation. It is important to prevent injury or trauma, even from the weight of the bed covers.
③ II, 1 & 2, B. Peripheral Vascular Disease.

86. Essential hypertension is also defined as primary hypertension. Secondary hypertension is caused by another condition, and malignant hypertension is progressively increasing hypertension that cannot be controlled.
③ I, 2, B. Hypertension.

87. Aerobic exercises are appropriate cardiovascular exercises that actually improve cardiovascular function, not cause hypertension. The others are predisposing factors for hypertension.
② I, 2 & 4, B. Hypertension.

88. With severely increased blood pressure, blurred vision and tinnitus are common problems. The other symptoms listed would not occur with hypertension.
① I & III, 2 & 4, B. Hypertension.

89. When the patient begins antihypertensive therapy, one effect is orthostatic changes. Checking the blood pressure in the three positions can indicate the presence of this side effect of treatment. Once the patient has adjusted to the medication, it should be taken weekly or monthly, depending on the physician's orders.
④ III, 1 & 4, B. Hypertension.

90. Milk is naturally high in sodium. Cream of Wheat, despite the name, does not contain milk or cream.
④ II, 4, F. Hypertension.

91. Exercise that is not too strenuous is important for improving the cardiovascular system. Walking is a good exercise for the nonactive person to begin with.
② II, 2 & 4, B. Hypertension.

92. Many antihypertensives act as diuretics and cause potassium to be lost. The nurse needs to know if the patient needs to be taught a high potassium diet. Antihypertensives would not cause hypernatremia.
③ II, 2 & 4, B. Hypertension.

93. Congestive heart failure is often caused by hypertension. Cirrhosis is possible, but uncommon.
① I, 2, B. Hypertension.

94. Fresh vegetables are low in cholesterol. Broiled chicken is low only if the skin is removed. Tuna salad and rolls are fairly high in cholesterol.
③ II, 4, F. Hypertension.

95. Left-sided heart failure results in a build up of pressure and fluid in the pulmonary system. This can lead to pulmonary edema and orthopnea. The other symptoms are not associated with left-sided failure.
③ I, 2, B. CHF.

96. When the patient suffers from CHF, there is a decrease in oxygen to the tissues. This results in a feeling of tiredness and fatigue.
① I, 2, B. CHF.

97. Lasix causes diuresis, resulting in a loss of both potassium and sodium. This can lead to a depletion of these electrolytes.
④ IV, 2, B. CHF.

98. Diuretics work by increasing the urine output and thereby decreasing the blood volume.
② IV, 2, B. CHF.

99. Digoxin slows the heart rate and increases the force of contractions. A side effect can be that the heart rate slows down too much. To prevent this, the nurse should check the apical pulse before administration. If the pulse is below 60, the medication is held and the physician notified.
① III, 1 & 2, B. CHF.

100. As above, digoxin slows the heart rate and strengthens the contractions.
① III, 2 & 4, B. CHF.

101. With congestive failure, breathing can be difficult as the lungs fill with fluid. The patient will be much more comfortable sitting up to breathe.
④ III, 1 & 2, B. CHF.

102. The pulse pressure is the difference between the systolic and diastolic blood pressure. This can reflect a number of different changes in cardiac function and even in intracranial pressure.
③ III, 1 & 2, B. CHF.

103. The fluid restrictions associated with CHF can be quite severe, as low as 1000 mL/day. To manage a restriction of this severity, it is vital
①

104. Lemon juice is a good seasoning substitute for
① salt because it adds a great deal of flavor to
food while adding no salt. The other options
are all high in salt themselves.
III, 4, B & F. CHF.

that dietary and nursing plan together so that
the patient has maximum comfort.
II, 1 & 2, B. CHF.

105. Treatment for congestive heart failure is for
④ the rest of the patient's life, because the heart
can never be cured of its failure. Congestive
heart failure is controllable as the heart compensates.
III, 4, B. CHF.

106. Flu-like symptoms are common early in leu-
① kemia. As the blood counts begin to drop,
fatigue is a common early symptom. The
other symptoms occur much later.
I, 1 & 2, B. Leukemia.

107. A bone marrow biopsy is the most accurate
④ test for diagnosing leukemia, because it is the
one test that allows the malignant cells to be
collected and tested. Leukemia is cancer of the
bone marrow.
I, 2, B. Leukemia.

108. Chemotherapy kills all rapidly dividing cells,
① both normal and malignant. In order to kill
the cancer within the bone marrow, drugs
must be given in high doses. These doses will
also kill normal cells within the marrow, leading to bone marrow depression.
IV, 2, B. Leukemia.

109. Leukemia causes an abnormal proliferation of
③ immature and useless white blood cells
(WBCs) that are ineffective in combating infections. The chemotherapy further deletes
the WBCs, leaving the patient even more vul-
nerable to infection.
II & III, 1, B & D. Leukemia.

110. An enlarged spleen, a lymphatic organ, is a
④ common problem with leukemia. Radiation is
an effective way to treat this enlargement.
III, 2, B. Leukemia.

111. The low platelet count can occur with therapy
② and makes bleeding likely. Forceful nose-
blowing could cause bleeding.
III, 2 & 4, B & D. Leukemia.

112. It is important to do a culture and sensitivity
① test before antibiotics are started. Once antibiotics are started, this alters the bacteria. Postural drainage may help to obtain the specimen, but is not required. Coughing should
never be stimulated right after a patient eats,
because it may cause vomiting.
III, 1 & 2, B. Pneumonia.

113. Sputum related to pneumonia is often rust
④ colored. It may also be green or yellowish.
I, 2, B. Pneumonia.

114. Chilling is associated with the end of a tem-
① perature spike. Shivering is an attempt by the
body to lower the temperature.
I, 2, B. Pneumonia.

115. Aspirin is both an antipyretic that treats fever
③ and a nonsteroidal antiinflammatory that
treats muscle aches. The other medications
treat one or the other.
III, 2, B. Pneumonia.

116. Allergies to penicillin are common and can be
③ very severe. It is vital to assess the patient for
a history of allergies to penicillin or cephalosporins. A skin rash is often the first sign of an
allergic reaction.
I & III, 1 & 2, B. Pneumonia.

117. Increasing fluid intake and humidifying the
④ air help to liquify thick and tenacious sputum
and to increase the patient's ability to cough
up sputum.
III, 1 & 2, B. Pneumonia.

118. Awareness of the loss develops gradually
④ over several weeks to months after the loss.
The behaviors in #1 and #2 should not last
this long, and preoccupation with the image
of the lost person is normal.
I, 3, G. Grieving.

119. It is not normal to avoid all contact with others
① when grieving. The other behaviors are part
of normal grieving.
I, 3, G. Grieving.

120. It is very important to allow the patient to
③ express all feelings so that they grieve. Negative feelings are appropriate in a grieving patient. The other interventions would be inappropriate.
III, 3, G. Grieving.

Practice Test

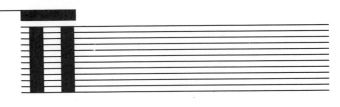

Questions

121. The normal fasting blood glucose range (mg) per 100 mL of venous blood is:

  ① 60–80
  ② 80–120
  ③ 100–150
  ④ 100–200

122. When a *nondiabetic* person is given oral glucose for a glucose tolerance test, his or her blood glucose level will return to normal in approximately how many hours?

  ① 1
  ② 2
  ③ 4
  ④ 6

123. Before beginning to teach the new diabetic, it is important to:

  ① Be sure the diabetes is severe enough to require teaching
  ② Determine if the patient has accepted the illness before teaching begins
  ③ Assess how the patient is accepting the illness
  ④ List all the best ways of caring for his or her illness

124. One of the most important factors in controlling diabetes is the diet. If the intake of carbohydrates is more than what can be used or stored, the patient will eventually go into:

  ① Ketoacidosis
  ② Shock
  ③ Hypoglycemia
  ④ Metabolic alkalosis

125. It is important to eat all the food on the prescribed diabetic diet. If the patient is taking insulin and eats too little food, which of the following will occur?

  ① Hyperinsulinism with resultant hypoglycemia
  ② Diabetic coma

  ③ Hyperglycemia
  ④ Hypoinsulinism with resultant hyperglycemia

126. If the patient inquires about eating *dietetic* cookies that are sold in the supermarket, you would reply:

  ① "Dietetic and diabetic are the same; therefore, these foods can be eaten."
  ② "The foods can be eaten, providing the fats, proteins, and carbohydrates are counted in the diet."
  ③ "These foods are for people who wish to lose weight and are not intended for diabetics."
  ④ "There is no real nutritional value to these products."

127. When teaching the diabetic, the nurse should explain that any slight illness is an indication that the patient should:

  ① Increase insulin dose
  ② Decrease insulin dose
  ③ Eliminate $\frac{1}{2}$ the carbohydrates in diet
  ④ Test urine or blood sugar more frequently

128. The individual best able to manage his or her diabetes is one who:

  ① Takes insulin regularly
  ② Does not spill sugar in urine
  ③ Understands the disease
  ④ Is diagnosed as diabetic while still young

129. Oral hypoglycemic agents are of value only if the:

  ① Patient is young
  ② Fasting blood sugar (FBS) is initially below 100
  ③ Patient is able to produce some insulin
  ④ Patient is not obese

Monica Helms, age 56 years, saw her physician because of a lump she discovered in her right breast. After a breast biopsy revealed malignancy, she was admitted for a modified radical mastectomy.

130. A drain has been inserted in Mrs. Helms's incision and connected to a Hemovac suction device. Unless the doctor orders otherwise, suction drains are usually:

① Emptied every 2 hours
② Emptied every 4 hours
③ Emptied every shift and prn
④ *Not* emptied unless there is a specific order

131. The nurse frequently performs a circulation check on the patient's hands because:

① The patient is not very active, so circulation to the fingers decreases
② Edema in the axillary region may constrict blood flow to the hands
③ If the IV infiltrates, there may be pressure on the radial artery, thus diminishing blood supply to the fingers
④ If the incisional sutures are too snug, they can obstruct blood flow to the fingers

132. Mrs. Helms has a pressure dressing over the surgical area. When checking the dressing for hemorrhage, the nurse should:

① Remove the uppermost layers of the dressing
② Turn the patient frequently in order to assess for bleeding
③ Remove the entire dressing to observe the operative site
④ Maintain the patient on her unoperative side so that bleeding can be observed readily

133. An intravenous fluids line for Mrs. Helms should be placed in:

① The affected arm
② The hand
③ The unaffected arm
④ The subclavian vein

134. In what position should Mrs. Helms's arm on the affected side be placed?

① Abducted
② Supported on two pillows
③ Flexed 20 degrees
④ Elevated with the wrist higher than the shoulder

135. Mrs. Helms may be taught postoperative exercises as ordered by her surgeon. The purpose of these exercises is to:

① Help in her ambulation

② Help her relax
③ Enable her to comb her hair
④ Avoid limitation of movement

John, age 50 years, visits a local vision clinic, complaining of headaches at intervals, blurring of his vision, and seeing rainbows or halos around lights. A diagnosis of glaucoma is made.

136. The nurse explains to John that glaucoma is:

① A disease of the eye resulting from an infection in the anterior chamber
② A disorder involving the vitreous humor and retina
③ Absence of aqueous humor in the anterior chamber
④ A condition of increased intraocular pressure

137. The symptoms of glaucoma occur because:

① The pupil is contracted
② The lens cannot accommodate
③ Aqueous humor is produced faster than it is drained away
④ The vitreous humor is increased

138. Eye drops are prescribed for John. He asks the nurse how long he will have to continue using them. The nurse tells him that eye drops for glaucoma should be continued:

① Until the predisposing condition is corrected
② For the rest of his life
③ For about 6 months to a year
④ Until the blockage is eliminated

139. The nurse also cautions John to contact the doctor prior to taking over-the-counter medications that contain:

① Miotics
② Mydriatics
③ Vasodilators
④ Antiseptics

140. The nurse explains the proper method of eye drop administration to John by stating that he should instill the eye drops:

① Directly onto the cornea
② In the inner aspect of the eye
③ Into the inner canthus
④ Into the upper portion of the eye

141. A 6-month-old suspected of having cerebral palsy would most likely exhibit:

① Delay or failure to control head and roll over
② Frequent episodes of seizure activity
③ Visual or hearing deficits
④ Frequent respiratory infections

142. The parents of an infant diagnosed with cerebral palsy ask the nurse how severe a handicap their child will have. The best response by the nurse is:

① "With early and vigorous therapy, he may have only mild problems."
② "It's hard to tell so early; some mental retardation is expected."
③ "Children with CP vary in symptoms and severity but can be helped with treatment."
④ "No one can really tell how much disability there will be until the child starts school."

143. Children with CP are often at risk for nutritional deficits because they have:

① Difficulties controlling the muscles of chewing and swallowing
② Restricted sense of taste and are picky eaters
③ GI impairment which decreases absorption of nutrients
④ Frequent episodes of vomiting related to muscle spasticity

144. A high school sophomore, Shirley has not been selected for a favored school team. She is suddenly neglecting her studies and appearance, and is disinterested in the world around her. As the nurse in her school, your best action would be to:

① Establish regular appointments for her to see you to talk over problems.
② Encourage her not to discuss her problems with her peer group.
③ Recommend mental health intervention if her withdrawal continues.
④ Allow her to find her own time to talk about her feelings.

145. After exhibiting depressive behavior, Shirley suddenly becomes more active and begins to give away her prized pictures and audio cassettes, among other things. What might you suspect from her behavior?

① That she has begun to abuse illicit drugs
② That her behavior is more typically adolescent now
③ That she may be pregnant
④ That she is considering suicide

Mrs. Ruth Lamb, age 68 years, has had a stroke that left her unable to help herself. She is primarily bedridden.

146. Which of the following *best* describes the psychological effect of inactivity that many older patients such as Mrs. Lamb experience?

① Abnormal talkativeness
② Hallucinations
③ Lack of normal initiative
④ Lack of normal inhibition

147. The nurse encourages Mr. Lamb to make a footboard for Mrs. Lamb's bed. She explains that the *primary* purpose for using a footboard for Mrs. Lamb is to help prevent:

① Bedsores
② Foot drop
③ Knee contractures
④ Edema in the feet

148. The nurse moves Mrs. Lamb's knee through range of motion, but the patient begins to complain of *considerable* discomfort. Which of the following courses of action should the nurse take?

① Stop the exercise and inform the physician
② Continue with the exercise but at a slower pace
③ Stop the exercise and begin again after the patient has had a few minutes of rest
④ Explain to the patient that she will experience discomfort when the exercise is done properly

149. The nurse uses trochanter rolls for Mrs. Lamb while she is in bed. Trochanter rolls are used *primarily* to help prevent:

① Flexion of the knees
② Extension of the hips
③ Hyperextension of the feet
④ External rotation of the legs

The nurse is teaching Mr. and Mrs. Lamb about the possible complications of inactivity. She explains that each system of the body may be affected.

150. A danger affecting the circulatory system when a patient is immobile is:

① The formation of blood clots
② The development of air emboli
③ An increased alkalinity of the blood
④ An excessive white blood cell formation

151. In order to prevent the effects of immobility on the gastrointestinal system, the nurse suggests that Mrs. Lamb:

① Be given daily enemas
② Decrease her fluid intake
③ Increase roughage in her diet
④ Avoid stool softeners

152. A result *least likely* to develop from muscle disuse is:

① Contractures
② Muscular weakness
③ Decreased stamina
④ Hyperactive muscular responses

153. Which of the following electrolytes is lost in the *largest* amount when the patient requires a long period of bed rest?

① Sodium
② Calcium
③ Potassium
④ Bicarbonate

154. The *primary* cause of a decubitus ulcer is:

① Excessive perspiration
② Pressure on a body area
③ Poor nutrition and inadequate fluid intake
④ Inability to control voiding and defecating

155. The nurse explains to Mr. Lamb that Mrs. Lamb's position should be changed every:

① 1–2 hours
② 3–4 hours
③ 6 hours
④ 8 hours

Marie is a 14-year-old, single, primigravida high school student who has received no prenatal care.

156. Which of the following behaviors indicates that Marie may have been denying her pregnancy?

① Obtaining no prenatal care
② Considering adoption as an alternative
③ Making plans to finish high school
④ Not telling her parents about the pregnancy

157. When Marie is admitted in active labor, the nurse knows that:

① It is too late to teach breathing and relaxation exercises
② If teaching is to be done, Marie should be medicated first so that she will be more relaxed
③ Teaching should begin immediately with short, simple instructions
④ Teaching should be extensive to make up for no prenatal care

158. Marie notices that the fetal monitor indicates that her baby's heart rate is 148 beats per minute (bpm), and asks you if that is too fast. Your best response would be:

① "Yes, that is too fast. It is because you are so tense."
② "No, that is not too fast. The normal fetal heart beat is 120 to 160 beats every minute."
③ "It's okay, because the normal heart rate goes up to 200 beats every minute."
④ "That's great! It means that your baby is a girl."

159. Marie's pregnancy is considered high risk because of:

① Lack of prenatal care
② Her age
③ Her educational and marital status
④ All of the above

160. To monitor the frequency of Marie's contractions, the nurse should count the time from the:

① Beginning of one contraction to the beginning of the next contraction
② End of one contraction to the beginning of the next contraction
③ Beginning of the contraction to the end of the same contraction
④ Peak of one contraction to the peak of the next contraction

161. When Marie's cervix is 6 to 7 cm dilated, she is given meperidine (Demerol) 50 mg IM. The PN knows that Demerol will:

① Increase the intensity and durations of the contractions
② Prevent nausea during labor
③ Relieve discomfort and promote relaxation
④ Cause the cervix to dilate more rapidly

162. During delivery, an episiotomy is performed. An episiotomy is an incision:

① Into the abdomen to facilitate the delivery of the infant
② Into the cervix to prevent lacerations
③ Into the perineum to facilitate the delivery of the infant
④ Into the vagina to prevent lacerations of the reproductive tract

163. Which of the following indicates that Marie understands her postpartum teaching? She:

① Washes hands, does peri-care, and applies clean peri-pad back to front
② Washes hands, does peri-care, and applies clean peri-pad front to back
③ Washes hands and changes peri-pad four times a day
④ Showers twice a day and applies a clean peri-pad

164. Marie tells you that she plans to bottle-feed her infant. Your best response would be:

① "Your baby would do much better if you would breast-feed."
② "Holding and cuddling your baby during feeding is very important."
③ "That's a good idea. That way anyone can feed the baby."
④ "That's a good idea because you cannot breast-feed and go to school or have a job."

165. Marie is concerned about losing weight after the baby is born. Which of the following statements indicates that Marie understands her nutritional needs?

① "I won't eat any food between meals."
② "I won't eat any bread, potatoes, cereal or pasta."
③ "I guess I'd better not eat any pizza or fast food."
④ "Drinking milk with my pizza and salad will be a real change."

166. Before Marie is discharged, it will be important to discuss with her:

① Plans for the future and her support system
② Who got her pregnant and why
③ How unrealistic her ideas are about caring for her baby
④ The rules of society and morality so she will not get pregnant again

Mrs. Gonzales is admitted to the labor floor in active labor and vaginally delivers a healthy, 8-lb boy without complications.

167. In the recovery room, Mrs. Gonzales's lochia increases, and the fundus is firm but rising and displaced toward her left side. The most probable cause is:

① A full bladder
② Uterine atony
③ Lacerations of the reproductive tract
④ Uterine tetany

168. Mrs. Gonzales is breast-feeding her son and says she has uterine cramping. The PN knows that this is:

① A sign of retained placenta
② An indication that she should stop breast-feeding
③ Because the uterus is expelling clots
④ Because oxytocin is being released

169. Mr. and Mrs. Gonzales are concerned about how their 3-year-old daughter will respond to the new baby. The most helpful intervention would be to allow her daughter to:

① See the baby in the nursery
② Spend time alone with her mother
③ Spend time with the mother and new baby together
④ Phone her mother often

170. Routine postpartum assessment includes checking Homans' sign. A positive Homans' sign indicates:

① Thrombophlebitis
② Mastitis
③ Endometritis
④ Nephritis

Mrs. Mary Jones suspects that she is pregnant. She missed two menstrual periods and decides to go to the obstetrician's office to confirm her suspicions. The office visit confirms pregnancy.

171. Mrs. Jones has had one prior pregnancy, which terminated in a spontaneous abortion. The nurse identifies the patient on the history form as a:

① Multipara
② Multigravida
③ Nulligravida
④ Primigravida

172. The nurse working in the obstetrician's office is aware that Mrs. Jones's growing child is at which stage of human development?

① Embryonic
② Organogenic
③ Fetal
④ Zygotic

173. Mrs. Jones is a Seventh Day Adventist and a lacto-ovo-vegetarian. The practical nurse is concerned about Mrs. Jones's level of protein intake. The nurse's *first* action would be to:

① Refer Mrs. Jones to the dietician to assess her protein intake
② Explain to Mrs. Jones the importance of eating lean meats with her vegetables
③ Give Mrs. Jones a nutrition booklet that lists foods high in protein
④ Ask Mrs. Jones to list everything she normally eats each week

174. Mrs. Jones tells the nurse that she is experiencing heartburn. Which suggestion would be appropriate for the nurse to make?

① Lie down and rest after meals
② Avoid drinking milk with meals
③ Consume frequent, small meals throughout the day
④ Maalox will offer some relief

175. At 16 weeks' gestation, Mrs. Jones asks the nurse what the baby is like. Which of the following would be the best response by the nurse?

① "Your baby has not yet reached viability."
② "It is possible to distinguish the sex organs of your baby at this time."
③ "Your baby's organs are not yet formed."
④ "Because each pregnancy is different, it is difficult to know."

176. At about 20 weeks' gestation, which of the following statements made by Mrs. Jones is most important for the nurse to report to the obstetrician?

① "My nausea has decreased."
② "My heartburn is still present."
③ "I've noticed a dark line running up and down my abdomen."
④ "I think I felt my baby move for the first time today."

177. Which of the following is the most appropriate response by the nurse to explain Mrs. Jones's continuing heartburn?

① "Your stomach produces more acid during pregnancy."
② "Your growing uterus is pressing against the stomach."
③ "Your digestive processes are slowed and there is more regurgitation because of the pregnancy hormones."
④ "You are producing an excess of bile, which causes regurgitation of food."

178. During the third trimester, Mrs. Jones tells the nurse that she is experiencing backache. Which of the following nursing actions is appropriate?

① Suggest she take aspirin to relieve the pain
② Teach her breathing exercises
③ Apply ice to her lower back
④ Teach her pelvic rocking exercises

179. During the third trimester, Mrs. Jones complains of a thin, colorless drainage from her nipples. The nurse's best response would be:

① "This is a rare occurence."
② "Your breasts are producing colostrum, the substance before mature milk forms."
③ "You must be sure to cleanse your nipples once a day with soap and warm water."
④ "You must report that to your obstetrician."

180. At 32 weeks' gestation, Mrs. Jones says she has nocturia and frequency. The nurse's best response would be to:

① Ignore this, because it is expected
② Question Mrs. Jones about any other urinary symptoms
③ Suggest that Mrs. Jones decrease her overall fluid intake
④ Prepare Mrs. Jones for a glucose tolerance screen

Ms. Susan Kane is a 21-year-old single primigravida. She has been attending the local hospital's maternity clinic.

181. At 38 weeks' gestation, Ms. Kane complains, "I'm tired of being pregnant. I just want this to be over." The nurse responds based on her knowledge that the patient:

① Is reacting in a normal manner
② Will likely experience some difficulty bonding with her child

③ Does not actually mean what she says
④ Is a candidate for elective induction

182. During routine assessments, the nurse is aware that an expected physiological change in Ms. Kane's cardiovascular system would include:

① An increased blood volume
② A decreased fluid volume
③ An increased blood pressure
④ A decreased pulse rate

183. In addition to cardiac changes, physiologic changes in Ms. Kane's gastrointestinal system would include an increase in:

① Production of hydrochloric acid in the stomach
② Intestinal motility
③ Cardiac sphincter tone
④ Water reabsorption in the large intestine

184. Other expected physiological changes during Ms. Kane's pregnancy would include:

① Proteinuria
② A decrease in blood clotting factors
③ A decrease in white blood cells (WBCs)
④ Thyroid gland enlargement

185. Five days before the estimated date of confinement, Ms. Kane enters the hospital with contractions occurring every 10 to 12 minutes. During the admission process, she informs the nurse of a vaginal discharge containing blood-stained mucus. The nurse's best response would be:

① "I will tell your doctor because of the risk of hemorrhage during labor."
② "You shouldn't worry about that now. We will take good care of you."
③ "That is called show. It is the loss of the mucus plug in the mouth of the womb and is expected during early labor."
④ "I am not sure what is going on, but it is not serious."

186. Ms. Kane tells the nurse that her mother is her coach and they attended Lamaze classes together. The nurse is aware that these classes provide:

① For a labor and delivery free of analgesia and anesthesia
② An increased knowledge base of the labor and delivery process
③ For a pain-free labor and delivery process

④ No information related to cesarean delivery

Jane Smith is a 17-year-old unmarried primigravida at 12 weeks' gestation. She has sought prenatal care at the health department.

187. Of the following symptoms reported by Jane, which one would the nurse be most concerned about?

① Urinary frequency
② Nausea
③ Constipation
④ Vaginal bleeding

188. After Jane's examination, the clinic physician determines that she has some cervical dilatation, in addition to her other symptoms. The diagnosis would likely be recorded as:

① Complete abortion
② Threatened abortion
③ Imminent abortion
④ Cervical incompetence

189. The plan of care for Jane would likely include:

① Bed rest and observation
② Fleet enema and sitz baths
③ Vistaril IM every 3 hours as needed
④ Foley catheter and oral antibiotics as ordered

Carol Ingram, a 24-year-old gravida 2, para 1, has been admitted to an acute care facility. She is now at 10 weeks' gestation, and ectopic pregnancy is diagnosed.

190. Ms. Ingram's condition is best defined as:

① Loss of a pregnancy in which part of the products of conception have been expelled
② A gestation implanted outside the uterine cavity
③ An abnormal development of the chorionic villi
④ A fetal death in which the products of conception are retained for over 4 weeks

191. The hospital practical nurse will observe Ms. Ingram closely for:

① Passage of grape-like vesicles
② Sharp, unilateral pelvic pain
③ Signs of pulmonary edema
④ False labor

192. In light of her current diagnosis, the nurse is not surprised to see in Ms. Ingram's medical history:

① A previous episode of pelvic inflammatory disease
② An exposure to rubella during this pregnancy
③ A congenital cervical anomaly
④ A family history of hypertension

193. Ms. Ingram is scheduled for emergency surgery. Her surgeon performed a right salpingectomy. During her postoperative recovery, she asks the nurse, "Will I be able to have any more children?" The nurse's answer is based on her knowledge that Ms. Ingram will now:

① Have anovulatory cycles
② Be able to conceive as easily as before
③ May take longer to conceive
④ Be maintained on hormonal therapy and cannot conceive

Mrs. McCampbell is at 35 weeks' gestation. She has just been admitted through the local hospital's emergency room. At 6 AM, she awoke in a pool of bright red blood. She is diagnosed by ultrasound as having placenta previa.

194. Based on Mrs. McCampbell's diagnosis, the nurse would expect the patient to experience:

① A severe headache
② Continuous abdominal pain
③ A rigid abdomen
④ Abdominal pain only during labor contractions

195. Mrs. McCampbell's condition is the result of the placenta:

① Developing an anomaly involving the site of the umbilical cord attachment
② Imbedding deeply into the myometrium
③ Implanting low in the uterine cavity near the internal cervical os
④ Prematurely separating from the uterine wall

196. The obstetrician requests a double set-up in preparation for a vaginal examination of Mrs. McCampbell. The nurse knows:

① The anesthesia department will be needing two trays for the procedure
② She must be prepared for delivery of the baby by the cesarean and vaginal routes

③ She must double-drape the patient for the procedure
④ The physician will need two scrub nurses to assist him with the procedure

Forty-year-old Katherine Karnes is a trauma victim from an automobile accident. She is a gravida 2, para 1 at 36 weeks' gestation who sustained an abdominal injury from her seat belt. She is very anxious about the well-being of her fetus. An ultrasound scan reveals an abruptio placenta.

197. Because of Mrs. Karnes's diagnosis, on assessment the nurse would expect to find:

① A board-like, tender uterus
② Excessive amounts of dark red vaginal bleeding
③ Hypertension and brisk reflexes
④ A high fever and bounding pulse

198. Mrs. Karnes's obstetrical complication involves a:

① Placental detachment from the uterine wall
② Torn cervix
③ Malformation of the placenta
④ Ruptured placenta

Sally, age 28 years, has progressed to 26 weeks' gestation. Although she has had no personal history of hyperglycemia, the obstetrician just informed her that she has gestational diabetes.

199. Sally was so concerned over her newly diagnosed condition that she did not comprehend all of what her physician said during his explanations. After the physician left the examination room, Sally says to the attending nurse, "Won't I have to be on insulin the rest of my life?" The nurse's *best* response would be:

① "You will probably be taking tablets instead of insulin injections."
② "Your condition will go away after the delivery of your baby."
③ "There is a good possibility that you will continue on insulin indefinitely."
④ "I don't know, but there is no need to worry over that now."

200. The prenatal office nurse prepares a written plan of care for Sally. Which of the following would be *inappropriate* to include on her care plan?

① Discourage exercise
② Teach about nonstress test procedures
③ Teach blood glucose monitoring
④ Reinforce diet principles

201. Sally asks the office nurse, "Will I be able to breast-feed this baby with my condition?" The nurse's *best* reply is:

① "Breast-feeding will worsen your condition."
② "Your doctor will tell you when it is safe to breast-feed."
③ "Patients with your condition may breast-feed if they wish."
④ "It is likely that you will not feel like breast-feeding."

202. At 36 weeks' gestation, Sally says to the office nurse, "My friends in childbirth classes tell me I will probably have a cesarean section. Is this true?" The nurse's *best* response is:

① "Some patients with your condition tend to have large babies, which may require that they have a cesarean section."
② "You must not allow what they say to upset you."
③ "That is untrue and an old wives' tale."
④ "It is best to wait until you are in labor and ask your doctor that question."

203. The rationale for the nurse's response in the previous question is based on:

① Her role as a nurse to dispel old wives' tales
② Her knowledge that no one knows a patient's risk for cesarean section until she is in labor
③ Her role as a support person and patient educator
④ Her limitations to answer certain questions that should be referred to the obstetrician

204. Your patient had a cesarean section yesterday. She is recovering normally, but has experienced incisional pain relieved by Tylenol #3 every 6 hours. Because she has received this drug, she is more likely to have problems with:

① Pneumonia
② Urinary retention
③ Constipation
④ Thrombophlebitis

Mr. Jones, who was admitted for gastrointestinal bleeding, has been sleeping since admission 2 hours ago. He is now restless and complains of thirst.

205. Which of the following actions will the nurse do first?

① Give him a glass of milk
② Ambulate him in the room
③ Notify the physician
④ Take his vital signs

206. Mr. Jones had a gastrojejunostomy. Which portion of the postoperative care plan must be modified?

① Irrigate the nasogastric tube with normal saline
② Cough and deep breathing every 2 hours
③ Leg exercises every hour while awake
④ Encourage early ambulation

207. Mr. Jones begins a regular diet after several days. The nurse observes for symptoms of dumping syndrome, which include:

① Abdominal cramping and pain
② Bradycardia and indigestion
③ Sweating and pallor
④ Blurred vision and chest pain

208. Which of the following interventions would be appropriate to prevent dumping syndrome?

① Limit fluids at mealtime
② Have the patient sit up for 1 hour after meals
③ Restrict fiber in the diet
④ Encourage high carbohydrate meals

Mary Love is admitted with acute exacerbation of chronic obstructive pulmonary disease (COPD).

209. An early sign/symptom of COPD is:

① Dyspnea on mild exertion
② Barrel chest
③ Clubbing of the distal ends of fingers and toes
④ Cyanosis

210. Ms. Love is receiving oxygen at 1 L/minute by nasal prongs. High concentrations of oxygen could cause:

① Decreased respiratory rate
② Increased secretions in the respiratory tract
③ Increased episodes of coughing
④ Respiratory alkalosis

211. Aminophylline 500 mg IV in normal saline is ordered. This drug is given to:

① Liquify bronchial secretions
② Reduce anxiety
③ Relax bronchial muscles
④ Depress the cough reflex

212. Emphysema is a condition:

① Manifested by scar tissue of the bronchi and bronchioles
② Characterized by distention of the bronchioles and destruction of the alveolar walls
③ Caused only by smoking and air pollution
④ That affects the cilia of the respiratory passage

213. Discharge instructions for Ms. Love would *not* include which of the following?

① Avoiding persons with infections
② Not taking any over-the-counter drugs without physician approval
③ Avoiding large meals
④ Attending an exercise class at least three times a week

214. Ms. Love is taught to use pursed lip and diaphragmatic breathing to:

① Increase air space within the lungs
② Assist in eliminating carbon dioxide
③ Improve respiratory muscle tone
④ Conserve energy needed to breathe

215. Nerve receptors for thirst are located in the:

① Hypothalamus
② Adrenal glands
③ Brain stem
④ Cerebral cortex

216. Intracellular fluid is fluid that is contained:

① Between the cells
② In the blood stream
③ Outside the cells
④ Inside the cells

217. A situation that would *not* result in edema is:

① Congestive heart failure
② Hyponatremia
③ Cirrhosis of the liver
④ Renal failure

218. A nursing intervention that would not be appropriate for a patient with edema is:

① Monitor intake and output
② Weigh daily
③ Encourage oral fluids
④ Reduce high sodium foods

219. When thiazide diuretics are ordered to correct edema, the nurse should observe the patient for symptoms of:

① Hypernatremia
② Hypokalemia
③ Increased blood sugar
④ Lowered blood sugar

220. Mr. Elliot is dehydrated. Which of the following symptoms indicates the presence of dehydration?

① Loss of skin turgor
② Increased blood pressure
③ Lowered body temperature
④ Restlessness

221. Mr. Jay's serum sodium is 155 mEq. The nurse should assess him for:

① Poor skin turgor
② Hypotension
③ Bradycardia
④ Pitting edema

222. One common cause of decreased sodium in cardiac patients is:

① Administration of diuretics
② Inadequate fluid intake
③ Poor dietary intake
④ Decreased renal function

223. Your patient is suffering from severe hyperkalemia. The nurse expects that the physician will order:

① IV solution of Ringer's lactate
② Kayexalate enemas
③ A low sodium diet
④ Increased use of salt substitutes

224. An early symptom of hypokalemia is:

① Muscle cramping

② Cardiac irritability
③ Fatigue
④ Tetany

225. A disorder brought on by prolonged immobility is:

① Hyperkalemia
② Hyponatremia
③ Hypokalemia
④ Hypercalcemia

226. The nurse should observe a patient for symptoms of hypocalcemia following a:

① Cholecystectomy
② Thoracotomy
③ Thyroidectomy
④ Hysterectomy

227. An example of a hypotonic solution is:

① Ringer's lactate
② 5% dextrose in water
③ 0.45% saline solution
④ Dextran solution

228. A symptom of fluid overload would be:

① Increased urinary output
② Decreased blood pressure
③ Increased body temperature
④ Increased heart rate

229. The nurse should assess the site of IV insertion:

① At least once a shift
② Every 2 hours
③ Every time the tubing is changed
④ After each new solution is started

Jason Kane is brought to the emergency room with dyspnea and severe abdominal pain. He has a history of sickle cell disease.

230. A common precipitating factor of sickle cell crisis is:

① Tension
② Dehydration
③ Decreased food intake
④ Depression

231. The pain associated with sickle cell disease is due to:

① Muscle spasms in the affected area
② Pressure from the edema caused by fluid retention

③ Irritation of nerve endings of the mucous secreting glands
④ Occlusion of small blood vessels

232. The diagnostic test that will differentiate between sickle cell trait and sickle cell disease is a:

① Hemoglobin electrophoresis
② Sickle cell prep
③ Sickledex
④ Blood smears

233. Jason should be instructed to:

① Limit fluid intake
② Avoid wearing tight clothes
③ Keep his room cool at all times
④ Not take any immunizations

234. In discharge planning, Jason is taught that management of a mild crisis would not include which of the following?

① Increasing fluid intake
② Controlling fever with antipyretic medications
③ Getting adequate rest
④ Checking for blood in the urine

235. The most critical assessment of Jason's abdomen is for:

① Signs of splenomegaly
② Active bowel sounds
③ Generalized tenderness
④ Changes in skin color

236. If Jane is angry at her husband but yells at her son instead, she is using the defense mechanism of:

① Denial
② Reaction formation
③ Suppression
④ Displacement

237. Which of the following is an example of the defense mechanism compensation?

① An ungainly youth works hard for a scholastic scholarship instead of trying to play sports
② An angry husband yells at his wife
③ A woman reverts to an earlier developmental level when faced with intolerable stress
④ A young man with low grades says he never tried to make good grades anyway

238. Harold has been making rather questionable moves in business. When he is asked about his behavior he states that all successful businessmen have to engage in these sorts of behaviors. This is an example of what defense mechanism?

① Conversion
② Projection
③ Regression
④ Rationalization

239. Mark is a 25-year-old man in the hospital for major surgery. He has been very demanding of attention and even demanded that his mother should be allowed to spend the night at his bedside. This is an example of the use of what defense mechanism?

① Denial
② Projection
③ Conversion
④ Regression

240. A man who hates his father goes out of his way to be nice to him. This is an example of which defense mechanism?

① Compensation
② Repression
③ Reaction formation
④ Projection

Answers & Rationales

Guide to item identification (see pp. 3–5 for further details about each category)

I, II, III, or IV for the phase of the nursing process
1, 2, 3, or 4 for the category of client needs
A, B, C, D, E, F, or G for the category of human functioning
Specific content category by name; ie, cholecystectomy

121. 80–120 mg/100 mL venous blood; other answers are incorrect.
② I, 2, F. Diabetes/Endocrine.

122. Two hours; other answers are incorrect theoretical concepts.
② I, 2, F. Diabetes/Endocrine.

123. The patient's degree of acceptance of his illness affects the nurse's teaching plan, because it influences how and where she begins her teaching. All diabetics need knowledge of their illness, because it helps them to accept their new lifestyle. Ways of caring for the illness are part of the teaching plan and must be individualized to the patient's lifestyle.
③ I, 4, F. & G. Endocrine/Diabetes.

124. Incomplete metabolism of carbohydrates and fats causes production of ketones and resultant acidosis and elevated blood sugar. Other choices are incorrect concepts.
① IV, 2, F. Endocrine/Diabetes.

125. Insulin lowers blood sugar. Appropriate balanced intake of carbohydrates, proteins and fats is essential to maintain a stable blood sugar level. If food intake is not adequate after administration of insulin, the insulin level is increased and the blood sugar is decreased.
① IV, 2 & 4, F. Endocrine/Diabetes.

126. The value of all foods ingested must be counted in the diet. Dietetic foods have a lower sugar content and are therefore lower in calories, but must still be counted. Other choices represent incorrect theoretical concepts.
② III, 4, F. Endocrine/Diabetes.

127. Illness influences metabolic rate and may increase or decrease blood sugar levels depend-
④ ing on many factors including appetite, fever, and altered activity. This assessment is imperative prior to any intervention relative to food or insulin intake.
III, 2 & 4, F. Endocrine/Diabetes.

128. The patient who understands the disease is better able to adapt to lifestyle changes and maintain control of the disease. This supercedes all other choices.
③ IV, 2, F. Endocrine/Diabetes.

129. Oral hypoglycemic agents stimulate the islets of Langerhans in the pancreas to produce insulin. Other choices are incorrect theoretical concepts.
③ II, 2, F. Endocrine/Diabetes.

130. Suction drains must be emptied whenever they are becoming full in order to maintain suction of drainage. They must be emptied at least every shift in order to evaluate output.
③ III, 1 & 2, A & D. Breast Cancer.

131. When the axillary area is surgically explored and lymph nodes are removed, edema frequently results, which causes pressure on the axillary and brachial arteries. Inactivity alone does not cause the circulation to the fingers to diminish. The IV should not be started in the arm on the affected side because of potential circulatory problems. Snug incisional sutures do not obstruct blood flow to the arteries because arteries are deep.
② I, 1 & 2, A, B & D. Breast Cancer.

132. The blood will flow by gravity to dependent areas. Dressings are not removed to assess for hemorrhage, and the patient's position should be changed frequently.
② I, 1 & 2, A & D. Breast Cancer.

133. Circulation must be protected in the affected arm owing to removal of axillary lymph nodes.
③ III, 1 & 2, A & B. Breast Cancer.

134. The wrist must be higher than the shoulder for gravity to promote venous drainage back toward the heart. The other options are not specific enough.
④ III, 1 & 2, A & D. Breast Cancer.

135. There can be contractures of the shoulder because the pectoralis and axillary muscles have been cut.
④ III, 1 & 2, A & D. Breast Cancer.

136. Glaucoma is a condition of increased intra-ocular pressure.
④ III, 4, C. Glaucoma.

137. Glaucoma is a problem of increased produc-tion or obstruction in the outflow of aqueous humor.
③ III, 4, C. Glaucoma.

138. Miotics are used to decrease intraocular pres-sure by constricting the pupil and increasing outflow of aqueous humor. This medication must be continued for the rest of the patient's life to prevent vision loss.
② III, 2 & 4, C. Glaucoma/Medication Adminis-tration.

139. Mydriatics dilate the pupil to decrease the an-gle, slow the outflow of aqueous humor, and thus increase the intraocular pressure.
② III, 2 & 4, C. Glaucoma/Medication Adminis-tration.

140. Eyedrops are instilled into the inner canthus of the eye, being careful not to touch the drop-per to the eye.
③ III, 2 & 4, C. Glaucoma/Medication Adminis-tration.

141. The delayed acquisition of gross motor mile-stones is usually the primary complaint in the history of infants with CP.
① I, 2, C. Cerebral Palsy.

142. When talking to parents the nurse must re-member that CP varies from mild to severe.
③ III, 2 & 3, C & G. Cerebral Palsy.

143. Persistent oral reflexes, poor breathing pat-terns, tongue thrust, excessive opening of the mouth, and drooling make it difficult for the child to obtain adequate nutrition.
① II, 4, C. Cerebral Palsy.

144. A major part of the nurse's role when working with adolescents who are depressed would be to make appropriate referral when necessary.
③ III, 3, G. Suicidal Behavior.

145. Depression is found in two thirds of the cases of suicide. The nurse should be alert for any changes in behavior, as well as the giving away of personal belongings, which may sig-nal a suicide attempt.
④ I, 3, G. Suicidal Behavior.

146. Being inactive tends to perpetuate itself, caus-ing the patient to lose the initiative to do what she is capable of doing.
③ I, 2, E. Immobility/Older Adults.

147. Foot drop is a common result of immobility. A footboard keeps the foot in proper alignment and prevents foot drop.
② III, 4, E. Immobility.

148. ROM exercises should not cause considerable pain. The physician should be notified before continuing.
① IV, 2, E. Immobility.

149. Trochanter rolls are placed on the outside of the hips and legs, and prevent them from rolling outwardly.
④ III, 2, C. Immobility.

150. Without muscle movement, blood becomes static in the venous system, which in turn increases the likelihood of thrombi or emboli.
① I, 4, B & F. Immobility.

151. Immobility can lead to constipation related to decreased peristalsis. Increased bulk and roughage in the diet can help prevent this problem. Enemas should be avoided. Stool softeners are suggested, along with increased fluid intake.
③ III, 4, E. Immobility.

152. Hyperactivity is not normally an effect of im-mobility.
④ II, 2 & 4, E. Immobility.

153. Calcium is lost in large amounts from the bones, leading to disuse osteoporosis.
② II, 2 & 4, E. Immobility/Fluid & Electrolytes.

154. Pressure on an area decreases circulation, re-sulting in cell death. #1, #3, and #4 are con-tributing factors, but not the primary cause.
② I, 2 & 4, E. Immobility.

155. This is usually adequate to prevent break-down. #2, #3, and #4: time periods are too long.
① III, 2 & 4, E. Immobility.

156. Denial is a primary defense mechanism, espe-cially among younger adolescents. It is char-acterized by the inability or unwillingness to acknowledge pertinent information.
① I, 3 & 4, A & G. Labor and Delivery.

157. In anxiety-producing situations, concentra-tion is diminished, so communication should be short and simple. Medication would simply further interfere with concentration.
③ III, 3 & 4, A & G. Labor and Delivery.

158. The normal FHR is 120 to 160 bpm. It is impor-
② tant to give the patient correct information so
that she will not be so anxious. The other
answers are untrue and would not be therapeutic.
III, 3 & 4, A & G. Labor and Delivery.

159. The teenager is at risk for all of these reasons.
④ I & II, 4, A. Labor and Delivery.

160. Contractions are measured from the begin-
① ning of one contraction to the beginning of the
next contraction.
I, 4, A. Labor and Delivery.

161. Demerol is a narcotic analgesic that can be
③ given for pain during the active phases of
labor.
III & IV, 2 & 4, A. Labor and Delivery.

162. An episiotomy is an incision made into the
③ perineum prior to delivery. It is done to facilitate the delivery of the baby and to prevent
tearing when the baby is delivered.
I, 4, A. Labor and Delivery.

163. Handwashing is imperative; it is the most ba-
② sic form of hygiene and infection prevention.
All perineal care should be done from front to
back.
IV, 4, A. Postpartum.

164. The patient's decision should be supported.
② Bonding and attachment are encouraged by
frequent, loving contact with the parent. It is
not necessary to breast-feed the infant in order to bond.
III, 3 & 4, A & G. Postpartum.

165. Answers #1, #2, and #3 indicate a lack of
④ nutritional knowledge. Nutritional intake
must provide sufficient calories and a wide
variety of nutrients to meet the adolescent's
own growth needs.
IV, 4, A & F. Postpartum.

166. Consideration must be given to identifying
① and supporting the adolescent's need for a
lifestyle that is both realistic and satisfying.
II, 4, A. Postpartum.

167. These are the typical signs of a full and dis-
① tended bladder. When the bladder becomes
distended, it displaces the uterus.
I, 4, A. Postpartum.

168. Breast-feeding stimulates the body to release
④ oxytocin. Oxytocin causes the uterine contractions that she is feeling.
I, 4, A. Postpartum.

169. Sibling visitation with the parents and new
③ baby help the older child (children) adjust to
this major change.
III, 3 & 4, A. & G. Postpartum.

170. A positive Homans' sign is indicative of
① thrombophlebitis. Thrombophlebitis is one of
the complications that can occur postpartum.
I, 2 & 4, A & B. Postpartum.

171. Mrs. Jones is a multigravida because of her
② one prior pregnancy, but not a multipara because the prior pregnancy was terminated before viability. Nulligravid means never having been pregnant; primigravid means
pregnant for the first time.
I, 4, A. Prenatal Care.

172. The fetal stage begins at the end of 8 weeks,
③ which has passed by the second missed period. The embryonic or organogenic stage
ends at the end of 8 weeks. The zygotic stage
ends at implantation.
I, 4, A. Fetal Development.

173. The nurse should first assess if Mrs. Jones has
④ an adequate protein intake by gathering data
about her diet. Mrs. Jones's religious preferences should be respected. It may be a bit
premature to refer to the dietician or even
promote a change in her diet.
I, 1 & 4, A & F. Prenatal/Nutrition.

174. Heartburn can be caused by increased pres-
③ sure of the growing uterus on the stomach.
Measures to deal with heartburn include
small frequent meals, drinking milk before
and during meals, and sitting up an hour after
meals. Over-the-counter drugs should be
taken during pregnancy only under advice of
a physician.
III, 1 & 4, A & F. Prenatal Care.

175. The sex organs are distinguishable by 16
② weeks' gestation, the fetus has reached viability, and all organs have completed their formation.
III, 4, A. Fetal Development.

176. Quickening is important to note for assessing
④ gestational age.
I, 4, A. Fetal Development.

177. ③ This is the physiological basis for heartburn of pregnancy. Acid secretion is decreased during pregnancy and bile secretion is not the cause for regurgitation.
III, 4, A. Prenatal Care.

178. ④ Pelvic rocking exercises will strengthen muscle tone and provide muscle tension relief.
III, 4, A. Prenatal Care.

179. ② This is an accurate explanation to Mrs. Jones and helps to allay her anxiety. Soap on the nipples is drying and not recommended.
III, 3 & 4, A & G. Prenatal Care.

180. ② The nurse should ascertain if other symptoms indicative of UTI are present. This symptom is often encountered in the third trimester, but overall fluid intake should not be decreased. A glucose tolerance screen is not warranted just because of this symptom.
I, 1 & 4, A. Prenatal Care.

181. ① This is expected as term approaches and not indicative of future bonding difficulties or an induction.
I, 3, A. Prenatal Care.

182. ① Increased blood volume is a normal physiologic adaptation to pregnancy in the last two trimesters. Pulse usually increases slightly; blood pressure should not increase.
I, 4, A. Prenatal Care.

183. ④ Increased water reabsorption in the large bowel is expected during pregnancy, hydrochloric acid production is decreased, intestinal motility and cardiac sphincter tone is decreased.
I, 4, A & F. Prenatal Care.

184. ④ Thyroid gland enlargement is expected, blood clotting factors and WBCs increase, and proteinuria is abnormal.
I, 4, A. Prenatal Care.

185. ③ The patient is describing bloody show, a normal finding during labor. The nurse should explain the process to the patient without discussing risk of hemorrhage, which is not applicable to the situation.
III, 3 & 4, A & G. Labor & Delivery.

186. ② This is the main function of Lamaze classes, not to eliminate pain or need for pain relief.

Most classes provide information about cesarean delivery.
II, 4, A. Labor & Delivery.

187. ④ Bleeding could indicate threatened abortion. The other symptoms are expected.
I, 2, A. Prenatal Complications.

188. ③ Once dilatation occurs, abortion is imminent or inevitable. Threatened abortion is bleeding only without dilatation. Cervical incompetence is usually not associated with bleeding or cramping.
I, 2, A. Prenatal Complications.

189. ① Bed rest and observation are standard for imminent abortion. The other actions are not usually implemented.
II, 1 & 2, A. Complications of Pregnancy.

190. ② Ectopic pregnancy is one implanted outside the uterus. The others options describe other complications of pregnancy.
I, 2, A. Complications of Pregnancy/Ectopic Pregnancy.

191. ② This is a symptom of a ruptured ectopic pregnancy. The others are unrelated to her particular situation.
I, 2, A. Complications of Pregnancy/Ectopic Pregnancy.

192. ① Pelvic inflammatory disease is associated with scarring of fallopian tubes, which often causes ectopic pregnancy. The other options are not directly related to her condition.
I, 2, A. Complications of Pregnancy/Ectopic Pregnancy.

193. ③ With one tube gone, Mrs. Ingram's chances of future pregnancy are decreased. She will continue to ovulate, and will not be on hormonal therapy in the absence of other problems.
II, 2 & 4, A. Complications of Pregnancy/Ectopic Pregnancy.

194. ④ Placenta previa is usually not painful or associated with a rigid abdomen unless labor is present.
I, 2, A. Complications of Pregnancy/Placenta Previa.

195. ③ A low-implanted placenta; the others do not describe the condition.
I, 2, A. Complications of Pregnancy/Placenta Previa.

196. ② A double set-up requires being ready for a vaginal and a cesarean delivery. The other answers are not specific.
II, 2, A. Cesarean Section.

197. ① A board-like tender uterus is characteristic of abruptio placenta; bleeding may be hidden.
I, 2, A. Abruptio Placenta.

198. ① This describes abruptio placenta. The other options are inaccurate.
I, 2, A. Abruptio Placenta.

199. ② Gestational diabetes is present only during pregnancy; the condition subsides after delivery.
III, 2 & 3, A & G. Complications of Pregnancy/Gestational Diabetes.

200. ① All other actions are appropriate. Moderate exercise helps to maintain normal glucose levels.
II, 2, A. Complications of Pregnancy/Gestational Diabetes.

201. ③ Breastfeeding is encouraged because it decreases the diabetic state. Only if ketonuria develops would it be discontinued for a time.
III, 2 & 4, A. Complications of Pregnancy/Gestational Diabetes.

202. ① This statement is true and answers the question accurately and in a straightforward manner.
III, 3, A & G. Complications of Pregnancy/Gestational Diabetes.

203. ③ The nurse is responding based on knowledge of the patient's condition and her role as a patient educator.
III, 3, E. Complications of Pregnancy/Gestational Diabetes.

204. ③ Tylenol #3 contains 30 mg of codeine. Codeine has constipation as a major side effect. A stool softener is often given with it to prevent this.
II, 1, A. Medications.

205. ④ A change in vital signs will occur with internal bleeding; therefore, vital signs should be taken first, because notification of the physician includes all of the assessment data. #2 is inappropriate because activity will increase bleeding. The milk may increase nausea and vomiting.
I, 2, F. Upper GI.

206. ① The nurse never irrigates or repositions the nasogastric tube after gastric surgery.
II, 1, F. Upper GI.

207. ③ Symptoms of dumping syndrome include vertigo, increased heart rate, sweating, pallor, palpitation, and the desire to lie down.
I, 2, F. Upper GI.

208. ① Gastric emptying can be delayed by not taking fluids with meals, by eating in a recumbent or semirecumbent position, or by lying down after meals.
III, 2, F. Upper GI.

209. ① Dyspnea with mild exertion is an early symptom of the hypoxia associated with COPD. The other options listed are late symptoms of COPD.
I, 2, B. COPD.

210. ① The COPD patient has a chronically high CO_2 level, so that this is no longer a stimulus for respiration. The COPD patient's stimulus for breathing is hypoxia. If the patient receives too much oxygen, the stimulus for respiration is lost and the respiratory rate drops.
IV, 2, B. COPD.

211. ③ Aminophylline is a smooth muscle relaxant that promotes relaxation of the bronchial smooth muscles. As COPD becomes worse, the medication will become less and less effective.
IV, 2, B. COPD.

212. ② Emphysema is characterized by air trapping. As the air is trapped in the alveoli, the bronchioles and alveoli become distended and "blebs" or air pockets are formed.
IV, 2, B. COPD.

213. ④ Once the patient has symptomatic COPD, exercise must be limited. The other options are instructions that are important for the patient to follow.
III, 2 & 4, B. COPD.

214. ② With COPD, the air becomes trapped in the alveoli; therefore, an increase in carbon dioxide occurs. Pursed lip and diaphragmatic breathing increase the outflow of air, helping to remove some of the air trapped in the alveoli.
III, 2 & 4, B. COPD.

215. One of the functions of the hypothalamus is to control thirst.
① I, 2, B. Fluid and Electrolytes.

216. The intracellular fluid is that which is contained within the cells. The fluid outside the cells is referred to as extracellular fluid.
④ I, 2, B. Fluid and Electrolytes.

217. A low serum sodium, unless it is dilutional hyponatremia, is not associate with edema. Usually, when sodium is low, so is water. All the other options cause edema.
② IV, 2, B. Fluid and Electrolytes.

218. Edema is a condition in which the patient has too much fluid in the body, usually in the third space. The patient with edema is usually on fluid restriction, so that further water retention can be limited. Sodium is reduced because it holds water in the body.
③ III, 2, B. Fluid and Electrolytes.

219. Thiazide diuretics work by causing potassium to be lost through the kidneys along with the excessive water. When these diuretics are used, the patient is usually directed to increase the potassium in the diet.
② I, 2, B. Fluid and Electrolytes.

220. Dehydration is characterized by loss of skin turgor, hypotension, conservation of urine, and an elevated temperature.
① I, 2, B. Fluid and Electrolytes.

221. An increased serum sodium leads to the retention of water in the body to dilute it. When the patient has hypernatremia, he or she will also exhibit edema. With a high serum sodium, pitting edema is seen.
④ I, 2, B. Fluid and Electrolytes.

222. Diuretics act by causing loss of potassium or sodium. As these electrolytes are lost, loss of water also occurs. Because cardiac patients often exhibit hypertension or CHF, they typically receive diuretic medications.
① I, 2, B. Fluid and Electrolytes.

223. A severely increased serum potassium predisposes the patient to the development of potentially fatal cardiac arrhythmias. It is important, therefore, to lower the serum potassium rapidly. Kayexalate can be given either orally or by enema. It acts to bind the excessive potassium and causes it to be excreted through the feces.
② II, 2, B. Fluid and Electrolytes.

224. A low serum potassium produces muscle weakness and accompanying fatigue.
③ I, 2, B. Fluid and Electrolytes.

225. When a patient is immobilized for any prolonged period of time, calcium is released from the bone, leading to hypercalcemia.
④ IV, 2, B. Fluid and Electrolytes.

226. The parathyroid glands lie directly posterior to the thyroid gland. The parathyroids control calcium metabolism. When a thyroidectomy is performed, the parathyroids are often incidently removed, damaged or, at least, traumatized and edematous from the surgery. This leads to altered calcium metabolism, usually reversible after healing occurs.
③ I, 2, B. Fluid and Electrolytes.

227. 0.9% or normal saline is an isotonic solution, which means that it is the same concentration as blood, used IV. Hypotonic means that the solution is less concentrated than the blood; 0.45% saline is less concentrated.
③ III, 2, B. Fluid and Electrolytes.

228. When there is a fluid overload, the workload of the heart and circulatory system is dramatically increased. To compensate for this problem, the heart rate increases.
④ I, 2, B. Fluid and Electrolytes.

229. The IV site should be assessed every shift for problems such as infiltration or inflammation. The dressing over the site is usually changed every 48 to 72 hours.
① I, 1, B. Fluid and Electrolytes.

230. Dehydration leads to hemoconcentration, which can precipitate sickle cell crisis because of the abnormal shape of the red blood cells.
② I, 2, B. Sickle Cell Anemia.

231. The abnormally shaped, "sickled" red blood cells clog small vessels, leading to occlusion and ischemia.
④ I, 2, B. Sickle Cell Anemia.

232. To differentiate the trait from the disease, the hemoglobin electrophoresis is necessary. The other tests are not that specific.
① I, 2, B. Sickle Cell Anemia.

233. Occlusion of vessels is a common problem with this disorder, so nothing that will increase the risk of this should be done.
② III, 2 & 4, B. Sickle Cell Anemia.

234.
④
This is not a problem of mild crisis. The other actions are appropriate.
III, 2 & 4, B. Sickle Cell Anemia.

235.
①
The abnormal-shaped cells can become trapped in the spleen, causing enlargement. As the spleen becomes enlarged, even more red blood cells and platelets are destroyed.
I, 2, B. Sickle Cell Anemia.

236.
④
The description is of displacement or moving anger from the correct object to a safer object. The other options refer to other defense mechanisms.
I, 3, G. Defense Mechanisms.

237.
①
When a person is unable to excel in one area, he or she often overcompensates by focusing all energies in another area. The other options refer to other defense mechanisms.
I, 3, G. Defense Mechanisms.

238.
④
Rationalization refers to blaming others for problems of one's own making, rather than accepting the consequences of one's own actions. The other options refer to other defense mechanisms.
I, 3, G. Defense Mechanisms.

239.
④
When a patient is faced with a very stressful situation, the patient often retreats to a more comfortable level of development temporarily. The other options refer to other defense mechanisms.
I, 3, G. Defense Mechanisms.

240.
③
Feelings that are unacceptable to the individual on a conscious level are often hidden from the self by overemphasizing the opposite feelings. The other options refer to other defense mechanisms.
I, 3, G. Defense Mechanisms.

Analysis of Questions in Practice Tests I and II

PHASES OF THE NURSING PROCESS

Assessment

1, 4, 5, 6, 9, 10, 12, 15, 22, 23, 25, 28, 29, 30, 31, 32, 37, 53, 57, 59, 60, 63, 64, 65, 66, 67, 69, 71, 75, 76, 79, 80, 81, 83, 84, 86, 87, 88, 95, 96, 106, 107, 113, 114, 116, 121, 122, 123, 131, 132, 138, 141, 144, 146, 152, 154, 156, 160, 162, 167, 168, 170, 171, 172, 173, 176, 180, 181, 182, 183, 184, 187, 188, 190, 191, 192, 194, 195, 197, 198, 205, 207, 209, 215, 216, 219, 220, 221, 222, 224, 226, 228, 229, 230, 231, 232, 235, 236, 237, 238, 239, 240.

Planning

13, 14, 33, 43, 48, 49, 56, 61, 62, 85, 90, 91, 92, 94, 103, 109, 129, 143, 152, 153, 159, 166, 186, 189, 193, 196, 200, 204, 206, 223.

Implementation

2, 3, 7, 8, 11, 15, 16, 17, 18, 19, 20, 24, 26, 27, 34, 36, 38, 39, 40, 41, 42, 44, 45, 46, 47, 50, 51, 52, 54, 55, 58, 68, 73, 74, 77, 78, 82, 88, 89, 90, 93, 99, 100, 101, 102, 104, 105, 109, 110, 111, 112, 115, 116, 117, 126, 127, 130, 133, 134, 135, 136, 137, 139, 140, 142, 145, 147, 149, 150, 151, 153, 154, 155, 157, 158, 161, 164, 174, 175, 177, 178, 179, 177, 178, 179, 185, 199, 201, 202, 203, 208, 213, 214, 218, 226, 227, 233, 234.

Evaluation

21, 35, 70, 72, 91, 97, 98, 100, 105, 108, 124, 125, 128, 148, 156, 159, 161, 163, 165, 210, 211, 212, 214, 217, 225.

CATEGORIES OF CLIENT NEEDS

Safe, Effective Care Environment

13, 14, 15, 18, 19, 33, 34, 36, 39, 40, 41, 43, 44, 45, 48, 49, 50, 51, 52, 74, 79, 80, 81, 83, 84, 85, 87, 88, 89, 99, 101, 102, 103, 106, 109, 111, 112, 116, 117, 130, 131, 132, 133, 134, 135, 117, 173, 174, 189, 206, 214, 217, 220, 223, 228, 229, 234, 235.

Physiologic Integrity

1, 2, 4, 5, 6, 7, 8, 9, 10, 11, 12, 13, 14, 15, 16, 17, 18, 21, 22, 23, 24, 25, 26, 33, 34, 36, 37, 38, 39, 40, 41, 42, 43, 44, 45, 46, 47, 48, 49, 53, 54, 55, 57, 58, 59, 61, 62, 63, 65, 66, 67, 84, 85, 86, 87, 88, 91, 92, 93, 95, 96, 97, 98, 99, 100, 101, 102, 103, 106, 107, 108, 110, 111, 112, 113, 114, 115, 116, 117, 121, 122, 124, 125, 127, 128, 129, 130, 131, 132, 133, 134, 135, 138, 139, 140, 141, 142, 148, 149, 152, 153, 154, 155, 161, 170, 187, 188, 189, 190, 191, 192, 193, 194, 195, 196, 197, 198, 199, 199, 200, 201, 202, 204, 205, 207, 208, 209, 210, 211, 212, 213, 214, 215, 216, 217, 218, 219, 220, 221, 222, 223, 224, 225, 226, 227, 228, 230, 231, 232, 233, 234, 235.

Psychosocial Integrity

19, 20, 27, 56, 60, 64, 68, 142, 144, 145, 146, 156, 157, 158, 164, 168, 179, 181, 185, 193, 202, 203, 236, 237, 238, 239, 240.

Health Promotion and Maintenance

3, 6, 23, 24, 28, 29, 30, 31, 32, 68, 69, 70, 71, 72, 73, 74, 75, 76, 77, 78, 82, 87, 88, 89, 90, 91, 92, 94, 100, 104, 105, 111, 123, 125, 126, 127, 136, 137, 138, 139, 140, 143, 147, 150, 151, 152, 153, 154, 155, 157, 158, 159, 160, 161, 162, 163, 164, 165, 166, 167, 168, 169, 170, 171, 172, 173, 174, 175, 176, 177, 178, 180, 181, 182, 183, 184, 185, 186, 193, 201, 213, 214, 233, 234.

The Nursing Process and Basic Skills

3

I. THE NURSING PROCESS

A. Assessment

1. Collection of data about patients to aid in the planning, implementing, and evaluating of patient care
2. Methods
   a. observe patient and environment
   b. perform physical examination, including procedures such as vital signs, height, weight, and other objective data
   c. communicate with patient to obtain an accurate and complete history
   d. collect all laboratory specimens ordered

B. Planning

1. The act of setting reasonable goals and priorities designed to meet client needs
2. Must be based on the patient's assessed needs
3. Becomes basis of nursing interventions

C. Implementation

1. Provision of nursing care designed to meet established goals
2. Includes both physical and psychosocial care of patients and their environment
3. Recording/documentation of all pertinent data is an important part of nursing care

D. Evaluation

1. Identifying whether established goals set for each patient were accomplished; whether nursing care was effective in meeting goals
2. Evaluation should always lead to revision of the plan of care so that unmet needs are met and effective interventions are continued

II. BASIC SKILLS

A. Skills Related to Sexuality

1. Privacy
   a. always drape patient who is potentially exposed for examination
   b. draw curtain or close door when patient might be exposed
2. Perineal care
   a. always wipe or wash from front to back
   b. daily cleanse area with soap and water in both men and women
   c. type of solutions used for cleansing varies and may require a physician's order
   d. change and remove soiled perineal pads front to back
3. Vaginal douche
   a. done to cleanse vagina
   b. patient should void first
   c. patient is placed on bedpan in dorsal recumbent position with knees flexed
   d. solution varies from soap solution to vinegar in warm water
   e. irrigation administered under low pressure to avoid trauma; hold container just above patient's hips
   f. nozzle is inserted with solution running and is pointed down and back into vagina
   g. rotate nozzle gently to clean all vaginal folds
4. Pap smear
   a. test to detect changes in cervix that are either premalignant or malignant
   b. performed on women beginning at age 18 years or earlier if they are sexually active
   c. frequency of examination yearly in high-risk women and then according to doctor's decision in others; guidelines vary
   d. must refrain from douching 24 hours prior to test
   e. patient in lithotomy position; drape carefully
   f. when doctor scrapes tissue from cervix, apply to glass slide and spray with fixative agent
5. Breast self-examination
   a. systematic observation and palpation of breasts to detect cysts or tumors

b. should be done by women over age 20 years, monthly about 1 week following menstrual period

c. encourage correct technique

6. Testicular self-examination
   a. systematic observation and palpation of testicles to detect tumors
   b. should be done monthly by men between age 20 and 40 years
   c. encourage correct technique

B. Skills Related to Oxygenation

1. Ace bandages/TED hose/compression stockings
   a. used to encourage venous return from extremities and prevent thrombi formation
   b. pressure should not be great enough to interfere with circulation
   c. should be worn while patient is in bed
   d. remove every 8 hours to check for undue pressure on skin
   e. apply with patient lying in bed
2. Heat and cold application
   a. heat application
      (1) produces muscle relaxation
      (2) promotes suppuration
      (3) helps localize infections
      (4) increases metabolic rate
      (5) increases local blood flow to relieve circulatory congestion
   b. apply heat and cold only with doctor's order
   c. K-pads have exact temperature settings
   d. monitor closely for redness, pain, and swelling, prevent burning
   e. cold application
      (1) constricts blood vessels and reduces blood flow
      (2) aids in control of hemorrhage
      (3) reduces inflammatory process
      (4) prevents suppuration
   f. fill ice packs about 2/3 full of ice; remove all air
   g. cover pack before application
   h. refill about every 2 hours; remove periodically to maintain circulation
   i. monitor skin closely for excess cold; white, mottled skin, numbness
   j. monitor body temperature
3. Coughing and deep breathing
   a. done to effectively remove secretions from the respiratory tract
   b. improves oxygenation by preventing atelectasis
   c. method of effective coughing and deep breathing
      (1) sit patient up in high Fowler's position
      (2) splint abdomen or chest with pillows or

hands, if necessary, to prevent incisional pain

(3) request deep inspiration through mouth several times

(4) bend patient forward and instruct to contract thorax and abdomen to forcibly expel air

d. medicate for pain prior to coughing to improve effort

e. encourage in pre- and postoperative patients and those with decreased mobility

4. Vaporizer/nebulizer
   a. provision of air with a high humidity to
      (1) sooth irritated mucous membranes
      (2) provide extra moisture to respiratory tract
      (3) liquify thick secretions
      (4) loosen crusts on mucous membranes
      (5) administer medications directly to respiratory tract
   b. administered by a wide variety of equipment
   c. possibility of bacterial growth in warm water reservoir
   d. monitor for bronchospasms and overhydration
5. Blow bottles/Triflow
   a. used to encourage deep breathing and coughing
   b. patient exhales against pressure of water or balls in Triflow
   c. should be done hourly while awake
6. Inspiratory/incentive spirometer
   a. helps patient to inspire deeply, thereby expanding lung capacity
   b. with lips sealed over mouthpiece, patient takes a deep breath, holds 3 seconds, then exhales slowly
   c. encourage patient to use hourly while awake
7. Intermittent positive pressure breathing (IPPB) treatments
   a. administration of higher-than-ambient pressures and higher-than-patient's normal tidal volume to force oxygen into respiratory tract
   b. IPPB used to
      (1) promote deep breathing in patients with decreasing levels of consciousness
      (2) mobilize secretions through stimulation of coughing
      (3) increase O_2 intake and CO_2 removal
      (4) produce mechanical bronchodilation
      (5) administer aerosol medications
      (6) prevent atelectasis by hyperinflation of alveoli
      (7) decrease work of breathing temporarily
   c. should only be administered by trained personnel
8. Postural drainage
   a. technique of positioning patient so that gravity

assists with the drainage of secretions from the lobes of the lungs

b. improves removal of secretions when combined with clapping and vibration over affected areas of lungs

c. position patient so that gravity helps to drain affected areas of lung

9. Suctioning
   a. mechanical aspiration of secretions from the tracheobronchial tree, when patient unable to remove
   b. tracheal suctioning is a sterile procedure; oral or nasal suctioning is a clean procedure
   c. administer O_2 in high levels before and after suctioning
   d. apply suction after inserting the catheter
   e. do not suction for more than 10 seconds continuously
   f. withdraw catheter slowly with rotating motion

10. Sputum specimen
    a. performed to inspect sputum for infective agents or malignancy
    b. best obtained in morning before breakfast
    c. use proper container, sterile for culture, and with preservative for cytology
    d. have patient breathe deeply to induce cough
    e. avoid contamination of inside of container

11. Tracheostomy care
    a. monitor patient closely for signs of obstruction of tube
    b. suctioning and cleaning of tracheostomy: sterile procedure
    c. monitor and maintain skin around stoma
    d. always provide humidified air

12. Oxygen administration
    a. used to treat hypoxemia, low blood oxygen; determined by blood gas analysis or pulse oximeter
    b. can be given in many concentrations and through many devices
       (1) ordered in L/minute
       (2) various devices provide higher or lower concentrations; mask higher, nasal cannula lower
    c. post signs against smoking because oxygen supports combustion
    d. avoid high levels of oxygen in patients with chronic obstructive pulmonary disease (COPD) or over long times for any patient

13. CPR (see pp 148)

14. Intake and output
    a. must be measured accurately to determine patient's fluid balance
    b. learn volumes of containers commonly used for fluids
    c. measure urine, liquid feces, and other bodily drainage for accurate output

C. Skills Related to Sensory/Perception

1. Eye/ear irrigations
   a. use of a large volume of therapeutic agent to wash or flush the eye or ear
   b. to flush eye
      (1) use sterile technique when irrigating eye; treat each eye separately
      (2) position patient to drain fluids and any foreign bodies from eye
      (3) expose conjunctival sac and direct irrigation from inner canthus toward outer angle
      (4) use little force when irrigating
   c. to flush ear
      (1) draw auricle down and back for children and up and back for adults to straighten ear canal
      (2) tilt patient's head so ear to be treated is uppermost
      (3) direct stream toward wall of ear canal, not eardrum

2. Level of consciousness (LOC)
   a. describe what patient is doing or is able to do; avoid labels
   b. assess orientation to person, place, and time
   c. test reflexes, especially protective reflexes (gag and corneal)
   d. test neuromuscular function to determine purposeful activities

3. Neurological assessment
   a. pupil reactions
      (1) normal pupils are equal, round, react to light with accommodation (PERRLA)
      (2) size and shape
      (3) speed of reaction to light
      (4) equality of pupil size and reaction
   b. eye movements, ability to follow finger vs. erratic and uncontrolled movement
   c. movement of extremities
      (1) voluntary and purposeful
      (2) equality of strength and movement
   d. reflexes, normal reponses and equal on both sides of the body
   e. vital signs
   f. level of consciousness

4. Protective devices/restraints
   a. protectors used to prevent patients from harming either themselves or others
   b. require physician's order
   c. select the least restrictive device of proper type and size
   d. investigate all alternatives to eliminate the precipitating problem before resorting to restraints
   e. use restraints as a last resort and only on a short-term basis

f. involve the patient (if possible) and the family in the decision making

g. document need for restraints clearly on chart

h. assess the patient frequently for
    (1) damage to tissue under restraint
    (2) damage to other body parts such as shoulder dislocation
    (3) problems related to immobility
    (4) damage to joints
    (5) safety; patient may be unable to call for help, reach water, or relieve pressure on areas; anticipate needs

i. check every hour, release × 15 minutes and reapply at least every 2 hours

j. avoid patient isolation, encourage interaction

k. maintain restraint record per institutional policy

l. reevaluate need for restraints frequently

5. Pain control
   a. assessment of pain
      (1) history of pain development and occurrence
      (2) location of pain
      (3) nature of pain: onset, intensity, depth, radiation, duration, quality
      (4) physical signs: grimacing, crying, change in vital signs, restlessness, insomnia
      (5) what relieves pain
      (6) associated symptoms: nausea, restlessness, constipation
   b. methods of controlling pain
      (1) medication
          (a) narcotic analgesics: oral, parenteral, rectal, transdermal, intrathecal
          (b) nonnarcotic analgesics: oral most common
      (2) noninvasive methods
          (a) relaxation exercises
          (b) repositioning
          (c) therapeutic interaction with patient
          (d) rhythmic breathing
          (e) heat and cold applications, as ordered
          (f) cutaneous stimulation, back rubs
          (g) diversional activities

D. Skills Related to Protective Functions

1. Culture and sensitivity specimens
   a. culture identifies infective organisms from multiple body sites and fluids
   b. sensitivity identifies drugs that should effectively combat the identified microorganism
   c. requires sterile container and sterile collection techniques
   d. collect specimen before beginning antibiotics

e. antibiotic treatments based on results

2. Hygiene needs
   a. bed bath
      (1) avoid chilling or exposure
      (2) water should be between 105°F and 115°F
      (3) change bath water frequently, as needed
      (4) use soap sparingly to avoid drying skin; rinse well
      (5) assess skin during bath
      (6) soak hands and feet in warm water
   b. skin care
      (1) use oils and lotions to restore natural oils to skin
      (2) massage skin gently
      (3) turn and reposition patient frequently
      (4) assess for reddened or broken areas
      (5) keep bed linen clean, dry, and wrinkle-free
      (6) use special beds or mattresses to avoid skin breakdown in high-risk patients
      (7) wash and clean patient thoroughly after using bedpan
   c. oral care
      (1) brush teeth before meals, if necessary, and after
      (2) use mouthwashes unless mouth ulcers or dry mucous membranes are present (mouthwashes contain alcohol)
      (3) provide mouth care to unconscious patients every 2 hours
      (4) remove dentures for thorough cleaning and examine gums underneath for sores
      (5) keep unused dentures in container labeled with patient's name
   d. hair care
      (1) needs daily brushing and periodic shampooing if possible
      (2) apply alcohol or vinegar to hair to help remove matting or tangles
      (3) braid long hair to prevent tangling
      (4) never cut a patient's hair without permission

3. Bed making
   a. types of beds
      (1) unoccupied: top covers fan-folded to bottom of bed and ready for patient
      (2) occupied: made with the patient in the bed; turn patient from side to side
      (3) surgical: prepared for a patient returning from surgery; top covers not tucked in but fan-folded to side or bottom
   b. linen must be tightly pulled to avoid wrinkling
   c. do not shake out linens, to avoid spreading of dust and microorganisms
   d. avoid holding linens close to nurse's clothing
   e. complete one side of the bed at a time
   f. use good body mechanics to avoid injury or straining

4. Positioning and body alignment
   a. patient positioning (Fig. 3-1)
      (1) prone: lying flat in bed on abdomen (Fig. 3-1A)
      (2) semi-Fowler's: head of bed raised 45 degrees
      (3) supine: lying flat on back (Fig. 3-1B)
      (4) high Fowler's: head of bed elevated to a 90-degree position with patient's knees slightly flexed (Fig. 3-1C)
      (5) knee-chest: patient on knees with shoulders flat on bed
      (6) Sims': on left or right side with opposite hip and knee acutely flexed, patient slightly forward (Fig. 3-1D)
      (7) lithotomy: patient on back with legs widely separated, thighs acutely flexed to abdomen and feet in stirrups
      (8) orthopneic: patient fully upright leaning over padded overbed table, resting head on arms
      (9) Trendelenburg: head lower than feet and legs (Fig. 3-1E)
      (10) reverse Trendelenburg: head elevated, feet and legs lower
   b. alignment
      (1) always prevent pressure on bony prominences
      (2) use pillows and blanket rolls to position patient for comfort
5. Wound care
   a. sterile dressing: used to protect wound from contaminants
      (1) wash hands
      (2) assemble sterile equipment and field
      (3) remove old dressing wearing gloves

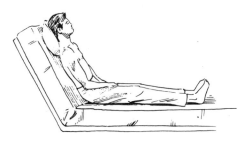

A Prone position.

FIGURE 3–1. *A*, Prone position. (From Rambo, B. J., and Wood, L. A.: Nursing Skills for Clinical Practice. 3rd ed. Philadelphia, W. B. Saunders Company, 1982.)

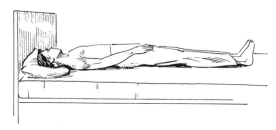

B Supine position.

FIGURE 3–1. *B*, Supine position. (From Rambo, B. J., and Wood, L. A.: Nursing Skills for Clinical Practice. 3rd ed. Philadelphia, W. B. Saunders Company, 1982.)

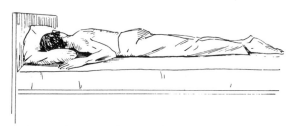

C Fowler's position.

FIGURE 3–1. *C*, Fowler's position. (From Rambo, B. J., and Wood, L. A.: Nursing Skills for Clinical Practice. 3rd ed. Philadelphia, W. B. Saunders Company, 1982.)

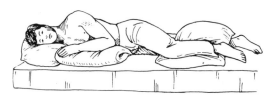

D Sims' position.

FIGURE 3–1. *D*, Sims' position. (From Rambo, B. J., and Wood, L. A.: Nursing Skills for Clinical Practice. 3rd ed. Philadelphia, W. B. Saunders Company, 1982.)

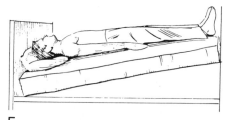

E Trendelenburg position

FIGURE 3–1. *E*, Trendelenburg position. (From Rambo, B. J., and Wood, L. A.: Nursing Skills for Clinical Practice. 3rd ed. Philadelphia, W. B. Saunders Company, 1982.)

(4) carefully note drainage for later charting

(5) place old dressing in watertight container and dispose of properly

(6) carefully assess wound

(7) put on sterile gloves

(8) cleanse wound per institutional policy or physician order from clean area to dirty

(9) apply sterile dressing

(10) anchor securely with tape or binder

  b. wet-to-dry dressings

(1) similar to sterile

(2) done to cleanse wound and remove debris

(3) sterile saline usually used to moisten dressing

(4) avoid saturating dressing to avoid leakage

(5) cover with dry sterile sponges to increase wicking action

(6) secure dressing

6. Bandages and binders

  a. types of and uses for bandages

(1) circular: holds dressings in place

(2) spiral: immobilizes part of extremity or decreases swelling

(3) figure-of-eight: applies pressure, supports or immobilizes joint, shapes stump

(4) triangular: sling to hold forearm immobile

  b. Montgomery straps

(1) consists of two large pieces of tape with cloth straps that tie over dressing to immobilize it

(2) used for frequently changed dressings to prevent constant retaping

  c. abdominal or chest binders

(1) apply tightly enough to support chest or abdomen

(2) avoid an overtight binder that prevents adequate chest expansion

  d. scultetus or "many-tailed" binder

(1) made of rectangular cloth with many long tails attached

(2) used either for support or to hold dressings in place

(3) apply while patient supine

(4) starting at bottom of binder, bring each tail across abdomen, pulling taut

(5) overlap tails at slight upward angle

(6) anchor each tail with next one

(7) pin final tail in place

  e. T binder: used to secure rectal or perineal dressings

7. Isolation precautions

  a. universal or body fluid precautions: used with all patients

(1) gloves worn for any contact with body fluids

(2) gown and mask with goggles worn if potential contamination from body fluids

such as hemorrhaging patient in emergency room

(3) separate disposal of sharps without breaking; do not recap needles

  b. strict isolation: used for airborne and contact spread of highly contagious pathogens

(1) private room

(2) gown, gloves, and mask when entering room

(3) double bag linens, disposable eating utensils, dishes and cups, trash and other contaminated articles

(4) flush urine and feces down toilet in room

(5) keep a stetescope and a glass thermometer in the room

(6) hand washing after patient contact

  c. respiratory isolation: used with airborne pathogens

(1) private room

(2) wear mask when entering room

(3) hand washing after patient contact

(4) double bag contaminated articles

  d. drainage secretion precautions

(1) private room preferable, if excessive drainage

(2) wear gown and gloves for direct contact, mask if excessive secretions

(3) double bag linens and dressings and other contaminated articles

(4) hand washing after patient contact

  e. enteric precautions: used for infections spread through fecal contact

(1) private room for children or uncooperative adults

(2) wear gown for direct contact

(3) wear gloves for contact with fecal material; ie, bedpans or cleaning up patient

(4) double bag linens, dressings, use disposable dishes

(5) flush feces down toilet immediately

  f. blood precautions: used for blood-borne infections

(1) dispose of all blood-contaminated equipment separately, double-bag

(2) dispose of sharps in container without breaking, do not recap needles

(3) flush urine and feces down toilet immediately

8. Care of the dying

  a. psychosocial issues

(1) patient's need to know of impending death

(2) PN's attitude toward death influences care of dying

(3) cultural or ethnic responses to dying

(4) patient and families ability to cope with dying

(5) patient's reactions to dying, described by Kubler-Ross (1975)
   (a) denial
   (b) anger: difficult for PN and family to handle
   (c) bargaining
   (d) depression: difficult for PN and family to handle
   (e) acceptance
(6) all actions should be directed at opening communication with patient

b. spiritual needs
   (1) provide clergy for patient as appropriate
   (2) allow patient to participate in appropriate religious practices
   (3) provide for family comfort and time with patient

c. physical changes of approaching death
   (1) facial muscles relax, cheeks flaccid, dentures do not fit, mumbling speech
   (2) pale, ashen skin that is cool and clammy
   (3) sight gradually fails
   (4) hearing believed to be sense retained longest
   (5) muscles become flaccid
   (6) respirations become irregular, rapid and shallow or very slow, Cheyne-Stokes—periods of hyperpnea regularly alternate with periods of apnea
   (7) pulse becomes weak, irregular, and thready
   (8) mental status varies from clarity to coma
   (9) reflexes decreased or absent
   (10) bowel and bladder retention or incontinence

d. nursing care
   (1) all care directed at patient comfort and safety
   (2) provide for relief of unpleasant symptoms
   (3) maintain good hygiene and oral care
   (4) turn patient frequently and position for maximum comfort
   (5) keep linens fresh and dry
   (6) allow family sufficient time with patient
   (7) support patient and family as needed
   (8) continue pain medications and treatments as appropriate

e. postmortem care
   (1) performed after the physician pronounces the patient dead
   (2) position patient flat in bed in a natural position with one pillow under head
   (3) close eyes
   (4) return dentures to mouth as soon as possible and close mouth
   (5) clean body and remove all tubes per institutional policy
   (6) allow family time with body after it is prepared
   (7) wrap in shroud and label body per policy
   (8) remove body to morgue or funeral home per policy
   (9) pack all belongings, give to family, and document in chart
   (10) complete institutional death record

9. Discharging patients
a. done only after written physician's order
b. nursing care
   (1) help patient gather all belongings
   (2) review discharge instructions, prescriptions, and follow up appointments
   (3) help patient obtain transportation from family or contact social service if assistance needed
   (4) accompany patient to exit per institution policy
   (5) chart information per policy

E. Skills Related to Mobility

1. Rest and sleep
a. position patient in individualized comfort position
b. maintain quiet and darkness to help with sleep
c. provide comfortable environment, blankets or cooling as needed
d. promote relaxation
   (1) warm bath
   (2) back rub
e. avoid overuse of prescribed sleep agents

2. Body mechanics
a. lifting or moving
   (1) feet apart to width of shoulder
   (2) move object to be lifted close to body before lifting
   (3) keep back slightly flexed
   (4) contract abdominal and lumbar muscles during lifting
   (5) use shoulder and arm muscles to pull
   (6) flex knees slightly and then straighten as object lifted

b. transfering patient from bed to stretcher
   (1) use at least two or three people
   (2) use drawsheet to move patient
   (3) move patient toward edge of bed
   (4) adjust stretcher next to bed at level of bed
   (5) lock both bed and stretcher
   (6) reach across stretcher and using drawsheet, pull patient toward you, first to edge, then to center of stretcher

c. assisting patient from bed to chair
   (1) lower bed to lowest position

(2) move chair close to bed and firmly anchor or lock wheelchair

(3) help patient to sitting position, then to side of bed with legs dangling

(4) face patient, maintain wide base of support, hands around patient's lower chest

(5) keep patient's knees between your legs to prevent falls

(6) have patient lean forward and place hands on PN's shoulders, not neck

(7) pull patient to standing position

(8) pivot patient and lower into chair or wheelchair

d. positioning patient up in bed

(1) adjust bed height to below your waist

(2) position the patient flat in bed

(3) stand at side of bed with feet pointed in direction you are to move patient

(4) reach under patient's shoulders and back to slide patient without lifting

(5) have patient bend knees and use feet to push self up if possible

(6) use draw sheet, if possible, to avoid shearing force on patient's back

e. turning patient

(1) patient should be turned every 2 hours while in bed

(2) adjust bed to mid or upper thigh level

(3) lower bed rail on the side where you are standing

(4) cross patient's arms on chest and cross legs

(5) reach across patient, placing your hands on the patient's far shoulder and hip, or use a draw sheet

(6) turn patient toward you using your whole body

(7) put pillow(s) behind patient's back and between legs, raise side rail

3. Range of motion (ROM) exercises

a. definitions

(1) passive: movement of patient's joints through complete range of mobility when patient is unable to perform this activity independently

(2) active: patient moves joints through complete range of mobility independently

b. always exercise only to limit of mobility or pain

c. support limb by cupping or cradling extremity to avoid stress on joints

d. often done easily during bath

F. Skills Related to Metabolism/Elimination

1. Feeding patients

a. place tray so patient can see food being served

b. if possible, raise head of bed to ease swallowing

c. prepare foods, but allow patient as much independence as possible

d. use straws for fluids and allow patient to eat finger foods independently

e. offer food in small amounts

f. vary foods being offered or ask patients what they want next

g. alternate liquids with solid foods

h. blind patients: describe what foods offered and position of foods on plate

i. always strive to make mealtimes pleasant to promote a good appetite

2. Nasogastric (NG) tubes

a. used to either drain gastric contents or to administer tube feedings

b. NG tubes (Levin, Salem Sump, Miller-Abbott, Cantor) may be connected to continuous or intermittent suction

c. check proper tube placement before irrigating

(1) aspirate stomach contents with a syringe

(2) inject 10 mL of air into tube while listening with stethoscope for whooshing sound over stomach

d. irrigate with normal saline at intervals to prevent clogging

e. note and chart amount, color and consistency of drainage at end of shift, being sure to subtract irrigating solution

f. provide mouth care every 2 hours

3. Tube feedings

a. done through nasogastric or gastrostomy tube for patients unable to swallow or take in sufficient nutrients

b. feedings either continuous at slow drip rates or intermittently throughout the day and night

c. many prepared solutions avilable; also may be made by dietary department

d. always serve feedings at room temperature to prevent cramping

e. give feedings by gravity infusion; never force the feeding under pressure

f. raise head of bed during feedings and maintain elevated position for 45 minutes following feeding

g. administer feedings slowly to prevent nausea and overdistention of stomach

h. follow feedings with prescribed amount of water

i. aspirate stomach contents 1 hour after feeding, as ordered, to check for residual feedings left in stomach

j. provide patient with emotional support, because inability to eat independently is often distressing

k. administer mouth care every 2 hours

4. Assisting with normal bowel function
   a. assess each patient's normal bowel pattern and attempt to maintain it
   b. encourage adequate intake of fluids unless contraindicated, and fiber to prevent constipation, often associated with decreased mobility
   c. if possible, have patient sit on toilet, commode, or bedpan for natural position for defecation
   d. tell patient not to ignore urge to defecate
   e. provide privacy
   f. help cleanse patient after defecation
   g. monitor amount, color, and consistency of stool
5. Rectal tubes
   a. insert to relieve distention due to flatus
   b. lubricate tube before inserting 2–4 inches into rectum
   c. position patient in left lateral Sims' position
   d. tape in place and leave no longer than 30 minutes
   e. report and record results
6. Enemas
   a. cleansing
      (1) can be tap water, mixture of soap and water, or saline
      (2) temperature of solution should be no more than 105°F
      (3) administer 500–1000 mL of fluid
      (4) position patient in left lateral Sims' position
      (5) hold fluid container about 18 inches above anus
      (6) lubricate tube and insert 3–4 inches
      (7) if cramping occurs, stop and have patient take deep breaths until cramping passes
      (8) observe results and record amount of feces
      (9) if ordered "until clear," return should eventually be free of feces; no more than three enemas unless specified by physician
   b. Oil retention
      (1) given to soften feces in order to ease defecation
      (2) oil heated to 100°F
      (3) use only about 100 mL; encourage patient to try to retain it for 30 minutes
      (4) may require cleansing enema afterwards
      (5) commercially prepared prefilled enemas available
7. Manual extraction of impaction
   a. apply gloves and adequately lubricate index finger
   b. position patient in left lateral Sims'
   c. gently insert finger into hardened stool and break off small pieces and remove
   d. assess patient's condition throughout, stop if patient's vital signs change or if discomfort experienced
   e. place patient on bedpan following procedure to allow evacuation of remaining stool
8. Stool specimens
   a. to determine presence of blood, ova, and parasites, or microorganisms
   b. all specimens except for blood require sterile container, and collection must be sent to laboratory warm and fresh
9. Colostomy irrigation
   a. done to empty bowel and regulate the passage of feces and flatus
   b. presently not considered a necessary procedure in colostomy management
   c. not all patients require irrigation to regulate defecation
   d. irrigation takes about 45 minutes and is best done at patient's established routine time
   e. irrigation done daily or every other day
   f. equipment and procedure same as for enema administration
   g. irrigation done with warm normal saline or tap water
   h. special ostomy pouch worn for irrigation to collect fecal drainage
   i. record results of irrigation
10. Assisting with urinary elimination
   a. altered patterns of urinary elimination
      (1) incontinence: inability to control voiding
      (2) retention: inability to void
      (3) dysuria: painful urination
      (4) polyuria: excessive urination
      (5) oliguria: output less than 400 mL/day
      (6) anuria: no urine output
   b. offer bedpan or urinal at regular intervals or leave within patient's reach
   c. provide patient privacy
   d. encourage patient to sit or stand, if able, to promote ease of voiding
   e. if patient has difficulty voiding
      (1) run water in his or her hearing
      (2) place patient's hand in basin of warm water
      (3) pour warm water over perineum
   f. help patient wash hands after voiding
11. Catheters
   a. purposes
      (1) to obtain sterile urine specimens
      (2) to relieve retention
      (3) to keep bladder decompressed
      (4) to measure residual urine following voiding
      (5) to irrigate bladder or instill medication
   b. "straight" catheters inserted for single bladder decompression and then removed

c. Foley catheter inserted and left in for length of time ordered

d. general principles of catheterization
   (1) use sterile procedure
   (2) use smallest size possible to avoid trauma
   (3) explain procedure to patient before beginning
   (4) provide privacy, position patient
   (5) put on sterile gloves and set up sterile field
   (6) cleanse the urinary meatus front to back for women and in a circular motion for men
   (7) lubricate catheter well before inserting
   (8) insert catheter about 3–4 inches in women and 6–8 inches in men
   (9) if using indwelling catheter, fill balloon with 5–10 mL of sterile water and anchor with tape to thigh, straight for women and at right angle in men, and connect to drainage tubing and bag

e. removal of indwelling catheter
   (1) position patient and provide for privacy
   (2) withdraw water from balloon port with syringe
   (3) release tape, have patient take deep breath, and remove catheter with steady, gentle pull
   (4) monitor patient for voiding within 8 hours after removal
   (5) encourage fluid intake to improve output
   (6) warn patient that some burning may occur with first voiding

12. Urine specimens
    a. sterile specimen collected by straight catheterization
    b. voided specimen
       (1) wash perineal area well first
       (2) collect mid-stream specimen by having patient start voiding, stop voiding and restart voiding into sterile container
    c. clean specimen collected for urinalysis
    d. single specimen or up to 24-hour specimens may be collected

e. container and preservative dependent on type of specimen collected

f. 24-hour specimens: discard first void and record time; collect all urine for next 24 hours

g. double-voided specimen: patient empties bladder; collect next voided specimen. Done when testing for sugar and acetone

13. Bladder irrigation
    a. must be done using aseptic technique
    b. can be done as manual irrigation using syringe or constant bladder irrigation (CBI), using an intravenous-type set-up
    c. done to clear catheter of obstructions, remove clots from urine, wash the bladder with medication, or decrease bleeding from bladder or prostate, usually after surgery
    d. can be done without disconnecting catheter if three-way Foley used
    e. amount and type of solution determined by doctor's orders
    f. account for amount of solution on output record

BIBLIOGRAPHY

Brunner, L.S., and Suddarth, D.S. (1988). *Textbook of medical-surgical nursing, 2nd ed.* Philadelphia: J.B. Lippincott Co.

Hood, G., and Dincher, J.R., (1988). *Total patient care: Foundations and practices.* St. Louis: C.V. Mosby Co.

Kubler-Ross, E. (1975). *Death: The final stage of growth.* Englewood Cliffs, NJ: Prentice-Hall.

Long, B., and Phipps, W. (1988). *Essentials of medical-surgical nursing, 2nd ed.* St. Louis: C.V. Mosby Co.

Miller, B.F., and Keane, C. (1983). *Encyclopedia and dictionary of medicine, nursing, and allied health, 3rd ed.* Philadelphia: W.B. Saunders Co.

Milliken, M.E., and Campbell, G. (1984). *Essential competencies for patient care.* St Louis: C.V. Mosby Co.

Perry, A.G., and Potter, P.A. (1990). *Clinical nursing skills and techniques, 2nd ed.* St. Louis: C.V. Mosby Co.

Potter, P.A., and Perry, A.G. (1989). *Fundamentals of nursing: Concepts, process, and practice, 2nd ed.* St. Louis: C.V. Mosby Co.

Sorensen, K., and Luckmann, J. (1986). *Basic nursing: A psychophysiologic approach, 2nd Ed.* Philadelphia: W.B. Saunders Co.

Thompson, J.M., et al. (1989). *Mosby's manual of clinical nursing, 2nd ed.* St. Louis: C.V. Mosby Co.

Questions

In practice, using the nursing process involves a systematic, organized method of collecting information about a patient's needs and using the information obtained to meet those needs in an appropriate and effective way.

1. What four major steps are utilized in the nursing process?

① Planning; assessment; implementation; evaluation
② Assessment; planning; implementation, evaluation
③ Assessment, nursing diagnosis, intervention; evaluation
④ Nursing diagnosis; planning; implementation; evaluation

2. Although terminology differs, the steps in the nursing process and in the problem-solving approach to nursing care are quite similar. Stating the patient's problem correlates with which step in the nursing process?

① Planning
② Assessment
③ Intervention
④ Coming to a conclusion

3. When a soapsuds enema is given, the soapsuds have the effect of:

① Soothing the mucosal lining of the colon
② Cleansing the intestinal tract of bacteria
③ Allowing easier passage of feces
④ Irritating the mucosal lining of the colon

4. An oil retention enema is primarily given to:

① Stimulate peristalsis
② Soften fecal material
③ Cleanse the bowel before a diagnostic test
④ Relieve distention from flatus

5. When heating the oil for an oil retention enema, the nurse must remember that:

① Oil should not be heated to more than 100°F, because it retains heat longer than water
② Oil must be heated to over 100°F for it to flow freely through the rectal tube
③ Oil will mix with water only after it has been heated

④ Oil does not conduct heat as well as water, so it must be heated to more than 100°F.

6. Before administering an oil retention enema, the nurse should tell the patient to:

① Try to go to the bathroom before the enema is given
② Expel the enema as soon as possible after it is given
③ Hold it until the urge to defecate is strong
④ Hold it for at least an hour

7. The amount given for an oil retention enema is usually:

① 500 mL
② 300 mL
③ 100 mL
④ 10 mL

8. To decrease the patient's urge to defecate, the nurse should insert a rectal suppository:

① Very quickly
② Well beyond the sphincter
③ At least 2 inches into the rectum
④ Only at body temperature

9. When applying a dressing to the rectal area, the nurse should use a:

① A Velcro binder
② Scultetus binder
③ T-binder
④ Straight binder

10. The patient who requires frequent dressing changes will experience fewer skin problems if the nurse applies:

① Wide strips of adhesive tape
② A tight abdominal binder
③ A T-binder
④ Mongomery straps

General principles to follow when applying an Ace bandage to an extremity are presented in the following questions.

11. A disadvantage associated with a circular bandage is:

① Permitting movement
② Increasing circulation
③ Causing a tourniquet effect
④ Increasing temperature

12. The advantage of using a figure-of-eight bandage is:

① Decreasing temperature
② Decreasing circulation
③ Preventing a tourniquet effect
④ Restricting movement

13. The foot and hand should be included in the Ace wrap in order to:

① Prevent edema
② Permit movement
③ Cause blanching
④ Decrease pain

14. The toes and fingers should *not* be included in Ace wraps in order to:

① Improve circulation
② Permit circulation check
③ Allow movement
④ Decrease pain

When the implementation component of the nursing care plan is developed, the format is based on principles presented in the following questions.

15. The term implementation refers to the:

① Measurement of the effectiveness of the nursing care plan in meeting patient needs
② Management and performance of the nursing care plan
③ Systematic approach to data collection and analysis
④ Link between the identification of patient needs and the actual performance of health care activities

16. Performance of nursing care designates that the nurse:

① Delegates the responsibility for some nursing actions to others
② Is responsible for all the nursing care of every assigned patient
③ Limits interaction with the patient
④ Assesses in the beginning of the nursing process

17. Documentation for nursing care needs to be:

① Written qualitatively
② Read by the patient
③ Reported verbally to the doctor
④ Written after each nurse–patient interaction

18. Documentation is an important source for:

① Proving what procedural skills the nurse can perform
② Recording the nurse's verbal responses to the patient
③ Recording the patient's response to treatment
④ Specifying the responsible person for each procedure

19. The purpose of recording information throughout a patient's stay is to:

① Establish the same format in all hospitals
② Eliminate interpersonal relationships among the health care personnel
③ Aid the nurse in coordinating and directing continuous care for each patient
④ Protect the patient from being sued

20. A sterile urine specimen should be obtained by:

① Having the patient void in a sterile bedpan
② Straight catheterizing the patient
③ Cleansing the external genitalis before the patient voids
④ Obtaining a mid-stream voided urine

21. For a clean urine specimen, the nurse should:

① Give the patient a clean urine cup to void into
② Straight catheterize the patient
③ Cleanse the external genitalia before the patient voids
④ Have the patient drink a full glass of water first

22. To collect a 24-hour urine specimen correctly, the nurse should:

① Discard the first void and save all urine for 24 hours
② Save the first and last void in a 24-hour period
③ Randomly collect a single specimen during a 24-hour period
④ Collect all urine from the first void at 7 AM for 24 hours

23. In order to assure an accurate result when testing the urine for sugar and acetone, the nurse should:

① Keep the patient NPO for 4 hours
② Withhold all fluids for at least 1 hour prior to the test
③ Cleanse the external genitalia before the patient voids

④ Have the patient void, drink water, and then void again in 30 minutes

24. The optimum time to collect a sputum specimen is:

   ① At bedtime
   ② Early morning
   ③ After lunch
   ④ In the mid-morning

25. A sputum specimen must contain material from the:

   ① Lungs and bronchi
   ② Nasal secretions
   ③ Lining of the trachea
   ④ Salivary glands

26. When collecting a stool specimen for ova and parasites, it is important to remember that the specimen must be:

   ① Refrigerated until examined
   ② In a sterile container
   ③ In an airtight container
   ④ Warm until examined

27. When collecting a specimen for culture and sensitivity, the nurse must remember that the specimen will be:

   ① Potentially contaminated with pathogenic bacteria
   ② A urine or stool specimen
   ③ A large amount, usually 500 mL
   ④ Collected only by an RN

28. The container for a specimen collected for a culture must be:

   ① Covered with a sterile gauze
   ② Plugged with cotton
   ③ Filled completely
   ④ Checked for cracks before it is used

29. After the specimen for culture is obtained, the container must be:

   ① Kept warm until sent to the laboratory
   ② Taken to the laboratory promptly
   ③ Refrigerated until it can be sent to the laboratory
   ④ Wrapped in a sterile wrapper

30. Which of the following would *not* be the responsibility of the LPN/LVN in obtaining a culture specimen?

   ① Instruct the client what is to be done
   ② Accurately label the specimen container
   ③ Determine the type of test to be done
   ④ Avoid contaminating the specimen

Answers & Rationales

Guide to item identification (see pp. 3–5 for further details about each category)

I, II, III, or IV for the phase of the nursing process
1, 2, 3, or 4 for the category of client needs
A, B, C, D, E, F, or G for the category of human functioning
Specific content category by name; ie, cholecystectomy

1. ② The nursing process consists of four basic steps performed in a specific order for the purpose of obtaining maximum benefit to the patient.
I, 1, G. Nursing Process

2. ② Both assessment and stating the patient's problem require collection and organization of data from a variety of sources in order to plan care based on patient needs.
III, 1, G. Nursing Process.

3. ④ Soapsuds irritate the lining of the intestine, leading to increased peristalsis and bowel evacuation.
I, 1, F. Enema.

4. ② The oil retention enema is given to soften the feces with the oil and to lubricate the lining of the bowel.
IV, 1, F. Enema.

5. ① Oil retains heat longer than water, and there is a greater risk of injury if it is heated too much.
III, 1, F. Enema.

6. ③ It is important for the patient to hold the oil as long as possible for the maximum effect.
III, 1, F. Enema.

7. ③ An oil retention enema requires that only a very small amount of oil be given to achieve the maximum effect.
III, 1, F. Enema.

8. ② Unless the suppository is inserted well past the sphincter, the patient will feel the urge to defecate.
III, 5, F. Suppository.

9. ③ A T-binder is used to hold a rectal dressing in place.
III, 1, D. Dressings.

10. ④ Montgomery straps allow the dressing to be changed without constantly removing tape.
III, 1, D. Dressings.

11. ③ A circular bandage applied too tightly creates a tourniquet effect which would prevent adequate circulation and probably cause necrosis.
IV, 1, F. Bandages.

12. ③ Circulation needs to be maintained while supporting the muscles to prevent edema.
IV, 1, F. Bandages.

13. ① If the foot and hand were not included in an Ace wrap, a tourniquet effect could possibly form, which would decrease the blood supply and promote edema formation.
IV, 1, F. Bandages.

14. ② Visibility is necessary to insure that proper circulation is maintained.
III, 1, F. Bandages.

15. ② Implementation is assigning the workload to appropriately trained personnel and the performance of skills according to procedure.
III, 1, G. Nursing Process.

16. ① No one nurse can do everything for all patients; it is a team coordinated effort.
III, 1, G. Nursing Process.

17. ④ Documentation proves what observation was made, when it was made and by whom.
IV, 1, G. Documentation.

18. ③ Documentation is an ongoing written communication concerning a patient.
IV, 1, G. Documentation

19. ③ Implementation is based on the continual assessment of changes noted in documentation.
IV, 1, G. Nursing Process.

20. ② The only way to obtain a sterile specimen is with a catheter; a voided specimen is always contaminated.
III, 2. Urine Specimen.

21. ③ A clean specimen requires that the nurse clean the patient's external genitalia with an antiseptic solution before voiding.
III, 2, F. Urine Specimen.

22. A 24-hour specimen is collected by discarding
① the specimen that has been sitting in the bladder, the first void, and then collecting all urine voided in a 24-hour period, including having the patient void the last specimen exactly 24 hours later.
III, 2, F. Urine Specimen.

23. The first void contains urine that has been in
④ the bladder for an indeterminate time. Having the patient void and then drink and revoid gives a picture of the patient's current status.
III, 2, F. Urine Specimen.

24. The most sputum will be available first thing in
② the morning. Also, these specimens are most likely to contain cells and bacteria.
III, 2, B. Specimens/Basic Skills.

25. In order to test the specimen, there must be
① actual material from the lungs and bronchi.
III, 2, B. Sputum Specimens.

26. In order for ova and parasites to survive until
④ testing, the stool must be kept warm.
III, 2, F. Stool Specimens.

27. A culture and sensitivity is done when infection
① is suspected, so there is a good chance the specimen will contain a large number of potentially pathogenic organisms.
III, 2, D. Culture and Sensitivity.

28. A culture and sensitivity specimen must be collected in an intact sterile container.
④ III, 2, D. Culture and Sensitivity.

29. In order to obtain accurate results, the specimen should be taken to the laboratory
② promptly.
III, 2, D. Specimens/Basic Skills.

30. The LPN is responsible for all actions except
③ determining the actual test to be done. This action is solely the responsibility of the physician.
III, 2, D. Diagnostic Tests/Basic Skills.

Medication Administration

4

I. OVERVIEW OF PHARMACOLOGY

A. Names of Drugs

1. Chemical name: description of drug using nomenclature of chemistry
2. Generic name
   a. name assigned by government to drug
   b. also known as nonproprietary name
   c. universal drug name
3. Trade name
   a. created by drug companies to sell a product
   b. also known as proprietary or brand name
   c. generic drug may have many trade names

B. Drug Information Sources

1. Nursing drug books
   a. many different books available
   b. both pharamacology texts and drug handbooks
   c. focus on nursing implications of drugs
2. *Physician's Desk Reference*
   a. published yearly
   b. similar to drug inserts supplied by manufacturers
   c. easy to find drug by brand name
3. *Drug Facts and Comparisons*
4. United States Pharmacopeia (USP) and National Formulary (NF)
   a. revised every 5 years, with supplements in between
   b. establishes legal standards for drugs
5. Package inserts
   a. supplied by manufacturer
   b. regulated by Food and Drug Administration (FDA)

C. Drug Legislation and Regulation

1. FDA maintains strict control of all drugs for use in humans
2. Food, Drug, and Cosmetic Act
   a. first legislation to regulate drug safety
   b. ensures that drugs are safe and effective
   c. requires physician's prescription for dispensing of drugs

3. Controlled Substances Act
   a. sets rules for manufacture and distribution of drugs that have potential for abuse
   b. sets categories into which various controlled substance are divided
      (1) Schedule I: drugs with a high potential of abuse and not approved for medical use
      (2) Schedule II: drugs with a high potential for abuse but have been approved for medical use
      (3) Schedule III: drugs with a lower potential for abuse but have high risk of psychological dependence and low to moderate potential of dependence
      (4) Schedule IV: drugs with some potential for abuse
      (5) Schedule V: drugs with very little potential for abuse, often in combination with small amounts of controlled substances; some may be dispensed without prescription

D. Sources of Drugs

1. Chemicals
2. Plants
3. Animal products
4. Food substances
5. Microorganisms

E. Forms of Drugs

1. Liquid
   a. solution: drug dissolved in a liquid, usually water
   b. suspension: drug in finely divided, undissolved state dispersed in a liquid substance
   c. elixir: solutions containing alcohol, sugar, and water
   d. emulsion: suspension of fat globules and water
   e. tincture: drugs dissolved in alcohol alone or plus water
   f. lotion: liquid suspension or dispersion of drug for topical use
   g. liniment: drug in oily, soapy, or alcohol mixture applied to skin as counterirritant

69

2. Solid or semisolid drug forms
   a. capsule
      (1) liquid or solid drug inside gelatinous capsule that dissolves after swallowing
      (2) sustained release form: drug in small particles coated with substances to vary solubility, contained inside capsule; released slowly, should not be crushed
   b. tablet: solid form of drug pressed into various sizes and shapes
      (1) buccal: solid form that dissolves when held between cheek and gum and directly absorbed by oral mucosa
      (2) sublingual: solid form that dissolves when held under tongue and directly absorbed by oral mucosa
      (3) enteric coated: drug coated with substance that delays release of drug until it reaches intestine, should not be crushed
   c. suppository: drug mixed in soft material that melts at body temperature when inserted into body orifice
   d. ointment: semisolid preparation, usually fatty substance, for external application
   e. troche or lozenge: drug incorporated into mass made of sugar and mucilage or fruit base made to dissolve in mouth

F. Pharmacokinetics: Study of Drug Movement Throughout Body

1. Absorption
   a. movement of drug from site of administration into blood stream
   b. drugs must first be dissolved
   c. affected by
      (1) rate at which drug dissolves
      (2) surface area exposed to dissolved drug
      (3) blood flow to site of drug absorption
      (4) how fat soluble drug is (more fat soluble, faster absorption)
2. Distribution
   a. movement of drug throughout body
   b. affected by
      (1) blood flow through tissues, to move drug
      (2) ability of drug to leave vascular system
      (3) ability of drug to enter cells
3. Metabolism
   a. enzymatic alteration of drug structure; also know as biotransformation
   b. usually occurs in liver
   c. prepares the drug either for action or excretion
   d. affected by
      (1) age of patient; under 1 year old, liver not fully functional
      (2) liver function

---

      (3) nutritional status
      (4) competition of two drugs for same enzymes
      (5) time administered
4. Excretion
   a. removal of drugs from body
   b. usually occurs through kidneys and urine
   c. affected by renal function
   d. some excretion through nonrenal sources
      (1) breast milk
      (2) bile and feces
      (3) lungs
      (4) skin

G. Factors Affecting Drug Action

1. Dose of drug and route of administration
2. Patient age
   a. newborns and infants with immature systems for metabolism and excretion
   b. elderly may have deterioration of systems affecting pharmacokinetics
3. Diet: some foods may alter action of drugs
4. Other drugs
   a. additive effects: two drugs taken together lead to increased effect
   b. potentiation: effect of two drugs greater than sum of effects if drugs taken separately
   c. antagonism: one drug acts on another to decrease its effectiveness
5. Body size: both height and weight affect dose of drug needed
6. Pregnancy
7. Disease processes

H. Reactions to Medication

1. Intended effect: that effect for which drug was designed
2. Side effect: drug effect other than that intended
3. Local effect: action of drug limited to area of application
4. Systemic effect: potential effect on any body system resulting from absorption of drug into blood
5. Adverse effects
   a. idiosyncratic reaction: unusual or unexpected reaction to a drug
   b. allergic reaction: stimulation of antibodies in reaction to foreign antigen
   c. untoward reaction: one harmful to one or more body systems
   d. teratogenic effect: drug that causes fetal abnormalities when given to pregnant patient
   e. dependency: physical or psychologic need for further doses of drug
6. Tolerance: drug given over a period of time no

longer producing same effect, requires larger doses to achieve same effect

II. COMMON CATEGORIES OF DRUGS
(SEE EACH SECTION FOR MORE DETAILS ON SPECIFIC DRUGS)

A. Drugs Affecting Sexuality

1. Uterine smooth muscle stimulants
   a. description: drugs that stimulate uterine smooth muscle, especially gravid uterus; sensitivity of uterus increases during gestation and increases sharply before parturition
   b. uses: for initiation and improvement of uterine contractions for term or preterm delivery in maternal or fetal distress situations; postpartum to control postpartum bleeding or hemorrhage; nasal oxytocin indicated for initial letdown of milk
   c. side effects: fetal bradycardia, anaphylaxis, hemorrhage, nausea, vomiting, uterine hypertonicity, rupture of uterus, water intoxication
   d. nursing implications: obtain good obstetric (OB) history; do not administer IV without physician available; have $MgSO_4$ on hand to treat tetany; use infusion pump with IV; monitor mother and fetus continually during administration; monitor for postpartum bleeding; monitor uterine contractions
   e. example: oxytocin (Pitocin)
2. Beta-receptor antagonist
   a. description: drugs that have an antagonistic effect on B_2 adrenergic receptors such as those in uterine smooth muscle
   b. uses: management of preterm labor in suitable patients; safe and effective under 20 weeks' gestation
   c. side effects: dose-related alterations in maternal and fetal heart rates and maternal blood pressure; palpitations; tremors; nausea; vomiting; headache; erythema; malaise
   d. nursing implications: check maternal vital signs and monitor fetus; monitor uterine contractions; run as IV piggyback; use IV infusion pump; teach patient use of oral form; keep in left lateral position during IV administration
   e. example: ritrodrine hydrochloride (Yutopar)
3. Hormones
   a. androgens
      (1) description: drugs that produce anabolic and androgenic effects
      (2) uses: replacement therapy for males; to treat dysmenorrhea and menopause in women; treatment of inoperable breast cancer in certain women

      (3) side effects: *males*—impotence, gynecomastia, epididymitis, bladder irritation; *females*—hirsutism, amenorrhea, masculinization; *both*—nausea, vomiting, diarrhea, fluid retention
      (4) nursing implications: warn patient about possible changes in sexual characteristics; use with caution in patients on oral anticoagulants; monitor input and output (I&O); check for edema; monitor calcium levels
      (5) example: testosterone propionate
   b. estrogens
      (1) description: acts by inhibiting pituitary activity; increases tone of breasts and genitourinary (GU) structures and insures proper menstrual flow in premenopausal women
      (2) uses: postmenopausal syndrome, amenorrhea due to ovarian failure, suppression of lactation; prostatic cancer in men
      (3) side effects: nausea, vomiting, anorexia, abdominal distention and bloating, spotting, menstrual changes, fluid retention, depression, hypercalcemia, migraines, breast tenderness and enlargement, reduced glucose tolerance, possible uterine cancer, hypersensitivity; males have similar side effects but also development of female secondary sexual characteristics
      (4) nursing implications: contraindicated in pregnancy, some breast cancers, thrombophlebitis, thyroid and liver disease; use cautiously in patients with hypertension (HTN), migraines, diabetes mellitus (DM), and asthma; monitor for edema and congestive heart failure (CHF); watch for depression
      (5) example: diethlystilbestrol (DES)

B. Drugs Affecting Oxygenation

1. Antihypertensives
   a. description: drugs that act to reduce blood pressure through wide variety of mechanisms
   b. uses: control of moderate to severe hypertension
   c. thiazide diuretics
      (1) side effects: hypokalemia, hyponatremia, hyperuricemia, hyperglycemia, orthostatic hypotension
      (2) nursing implications: maintain K^+ level; teach high K^+, low Na^+ diet; monitor I&O, blood pressure
      (3) example: hydrochlorothiazide (Hydrodiuril)
   d. loop diuretics
      (1) side effects: orthostatic hypertension, hy-

pokalemia, hyponatremia, constipation, urinary frequency
    (2) nursing implications: maintain K^+ level; give in early morning to prevent nocturia; weigh patient to monitor fluid loss; give with food to reduce GI distress; encourage high potassium diet
    (3) example: furosemide (Lasix)
  e. potassium-sparing diuretic
    (1) side effects: hyponatremia, hyperkalemia, GI disturbances, allergic reactions
    (2) nursing implications: monitor K^+ intake to insure excess not ingested; monitor I&O, blood pressure
    (3) example: spironolactone (Aldactone)
  f. sympathetic-inhibiting agents
    (1) side effects: orthostatic hypotension, depression, drowsiness, GI disturbances, impotence (Aldomet), bradycardia, sodium and water retention
    (2) nursing implications: caution patient to change position slowly; monitor for side effects altering compliance; maintain low Na^+ diet; restrict alcohol use (may increase hypotension)
    (3) example: methyldopa (Aldomet)
2. Cardiac glycosides
  a. description: drugs that act directly on myocardium to increase force of contraction; cardiac output increased while heart rate slowed
  b. uses: congestive heart failure (CHF), dysrhythmias (especially those with increased rate), cardiogenic shock with pulmonary edema
  c. side effects: dysrhythmias, heart block, bradycardia, GI upset, muscle weakness, diplopia
  d. nursing implications: take apical pulse prior to administration; if above 120 or below 60, hold medication and notify physician; monitor for toxicity and hypokalemia if patient also on diuretics; teach patient to check pulse rate at home, eat high potassium K^+ diet if on diuretics
  e. example: digoxin (Lanoxin)
3. Vasodilators
  a. description: drugs that act on blood vessels to cause increase in diameter, thereby improving blood flow; most effective in dilating coronary arteries and less effective in dilating peripheral vessels
  b. uses: antianginal, some action on cerebral and peripheral circulation
  c. side effects: generalized vasodilation (headache, flushing, orthostatic hypotension, tachycardia)
  d. nursing implications: know correct form and schedule of administration; eg, prn vs. regu-

lar, oral, sublingual, chewable, or transdermal
  e. types and examples: nitrites/nitrates, nitroglycerin (Nitro-Bid); calcium channel blockers, verapamil (Calan), cerebral vasodilators: dipyridamole (Persantine); peripheral vasodilators, isoxsuprine HCl (Vasodilan)
4. Anticoagulants
  a. description: drugs that act to prevent blood clotting; parenteral forms act by inhibiting formation of prothrombin activator, which then diminishes conversion of prothrombin to thrombin; also form plasma antithrombin and block activation of fibrin-stabilizing factor; oral forms block synthesis of vitamin K-dependent clotting factors in liver; neither form has any effect on existing clots
  b. uses: prevention and treatment of thromboses; parenteral drugs can also be used to prevent clotting of blood outside body
  c. side effects: hemorrhage
  d. nursing implications: avoid use of any other product that increases anticoagulation or causes bleeding (eg, aspirin); teach patient safety precautions to avoid bleeding (eg, soft toothbrush, electric razor); monitor laboratory tests. Parenteral: partial thromboplastin time (PTT); oral: prothrombin time (PT)
  e. types and examples: parenteral, heparin; oral, warfarin (Coumadin)
5. Anticoagulant antagonists
  a. description: drugs that act as antagonists to block action of anticoagulants
  b. uses: overdose of anticoagulants; bleeding; hypoprothrombinemia
  c. side effects; flushing, GI upset, allergic reactions
  d. nursing implications: monitor patient during administration, assess effectiveness by noting decrease in bleeding
  e. examples: parenteral, protamine sulfate; oral, vitamin K (Aqua-Mephyton)
6. Bronchodilators—xanthine derivatives
  a. description: drugs that relax bronchial smooth muscle and inhibit release of histamine and slow-release substance A (SRS-A) from mast cells; mild diuretics and cardiac stimulants
  b. uses: symptomatic relief of asthma and bronchial spasms
  c. side effects: GI upset, nausea, nervousness, frequency, diarrhea, insomnia, tachycardia, palpitations, esophageal reflux
  d. nursing implications: use with caution in patients with hypertension, tachycardia, hypoxemia, glaucoma, hyperthyroidism, benign prostatic hypertrophy (BPH), diabetes; monitor for central nervous system (CNS) symptoms; give with food or antacids; patient

should avoid smoking, maintain upright position after meals

    e. example: theophylline (Theo-Dur)

7. Cough preparations

  a. Expectorants

    (1) description: drugs that facilitate removal of thick mucus from lungs and act as soothing demulcent by stimulating secretion of lubricant

    (2) uses: facilitate productive cough

    (3) side effects: nausea, vomiting, GI irritation, drowsiness

    (4) nursing implications: instruct patient not to use >1 week without seeing physician; use high fluid intake and humidity to loosen secretions; do not follow with water, except potassium iodide

    (5) example: guaifenesin (Robitussin)

  b. antitussives

    (1) description: drugs that suppress cough reflex

    (2) uses: to treat nonproductive coughs

    (3) side effects: dizziness, sedation, sweating, nausea, dry mouth, urinary retention, constipation

    (4) nursing implications: never use in patients with productive coughs; administer with caution in patients with asthma, COPD, cardiac disease, convulsions, renal or hepatic disease; if cough continues more than 1 week, patient should see doctor

    (5) example: codeine

8. Antibiotics

  a. group of drugs that are either bacteriostatic (inhibiting or arresting growth of microorganisms) or bacteriocidal (killing of microorganisms); terms antibacterial, antimicrobial, antiinfective, and antiseptic are often used synonymously with antibiotic

  b. Penicillins

    (1) uses: treatment of common infections caused by penicillin-sensitive microorganisms

    (2) side effects: allergic reactions including anaphylaxis; diarrhea; development of resistant organisms; superinfection; GI distress

    (3) nursing implications: watch closely for rash or early signs of allergic reactions; check all patients for allergy before giving; obtain appropriate culture and sensitivity before starting drug; teach patient to take full course of drugs as ordered

    (4) example: ampicillin (Polycillin)

  c. Aminoglycosides

    (1) uses: treatment of gram-negative infections (often nosocomial or iatrogenic); effective in treating serious, systemic, gram-negative infections

    (2) side effects: ototoxicity, nephrotoxicity, superinfections; allergic potential small

    (3) nursing implications: monitor closely for hearing changes; monitor renal function; watch for development of superinfection

    (4) example: gentamicin (Garamycin)

  d. Cephalosporins

    (1) uses: treatment of septicemia and most systemic infections; effective against some penicillin-resistant organisms

    (2) side effects: allergic reactions ($\frac{2}{3}$ of penicillin-sensitive patients are also cephalosporin sensitive), superinfection, nephrotoxicity with higher doses, phlebitis at IV site, diarrhea

    (3) nursing implications: monitor known penicillin-sensitive patients closely for allergies; give IV preparations over 30 minutes to reduce phlebitis; give oral preparations 1 hour before or 2 hours after meals for maximum effectiveness; monitor for superinfection, especially oral or vaginal fungal infections

    (4) example: cephalothin (Keflin)

  e. Tetracyclines

    (1) uses: effective against wide variety of pathogens, including many of those causing diarrhea and pneumonia; used to control acne

    (2) side effects: diarrhea, nausea, vestibular disturbances (minocycline), hypersensitivity reactions, GI upset, permanent discoloration of teeth (especially in children), impairment of bone growth, superinfection

    (3) nursing implications: check for symptoms of hypersensitivity; do not give to pregnant women or children under age 8 years; do not administer with milk or antacids; give with sufficient water; watch for superinfection

    (4) examples: tetracycline (Achromycin)

9. Antitubercular agents

  a. description: drugs that act specifically on tubercular bacillus to inhibit growth of organism and cause it to become walled off; made up of first-line drugs (most effective with fewest side effects) and second-line drugs (more side effects and less effective)

  b. uses: to treat tuberculosis (TB) and for TB prophylaxis

  c. side effects: isoniazid (INH)—peripheral neuropathy, GI distress, hepatic toxicity, agranulocytosis, hemolytic anemia; rifampin (Rifadin)—red-orange urine and secretions,

GI distress, liver dysfunction, hematologic reaction; ethambutol HCl (Myambutol)—loss of visual acuity, disturbance of color discrimination, dermatitis, GI symptoms, elevated liver function tests, precipitation of gout

d. nursing implications: emphasize importance of finishing medication; instruct patient about side effects; monitor drug dosage, liver and renal function; administer pyridoxine to prevent peripheral neuropathy from INH; administer INH on empty stomach or 1 hour prior to intake of antacids to increase absorption; monitor visual acuity and color discrimination

e. examples: first-line drugs—isoniazid (INH) and pyridoxine (Vitamin B_6), rifampin (Rifadin), ethambutol (Myambutol); second-line drugs—para-aminosalicylic acid (PAS), streptomycin

10. Iron preparations
   a. description: acts to build hemoglobin in iron deficient patients
   b. uses: iron deficiency anemia; prophylactically in pregnancy, childhood, menopause, and heavy menses
   c. side effects: nausea, vomiting, GI distress, constipation, headache, lethargy; do not use in patients with cirrhosis, peptic ulcers, or ulcerative colitis
   d. nursing implications: do not give tetracycline or antacids; use straw with solutions to avoid staining teeth; warn patient that stools will turn black; give with meals to prevent GI distress; increase iron in diet; give IM Z-track
   e. examples: ferrous sulfate (Feosol), iron dextran (Imferon)

C. Drugs Affecting Perception

1. Analgesics
   a. non-narcotic
      (1) description: drugs that act to decrease pain, often through anti-inflammatory actions without side effects of narcotics; major drugs either salicylate (aspirin) or para-aminophenols (acetaminophen)
      (2) uses: for relief of mild to moderate pain
      (3) side effects: *salicylate:* salicylism (headache, nausea, vomiting, palpitations, hyperventilation), hypersensitivity, GI distress and bleeding, anticoagulant effect, liver damage; *acetaminophen:* hypersensitivity, CNS stimulation, liver and renal damage, palpitations
      (4) nursing implications: avoid use of salicylate in patients with GI disorders, anti-inflammatory or anticoagulant therapy, or history of aspirin sensitivity; avoid overuse; keep supply away from children; monitor liver and renal function; warn patient to avoid over-the-counter medicines that contain "hidden" aspirin
      (5) examples: *salicylate:* acetylsalicylic acid (aspirin); *para-aminophenols:* acetaminophen (Tylenol)
   b. narcotics
      (1) description: drugs that act to decrease pain by inhibiting transmission of pain impulses, reducing cortical responses to pain stimuli, or altering activity in pain-perception center of brain
      (2) uses: treatment of moderate or severe pain
      (3) side effects: drowsiness, dizziness or lightheadedness, euphoria, respiratory depression, constipation, urinary retention, hypersensitivity, hypotension
      (4) nursing implications: monitor effectiveness of analgesia; watch for hypotension and respiratory depression; monitor I&O, bowel movements; watch for possible tolerance and dependence
      (5) examples: morphine sulfate, meperidine (Demerol)

2. Miotic-cholinergics
   a. description: drugs that mimic effects of cholinergic nerve stimulation and produce response similar to acetylcholine
   b. uses: glaucoma (miotic), urinary retention, postoperative abdominal distension, myasthenia gravis, antidote for curare
   c. side effects: headache, conjunctival hyperemia (otic), urinary urgency, severe hypotension, bronchospasms, respiratory paralysis, cholinergic crisis
   d. nursing implications: administer miotic preparations on time; note CNS irritability; monitor vital signs; have atropine available as antidote; avoid IM or IV use, may cause vascular collapse
   e. examples: *direct-acting cholinomimetic:* bethanechol (Urecholine), pilocarpine (Isopto Carpine); *indirect-acting cholinomimetic:* physostigmine sulfate (Eserine Sulfate)

3. Carbonic anhydrase inhibitors
   a. description: drugs that increase urine output by blocking carbonic anhydrase in kidneys; also decrease production of aqueous humor
   b. uses: to treat glaucoma, edema not responding well to single-drug therapy, adjuvant to anticonvulsant therapy for epilepsy
   c. side effects: paresthesia, lethargy, anorexia, tinnitus, headache, hypokalemia, hyponatremia, ureteral colic, metabolic acidosis
   d. nursing implications: use cautiously in patients

with respiratory acidosis, diabetes and gout; monitor Na$^+$ and K$^+$ levels; watch for hypersensitivity; monitor visual improvement
  e. Example: acetazolamide (Diamox)
4. Barbiturates
  a. description: drugs that act by reversibly depressing activity of all excitable tissues; CNS is particularly sensitive; sleep induced has decreased rapid eye movement (REM) time
  b. uses: sedation, sleeplessness, anticonvulsant (phenobarbital), general anesthesia adjunct
  c. side effects: drowsiness, lethargy, headache, depression, hangover, hypersensitivity, blood dyscrasias
  d. nursing implications: warn patient about potential drug interactions, especially other CNS depressants; use other means to promote sleep; avoid overuse or dependence; monitor for overdose
  e. example: secobarbital (Seconal)
5. Nonbarbiturates
  a. description: drugs that act by increasing nonrapid eye movement (NREM) sleep while decreasing REM sleep by depressing subcortical levels in CNS
  b. uses: sleeplessness, preoperative sedation
  c. side effects: nausea, vomiting, constipation, hangover, headache, rash, urinary frequency
  d. nursing implications: use with care with elderly, COPD, depressed patients; avoid other CNS depressants; use natural methods to induce sleep; monitor for overuse or abuse
  e. example: flurazepam (Dalmane)
6. Minor tranquilizers (benzodiazepines)
  a. description: drugs that act selectively as presynaptic inhibitors of neural pathways throughout CNS; have similar activities to CNS depressants but more selectively
  b. uses: to treat anxiety, preoperative sedation, status epilepticus, acute alcohol withdrawal syndrome, mild muscle relaxant
  c. side effects: confusion, headache, agitation, oversedation, drowsiness, constipation, decreased libido, urinary retention, hypersensitivity; may be habit forming
  d. nursing implications: avoid use with alcohol or CNS depressants; food and antacids decrease absorption; avoid overuse and abuse; withdraw drugs slowly, assess mood and affect
  e. example: diazepam (Valium)
7. Major tranquilizers
  a. description: drugs that produce strong antipsychotic effects, possibly by blockade of postsynaptic dopamine receptors in brain; act on hypothalamus and reticular formation to produce strong sedation; strong alpha-adrenergic effect and weak anticholinergic effect
  b. uses: to control manic phase of manic-depressive illness; to treat severe nausea/vomiting; severe anxiety and agitation; intractable hiccoughs
  c. side effects: laryngospasms, dyspnea, extrapyramidal syndrome, agranulocytosis, jaundice, photosensitivity, orthostatic hypotension, tachycardia, sedation, constipation, dry mouth, tardive dyskinesia (abnormal facial grimaces and movements of the lips, tongue, and jaw)
  d. nursing implications: avoid other CNS depressants; monitor for development of extrapyramidal syndrome, liver function changes, signs of blood dyscrasias; check blood pressure; watch for constipation; do not give with antacids; teach about orthostatic changes
  e. example: chlorpromazine (Thorazine)

D. Drugs Affecting Protective Functions

1. Antineoplastics
  a. description: a wide variety of drugs that act to destroy rapidly dividing cells; classified as "cell-cycle specific" (those that attack cells at specific point in process of cell division) or "cell-cycle nonspecific" (those that act at any time during cell division)
  b. alkylating agents
    (1) uses: leukemias, lymphomas, multiple myelomas
    (2) side effects: bone-marrow depression, nausea/vomiting, vesicant action if extravasated, alpecia, hemorrhagic cystitis
    (3) nursing implications: monitor blood counts closely; teach patient safety precautions concerning low counts; avoid any contact with skin; prevent nausea
    (4) example: cyclophosphamide (Cytoxan)
  c. antimetabolites
    (1) uses: leukemias, testicular cancer, ovarian cancer, colon tumors
    (2) side effects: GI ulceration, stomatitis, bone-marrow depression, nephrotoxicity, ototoxicity, anaphylaxis
    (3) nursing implications: give leucovorin as ordered to prevent toxicity from methotrexate; hydrate well; monitor blood counts closely; watch for GI bleeding
    (4) example: methotrexate (Mexate)
  d. antitumor antibiotics
    (1) uses: to treat breast, ovarian, testicular, and lung cancer, leukemia and lymphoma
    (2) side effects: bone marrow depression, severe tissue necrosis with extravasation,

nausea/vomiting, cardiotoxicity, alopecia, stomatitis, red discoloration of urine
  (3) nursing implications: avoid extravasation; maintain adequate food and fluid intake; monitor cardiac function and blood counts
  (4) example: doxorubicin (Adriamycin)
e. vinca alkaloids
  (1) uses: to treat testicular, lung, ovary and breast cancers, leukemia and lymphoma
  (2) side effects: neurotoxicity, constipation, depression, mild bone marrow depression, alopecia, inflammation with extravasation
  (3) nursing implications: monitor for sensory or motor changes; administer stool softeners; administer IV slowly
  (4) example: vincristine (Oncovin)
f. hormones
  (1) uses: to treat hormone-dependent tumors such as breast and prostate cancers
  (2) side effects: minimal bone marrow depression, mild hypoglycemia, nausea, hypercalcemia in women with bone metastasis
  (3) nursing implications: monitor menstrual function; monitor blood calcium levels
  (4) example: tamoxifen (Nolvadex)

E. Drugs Affecting Mobility

1. Antiinflammatory drugs
  a. nonsteroidal
    (1) description: large group of drugs with antiinflammatory and often analgesic properties; act to reduce symptoms of inflammation such as redness, swelling, fever, and pain
    (2) uses: to treat mild to moderate pain due to inflammatory conditions; symptomatic relief of arthritic conditions
    (3) side effects: GI irritation, ulcers, bleeding, dyspepsia, bone-marrow depression, headache, dizziness, bowel changes, allergy
    (4) nursing implications: take with food or antacid to decrease GI distress; monitor blood counts; watch for GI bleeding; monitor for aspirin allergy; do not administer aspirin or other antiinflammatories
    (5) examples: ibuprofen (Motrin)
  b. steroids
    (1) description: drugs that block inflammatory, allergic, and immune responses by a variety of processes including both naturally occurring and synthetic glucocorticoids
    (2) uses: replacement for primary or secondary adrenocortical insufficiency; to treat wide variety of inflammatory, allergic/autoimmune disorders including rheuma-

toid disease, collagen disease, allergic reactions, dermatological responses, ophthalmic problems, ulcerative colitis, Crohn's disease, neoplasms
    (3) side effects: salt and water retention, GI ulceration from increased HCl secretion, hypertension (HTN), congestive heart failure (CHF), hirsutism, striae, impaired wound healing, fat redistribution, decreased growth in children, protein catabolism, osteoporosis, emotional lability, leukopenia, increased susceptibility to infection, sterility, cataracts, diabetes, hypokalemia
    (4) nursing implications: warn patient about need to avoid infections and increased need for steroids during times of physical and emotional stress; monitor decreased response to stress and side effects; help patient learn to minimize side effects as much as possible (low salt, high K+, low carbohydrate diet, for example); give with antacid or histamine receptor antagonist; give on diurnal schedule (high in AM); stress need for patient to strictly adhere to medication regime; offer support to patient's experiencing changes in body image; suggest Medic Alert
    (5) examples: dexamethasone (Decadron), cortisone acetate (prednisone)
2. Skeletal muscle relaxants
  a. description: drugs that act by interfering with nerve impulses in muscle tissues; CNS depressants with sedative properties; act on spinal and supraspinal sites to decrease frequency and amplitude of muscle spasms
  b. uses: acute painful muscle spasms, muscle tension and pains associated with anxiety; to treat spastic disorders such as multiple sclerosis
  c. side effects: headache, lethargy, dizziness, nausea/vomiting, hypotension, blurred vision, hypersensitivity, hypotonia
  d. nursing implications: give with meals; avoid orthostatic changes; warn about drowsiness; warn urine may change color; avoid alcohol or other CNS depressants; use cautiously with elderly and patients with seizure disorders; withdraw drugs slowly
  e. examples: methocarbamol (Robaxin), baclofen (Lioresal)
3. Anticonvulsants
  a. description: a wide variety of drugs that act to decrease nerve cell excitability in various ways
  b. uses: treatment of epilepsy and other seizure disorders
  c. side effects: GI irritation, dizziness, apathy, nervousness, ataxia, gum hyperplasia, blurred vision

d. nursing implications: teach patient to comply with consistent medication regime; avoid use of alcohol; warn patient about drowsiness or decreased alterness; give with meals to decrease GI distress

e. types and examples: *barbiturates:* phenobarbital; *hydantoins:* phenytoin (Dilantin)

4. Antiparkinson agents
   a. description: drugs that increase level of dopamine in CNS; often given in conjunction with anticholinergics, because cholinergic activity increased when deficit of dopamine exists
   b. uses: control of symptoms of Parkinson's disease
   c. side effects: nausea/vomiting, anorexia, orthostatic hypotension, dry mouth, dysphagia, ataxia, headache, insomnia, anxiety, hypertension, urinary retention
   d. nursing implications: use cautiously in patients with cardiovascular, respiratory, endocrine or hepatic disease, peptic ulcers, wide-angle glaucoma, diabetes and psychoses; watch blood pressure
   e. example: levodopa and carbidopa (Sinemet)

F. Drugs Affecting Metabolism

1. Antiemetics
   a. description: drugs that act to treat and prevent nausea and vomiting; most act by inhibiting chemoreceptor trigger zone (CTZ) or by depressing vestibular apparatus in inner ear
   b. uses: prevention and treatment of nausea and vomiting; motion sickness
   c. side effects: drowsiness, dry mouth, flushing, hypotension, restlessness, fatigue, extrapyramidal effects (parkinsonism, akathisia, tardive dyskinesia, dystonia)
   d. nursing implications: monitor I&O, blood pressure; when patient on long-term phenothiazine therapy, monitor for liver disease and extrapyramidal symptoms; warn patient about drowsiness; monitor effectiveness; use preventively
   e. types and examples: *phenothiazines:* prochlorperazine (Compazine); *nonphenothiazines:* trimethobenzamide (Tigan)

2. Antidiarrheals
   a. description: drugs that act to reduce liquidity of feces; local agents act within bowel to soothe intestinal tract and increase absorption of water, electrolytes, and nutrients; systemic agents act systemically to inhibit peristaltic reflex and reduce GI motility
   b. uses: treatment of acute and chronic diarrhea
   c. side effects: nausea/vomiting, acute glaucoma

(Lomotil), headache, drowsiness, hypersensitivity, nystagmus

   d. nursing implications: identify cause of diarrhea and eliminate cause; do not use Lomotil in patients with glaucoma or benign prostatic hypertrophy (BPH); avoid overuse; prevent constipation; protect drugs from light and moisture
   e. types and examples: *local:* kaolin and pectin (Kaopectate); *systemic:* diphenoxylate HCl with atropine (Lomotil)

3. Laxatives
   a. description: drugs that facilitate evacuation of bowel by wide variety of mechanisms
   b. uses: treatment of constipation; preparation for certain diagnostic tests
   c. nursing implication: suggest alternate methods to promote bowel movements: diet, fluids, exercise, etc; time administration according to action; do not use if obstruction suspected; give adequate fluids
   d. types and examples: *irritants:* biscadoyl (Dulcolax); *bulk formers:* psyllium (Metamucil); *saline/osmotic:* MgOH (milk of magnesia); *emollients:* sodium sulfosuccinate (Colace); *lubricants:* mineral oil

4. Hypoglycemics
   a. description: drugs that act to either stimulate islet cells in pancreas to secrete more insulin (oral) or act as insulin replacement when pancreatic function ceases (parenteral)
   b. uses: treatment of diabetes mellitus
   c. side effects: hypoglycemic reactions, GI distress, neurological symptoms, alcohol intolerance (oral), allergic reactions
   d. nursing implications: know onset and duration of action for each agent and teach to patient; monitor for and teach patient to monitor for hypoglycemic reactions; stress compliance with total diabetic regime; check for pork or beef allergy; teach patient insulin self-administration, site rotation, care of equipment, proper storage, glucose and urine self-testing
   e. examples: *oral agents:* acetohexamide (Dymelor); *insulins:* rapid-acting, regular insulin; intermediate-acting, insulin suspension (NPH); long-acting, protamine zinc (PZI)

5. Sulfonamides
   a. description: drugs that are bacteriostatic against both gram-positive and gram-negative organisms; drugs excreted unchanged and undissolved and dissolve well in urine; therefore excellent for treating urinary tract infections (UTIs)
   b. uses: urinary tract infections, acute otitis media, ulcerative colitis, chronic bronchitis
   c. side effects: GI distress, allergic reactions,

headache, peripheral neuritis, hearing loss, crystalluria, hypoglycemia

   d. nursing implications: administer with large amounts of fluid; monitor serum glucose levels (may produce false-positive urine glucose); monitor for allergies; check I&O; maintain alkaline pH because drugs more soluble in alkaline urine; teach patient to take full course of drugs

   e. examples: cotrimoxazole (Bactrim, Septra), sulfisoxazole (Gantrinsin)

6. Anticholinergics
   a. description: drugs that act as competitive antagonists at cholinergic-receptor sites, thereby blocking action of acetylcholine
   b. uses: to produce mydriasis; preoperative to decrease salivation and prevent laryngospasms and bradycardia; decrease GI motility; antiparkinsonian; decrease nasopharyngeal and bronchial secretions
   c. side effects: blurred vision, photophobia, urinary hesitancy, increased intraocular pressure, palpitations, flushing, tachycardia, dry mouth, allergic reactions, restlessness
   d. nursing implications: contraindicated in patients with glaucoma, GI obstruction, BPH, renal or hepatic disease; caution patient against driving; warn about usual side effects; monitor vital signs; give 30 minutes before meals
   e. examples: atropine; propantheline bromide (Pro-Banthine)

7. Antacids
   a. description: drugs that act to neutralize HCl and provide protective coating on lining of stomach
   b. uses: to treat duodenal ulcers; reduce gastric acid concentration and prevent stress ulcers; prevent ulcer recurrence; relieve flatus (simethicone)
   c. side effects: aluminum—constipation; magnesium—diarrhea
   d. nursing implications: check bowel movements; watch for rebound acidity and ulcer recurrence when drug discontinued
   e. types and examples: *aluminum:* Amphojel; *magnesium:* milk of magnesia; *aluminum and magnesium:* Maalox, Gelusil

8. Histamine H_2 receptor antagonist
   a. description: drugs that decrease gastric acid secretion, total acidity and pepsin activity
   b. uses: to prevent and treat duodenal ulcers; reduce gastric acid secretion and concentration; prevention of stress ulcers; prevention of ulcer recurrence
   c. side effects: diarrhea, dizziness, rash, gynecomastia, alopecia, neutropenia, impotence, bradycardia, headache

   d. nursing implications: do not give within 1 hour of antacids; monitor for relief of symptoms; does not cause rebound acidity when discontinued
   e. types and examples: cimetidine (Tagamet), ranitidine (Zantac)

9. Antithyroid drugs
   a. description: drugs that interfere with uptake of iodine and block synthesis of thyroxine (T4) and triiodothyronine (T3); does not interfere with release and use of stored thyroid; takes days or weeks for effect to be seen; hormone reduction leads to increased thyroid-stimulating hormone (TSH), which leads to hyperplasia and increased vascularity of gland; euthyroidism occurs in 6 to 12 weeks
   b. uses: to establish euthyroidism preoperatively; palliative care of toxic goiter
   c. side effects: nausea, vomiting, diarrhea, loss of taste, skin changes, headache, dizziness, drowsiness, lymphadenopathy, hypersensitivity, agranulocytosis, hypothyroidism
   d. nursing implications: monitor blood counts; should not be used in last trimester of pregnancy or during lactation; report any symptoms of infection; urge continued compliance because of slow response
   e. example: propylthiouracil (PTU)

10. Thyroid drugs
   a. description: synthetic thyroid preparation of controlled potency; contains T4, which is converted to T3; acts as replacement for thyroid hormone
   b. uses: to treat hypothyroidism
   c. side effects: rare; hyperthyroidism, tremors, hunger, weight loss
   d. nursing implications: use with caution in patients with acute myocardial infarctions (MIs), hypertension, renal insufficiency, diabetes, and elderly or pregnant patients; give a single dose in AM; watch for adverse effects early in treatment; monitor for improvement of symptoms
   e. example: levothyroxine sodium T4 (Synthroid)

III. PRINCIPLES OF MEDICATION ADMINISTRATION

A. Five Rights of Medication Administration and Safety

1. Right drug
2. Right dose
3. Right route
4. Right time
5. Right patient

B. Methods to Ensure Five Rights Followed

1. Do not administer any drug you are not familiar with; look it up first
   a. know intended action and uses for drug; does it fit this patient's diagnosis?
   b. know side and toxic effects
   c. know safe dosage range for patients of this age, weight, and health status
   d. be familiar with allergies and possible idiosyncracies
   e. know possible interactions with other drugs or foods
   f. be aware of any special precautions associated with drug
2. Be sure that drug ordered is what is given
   a. compare drug card to physician's order
   b. check label three times
      (1) when container taken from shelf or medication cart
      (2) before drug is poured
      (3) when container is replaced in cabinet or empty container discarded
3. Always keep medication card with drug and check it against patient's arm band to insure right patient is receiving right drug
4. Never take medication from an unmarked container or one with an illegible label (return to pharmacy for identification and correct relabeling)
5. Check to be sure that medication is being given by right route
6. Watch patient take medication, do not leave it at bedside or in patient's room
7. If the medication cannot be given for any reason, chart why it was not given and notify physician
8. Never leave your medication tray unattended
9. Administer medications at correct time; no more than 30 minutes before or 30 minutes after appointed time

C. Routes of Administration

1. Oral: po—by mouth
2. Injection
   a. subcutaneous: sc—under the skin; also called hypodermic
   b. intradermal: in between the layers of skin
   c. intramuscular: IM—into muscle tissues
   d. intravenous: IV—into a vein
3. Transdermal: onto the skin
4. Rectal: per rectum
5. Vaginal: per vagina
6. Inhalation: inhaled into respiratory tract
7. Sublingual: SL—placed under tongue until dissolved
8. Buccal: held against cheek until dissolved

D. Correct Methods of Medication Administration for Adults

1. Oral
   a. liquids
      (1) measured in ounces (oz), drams, minims, milliliters (mL), or cubic centimeters (cc)
      (2) hold container so that you are pouring away from label
      (3) position medicine cup at eye level; pour so bottom of meniscus at level of ordered dosage
      (4) never open a new bottle until the old one is empty
      (5) wipe lip of bottle before replacing cap
      (6) if medicine ordered in drops, use eye dropper provided with medication
   b. solid medications
      (1) only scored tablets may be broken; capsules and unscored tablets may never be broken
      (2) dissolve powders as ordered
      (3) crush pills only after checking safety of doing so; ie, never crush enteric coated tablets or spansules
2. Injections
   a. special points
      (1) maintain sterility of syringe and all its parts
      (2) carefully choose correct site for injection; measure site properly
      (3) always cleanse site of injection with disinfectant before injection
      (4) after needle inserted, draw back plunger except for intradermal injections; if blood returns, withdraw needle, discard medication contaminated with blood, and start over
   b. subcutaneous injections
      (1) given into any subcutaneous tissues, especially upper arm, thigh, and abdomen
      (2) use small gauge, #25, short needle, 3/4 inches
      (3) amount usually under 2 mL
      (4) administer at 90-degree angle
      (5) check carefully to insure that it is safe to administer drug by this route
   c. intradermal injections
      (1) usually given in inner part of forearm
      (2) use 3/8 to 1/2 inch #25-gauge needle
      (3) dosage usually under 1 mL
      (4) insert needle at 10- to 15-degree angle to skin
      (5) most often used for vaccines or skin tests

d. intramuscular injections
  (1) choose site and needle carefully
    (a) deltoid small muscle, little mass for injection
    (b) choose needle long enough to insert into muscle
  (2) position patient for best access to muscle chosen; ensure complete exposure so site can be properly palpated
e. intravenous therapy
  (1) assessment must be made at least each shift of the injection site, to insure that IV flowing properly and vein not inflammed
  (2) if vein inflammed or IV infiltrated
    (a) remove IV from vein
    (b) apply warm packs to area
    (c) notify physician
  (3) redress site of infusion per hospital policy
  (4) monitor type of fluids running and rate of infusion carefully and frequently
  (5) calculate IV rate: rate in drops/minute = amount of IV fluid (in mL) × drip factor/time (in minutes)
3. Ocular medications
  a. terminology; OD, right eye; OS, left eye; OU, both eyes
  b. have patient look up and instill drops into inner canthus
  c. do not touch the dropper to the eye
  d. have patient gently close eye, do not squeeze shut
  e. gently wipe excess away with clean tissue
4. Otic medications
  a. ear drops usually warmed to body temperature
  b. straighten adult ear canal by gently pulling lobe upward and backward, and children's ear canal by gently pulling lobe downward and backward
  c. have patient tilt head away from affected side
  d. after drops instilled, leave head tilted for a few minutes
  e. use a cotton ball to gently plug ear, if ordered
5. Transdermal medications
  a. medication that can be absorbed through intact skin
  b. check skin for irritation before application, do not apply over irritated skin
  c. apply measured dose or premeasured pad without rubbing medication into skin
  d. leave medication on skin, covered, for specified time
  e. apply to upper back, upper chest, or upper arms
6. Suppositories
  a. rectal
    (1) position patient in left lateral Sims' position

    (2) wear gloves for procedure
    (3) lubricate suppository and gloved index finger with water-soluble lubricant
    (4) insert suppository past rectal sphincter; if patient tense, encourage deep breaths
    (5) have patient hold suppository for required length of time (from 20 to 60 minutes)
  b. vaginal
    (1) wear gloves during procedure
    (2) have patient lie down with knees bent and slightly separated
    (3) insert foam or suppository into vagina
    (4) have patient lie down for required length of time

E. Pediatric Modifications for Correct Methods of Medication Administration

1. General principles
  a. correct drug therapy based on child's age, weight, and growth and development
  b. always approach child with assumption that child will take medication
  c. be honest with children and tell them about medication as appropriate for their developmental level
  d. administer distasteful medications with Jello or other tasteful food
  e. never call medication "candy" and never use medication as a threat
  f. calculate drug doses using one of following rules
    (1) body surface area: child's dose = body surface area (in square meters)/1.73 m² × adult dose
    (2) Clark's rule: child's dose = weight (in lb) ÷ 150 lb × adult dose
    (3) Young's rule: child's dose = age (in years) ÷ age (in years) + 12 × adult dose
    (4) Fried's rule: child's dose = age (in months) ÷ 150 × adult dose
2. Oral medication
  a. infants
    (1) give liquids through syringe without needle
    (2) insert syringe into infant's mouth and gently expel medication
    (3) medication can be mixed with baby food unless contraindicated
  b. toddlers: allow them to drink from cup if possible
3. Topical medications
  a. area may need to be covered to prevent child from rubbing medication off or spreading it

b. child may have to be restrained until medication dries

4. Injections
   a. infants and young children will have to be adequately restrained
   b. use gluteal or vastus lateralis sites for injections
   c. always talk to child and try to calm him or her without restraints if possible, but always restrain for safety

F. Modifications for Elderly Patients

1. Carefuly check for special precautions or warnings
2. Modify adult doses for elderly who weigh less than 150 lb
3. Check closely for drug interactions because elderly often on multiple medications
4. monitor closely for overmedication

5. In long-term care facilities, patients may be identified by pictures rather than arm bands

BIBLIOGRAPHY

Abrams, A.C. (1983). *Clinical drug therapy: Rationales for nursing practice*. Philadelphia: J.B. Lippincott Co.

Brown, M., and Mullholland, J.L. (1988). *Drug calculations, 3rd ed.* St. Louis: C.V. Mosby Co.

Clark, J.F., Queener, S.F., and Karb, V.B. (1990). *Pharamacological basis of nursing practice, 3rd ed.* St. Louis: C.V. Mosby Co.

Clayton, B.D. (1989). *Mosby's handbook of pharmacology in nursing, 4th ed.* St. Louis: C.V. Mosby Co.

Creighton, H. (1986). *Law every nurse should know, 5th ed.* Philadelphia: W.B. Saunders Co.

Govoni, L., and Hayes, J. (1988). *Drugs and nursing implications, 6th ed.* Norwalk, CT: Appleton and Lange.

Lehne, R., Crosby, L., Hamilton, D., and Moore, L. (1990) *Pharmacology for nursing care*. Philadelphia: W.B. Saunders Co.

Malseed, A.K., et al. (1982). *Pharmacology: Drug therapy and nursing considerations*. Philadelphia: J.B. Lippincott.

Pagliaro, L.A., and Pagliaro, A.M. (1983). *Pharmacologic aspects of aging*. St. Louis: C.V. Mosby Co.

Scherer, J.C. (1982). *Introductory clinical pharmacology, 2nd ed.* Philadelphia: J.B. Lippincott Co.

Questions

1. Which of the following medications may be ordered by the physician to reduce target symptoms seen in psychotic episodes?

   ① Valium
   ② Thorazine
   ③ Tofranil
   ④ Lithium

2. Which medication would the physician order to control extrapyramidal side effects?

   ① Cogentin
   ② Ativan
   ③ Mellaril
   ④ L-Dopa

3. Mrs. Davis is receiving Thorazine. What objective finding would indicate an early sign of tardive dyskinesia?

   ① Cogwheel rigidity at the elbow
   ② Drying of the mucous membranes
   ③ Akathisia of the lower extremities
   ④ Vermiform movements of the tongue

4. Medications administered in suppository form:

   ① Are always administered rectally
   ② Produce bowel evacuation
   ③ Have a base that melts at body temperature
   ④ Are soothing to mucous membranes

5. A medication consisting of a suspension of fat globules and water is classified as a(an):

   ① Emulsion
   ② Ointment
   ③ Tincture
   ④ Elixir

6. Tablets that are enteric coated are:

   ① Absorbed through the skin
   ② Dissolved by intestinal juices
   ③ Dissolved by gastric acid
   ④ Held in the mouth until dissolved

7. When administering a troche or lozenge, the nurse should instruct the patient to:

   ① Always dissolve it in water to protect the teeth
   ② Follow the medication with a full glass of water
   ③ Hold it in the mouth until dissolved
   ④ Take it on an empty stomach

8. Sustained release tablets are forms of drugs given to patients:

   ① Less frequently than regular tablets
   ② More often than gelatin coated capsules
   ③ For prevention of gastrointestinal (GI) irritation
   ④ Who need a delayed reaction because of hypersensitivity

9. When administering an antibiotic or a vaccine, the nurse must be alert for the possibility of:

   ① Overdosage and CNS depression
   ② Hypersensitivity and possible anaphylaxis
   ③ Signs of increasing infection
   ④ Orthostatic hypotension

10. Drugs that are administered to relieve pain are classified as:

    ① Analgesics
    ② Antipyretics
    ③ Hypnotics
    ④ Tranquilizers

11. Drugs that are administered to induce and maintain sleep are classified as:

    ① Analgesics
    ② Antipyretics
    ③ Hypnotics
    ④ Tranquilizers

12. A drug commonly used for the treatment of arthritis is:

    ① Phenobarbital
    ② Aspirin
    ③ Morphine sulfate
    ④ Codeine sulfate

13. Digoxin is an example of a cardiac glycoside that:

    ① Increases and strengthens the heart
    ② Raises the blood pressure
    ③ Slows the contraction of the heart
    ④ Slows and strengthens the heart

14. Before administering digoxin, the nurse must always:

    ① Check the patient's blood pressure
    ② Determine the patient's prothrombin time
    ③ Count the patient's apical pulse
    ④ Monitor the patient's radial pulse

15. The most common route used for administering nitroglycerin to treat acute angina is:

① Subcutaneous
② Intramuscular
③ Oral
④ Sublingual

16. Which of the following medications should *not* be followed by water?

① Cough syrups
② Antacids
③ Laxatives
④ Iron preparations

17. Before administering an antibiotic to a patient with a severe wound infection, the nurse must:

① First obtain a culture of the wound
② Hold the medication and recheck the order
③ First check the patient's temperature
④ Wait until the patient has had something to eat

18. Mr. Wilson, a patient with COPD, is receiving theophylline, which will act to:

① Relax the diaphragm and intercostals to increase chest expansion
② Decrease contraction of the smooth muscles of the bronchi
③ Increase the contraction of the bronchi and alveoli
④ Decrease the amount of mucus secretion from the bronchi

19. A nursing action to decrease reflux esophagitis, a side effect of theophylline, is:

① Administering the drug at bedtime
② Having the patient sit up after meals
③ Encouraging three large meals a day
④ Administering the medication with large quantities of water

20. While you are administering a rectal suppository, your patient asks, "Will I have a bowel movement after this suppository?" To answer this, the nurse must know that rectal suppositories are given to:

① Relieve constipation
② Treat hemorrhoids
③ The patient who cannot tolerate enemas
④ The patient for a variety of reasons, depending on the medication in the suppository

21. Iron preparations should be administered:

① At bedtime
② Before breakfast
③ With meals
④ Between meals

22. Pilocarpine, a miotic, causes:

① Dilation of the pupil
② Inhibition of bacteria in the eye
③ Local anesthesia to the pupil
④ Constriction of the pupil

23. Because of its action, the nurse knows that pilocarpine will be used to:

① Treat glaucoma
② Treat cataracts
③ Examine the retina
④ Prevent night blindness

24. Atropine, a mydriatic, causes:

① Dilation of the pupil
② Inhibition of bacteria in the eye
③ Local anesthesia to the pupil
④ Constriction of the pupil

25. Because of its action, the nurse knows that atropine will be used to:

① Treat glaucoma
② Treat cataracts
③ Examine the retina
④ Prevent night blindness

26. The classification of drugs used to treat the symptoms of an allergic reaction is:

① Antibiotic
② Antihistamine
③ Cholinergic
④ Sulfonamide

27. You notice that the label on the cough syrup bottle is difficult to read. Your most appropriate action is to:

① Return the drug to the pharmacy for relabeling
② Hold the medication and chart that it was not given
③ Make out a new label and apply it over the old one
④ Pour the medication, because you know what it is

28. You notice that the medication you are about to

administer has changed color since yesterday; you know that this means that:

① This is not uncommon and has no significance
② The drug can be given if you check first with the charge nurse
③ The drug should be held and charted as not given
④ The drug is not given, and a fresh supply is obtained and given

When you enter Mr. Smith's room to administer his 9 AM medications, you find that he and his wife are engaged in an argument about the cost of this hospitalization and the impact on their finances. When you offer him his medication, he refuses, stating, "Those pills make me sick to my stomach."

29. When charting the event, the nurse should write that the patient:

① Refused medication because it makes him sick
② Refused medication because upset by fight with wife
③ Refused medication, stating the pills made him sick to his stomach
④ Worried about the cost of hospitalization so refused to take medication

30. It is important to chart the patient's refusal of the medication to:

① Prove that this is a difficult patient
② Cover yourself in case there is trouble later
③ Notify the doctor of the patient's refusal to take the drug
④ Warn the other nurses that he is uncooperative

31. When you are charting later that day, you make an error. The proper way to correct an error is to:

① Cross it out with multiple lines and initial it as an error
② Use correction fluid and erase it
③ Ask the charge nurse to co-sign it as an error
④ Draw a single line through it and write the word "error" above it and initial it

32. It is important that the nurse is able to convert from pounds to kilograms, because medication dosages are based on kilograms of body weight. A 106-lb woman weighs approximately:

① 52 kg
② 48 kg
③ 42 kg
④ 36 kg

Answers & Rationales

Guide to item identification (see pp. 3–5 for further details about each category)

I, II, III, or IV for the phase of the nursing process
1, 2, 3, or 4 for the category of client needs
A, B, C, D, E, F, or G for the category of human functioning
Specific content category by name; ie, cholecystectomy

1. "Chlorpromazine (Thorazine) reduces psychotic symptomatology. Essentially, the client's behavior becomes more socially acceptable. Target symptoms most likely to improve from the use of antipsychotic drugs include hallucinations." (Bauer & Hill, 1986:128)
② III, 2 & 3, G. Psychiatric Medications.

2. "Pseudoparkinsonism is drug-induced . . ." "Antiparkinson agents, such as Cogentin, Artane, and Benadryl, relieve symptoms." (Bauer & Hill, 1986:129)
① III, 2 & 3, G. Psychiatric Medications.

3. "The health provider is encouraged to check the client's tongue regularly for vermiform (wormlike) movements, which are often the first sign of tardive dyskinesia." (Bauer & Hill, 1986:129)
④ I, 2 & 3, G. Psychiatric Medications.

4. Suppositories may be given vaginally, orally or rectally. They contain medication in a base that melts at body temperature.
③ III, 2, D. Medication Administration.

5. An emulsion is a suspension of fat in water that must be shaken before administration to mix the two.
① I, 2, D. Medication Administration.

6. Enteric-coated tablets resist dissolution by gastric acids but are made to dissolve in the basic intestinal secretions.
② I, 2, D. Medication Administration.

7. These medications are designed to act on the oral mucous membranes or upper throat, so they must be allowed to dissolve completely in the mouth. They should never be diluted with water, which would decrease their action.
③ III, 2, D. Medication Administration.

8. The action of these tablets is prolonged and gradual over time, allowing for less frequent administration.
① I, 2, D. Medication Administration.

9. These agents are often allergens in sensitive individuals, and anaphylaxis is always a risk.
② III & IV, 2, D. Medication Administration.

10. Analgesics, both narcotic and non-narcotic, are the drugs given for pain relief.
① I, 2, D. Medications/Analgesics.

11. Hypnotics is the class of drugs to which most sleeping pills belong. The other common class is sedatives.
③ I & IV, 2, C. Medications/Hypnotics.

12. Nonsteroidal antiinflammatories are the drugs of choice to treat arthritis.
② IV, 2, D. Medications/Antiinflammatories.

13. Digoxin acts by strengthening the contraction of the heart to improve cardiac output. It also slows the rate, making each beat more efficient and effective.
④ IV, 2, B. Medications/Cardiac.

14. Digoxin slows the heart rate as part of its action; however, an early symptom of overdose or toxicity is abnormal slowing of the heart. Digoxin should not be given without checking with the doctor if the apical pulse is <60 or >120.
③ III, 2, B. Medications/Cardiac.

15. Nitroglycerin for acute angina is needed immediately. The most rapid absorption is through the mucous membranes under the tongue.
④ III, 2, B. Medications/Cardiac.

16. Cough syrups are intended to coat the throat with a soothing medication and therefore should never be followed with water.
① III, 2, B. Medications/Expectorants.

17. If antibiotics are started before the culture is obtained, an accurate culture is impossible. Whenever possible, the culture should be obtained before the drugs are started.
② III, 2, D. Medications/Antibiotics.

18. The action of theophylline, a bronchodilator, is to relax the bronchial smooth muscles.
① IV, 2, B. Medications/Bronchodilators.

19. Sitting up after meals helps the food remain in

② the stomach and not reflux into the esophagus.
IV, 2, B. Medications/Bronchodilators.

20. ④ Any form of medication that can be absorbed through mucous membranes can technically be administered rectally. The nurse must find out why a medication is being given in order to give the patient an accurate explanation.
III, 1, F. Medication Administration.

21. ③ Iron is very irritating to the gastrointestinal tract, and administering it with food decreases this.
II, 1, F. Medications/Iron.

22. ④ Miotics constrict the pupil.
I, 2, C. Medications/Optic.

23. ① In order to increase the outflow of the humor in the eye, the canal of Schlemm must be open. Constricting the pupil increases the angle and therefore the outflow.
IV, 2, C. Medications/Optic.

24. ① Mydriatics dilate the pupil.
I, 2, C. Medications/Optic.

25. ③ In order to examine the retina better, atropine will be given to dilate the pupil.
II, 2, C. Medications/Optic.

26. ② Antihistamines counter the histamine produced by an allergic reaction.
IV, 2, D. Medications/Antihistamines.

27. ① The only person legally licensed to label medication is the pharmacist.
III, 2, D. Medication Administration.

28. ④ That drug should not be given because a color change may indicate an alteration in the chemical composition of a drug as a result of age, light or moisture. A new supply should be obtained and administered as ordered.
III, 2, D. Medication Administration.

29. ③ This is the most objective statement of the incident. When charting, the nurse should avoid subjective statements.
III, 1 & 2, G. Medication Administration.

30. ③ Charting is an important way to document accurately and objectively the patient's responses to therapy.
IV, 2, G. Medication Administration.

31. ④ The correct way to alter the legal chart record is to cross out the error with a single line, write "error" and initial it.
III, 1, G. Medication Administration.

32. ② The conversion is 2.2 pounds per kilogram.
III, 2, D. Medication Administration.

Diet Therapy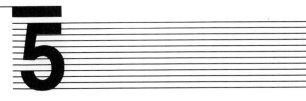

I. PRINCIPLES OF NORMAL NUTRITION

A. Requirements

Vary according to age, sex, activity level, state of health, and climate

B. Optimal Nutrition

1. Intake matches energy expenditure
2. Proper amounts of each essential nutrient

C. Essential For

1. Normal growth, development, organ function
2. Maintenance of bodily function
3. Optimal activity status
4. Resistance to infection
5. Repair of injuries to cells and tissues

D. Nutritional Deficiencies, of Either Calories or Specific Nutrients

1. Primary deficiencies: inadequate intake
2. Secondary deficiencies
   a. interference with ingestion, digestion, absorption, or usage of proper nutrients
   b. increased requirements as a result of stress or illness

E. Six Prime Nutrients

1. Fats
2. Proteins
3. Carbohydrates
4. Minerals
5. Vitamins
6. Water

F. Contents of Four Basic Food Groups (Table 5-1)

1. Milk group
   a. provides adequate amounts of calcium and riboflavin
   b. also contains protein, carbohydrates, phosphorus, thiamine, vitamin D, and possibly vitamin A
   c. whole milk has higher amounts of fat than skim or low fat milk
2. Vegetable and fruit group
   a. contain sugar, starch, cellulose, and varying amounts of vitamins and minerals
   b. primary source of vitamin C
      (1) citrus fruits
      (2) tomatoes
      (3) broccoli
      (4) Brussels sprouts
      (5) green and red peppers
   c. dark green and deep yellow vegetables are good sources of vitamin A
   d. leafy green vegetables are a good source of iron
   e. potatoes are high in iron, thiamine, and vitamin C
3. Meat/egg/legume group
   a. source of protein, iron, thiamine, niacin, fat, phosphorus, and riboflavin
   b. liver is an excellent source of iron and vitamin A
   c. saltwater seafood contains iodine
   d. eggs are high in protein, iron, thiamine, phosphorus, and riboflavin, with yolk high in vitamin A and fat (cholesterol)
   e. legumes contain protein, but of lower quality than that in meat, eggs, or fish
   f. nuts high in protein, iron, thiamine, riboflavin, and niacin
4. Cereal and bread group
   a. contain starch and incomplete proteins
   b. whole grain cereals contain cellulose
   c. grains often enriched to become good sources of iron, thiamine, riboflavin, and niacin

G. Vitamins

1. Fat-soluble vitamins
   a. vitamin A
      (1) requirements: men—5000 IU; women—4000 IU; pregnancy—+1000 IU; lactation—+2000 IU
      (2) functions: purple vision development, which allows vision in dim light; normal growth and development of bones and teeth; formation and maintenance of skin and mucous membranes

TABLE 5–1. Four Basic Food Groups

Group	Sources of nutrients
Milk	All forms of milk: yogurt, cheeses, cottage cheese, pudding, ice cream
Fruits/Vegetables	All fruits such as apples, oranges, peaches, pears, melons, apricots, and so on; vegetables include dark green and yellow vegetables such as carrots, squash, sweet potatoes, broccoli, Brussels sprouts, lettuce, and so on
Cereal/Breads	Whole grain and enriched, or restored grains such as rice, wheat, rye, oats, barley, and corn and any baked goods made from these such as breads or pasta
Meat and other high-protein foods	All meats such as beef, pork, lamb, poultry, veal; eggs, nuts, fish, legumes, lentils, dried beans

      (3) sources: liver, egg yolks, fortified dairy products, dark green and yellow vegetables
  b. vitamin D
      (1) requirements: age 19–22 years—300 IU; after 22 years—200 IU; pregnancy or lactation—+200 IU
      (2) functions: helps maintain optimal level of calcium and phosphorus for normal bone mineralization
      (3) sources: fortified milk and breakfast cereals, egg yolks, sardines, liver, salmon, and tuna fish (fish oils)
  c. vitamin E
      (1) requirements: men—10 mg; women—8 mg; pregnancy—+2 mg; lactation—+3 mg
      (2) functions: antioxidant that protects vitamin A and polyunsaturated fatty acid (PUFA); protects cell membrane
      (3) sources: vegetable oils, wheat germ, leafy vegetables, corn, nuts, and soybeans
  d. vitamin K
      (1) requirements: 70—140 μg
      (2) function: essential for formation of clotting factor prothrombin; salicylates interfere with vitamin K production
      (3) sources: green leafy vegetables, egg yolks, and liver
2. Water-soluble vitamins
  a. vitamin C
      (1) requirements: men and women—60 mg; pregnancy—+20 mg; lactation +40 mg
      (2) function: antioxidant; essential in formation of collagen; strengthens mucous membranes; enhances absorption of iron in gut; converts folic acid to active form; involved in metabolism of selected amino acids
      (3) sources: green vegetables, citrus fruits, potatoes, tomatoes, and cabbage
      (4) relatively unstable vitamin
  b. thiamine (vitamin B_1)
      (1) requirements: men and women—5 mg/1000 calories; pregnancy—+0.4 mg/1000 cal; lactation—+0.5 mg/1000 cal
      (2) function: carbohydrate metabolism; normal function of central nervous system (CNS)
      (3) sources: pork, liver, organ meats, whole and enriched grains, legumes, potatoes, eggs, and milk
  c. riboflavin (vitamin B_2)
      (1) requirements: men and women—0.6 mg/1000 cal; pregnancy—+0.3 mg/1000 cal; lactation—+0.5 mg/1000 cal
      (2) functions: fat, carbohydrate, and protein metabolism
      (3) sources: dairy products, organ meats, eggs, enriched grains, and green leafy vegetables
  d. niacin (vitamin B_3)
      (1) requirements: men and women—6.6 mg/1000 calories; pregnancy—+2 mg/1000 cal; lactation—+3 mg/1000 cal
      (2) function: fat, carbohydrate, and protein metabolism
      (3) sources: organ meat, poultry, lean meats, peanut butter, whole and enriched grains, dried beans and peas, and nuts
  e. pyridoxine (vitamin B_6)
      (1) requirements: men—2.2 mg; women—2 mg; pregnancy—+0.6 mg; lactation—+0.5 mg
      (2) functions: metabolism of amino acids; blood formation; maintenance of nervous system; conversion of tryptophan to niacin
      (3) sources: wheat germ, yeast, organ meats, pork, egg yolks, whole grain cereals, corn, potatoes, and bananas
  f. folic acid (folacin)
      (1) requirements: men and women—400 μg; pregnancy—+400 μg; lactation—+100 μg
      (2) functions: amino acid metabolism; proliferation of cells; blood formation
      (3) sources: green leafy vegetables, organ meats, eggs, milk, yeast, wheat germ, and kidney beans
  g. cobalamin (vitamin B_{12})
      (1) requirements: men and women—3 μg; pregnancy—+1 μg; lactation—+1 μg
      (2) functions: RNA and DNA synthesis; blood formation; maintenance of nervous tissue; folic acid metabolism; fat, protein, and carbohydrate metabolism
      (3) sources: liver, kidney, fresh shrimp and oysters, milk, eggs, and cheese
  h. pantothenic acid
      (1) requirements: men and women—4–7 mg
      (2) function: fat, protein, and carbohydrate metabolism
      (3) sources: organ meats, egg yolks, salmon, fresh vegetables, yeast, and whole grains

i. biotin
   (1) requirements: men and women—100–200 μg
   (2) function: fat, protein, and carbohydrate metabolism
   (3) sources: organ meats, peanuts, mushrooms, milk, egg yolks, and yeast

H. Daily Balanced Diet (Table 5-2)

1. Calculation of calories for ideal body weight
   a. females: 100 lb for first 5 feet and add 5 lb for each inch over 5 feet
   b. males: 106 lb for first 5 feet and add 6 lb for each inch over 5 feet
   c. children: consult growth charts
   d. basal caloric need = 10 × ideal weight; add ideal weight × 3 for sedentary people; add ideal weight × 5 for moderately active people; add ideal weight × 10 for people with strenuous activity
   e. 1 lb body fat = 3500 calories; add or subtract for each lb to lose per week
2. Milk
   a. children under age 9 years: two or three servings
   b. children ages 9–12 years: three or more servings
   c. teenagers: four or more servings
   d. adults: two servings
   e. pregnant women: three or more
   f. nursing mothers: four or more
3. Vegetables and fruits
   a. four or more servings per day
   b. one good or two fair sources of vitamin C daily
   c. one good source of vitamin A per day

TABLE 5–2. Daily Balanced Diet

Meal Pattern	Sample Menu
Breakfast	
Fruit	½ cup orange juice
Cereal or breadstuff	1 cup oatmeal
Hot food	1 soft boiled egg
Beverage	Coffee or tea, 1 cup milk
Lunch	
Sandwich	Sandwich with 2 slices whole wheat bread, 2 oz chicken, mustard, lettuce and tomato
Salad	1 cup fruit salad
Dessert	1 cup yogurt
Beverage	Coffee or tea
Dinner	
Soup	½ cup tomato soup with crackers
Meat	2 oz broiled ground beef
Salad	Lettuce salad with low fat dressing
Vegetable	½ cup broccoli
Dessert	1 banana
Beverage	1 cup milk

4. Meats
   a. two or more servings per day
   b. meats lower in fat should be used
   c. number of eggs per week should be limited because of high cholesterol content
5. Breads and cereals
   a. four or more servings per day
   b. enriched products preferable

I. Special Nutritional Needs by Age

1. Infants
   a. higher protein and calorie requirements because of high rates of growth and activity
   b. breast milk provides all essentials
   c. solid food introduced at 5–6 months
2. Preschoolers
   a. growth rate erratic
   b. dietary needs fluctuate throughout period
   c. child learns lifetime eating habits, so offer wide variety of foods
   d. finger food best
   e. give foods in small amounts
   f. avoid refined sweets
3. School age
   a. growth rate increases gradually, requiring increased nutrients
   b. between-meal snacks are often a problem because of poor nutritional content
4. Adolescents
   a. tremendous growth spurt; usually increased activity
   b. girls
      (1) usually 10–13 years old
      (2) usually gain fat tissue
   c. boys
      (1) usually 13–16 years old
      (2) gain lean muscle tissue
5. Pregnancy
   a. increase
      (1) protein intake by 50%
      (2) calories
      (3) calcium, phosphorus, and vitamin D
   c. no need to limit salt excessively
   d. weight gain within medical recommendations, but not severely limited
6. Nursing mothers
   a. high protein with increased calories
   b. all nutrients need to be increased
   c. increased fluid intake very important
7. Elderly
   a. lower metabolic rate and decreased activity mean fewer calories needed
   b. decreased food intake

(1) senses of smell and taste decrease resulting in decreased appetite

(2) loss of teeth, poor-fitting dentures, and social isolation all impair eating

(3) decreased bowel motility leads to constipation, which lowers appetite

(4) diets low in protein, vitamin C, and calcium

(5) shopping and cooking may be impaired because of other disabilities

c. diet planning with older adults should take all these areas into consideration

II. THERAPEUTIC DIET MODIFICATIONS

A. Postsurgical Diets

1. Clear liquid
   a. tea or coffee without cream or milk, fat-free broth, and gelatin
   b. carbonated beverages may be allowed, although carbonation may increase gas in postsurgical patients
   c. nutritionally inadequate diet
2. Full liquids
   a. any food that is liquid at body temperature
   b. foods allowed include milk, cream, ice cream, juices without pulp, gelatin, strained soups, broth, tea, coffee, and carbonated beverages
   c. lacks some necessary nutrients
   d. provides some calories and liquids
3. Soft diet
   a. composed of easily chewed foods
   b. can be nutritionally adequate and high in calories
   c. includes most foods except fried, high fiber, and strongly flavored foods

B. Low Sodium Diets (Table 5-3)

1. Mild restriction
   a. 2–3 g (2000–3000 mg) of sodium daily
   b. minimal restrictions; no brine foods or those prepared with monosodium glutamate (MSG)
   c. no added table salt to food
   d. usually palatable and easily followed
2. Moderate restriction
   a. 1 g (1000 mg) sodium/day
   b. meat, milk, and bakery goods restricted
   c. no table salt added during or after cooking
   d. some vegetables omitted
3. Strict sodium restriction
   a. 0.5 g (500 mg) sodium
   b. used only for severe disease states such as severe congestive heart failure
   c. many foods not allowed; severe meat and egg restriction
   d. Not well accepted by patients

C. High or Low Potassium Diet (Table 5-4)

1. Typical adult intake from 2000 to 4000 mg per day
2. Restrictions required for patients with renal disease
3. Increased amounts needed for patients on potassium-wasting diuretics; better handled through dietary means rather than supplements

D. Low Cholesterol Diet (Table 5-5)

1. Moderate restriction: 300–500 mg/day
   a. increase polyunsaturated fats and decrease saturated fats

TABLE 5–3. Low Sodium Diets: Sodium Content of Four Basic Food Groups

Dairy products	
Naturally high	None
High in added sodium	Buttermilk, cheese and cottage cheese, milk products such as ice cream, malts, milk shakes, and sherbet
Low sodium	Skim, 2%, evaporated, and low sodium milk, and low sodium cheeses
Fruits and vegetables	
Naturally high	Spinach, celery, carrots, white turnips, greens, beets, and artichokes
High in added sodium	Glazed fruits, maraschino cherries, fruits with sodium preservatives, canned vegetables and juices, frozen vegetables with added salt
Low sodium	Fresh fruits and vegetables, frozen or canned vegetables and fruit without added sodium
Breads and cereals	
Naturally high	None
High in added sodium	Mixes, bread and rolls made from premixed dough, crackers, instant cereals, most dry cereals, self-rising flour, baking soda and powder, and egg whites
Low sodium	Low sodium breads, crackers, and cereals, puffed rice, puffed wheat, cornmeal, shredded wheat, barley, unsalted matzo, and rice
Meats	
Naturally high	Seafoods, shellfish, brain, and kidney
High in added sodium	Bacon, lunch meat, corned beef, chipped beef, hot dogs, sausage, salt pork, codfish, smoked meats and fish, kosher meats and chicken, egg substitutes, and peanut butter
Low sodium	Low sodium products, fresh fish such as bass, catfish, flounder, sole, trout, and tuna, and low sodium tuna and salmon

TABLE 5–4. High Potassium Foods

Dairy products
  Whole milk
  Evaporated and canned milk
  Condensed sweetened milk
Fruits and vegetables
  Baked potato with skin
  Asparagus
  Lima beans
  Green beans
  Beets
  Broccoli
  Brussels sprouts
  Lettuce
  Spinach
  Tomato
  Apricot
  Avocado
  Banana
  Oranges
  Dates
  Grapefruit juice
  Peaches
  Raisins
  Watermelon
Breads and cereals
  Barley
  Raisin bread
  Pumpernickel bread
  Whole wheat bread
  Bran flakes
  Buckwheat flour
  Angelfood cake
  Coffeecake
  Gingerbread
  Chocolate cake
  Fruitcake
Meats
  Lean meats
  Flounder
  Raw shrimp
  Legumes
  Sunflower seeds

TABLE 5–5. High Cholesterol Foods

High Cholesterol Foods in Descending Order (Highest to Lowest)

Organ meats—beef, pork, and lamb
Egg yolks
Shrimp
Lamb
Veal
Crab
Beef
Pork
Lobster
Chicken and turkey, dark meat with skin
Chicken and turkey, white meat with skin
Clams
Halibut
Tuna
Oysters
Salmon
Butter
Whole milk
Cheddar cheese
Ice cream
Half-and-half
Creamed cottage cheese
Light cream
Lard
Plain cottage cheese
Skim milk

  b. up to three egg yolks/week can be substituted for 3 oz of lean meat
  c. use lean meats, fish, and poultry
  d. use skim milk and low fat products
2. Strict restriction of 100 to 300 mg/day
  a. increase polyunsaturated fats and decrease saturated fats to a 2 : 1 ratio
  b. limit meat intake, use mostly fish, chicken, turkey, and veal
  c. eliminate egg yolks
  d. use only skim or low fat milk
3. Either diet may be associated with decreased calorie intake

E. Low Fat Diet (Table 5-6)

1. Reduction of all fats in diet
2. Foods should not be fried or prepared with added fat; baking, broiling, or boiling are appropriate cooking methods

3. Trim all visible fat from meats and remove skin from poultry
4. Lean meat and up to three egg yolks/week
5. No more than six servings of fat/day

F. High Calcium Diet (Table 5-7)

1. Recommend daily amount is about 800 mg/day for men and up to 1500 mg/day for women
2. Increased need with various endocrine disorders, osteoporosis, and pregnancy and lactation
3. Milk and milk products are the best source
4. Canned fish with bones is also good
5. Vitamin D is necessary for normal calcium absorption

G. Low Calorie, Reducing Diet (Table 5-8)

1. First, identify amount of calories to maintain weight
  a. restrict calories to promote 1- to 2-lb weight loss/week
  b. subtract 500 cal/day for each pound to be lost
2. Very important that balanced diet be maintained
3. Use supportive techniques to help patient maintain diet

TABLE 5–6. Fat Content of Foods

Low fat foods
  Lean meats
  Fish
  Skinless poultry
  Egg whites
  Egg substitutes
  Skim milk
  Low fat cheese
  Low fat yogurt
  All fresh fruits and vegetables except avocados
  Plain cereals
  Pasta
  Rice
  Enriched or whole grain breads
  Sherbet
  Fruit ices
  Gelatin
  Angel food cake
  Skim or low fat milk
High fat foods
  Butter
  Margarine
  Shortening
  Cold cuts
  Oil
  Mayonnaise
  Avocados
  Bacon
  Heavy cream
  Salad dressings
  Nuts
  Olives
  Fatty meats
  Whole milk
  Oil-packed fish
  Peanut butter
  Cheese
  Yogurt
  Ice cream
  Breads products prepared with added fats: waffles, muffins, pancakes, biscuits, sweet rolls, danishes
  Gravy
  Desserts
  Chocolate

TABLE 5–7. High Calcium Foods

Highest amounts
  Milk
  Milk products
  Green leafy vegetables
  Shellfish
  Cheese
  Mustard and turnip greens
  Clams
  Oysters
  Broccoli
  Cauliflower
  Cabbage
  Molasses
Lesser amounts
  Egg
  Carrot
  Celery
  Orange
  Grapefruit
  Figs
  Breads made with milk

TABLE 5–8. Low Calorie, Reducing Diet (1200 cal)

Breakfast
  ½ cup orange juice
  ½ cup bran flakes with raisins
  1 cup skim milk
  1 slice whole wheat toast
  Coffe/tea
Lunch
  Sandwich
    2 slices enriched bread
    2 oz ham
    1 oz cheese slice
    ½ medium tomato
    lettuce
  1 medium apple
  Coffee/tea
Dinner
  3 oz roast beef
  1 medium baked potato
  2 T low fat sour cream
  ½ cup broccoli
  1 cup skim milk
Snack
  1 small cucumber, sliced
  3–4 carrot sticks, 3-inches long

H. Diabetic Diet (Table 5-9)

1. American Diabetes Association (ADA) recommendations
   a. carbohydrates should provide 50%–60% of total calories
      (1) complex carbohydrates best choice, such as grains and vegetables
      (2) limit simple carbohydrates, such as sugar
   b. protein should provide 12%–20% of total calories
      (1) sources should be low in saturated fat and cholesterol
      (2) good, biologic value proteins should be used
   c. fats should provide 30%–38% of calories
      (1) limit saturated fats and cholesterol
      (2) slight increase in polyunsaturated fats
2. Number of calories allowed on diet may vary greatly
   a. may need calorie reduction if patient is obese
   b. calories may be to maintain weight and minimize insulin requirements
3. Foods allowed should be similar to a normal balanced diet for the specific patient
   a. major limitations in high refined sugars
   b. ethnic foods included in exchange lists

I. Low Protein Diet (Table 5-10)

1. Lowered protein in renal or liver disease
2. Goal to maintain nitrogen balance while keeping

TABLE 5–9. Diabetic Diet Exchange Lists

Milk exchanges
1 exchange = 12 g CHO, 8 g protein, and 80 cal (1 cup serving)
Skim or nonfat milk
Yogurt made from skim milk
Whole milk, contains 2 fat exchanges
Buttermilk, contains 2 fat exchanges
Yogurt, contains 2 fat exchanges

Vegetable exchanges
1 exchange = 5 g CHO, 2 g protein, and 25 cal ($\frac{1}{2}$ cup serving)
Asparagus
Bean sprouts
Beets
Brussels sprouts
Cabbage
Cauliflower
Celery
Eggplant
Green pepper
Greens
Mushrooms
Okra
Onions
String beans
Summer squash
Tomato
Turnips
Zucchini

Free vegetables (used as desired)
Cucumbers
Endive
Escarole
Lettuce
Parsley
Dill pickles
Radishes
Watercress

Fruit exchanges
1 exchange = 10 g CHO and 40 cal
Apple—1 small
Apple juice—$\frac{1}{3}$ cup
Unsweetened applesauce—$\frac{1}{2}$ cup
Apricots—2 medium
Banana—$\frac{1}{2}$ small
Blackberries—$\frac{1}{2}$ cup
Blueberries—$\frac{1}{2}$ cup
Raspberries—$\frac{1}{2}$ cup
Strawberries—$\frac{3}{4}$ cup
Cherries—10 large
Cider—$\frac{1}{3}$ cup
Dates—2
Fresh figs—1
Grapefruit—$\frac{1}{2}$
Grapefruit juice—$\frac{1}{2}$ cup
Grapes—12
Grape juice—$\frac{1}{4}$ cup
Mango—$\frac{1}{2}$ small
Cantaloupe—$\frac{1}{4}$ small
Honeydew—$\frac{1}{8}$ medium
Watermelon—1 cup
Nectarine—1 small
Orange—1 small
Orange juice—$\frac{1}{2}$ cup
Papaya—$\frac{3}{4}$ cup
Peach—1 medium
Pear—1 small
Persimmons, native—1 medium
Pineapple—$\frac{1}{2}$ cup
Pineapple juice—$\frac{1}{3}$ cup
Plums—2 medium
Prunes—2 medium
Prune juice—$\frac{1}{4}$ cup
Raisins—2 tbsp
Tangerine—1 medium

Bread exchanges
1 exchange = 15 g CHO, 2 g protein, and 70 cal
White, French, and Italian bread—1 slice
Whole wheat bread—1 slice
Rye or pumpernickel—1 slice
Bagel, small—$\frac{1}{2}$
English muffin, small—$\frac{1}{2}$
Plain bread roll—1
Hamburger bun—$\frac{1}{2}$
Frankfurter roll—$\frac{1}{2}$
Dried bread crumbs—3 T
Tortilla, 6-inch—1

Low fat items
Bran flakes—$\frac{1}{2}$ cup
Unsweetened cereal—$\frac{3}{4}$ cup
Puffed cereal—1 cup
Cooked cereal—$\frac{1}{2}$ cup
Cooked grits—$\frac{1}{2}$ cup
Cooked rice or barley—$\frac{1}{2}$ cup
Pasta, cooked—$\frac{1}{2}$ cup
Popcorn popped without butter—3 cups
Dry cornmeal—2 T
Flour—2$\frac{1}{2}$ T
Wheat germ—$\frac{1}{4}$ cup
Graham crackers—3
Matzo, 4 inches × 6 inches—$\frac{1}{2}$
Oyster crackers—20
Pretzels, 3$\frac{1}{8}$ inches long × $\frac{1}{8}$ inches diameter—25
Rye wafers 2 inches × 3$\frac{1}{2}$ inches—3
Saltines—6
Soda crackers, 2$\frac{1}{2}$ inches sq—4
Beans, peas, lentils (dried and cooked)—$\frac{1}{2}$ cup
Baked beans, no pork (canned)—$\frac{1}{4}$ cup
Corn—$\frac{1}{3}$ cup
Corn on cob—1 small
Lima beans—$\frac{1}{2}$ cup
Parsnips—$\frac{2}{3}$ cup
Green peas—$\frac{1}{2}$ cup
White potato—1 small
Mashed potato—$\frac{1}{2}$ cup
Pumpkin—$\frac{3}{4}$ cup
Winter, acorn, or butternut squash—$\frac{1}{2}$ cup
Sweet potato—$\frac{1}{4}$ cup

Prepared foods with added fat
Biscuit 2 inch diameters—1, contains 1 fat exchange
Corn bread, 2 inches × 2 inches × 1 inch—1, contains 1 fat exchange
Corn muffin, 2 inch dia.—1, contains 1 fat exchange
Crackers, round butter type—5, contains 1 fat exchange
Muffin, plain small—1, contains 1 fat exchange
Potatoes, french fried, 2 inches to 3$\frac{1}{2}$ inches—8, contains 1 fat exchange
Potato or corn chips—15, contains 2 fat exchanges
Pancake, 5 inches × $\frac{1}{2}$ inches—1, contains 1 fat exchange
Waffle, 5 inches × $\frac{1}{2}$ inches—1, contains 1 fat exchange

Meat exchanges
1 exchange lean meat × 7 g protein, 3 g fat, and 55 cal (1 oz serving)

Beef: Baby beef, chipped beef, chuck, flank steak, tenderloin, plate ribs, skirt steak, round (top and bottom), all cuts rump, spare ribs, and tripe
Lamb: Leg, rib, sirloin, loin (roast and chops), shank, and shoulder
Pork: Leg (whole rump, center shank), ham, smoked (center slices)
Veal: Leg, loin, rib, shank, shoulder, cutlets
Poultry: Meat, without skin, of chicken, turkey, Cornish hen, guinea hen, pheasant
Fish: Any fresh or frozen, clams, oysters, scallops, shrimp
Canned salmon, tuna, mackerel, crab, and lobster—$\frac{1}{4}$ cup
Drained sardines—3
Cheese containing less than 5% butterfat—1 oz

Table continued on following page

TABLE 5–9. Diabetic Diet Exchange Lists *Continued*

Cottage cheese, dry and 2% butterfat—$\frac{1}{4}$ cup
Dried beans and peas—$\frac{1}{2}$ cup; contains 1 bread exchange
1 exchange medium-fat meat = 7 g protein, 5 g fat, and 75 cal, and $\frac{1}{2}$ extra fat exchange (1 oz serving)
Beef: Ground (15% fat), corned beef (canned), rib eye, and round (ground commercial)
Pork: Loin (all cuts tenderloin), should arm, shoulder blade, boston butt, canadian bacon, and boiled ham
Liver, heart, kidney and sweetbreads (high cholesterol)
Cheese: Mozzarella, ricotta, farmer's, neufchatel
Creamed cottage cheese—$\frac{1}{4}$ cup
Parmesan cheese—3 T
Egg—1 (high cholesterol)
Peanut butter—2 T, contains 2 extra fat exchanges
1 exchange high-fat meat = 7 g protein, 8 g fat, and 100 cal and 1 extra fat exchange (1 oz serving)
Beef: Brisket, corned beef brisket, ground beef (more than 20% fat), hamburger (commercial), chuck (ground commercial), rib roasts, and club and rib steaks
Lamb: Breast
Pork: Spare ribs, loin (back ribs), pork (ground), country-style ham, deviled ham
Veal: Breast
Poultry: Capon, duck (domestic), and goose
Cheese: Cheddar
Cold cuts, $4\frac{1}{2}$ inches $\times \frac{1}{8}$—1 slice
Frankfurter—1 small
Fat exchanges
1 exchange = 5 g fat and 45 cal
Polyunsaturated fats
Margarine, soft, tub, or stick—1 tsp
Avocado, 4-inch diameter—$\frac{1}{8}$
Corn, cottonseed, safflower, soy, sunflower oil—1 tsp
Olive oil—1 tsp
Peanut oil—1 tsp
Olives—5 small
Almonds—10 whole
Pecans—2 large whole
Spanish peanuts—20 whole
Virginia peanuts—10 whole
Walnuts—6 small
Other nuts—6 small
Saturated fats
Margarine, regular stick—1 tsp
Butter—1 tsp
Bacon fat—1 tsp
Bacon, crisp—1 strip
Light cream—2 T
Sour cream—2 T
Heavy cream—1 T
Cream cheese—1 T
French dressing—1 T
Italian dressing—1 T
Lard—1 tsp
Mayonnaise—1 tsp
Salad dressing, mayonnaise type—2 tsp
Salt pork—$\frac{3}{4}$-inch cube
Principles of diabetic diet
1. Diet set by physician's order.
2. Diet based on patient's age, weight, type of diabetes, and type of hypoglycemic agent used.
3. Carbohydrates should provide 50%–60% of total calories
   a. Emphasize complex CHO
   b. Restrict simple CHO
4. Protein should provide 30%–38% of calories, use sources low in fat and cholesterol, increase polyunsaturated fats.
5. Include at least minimum servings of four basic food groups.
6. Increase fiber by using high-fiber foods or highly refined carbohydrates low in fiber.
7. Calculate grams of each nutrient, then convert to exchanges.

CHO, carbohydrate.

TABLE 5–10. Low Protein Diet

Grams of protein per exchange
   Milk— 8 g
   Vegetable—2 g
   Bread—2 g
   Meat—7 g
40-gram protein diet
   Lacks calcium, iron, riboflavin, and niacin. Omit peas, lima beans, and dried legumes.
   Sample pattern for 40-gram protein diet

BREAKFAST	LUNCH	DINNER
Fruit	Cheese, 1 oz	Meat, 2 oz
Cereal	Vegetable	Potato, butter
Bread, 1 slice	Bread, 1 slice	Salad, dressing
Butter	Salad, dressing	Bread, 1 slice
Milk, 1 cup	Butter	Butter
Beverage	Fruit	Vegetable
Sugar	Beverage	Fruit
	Sugar	Beverage
		Sugar

100-gram protein diet
   Nutritionally adequate diet. Still based on food exchanges. Sugar, fats, and fruits may be used as desired. Increase fluid intake as protein intake increases.

blood urea nitrogen (BUN) and serum ammonia levels as low as possible
3. 40 g protein usually lowest level; may range from 40 to 90 g
4. Limited amounts of protein of highest biologic value used
   a. protein containing essential amino acids
   b. high biologic proteins include foods such as eggs, milk, yogurt, meat, fish, poultry, tuna
   c. include breads, cereal, fruits, and vegetables

BIBLIOGRAPHY

Dudek, S.G. (1987). *Nutrition handbook for nursing practice.* Philadelphia: J.B. Lippincott Co.

Green, M.I., et al. (1987). *Nutrition in contemporary nursing practice.* New York: John Wiley & Sons.

Krause, M.V., and Mahan, L.K. (1984). *Food, nutrition, and diet therapy,* 7th ed. Philadelphia: W.B. Saunders Co.

Lewis, C.M. (1986). *Nutrition and nutritional therapy in nursing.* Norwalk, CT: Appleton & Lange.

Pipes, P.L. (1989). *Nutrition in infancy and childhood,* 4th ed. St. Louis: C.V. Mosby Co.

Poleman, C.R., and Capra, C.L. (1984). *Nutrition essentials and diet therapy,* 5th ed. Philadelphia: W.B. Saunders Co.

Robinson, C., and Lawler, M. (1986). *Normal and therapeutic nutrition.* New York: Macmillan.

Whitney, E.N., and Cataldo, C.B. (1983). *Understanding normal and clinical nutrition.* St. Paul: West Publishing Co.

Williams, S.R. (1988). *Basic nutrition and diet therapy,* 8th ed. St. Louis: C.V. Mosby Co.

Questions

1. The basis for a therapeutic diet is:

   ① Cultural preferences
   ② A well-balanced diet
   ③ Previous dietary habits
   ④ Financial income

2. A full liquid diet is one that contains:

   ① Clear liquids at body temperature
   ② Any liquid at body temperature
   ③ Only liquids that have residue
   ④ Only liquids that have no residue

3. To increase protein, and not fat to the diet one could add:

   ① Bread
   ② Egg
   ③ Nonfat milk
   ④ Vegetables

4. To best method of increasing dietary iron content is:

   ① Pork, apples, Karo, corn
   ② Liver, raisins, molasses, soy beans
   ③ Chicken, cranberry juice, honey, tomatoes
   ④ Fish, oranges, brown sugar, red beets

5. The minimum fat diet is often used for:

   ① Colitis
   ② Kidney stones
   ③ Gallbladder and cardiac conditions
   ④ Gout

6. Which of the following foods would be limited on a low cholesterol diet?

   ① Skim milk
   ② Eggs
   ③ Oranges
   ④ Peas

7. A low cholesterol diet includes foods that are primarily low in:

   ① Animal proteins and carbohydrates
   ② Sodium
   ③ Saturated fats
   ④ Plant sources

8. The prescribed diet for a patient with kidney disease would limit:

   ① Glucose
   ② Vitamins
   ③ Fats
   ④ Proteins

9. Patients with severe burns or chronic debilitating disease need an increase in:

   ① Protein
   ② Cellulose
   ③ Fat
   ④ Fried food

10. Cow's milk can be supplemented to be equivalent to human milk except in:

    ① Sugar content
    ② Vitamin level
    ③ Water amounts
    ④ Natural immunity

11. Low purine diets are indicated for:

    ① Atonic constipation
    ② Peptic ulcer
    ③ Celiac
    ④ Gout

12. Obesity is defined as the following percent above the ideal weight:

    ① 5%
    ② 10%
    ③ 20%
    ④ 25%

13. Which of the following foods should be excluded from a low-residue diet?

    ① Cooked vegetables
    ② Whole grain products
    ③ Broiled foods
    ④ White rice

14. Fats used in a diabetic diet should be mainly:

    ① Polyunsaturated
    ② Monounsaturated
    ③ Saturated
    ④ Hydrogenated

15. An example of complex carbohydrates is:

    ① A monosaccharide
    ② Flour
    ③ Corn syrup
    ④ A disaccharide

16. Bacon is included in the exchange group of:

① Bread
② Milk
③ Fat
④ Meat

17. When a diabetic patient dislikes a carbohydrate food served, the nurse should:

① Call the doctor
② Tell the patient to eat it anyway
③ Give the patient an orange to eat
④ Substitute another equal carbohydrate

18. Nutritional anemia may develop if the pre-school child's or infant's diet consists chiefly of:

① Milk
② Vegetables
③ Meat
④ Fruit

19. Vitamins are defined as:

① Inorganic compounds supplied in large amounts to serve as catalysts
② Elements that prohibit bacterial production
③ Organic substances needed in small amounts for growth and maintenance of life
④ Enzymes that prohibit the acid-base balance

20. If fats were completely excluded from the diet, the result would be a deficiency in:

① Vitamins A, D, E, and K
② All the vitamins
③ All the water soluble vitamins
④ Vitamins A and D

21. A deficiency of vitamin K results in:

① Poor bone formation
② Extreme irritability of the nerves
③ Muscle spasms
④ Delay in the clotting of blood

22. Night blindness may occur as a result of a deficiency of vitamin:

① C
② D
③ E
④ A

23. Whole grain cereals are considered nutritional breakfast food because they:

① Contain large quantities of protein
② Supply great amounts of glucose
③ Contain vitamin B complex
④ Are easily digested

24. When the strength of the walls of the capillaries is reduced, resulting in small hemorrhages, as is the case in bleeding gums, the diet contains too little:

① Vitamin E
② Vitamin A
③ Vitamin C
④ Vitamin B_6

25. The highest quantity of vitamin C is found in:

① Potatoes
② Cereals
③ Citrus fruits
④ Milk

26. Fish liver oils are an important source of:

① Riboflavin
② Vitamin D
③ Vitamin C
④ Thiamine

27. Scurvy is a deficiency disease resulting from an extreme lack of:

① Phosphorus
② Vitamin D
③ Vitamin C
④ Calcium

28. Hypervitaminosis is caused by the vitamins:

① A, D, E, and K
② A and D
③ B complex
④ C and D

29. The most unstable of all vitamins is:

① A
② C
③ Thiamine
④ Riboflavin

30. The following oil is not to be used in food preparation:

① Mineral
② Safflower
③ Sunflower
④ Soybean

31. Vitamin K production may be interfered with by:

① Diuretics
② Vitamin C
③ AquaMephyton
④ Salicylates

32. Vitamin B$_{12}$ is found in:

① Meat
② Breads
③ Fruits
④ Sugars

33. Daily selection of foods as recommended in the basic four food groups will:

① Make it easier to plan a reducing diet
② Always prevent malnutrition
③ Inform people about the basis of good nutrition
④ Help plan diets that satisfy minimum nutritional needs of most people

34. The basic four food groups consists of:

① Milk, lean meats; citrus fruit; green and yellow vegetables; and whole grain bread
② Milk and cheese; meat, poultry, fish and beans; vegetables and fruit; bread and cereal
③ Meat; milk; cereal; salads and fruit
④ Dairy; fish, chicken, beef; green and yellow vegetables; cereal

35. The reason why a food is placed in a particular group is:

① They are grouped according to the primary nutrients contributed to a diet
② To make it easier to plan a therapeutic diet
③ To keep foods that come from the same organic or inorganic source together
④ That it organizes the calculation of caloric values

36. Nutrients are substances needed by the body for maintaining life and growth. Essential nutrient groups include:

① Meats; breads and cereals; milk; citrus fruits
② Fats; carbohydrates; meats; calcium; sodium and water
③ Proteins; minerals; starches; vitamins; fats
④ Proteins; fats; carbohydrates; vitamins; minerals; water

37. The kilocalorie refers to a unit of measurement indicating the amount of fuel value provided for the body in a given quantity of food. Which nutrients can be converted into kilocalories?

① Fats, starches and vitamins
② Sugars and starches and minerals
③ Proteins, carbohydrates and fats
④ Vitamin and mineral supplements, fats and starches

Answers & Rationales

Guide to item identification (see pp. 3–5 for further details about each category)

I, II, III, or IV for the phase of the nursing process
1, 2, 3, or 4 for the category of client needs
A, B, C, D, E, F, or G for the category of human functioning
Specific content category by name; ie, cholecystectomy

1. ② Adaptation of a well-balanced diet provides the nutritional needs for a client.
III, 3, F. Nutrition.

2. ② A full liquid diet includes a clear liquid diet and all liquids with residue at body temperature.
I, 2, F. Nutrition.

3. ③ Nonfat milk increases protein without increasing other significant nutrients.
III, 2, F. Nutrition.

4. ② These foods have more iron content than the other choices.
III, 2, F. Nutrition.

5. ③ The gallbladder would need to produce additional bile to emulsify the fat. Fat increases the cholesterol level of the blood, which may cause atherosclerosis of the coronary vessels.
II & III, 2, F. Nutrition.

6. ② Egg yolks contain a high percentage of cholesterol.
III, 2, F. Nutrition.

7. ③ Foods low in saturated fats may contain polyunsaturated fats, which will reduce the level of saturated fats. These indirectly reduce the cholesterol level.
III, 2, F. Nutrition.

8. ④ Kidney dysfunctions retain the toxic byproducts of protein metabolism. A limited daily amount of protein, 40 g (normal, 70 g), is recommended.
II & III, 2, F. Nutrition.

9. ① Patients with severe burns and debilitating diseases metabolize protein at an increased rate, and daily amounts of protein exceeding the 70 g normal level are recommended.
II & III, 2, F. Nutrition.

10. ④ Natural immunity is transferred through the colostrum of breast milk.
IV, 2, F. Nutrition.

11. ④ Pyruvic acids are absorbed in the joints, especially the big toe. Diets low in purine (pyruvic acid) may diminish the symptoms of gout.
I, 2, F. Nutrition.

12. ③ Ten percent is considered overweight. Twenty percent is termed obesity.
I, 2, F. Nutrition.

13. ② Whole grain products contain more fiber than other foods.
III, 2, F. Nutrition.

14. ① Polyunsaturated fats reduce the level of saturated, monounsaturated fats and cholesterol, which may reduce weight and increase the efficiency of insulin.
III, 2, F. Nutrition.

15. ② Flour is a complex carbohydrate made from combined grains.
III, 2, F. Nutrition.

16. ③ Bacon is predominantely fat with a small amount of protein.
III, 2, F. Nutrition.

17. ④ Carbohydrate foods are interchangeable within the amount of grams, as long as the food is not out of limits for protein and fats.
III, 2, F. Nutrition.

18. ① Milk contains only a slight amount of iron. More than the normal volume of milk would have to be consumed to obtain the necessary amounts of iron.
I & IV, 2 & 4, F. Nutrition.

19. ③ Minerals are inorganic compounds, and vitamins are organic compounds needed in small amounts for growth and maintenance of life. Both are catalysts.
I & IV, 2 & 4, F. Nutrition.

20. ① A, D, E, and K are fat soluble vitamins, and small amounts of fats are necessary for their absorption and metabolism.
I & IV, 2 & 4, F. Nutrition.

21. Vitamin K is a necessary component of the clotting factor.
④ I & IV, 2 & 4, F. Nutrition.

22. Vitamin A is a component of rhodopsin (visual purple) affecting the rods and cones of the retina, permitting sight at night.
④ I & IV, 2 & 4, F. Nutrition.

23. Vitamin B complex is necessary for a sound nervous system and carbohydrate metabolism.
③ I & IV, 2 & 4, F. Nutrition.

24. Ascorbic acid (vitamin C) strengthens the mucous membranes.
③ I & II, 4, F. Nutrition.

25. Citrus fruits contain more ascorbic acid (vitamin C) than the other foods.
③ I, 4, F. Nutrition.

26. Vitamin D is a fat soluble vitamin found in fish liver. Other vitamins are water soluble.
② I & II, 4, F. Nutrition.

27. Vitamin C (ascorbic acid) promotes mucous membrane and tissue development.
③ I, 4, F. Nutrition.

28. A and D are fat soluble vitamins that are retained by the body, especially in the liver and skin.
② I, 4, F. Nutrition.

29. Vitamin C is the most unstable of all vitamins. This is one of the reasons for covering citrus juices after opening, when refrigerating.
② I, 4, F. Nutrition.

30. Mineral oil blocks the absorption of the fat soluble vitamins.
① I, 4, D. Nutrition.

31. Salicylates interfere with vitamin K production, which is a component of the clotting factor.
④ I & III, 4, F. Nutrition.

32. Meat contains vitamin B₁₂; the other foods contain glucose.
① I, 4, F. Nutrition.

33. The four food groups show how minimum daily requirements can be met.
④ II, 1, F. Nutrition.

34. The basic four food groups consist of: I. Milk and cheese; II. Meat, poultry, fish, legumes; III. Vegetables, fruit; IV. Bread and cereal.
② IV, 1, F. Nutrition.

35. Foods are grouped because they contain similar nutrients or according to their main contributions to the diet.
① I, 1, F. Nutrition.

36. Essential nutrients are divided into six categories. They are proteins, fats, carbohydrates, vitamins, minerals and water.
④ I, 1, F. Nutrition.

37. The body can use three nutrients for fuel: carbohydrates, fats, and proteins. Minerals and vitamins assist in regulatory functions.
③ I, 1, F. Nutrition.

Special Needs of Older Adults

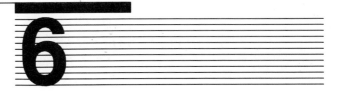

I. PHYSIOLOGIC ALTERATIONS RELATED TO AGING

A. Generalized Physiologic Changes

1. Decreased physical reserve
   a. diminishes recuperative powers
   b. homeostatic changes occur much more slowly
   c. cells and tissues less able to repair themselves, especially neurons, muscle, and kidney cells
   d. stress poses special problems with diminished reserves
2. Body systems begin to function less efficiently
   a. cardiovascular system
   b. nervous system
   c. endocrine system

B. Sensory System in General

1. Decreased efficiency
2. General decline of awareness of environmental stimuli
3. After age 75 years, three of five elderly have some sensory deficits

C. Nervous System Changes in General

1. Nervous transmission slows
2. Recent memory loss
3. Slower reaction time
4. Fine motor movement affected
5. Less able to react to painful stimuli
6. Impaired temperature regulation, more prone to hypo- and hyperthermia

D. Proprioception— Position Sense

1. Impaired
2. Balance and coordination affected, decreased
3. Increased risk of injury

E. Visual Changes

1. Loss of visual acuity, presbyopia
   a. decreases progressively greater in women than men
   b. leads to problems with close work
2. Arcus senilis, rings around corneal periphery, not pathologic
3. Cataracts
4. Altered color vision
   a. color transmission from green to violet decreases
   b. sensitivity to blue and possibly red decreases
5. Loss of accommodation
   a. rate diminishes
   b. after age 60 years, no further loss
   c. decreased adaptation to dark occurs
   d. vision strongly affected by glare
6. Reduced pupil size and reactivity
7. Depth perception less accurate
8. Glaucoma more common

F. Hearing Changes

1. Auditory threshold decreases
2. Unilateral or bilateral loss common over age 65 years
3. Greater loss of high frequency sounds
4. Lack of ability to discriminate volume or pitch; hard to understand speech
5. Long exposure to noise pollution of modern world increases hearing loss
6. Can lead to psychologic difficulties
7. May be mistaken for confusion or other mental status changes

G. Changes in Taste, Smell, Touch

1. Taste appears to change with aging
   a. often "picky" about foods
   b. increased preference for tart tastes
2. Smell seems to decrease with aging
3. Sense of touch decreased, affecting adaptation to environment

H. Metabolic Changes

1. Decreased enzyme secretion
2. Decreased nutrient and drug absorption
3. Decreased peristalsis
4. Often poor nutritional status
5. Changes in dentition
6. Decreased metabolic rate
7. Less ability to withstand stress, to maintain homeostasis
   a. Constipation common
8. Endocrine changes
   a. decrease response to stress
   b. most hormones normally decrease with aging

I. Cardiovascular Changes

1. Arteriosclerosis
2. Arterial blood pressure: rate of systolic increase greater than rate of diastolic increase
3. Baroreceptor sensitivity decreases
4. Circulation time increases
5. Decreased thirst mechanism may lead to dehydration, hemoconcentration, and decreased volume
6. Heart
   a. without disease, its pump function is relatively normal
   b. loses physiologic reserve
   c. decreased coronary artery blood flow
   d. difficulty maintaining homeostasis when stressed
   e. contractility
      (1) decreases
      (2) time prolonged, leading to increasing O_2 requirement
   f. stroke volume decreases
   g. cardiac output decreases
   h. electrocardiogram (ECG): usually shows no sign of change from aging alone
   i. atrial gallop common, even in absence of disease
7. Organ perfusion decreases
8. Peripheral vascular resistance increases
9. Postural hypotension
   a. happens fairly frequently
   b. increase with febrile diseases
   c. a side effect of many medications
10. Pulse pressure generally widens with age
11. Few changes in hemopoietic system
    a. anemia often associated with poor nutrition, not simply aging
    b. with decreased immunity white blood cells (WBCs) may decrease

J. Respiratory Changes

1. Decreased ventilatory volumes
2. Decreased capacity for gas exchange
3. Increased risk of disease
4. Decreased cough effectiveness

K. Genitourinary Function Changes

1. Benign prostatic hypertrophy with resultant urinary changes
2. Decreased blood flow to kidneys
3. Decreased control of urinary sphincter, incontinence may occur

L. Musculoskeletal Changes

1. Osteoporosis
2. Increase in fibrous connective tissue with stiffening
3. Arthritic changes
4. Muscle atrophy

M. Skin Changes

1. Decreased activity of oil and sweat glands
   a. increase in dry skin and itching
   b. decrease in perspiration leading to decrease in cooling effect
2. Increased skin fragility and susceptibility to trauma
3. Delayed wound healing
4. Decreased tone and elasticity causing wrinkles
5. Decreased hair and nail growth
6. Hair thinning and loss of color

II. PSYCHOLOGIC ALTERATIONS RELATED TO AGING

A. Retirement

1. May be difficult to live on fixed income
2. May alter self concept, if no longer breadwinner in family
3. New concerns about leisure time and what to do
4. Physical limitations may prevent enjoyment of these years
5. May be welcomed as new experience with growth potentials, especially if prepared for retirement in earlier years

B. Role Changes

1. May vary from independent one to dependent one
2. May be difficult to do without role of worker
3. May be that of widow or widower

C. Erikson's Stage of Ego Integrity vs. Despair

1. Successful adaptation shown through satisfaction with life and acceptance of eventual death
2. Unsuccessful adaptation shown by sense of failure and futility, desire to redo life, sense of worthlessness

D. Body Image Changes May Lead to Depression

1. Diminished strength
2. Actual physical changes of aging may alter appearance
3. May not see themselves as "old," but others identify them that way

E. Confidence in Cognitive Function Decreases

1. Slower response time
2. Slowed nerve impulse transmission
3. General intelligence not affected
4. Capacity to learn intact but learning may take longer and may require more repetition

F. Environment

1. Often lack control over changes in living arrangements
2. Limitations imposed by others increase
3. Likelihood that residence will change increases
4. Need for assistance with transportation increases

G. Financial Changes

1. Income usually decreases, often drastically
2. Usually on fixed income
3. Inflation adjustments restricted

H. Expectations for the Future

1. Less desire for new experiences
2. Planning impaired by decreased energy levels
3. Difficulty sustaining anticipation
4. Sense of decreased worth to others

I. Sexuality

1. Sexual function still present
2. Slowed or decreased capacity for orgasm
3. Slower to achieve erection, and decreased pressure of ejaculation
4. Vaginal dryness may require use of water-soluble lubricant or hormone therapy
5. Often decreased opportunities for intimacy
6. More women than men
7. Society seems to have negative feelings about sexual expression in elderly

III. LEGAL CONCERNS OF OLDER ADULTS

A. Legal Rights

1. Unchanged unless shown in courts to be incompetent
2. Right to refuse medical treatments
3. Entrance into nursing home does not mean automatic loss of rights
4. Encourage patient to obtain legal help as needed for financial matters, wills, and generalized legal counseling about his or her rights
5. Encourage patient to consider appropriate person to grant power of attorney, either limited or extended
6. Guardianship may be necessary to protect the older adult

B. Elder Abuse

1. Occurs much more frequently than previously imagined
2. May occur when living with children or in nursing home
3. Assess injuries in older adults for signs of abuse
4. Abuse can be physical or verbal
5. If abuse is suspected, it must be reported to proper authorities

IV. COMMON HEALTH PROBLEMS OF OLDER ADULTS

(See appropriate sections in chapter 7, *THE ADULT PATIENT*)

A. Cataracts

B. Glaucoma

C. Herpes Zoster

D. Parkinson's Disease

E. Alzheimer's Disease

F. Congestive Heart Failure

G. Peripheral Vascular Disease (PVD)

1. Stasis ulcers
2. Arterial occlusions

H. Chronic Obstructive Pulmonary Disease (COPD)

I. Anemia

J. Chronic Lymphocytic Leukemia (CLL)

K. Malignant Lymphomas

L. Benign Prostatic Hypertrophy (BPH)

M. Osteoarthritis

V. MEDICATIONS AND OLDER ADULTS

A. General Principles of Drug Therapy for Older Adults

1. Alterations in pharmacokinetics
   a. absorption often slower
      (1) decreased intestinal blood flow
      (2) delayed gastric emptying
      (3) increased gastric pH
      (4) multiple drugs ingested simultaneously may alter absorption of all or interact unfavorably
   b. distribution may be altered
      (1) lower fluid intake leads to increased plasma concentration of drugs
      (2) lean muscle mass decreased with increased body fat
      (3) fat-soluble drugs more dangerous because more accumulation in body fat
      (4) decreased serum proteins leads to problems with protein-bound drugs
   c. altered metabolism of drugs
      (1) liver function vital and decreased with age
      (2) blood flow to liver decreased
      (3) liver microsomal action decreased
   d. changes in elimination
      (1) renal function vital to drug elimination
      (2) approximately 50% loss of nephrons
      (3) decreased glomerular and tubular filtration
      (4) low fluid intake also decreased output
      (5) renal blood flow decreased
      (6) constipation may affect drugs eliminated through feces
   e. drug sensitivity
      (1) may suddenly develop new allergies
      (2) decreased T cells
      (3) increased permeability of blood–brain barrier
      (4) drug dosages often must be lowered to prevent problems
2. Drug interactions
   a. older adults, often with multiple chronic problems and multiple prescription and nonprescription drugs
   b. alcohol interacts with many medications, causing excessive effects, such as alcohol and sedatives
   c. drugs may interact with food
      (1) drugs may cause nutrients to be poorly absorbed
      (2) nutrients may interfere with drug actions

B. Other Problems

1. Older adults with limited resources may have problems affording drugs
2. Self-medication practices may be dangerous
   a. overuse of over-the-counter drugs
   b. may have difficulties remembering to take drugs
   c. often have multiple physicians and multiple medications
   d. may not understand dangers of increasing or decreasing dosages
   e. may not understand dangers of taking drugs ordered for their friends with similar problems

VI. NURSING PROCESS APPLIED TO THE SPECIAL NEEDS OF OLDER ADULTS

A. Assessment

1. Assess older adults level of development
2. Identify physiologic changes that have occurred and their effect on the patient
3. Identify psychologic changes that have occurred and their effect on the patient
4. Be aware of impaired communication potential, such as patient being hard of hearing, forgetful
5. Assess patient's level of functioning and independence
6. Find out what the patient's expectations are for this hospitalization
7. Take detailed medication and nutritional history

B. Planning

1. Identify reasonable goals with patient
2. Discuss possible outcomes with patient
3. Establish priorities

C. Implementation

1. Care related to general physiological changes
   a. decrease stress as much as possible
   b. monitor for changes in health status
   c. prevent injury through good safety precautions, because recuperative powers are less
      (1) provide adequate lighting
      (2) avoid hazards such as throw rugs and objects on floor
      (3) teach patient to rise from sitting or lying slowly
      (4) use of side rails and safety bars
2. Care related to sensory/perceptual changes
   a. allow longer for responses, because reaction time slower
   b. maintain body temperature; avoid extremes of heat or cold
   c. provide adequate pain medication
   d. monitor for development of cataracts or glaucoma; refer to physician if either develops
   e. monitor for hearing loss; refer to physician if this develops
   f. assess signs of confusion carefully; may be related to external causes
   g. orient to changes in environment
   h. monitor food intake
      (1) provide high-nutrition, appealing foods
      (2) find out patient likes and dislikes
      (3) provide socialization at mealtimes
      (4) frequent small feedings may be better tolerated
3. Care related to metabolic changes
   a. provide increased fluid and fiber to decrease constipation
   b. stool softeners may be necessary if stools are hard
   c. encourage activity and exercise
   d. provide consistent toileting
   e. monitor serum proteins for signs of malnutrition
   f. check for presence and condition of teeth
   g. assess ability to swallow
   h. monitor for hormonal deficiencies
      (1) increased antidiuretic hormone, observe for diluted urine and increased urine
      (2) decreased glucose tolerance, observe for frequent and excessive urination, excessive thirst, excessive eating, fatigue, visual blurring
      (3) hypothyroidism, observe for constipation, lethargy, dry skin, mental deterioration
4. Care related to cardiovascular changes
   a. remember increased systolic blood pressure is normal in aging adult
   b. monitor fluid intake carefully
   c. offer liquids frequently; make sure liquids are within reach; encourage intake
   d. monitor for signs of decreased organ perfusion, such as decreased urine output
   f. monitor for presence of anemia
   g. avoid abrupt position changes
   h. have patient avoid people with infections
5. Care related to respiratory changes
   a. turn, cough, and deep breathe if on bed rest and following surgery
   b. provide rest periods during exercise or increased activity
   c. assess for abnormal breathing patterns
   d. limit contact with people with respiratory infections
6. Care related to genitourinary (GU) changes
   a. monitor male patients for signs of benign prostatic hypertrophy (BPH)
   b. treat incontinence, if possible
      (1) encourage use of bedpan, urinal, etc., every 2 hours
      (2) respond to client's need to void promptly
   c. monitor output; urine often much more diluted
   d. observe for signs of urinary tract infection (UTI), such as confusion and urinary frequency
7. Care related to musculoskeletal changes
   a. prevent falls and monitor for fractures

b. encourage joint-sparing movements
c. treat arthritic changes as ordered
d. prevent pressure on bony prominences
e. encourage exercise, as tolerated
f. do not rush the patient
g. moist heat provides comfort; eg, showers
h. teach proper body mechanics

8. Care related to skin changes
   a. daily baths not necessary
   b. temperature of bath water no more than 105° F
   c. use superfatted soap or bath oil; avoid using soap, unless necessary
   d. apply emollient lotions to skin; avoid using alcohol or dusting powders
   e. discourage scratching, keep nails short
   f. turn patient on bed rest every 2 hours, using proper technique; establish turning schedule
   g. use pillows for proper positioning
   h. avoid friction when positioning patient
   i. provide for patient's safety to prevent skin trauma

9. Care related to psychosocial alterations
   a. assess developmental status and intervene if inappropriate
   b. watch for development of depression
   c. allow more time for learning activities
   d. encourage patient to remain as independent as possible
   e. be aware of financial difficulties and recommend social service involvement
   f. allow for appropriate sexual expression
      (1) provide privacy
      (2) allow couples to room together in extended care facilities, if possible
      (3) provide sexual counseling as needed
      (4) teach patients about expected changes in sexual functioning

10. Care related to legal concerns
    a. allow competent adults rights of decision making
    b. monitor for signs of elder abuse

11. Care related to common health problems (see appropriate sections in Chapter 7, *The Adult Patient*)

12. Care related to medications
    a. read precautions of all drugs before administering.

b. use drugs with care in patients with impaired liver function
c. monitor serum protein levels and administer drugs appropriately
d. monitor renal function and report changes to physician
e. encourage adequate intake to ensure drug excretion
f. monitor closely for idiosyncratic reactions to drugs
g. check for potential interactions between drugs when the patient is on multiple medications
h. check for possible food–drug interactions
i. teach patient principles of self-medication
   (1) provide patient with written reminders of teaching
   (2) teach patient importance of following medication prescription orders exactly
   (3) assess patient's ability to be dependable in self-medication

D. Evaluation

1. Decide if identified goals are met based on criteria
2. Identify changes required to meet unmet goals
3. Modify nursing care as necessary to meet established goals

BIBLIOGRAPHY

Brunner, L.S., and Suddarth, D.S. (1988). *Textbook of medical-surgical nursing, 2nd ed.* Philadelphia: J.B. Lippincott Co.

Ebersole, P., and Hess, P. (1990). *Toward healthy aging, 3rd ed.* St. Louis: C.V. Mosby Co.

Eliopoulos, C. (1987). *Gerontological nursing.* Philadelphia: J.B. Lippincott Co.

Hood, G., and Dincher, J.R., (1988). *Total patient care: Foundations and practices.* St. Louis: C.V. Mosby Co.

Kaluger, G., and Kaluger, M.F. (1988). *Human development: The span of life, 4th ed.* St. Louis: C.V. Mosby Co.

Lewis, C.B. (1985). *Aging: The health care challenge.* Philadelphia: F.A. Davis Co.

Long, B., and Phipps, W. (1988). *Essentials of medical-surgical nursing, 2nd ed.* St. Louis: C. V. Mosby Co.

Potter, P. A, and Perry, A. G. (1989). *Fundamentals of nursing: Concepts, process, and practice, 2nd ed.* St. Louis: C.V. Mosby Co.

Sorensen, K., and Luckmann, J. (1986). *Basic nursing: A psychophysiologic approach, 2nd ed.* Philadelphia: W.B. Saunders Co.

Questions

Mary Nelson, age 80 years, is admitted after falling at home and fracturing her femur. At the time of admission, she is very confused and disoriented.

1. On the basis of your knowledge of aging and her history, you may conclude that Mrs. Nelson is:

   ① Probably suffering from the trauma of the fall and will need time to adjust to the situation
   ② Behaving normally for her age and cannot be expected to show any improvement
   ③ In need of special attention and a lot of "babying" during her stay
   ④ Unable to control herself and will be totally dependent on the staff during her stay

2. Mrs. Nelson seems to confuse you with her daughter Anne during the first postoperative day and frequently calls you by her name. Your best response would be:

   ① Reassure her by telling her that Anne will visit soon even if you are not sure that she is coming in today.
   ② Tell her that Anne went home for a rest and will return and that in the meantime you will take good care of her.
   ③ Pretend that you are Anne and answer her questions so she will not be frightened
   ④ Tell her your name and explain that you are her nurse and will do anything you can to help her

3. Two days later Mrs. Nelson apologizes for being so much trouble for the nurses and says, "I don't know what is wrong; I always take care of myself. If I just hadn't broken my hip, I could take care of myself." The LPN realizes that she is probably:

   ① Expressing a desire to become more dependent
   ② Regressing into senility and childishness
   ③ Anxious that she is losing self-control and independence
   ④ Expressing guilt about her carelessness

4. It is important that Mrs. Nelson receive skin care daily but a daily bath is unnecessary for older adults because their:

   ① Activity level is decreased
   ② Sweat and oil glands are less active
   ③ Interest in hygiene is decreased
   ④ Body odor is diminished

5. Mrs. Nelson's diet in the hospital must include:

   ① Fewer calories, because she is less active
   ② More protein for adequate healing
   ③ More calories, because she is less active
   ④ Higher fat and carbohydrates for energy

6. You suggest to Mrs. Nelson that she wear a nice robe and apply some make-up before going to physical therapy. Your intervention is:

   ① Appropriate because she needs to clean herself up
   ② Inappropriate because she is unaware of her surroundings
   ③ Appropriate because it will increase her self-esteem
   ④ Inappropriate because make-up can be harmful to her skin

7. Because of decreased muscle tone in the digestive tract of elderly individuals, their diet should emphasize sufficient intake of:

   ① Cellulose and calcium
   ② Whole grain cereals, fresh fruits, vegetables and plenty of fluids
   ③ Increased amounts of meat and cheese
   ④ A bulk laxative daily with plenty of fluids

8. The term that applies to research and study of the aging process is:

   ① Gerontology
   ② Senility
   ③ Geriatrics
   ④ Bariatrics

9. Which of the following statements regarding aging is correct?

   ① Old age begins at 65 years
   ② People age in different ways and at different rates
   ③ The majority of old people live in retirement homes or in convalescent facilities
   ④ Elderly people generally lack the financial resources necessary for independent living

10. Characteristics that best describe the process of aging include:

① Increased flexibility in most situations and loss of rigidity of body parts
② Mental and physical deterioration
③ Inability to cope with the stress of everyday living
④ Decreased flexibility in some situations and increased rigidity of certain body parts

11. According to Erickson's stages of development, healthy aging would be characterized by:

① An acceptance of eventual death
② Reliving of past events
③ Refusal to retire well beyond normal retirement age
④ Reassessment of relationship with surviving spouse

12. Constipation is a common health problem in the elderly usually caused by:

① Decreased activity and poor eating habits
② Failure to use bulk laxatives daily
③ Too much residue in their diet
④ Decreased appetite

Celia Hill, age 68 years, has been admitted for evaluation of possible organic mental disorder. She is widowed and lives alone. Recently her family has become concerned by her neglect of personal hygiene, suspiciousness, and memory loss.

13. What kind of personality change is common in organic mental disorders?

① Docile, compliant personality
② Exaggeration of basic personality
③ Aggressive, uncooperative personality
④ Opposite of usual personality

14. What kind of group work can the practical nurse initiate for patients with organic mental disorders?

① Groups that focus on "here and now" issues
② Groups that focus on reasons for feelings
③ Groups that focus on reasons for behavior
④ Groups that focus on personality issues

15. Which is an example of using reminiscing to help bring Mrs. Hill to the present?

① "It sounds like you are lonely since your husband died 5 years ago. Tell me about him."

② "Your husband has been dead for 5 years. You're at The Happy Trails Mental Health Center now."
③ "Don't you remember? I told you yesterday that you were widowed 5 years ago."
④ "You need to accept that your husband is dead. He died of a heart attack 5 years ago."

16. Which of the following is appropriate recreational therapy for the patient?

① Individual physically active games
② Mind-stimulating games
③ Concrete, repetitious crafts
④ Noncompetitive team sports

17. Which of the following would be a physical change associated with the older adult between ages 75 and 80 years?

① Decreased response to physical stress
② Inability to carry out normal activities of daily living
③ Rapid progression of aging changes
④ Normal response time to stimuli

18. Older adults have a decrease in total body fluids, which can cause:

① Increased thirst
② Decreased risk of dehydration
③ Increase in urine output
④ Increased incidence of side effects from water-soluble drugs

19. Older adults are more susceptible to overdoses from fat-soluble drugs, because they have a/an:

① Decreased percentage of body fat
② Increased percentage of body fat
③ Decrease in renal function
④ Increase in bowel transit time

20. Respiratory changes in older adults include:

① Decrease in dead space
② Increased vital capacity
③ Decreased cough effectiveness
④ Increased respiratory rate

21. Which of the following is *not* an appropriate problem associated with skin changes in older adults?

① Increased ability for scar formation
② Dry cracking skin from decreased turgor
③ Decreased sweating due to decreased sweat glands
④ Increased risk of hypothermia

22. A normal visual change associated with aging is:

① Development of tunnel vision
② Decreased accommodation to light or dark
③ Loss of central vision
④ Decreased vision from clouding of the lens

23. The average number of calories a 65-year-old woman should eat daily to maintain an ideal body weight is about:

① 1000
② 1500
③ 2000
④ 2500

24. Which of the following is *not* a likely cause of nutritional problems in older adults?

① Difficulty chewing due to lost teeth
② Difficulty shopping for food
③ Decreased caloric needs
④ Social isolation during meals

25. Older adults are more prone to drug overdoses because:

① They have a lower fat content
② Their water content is proportionally high
③ They often forget to take their medication
④ Their serum albumin levels are lower

26. Your older patient is exhibiting severe confusion. The family says that the patient had been perfectly clear at home and never confused before. The most likely cause of the confusion is:

① Relocation trauma
② Alzheimer's disease
③ Organic brain syndrome
④ Related to medication

27. A common developmental task of the older adult is:

① Preparation of retirement
② Continued parenting of adult children
③ Preparation for death
④ Reassessment of roles within the family

28. Because old adults are more prone to accidents and fractures, the nurse should protect them by:

① Encouraging their families to put them in nursing homes
② Providing a safe environment for them
③ Keeping them confined to a chair; up only with help
④ Maintaining them on bed rest

Answers & Rationales

Guide to item identification (see pp. 3–5 for further details about each category)

I, II, III, or IV for the phase of the nursing process
1, 2, 3, or 4 for the category of client needs
A, B, C, D, E, F, or G for the category of human functioning
Specific content category by name; ie, cholecystectomy

1. ① Confusion often occurs in the elderly with trauma and a sudden, unexpected alteration in the environment.
I, 3, A & G. Older Adult/Fractured Hip.

2. ④ Never reinforce confusion by lying to a patient. Reorient the patient to reality when confusion occurs.
III, A & G. Older Adult/Fractured Hip.

3. ③ The patient was suffering from temporary confusion, but loss of independence is one of the greatest fears of older adults.
IV, 3, A & G. Older Adult/Fractured Hip.

4. ② The older adult does not need bathing daily owing to the decrease in function of the sweat and oil glands, but for the same reasons, they must have frequent skin care.
III, 2, A & D. Older Adult/Fractured Hip.

5. ② The older adult is often protein malnourished. Anyone suffering an injury will require more protein for healing.
I & III, 2, F. Older Adult/Fractured Hip.

6. ③ Wearing clothes of their own and good grooming help older adults maintain self-esteem.
III, 2, A & G. Older Adult/Fractured Hip.

7. ② In the elderly, constipation is a common problem attributable to decreased gastrointestinal muscle tone, which causes inability to move waste effectively through the system. Fresh fruits, vegetables and water provide bulk, which stimulates peristalsis.
II, 2 & 4, F. Older Adult.

8. ① Gerontology refers to research and study of the aging process.
I, 4, A. Older Adult.

9. ② The aging process is different for each person and is more related to feelings and behavior than to chronological age alone.
IV, 4, A. Older Adult.

10. ④ Aging involves the loss of ability to withstand change and increased rigidity of joints, muscles, lung tissue and so forth.
IV, 4, E. Older Adult.

11. ① It is healthy to begin to accept the inevitability of death.
I, 4, A & G. Older Adult.

12. ① Older adults experience a slowing of peristalsis because of their decreased activity. Fiber and bulk are often deficient in their diets.
IV, 4, F. Older Adult.

13. ② "The behavioral changes are usually closely related to the individual's basic personality but are more exaggerated." (Bauer & Hill, 1986:84) Organic Mental Disorder/Older Adult.
IV, 3, C & G. Older Adult.

14. ① Groups focusing on "here and now" issues offer a concrete basis for dealing with specific items the clients can grasp. Such groups are led by a wide spectrum of health providers who do not need special training in group dynamics.
II, 3, C & G. Organic Mental Disorder/Older Adult.

15. ① "Use the client's past memory to bring him to the present through reminiscing. For example, say, 'You are in a nursing home now. But tell me about the time that you had a farm.' In this way you are orienting the client to his present place while also allowing him to share with you his experiences of earlier years." (Bauer & Hill, 1986:85)
IV, 3, C & G. Organic Mental Disorder/Older Adult.

16. ③ "Concrete, repetitious crafts and projects breed familiarization and comfort." (Bauer & Hill, 1986:156)
III, 3, C & G. Organic Mental Disorder/Older Adult.

17. ① The major physical change experienced by the "middle" old is a decreased ability to respond to stress. They are still able to carry out normal activities of daily living, but do have a slightly slower response time. Aging is usually gradual.
I, 4, A & D. Older Adult.

18. Because older adults have a decrease in body
④ water, water-soluble drugs can become increasingly concentrated leading to an increase in side effects. Thirst is normally decreased, with an increased risk of dehydration. Urine output is usually decreased and concentrated.
I, 4, F. Older Adult.

19. Older adults have an increase in the percentage
② of fat in the body resulting in an increase in the amount of fat-soluble drugs that can be absorbed leading to possible overdose. Renal function should not affect these drugs and an increase in bowel transmit time would decrease their absorption leading to under dosing.
I, 4, F. Older Adult.

20. Older adults have an increase in dead space, a
③ decrease in vital capacity and little change in rate. A decrease in the effectiveness of the cough is the most common and potentially serious change.
I, 4, B. Older Adult.

21. There is a decreased ability to form granulation
① tissue in older adults, which impairs healing and scar formation.
I, 4, D. Older Adult.

22. Tunnel vision may be a sign of glaucoma, loss
② of central vision a retinal detachment and cloudy vision characteristic of cataracts. Decreased accommodation is the only normal visual change associated with aging.
I, 4, C. Older Adult.

23. The rule is that the caloric intake should de-
② crease about 7.5% per decade after age 25 years.

The normal caloric intake would be about 1500 calories from age 65 years on.
III, 4, F. Older Adult.

24. Older adults often need more calories than they
③ receive and more nutritious foods.
I, 4, F. Older Adult.

25. Many drugs that older adults take, such as car-
④ diac glycosides, are protein-bound drugs. The low serum albumin common in many older people means that higher levels of the drugs are in circulation, leading to overdose. Older adults have a higher percentage of fat, a low level of body water, and forgetting their drugs would lead to underdosing, not overdoses.
I, 4, F. Older Adult.

26. The most common cause of sudden acute con-
① fusion in this patient is probably due to relocation trauma associated with the change in the environment. Alzheimer's disease and organic brain syndrome occur gradually, and the family would have noticed some changes. There is no mention of medication administration and it *cannot* be assumed.
I, 4, G. Older Adult.

27. One of the common developmental tasks of
③ older adults is acceptance of and preparation for death. The other options are tasks of the middle-aged person.
II, 4, A. Older Adult.

28. If a safe environment is maintained, an older
② adult can remain independent and still be accident-free.
III, 4, D & E. Older Adult.

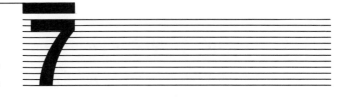

The Adult Patient

GROWTH AND DEVELOPMENT

■ Life Stages

I. THE MIDDLE AGED ADULT

A. Physiologic Alterations

1. Hormonal changes
   a. menopause (see p. 119)
      (1) cessation of reproductive ability
      (2) women are usually between age 40 and 50 years
      (3) Men usually between age 50 and 60 years, but symptoms not as pronounced
   b. benign prostatic hypertrophy in men begins usually by age 50 years
   c. decreasing hormonal production by both sexes may alter sexual function to some degree
2. Skeletal changes
   a. osteoporosis from decalcification of bones
      (1) women often lose up to 2 inches from shrinking of intervertebral discs
      (2) "dowager's hump" in cervical thoracic spine
   b. women are much more susceptible to hip and other bone fractures at age 55 years than are men
3. Skin changes
   a. cell atrophy and decreased repair
   b. body shrinks
   c. loss of subcutaneous tissue
4. Nerve conduction slows and muscle function decreases
   a. leads to increased muscle atrophy
   b. impaired heat and cold sensation
5. Vision
   a. presbyopia, decreasing accommodation
   b. glasses, often bifocals
6. Hearing
   a. decreased sensitivity to high-pitched sounds
   b. sound discrimination decreases
7. Cardiovascular changes
   a. decreased elasticity of vessels, especially coronary arteries
   b. rise in serum cholesterol in women after menopause, with increase in coronary heart disease
   c. cardiac output decreased
   d. glomerular filtration rate decreases
8. Metabolic changes
   a. altered nutritional needs
      (1) decreased basal metabolic rate
      (2) reduce calories by 7.5% per decade after age 25 years
      (3) maintain high fluid intake
   b. rest/activity
      (1) activity level relatively unchanged
      (2) some may develop new sense of energy
      (3) no reason to decrease activity or increase rest unless a disease state is present

B. Psychosocial Alterations

1. Cognitive changes
   a. reaction time usually unchanged
   b. ability to learn unchanged
   c. time for learning increases
   d. memory not impaired, but less able to memorize or remember new material
   e. problem solving abilities unchanged
2. Emotional development
   a. climacteric
   b. transitional period
      (1) prime of work life
      (2) role changes: children, spouse, own parents
      (3) time when goals are reached or never achieved
   c. Erickson's stage of generativity vs. self-absorption and stagnation
      (1) success means sense of parenthood and creativity, guiding new generation, establishing continuity
      (2) not necessarily biologic in nature
      (3) negativity shown through lack of acceptance of self and accomplishments, regression to earlier stages, self-absorption
3. Midlife crisis
   a. "empty nest" syndrome when children leave home
   b. change in roles
   c. upheaval, which may be internal or external
   d. time for reexamination of self, role, life, etc.
   e. healthier and constructive to work through positively
   f. reproductive ability lost in women

C. Common Health Problems

1. Fractures and dislocations are the leading types of injury
2. Sinusitis and upper respiratory infections are common
3. Hiatal hernia and esophagitis may be mistaken for myocardial infarction
4. Peptic ulcers, especially with increased stress
5. Angina pectoris
6. Essential hypertension
7. Hyperuricemia and gout
8. Type II diabetes mellitus (noninsulin-dependent diabetes mellitus)
9. Prostatitis, acute and chronic
10. Benign prostatic hypertrophy
11. Lumbosacral strain
12. Sexual dysfunction, of both physical and psychologic causes

II. THE OLDER ADULT
(SEE ALSO CHAPTER 6)

A. Physiologic Alterations

1. Nervous system changes
   a. nervous transmission slows
   b. recent memory loss
   c. slower reaction time
   d. sense of balance may decrease
   e. fine motor movement affected
   f. less able to react to painful stimuli
   g. impaired temperature regulation, more prone to hypo- and hyperthermia
   h. decreased tactile sensation
2. Visual changes
   a. normal
      (1) loss of visual acuity, presbyopia
      (2) arcus senilis (rings around corneal periphery) not pathologic
      (3) altered color vision
      (4) loss of accommodation
   b. pathologic
      (1) cataracts
      (2) glaucoma more common
3. Hearing changes
   a. unilateral or bilateral hearing loss common over age 65 years
   b. lack of ability to discriminate volume or pitch
4. Metabolic changes
   a. decreased enzyme secretion
   b. decreased nutrient and drug absorption
   c. decreased peristalsis
   d. often poor nutritional status
   e. loss of sense of taste and smell
   f. changes in dentition
   g. decreased metabolic rate
   h. less ability to withstand stress, to maintain homeostasis
   i. constipation is common
5. Cardiovascular changes
   a. arteriosclerosis
   b. decreased coronary artery blood flow
   c. hypertension common
   d. few changes in hemopoietic system
6. Respiratory changes
   a. decreased ventilatory volumes
   b. decreased capacity for gas exchange
   c. increased risk of disease
7. Genitourinary function changes
   a. benign prostatic hypertrophy with resultant urinary changes
   b. decreased blood flow to kidneys
   c. incontinence may occur, especially in women who had children with resultant perineal muscle weakness
8. Musculoskeletal changes
   a. osteoporosis
   b. increase in fibrous connective tissue with stiffening
   c. arthritic changes
   d. muscle atrophy

B. Psychosocial Alterations

1. Retirement
2. Role changes
3. Erickson's stage of ego integrity vs. despair
   a. successful adaptation shown through satisfaction with life and acceptance of eventual death
   b. unsuccessful adaptation shown by sense of failure and futility, desire to redo life, sense of worthlessness
4. Body image changes can lead to depression
5. Cognitive changes
   a. slower
   b. slowed nerve impulse transmission
   c. general intelligence not affected
   d. capacity to learn intact, but time longer and may require more repetition

C. Common Health Problems

1. Cataracts
2. Glaucoma
3. Herpes zoster
4. Parkinson's disease
5. Alzheimer's disease
6. Congestive heart failure
7. Peripheral vascular disease (PVD) with stasis ulcers and occlusions

8. Chronic obstructive pulmonary disease (COPD)
9. Anemia
10. Chronic lymphocytic leukemia
11. Malignant lymphomas
12. Benign prostatic hypertrophy
13. Osteoarthritis
14. Coronary artery disease (CAD)

■ Reproductive System in Women

I. NORMAL FUNCTION

A. Provide nourishment and protection for the developing fetus
B. To assist in the birth of the child through muscular contractions
C. To assist in the production of required hormones during pregnancy
D. To nourish the newborn child

■ Reproductive Changes and Disorders in Women

I. BREAST

A. Benign Tumors, Cysts

1. Assessment
   a. definition: painless or tender lumps in breast tissue
   b. incidence: most often occurs in women between ages 30 and 50 years
   c. predisposing factors
      (1) possible genetic link
      (2) diet high in caffeine
   d. signs and symptoms
      (1) enlargement of area in breast
      (2) pain when area pressed
   e. diagnostic tests
      (1) mammography: radiographic picture of breast tissue; no special preparation necessary except explanation to patient
      (2) biopsy: removal of section of tissue to be examined under microscope; procedure may be performed on outpatient basis or in hospital; explanation necessary
      (3) aspiration: fluid removed from the cyst using a needle and syringe; performed by the physician; explanation of procedure necessary
   f. usual treatment: excision or aspiration

B. Breast Carcinoma

1. Assessment
   a. definition: cancerous growth in breast tissue
   b. incidence
      (1) higher incidence in women with family history
      (2) higher in women over age 40 years
   c. predisposing/precipitating factors
      (1) genetic predisposition; mother, sister, or grandmother with breast cancer
      (2) age over 40 years
      (3) childless or first child after age 30 years
      (4) presence of other cancers (ovarian, endometrial)
   d. signs and symptoms
      (1) painless lump in breast
      (2) "dimpling" of skin
      (3) retraction of nipple
      (4) discharge from nipple
      (5) asymmetry of breasts
   e. diagnostic tests
      (1) biopsy
      (2) mammography
         (a) All women: yearly after age 50 years, baseline at age 35 years, and every other year after age 40 years
         (b) high-risk women: baseline at age 35 years and yearly after age 40 years
   f. usual treatments
      (1) chemotherapy: see explanation in discussion on cancer under "Immune Disorders."
      (2) radiation therapy
      (3) surgical procedure: mastectomy; lumpectomy; simple or modified radical mastectomy
2. Planning, goals/expected outcomes
   a. patient performs monthly breast self-examination correctly
   b. patient complies with breast self-examination (BSE)
   c. assist patient to alleviate emotional distress associated with breast disease
   d. assist in reducing complications of surgery and reducing recurrence of cancer
3. Implementation
   a. monthly breast self-examination techniques taught to patient; importance of early detection should be stressed
   b. palpation examination by physician should be performed on yearly basis
   c. mammography examination should be performed as ordered
   d. assist patient to verbalize fears related to breast disease and the diagnosis of cancer
   e. explain procedures and side effects as they relate to treatment

f. implement routine postoperative care and specific arm exercises to reduce postoperative complications

g. modify diet to decrease caffeine intake

4. Evaluation
   a. patient performs monthly breast self-examinations
   b. patient maintains regular check-up appointments
   c. patient fully recovers from any surgical procedures without complications
   d. patient performs postoperative exercises as instructed
   e. patient verbalizes feelings related to body image
   f. referrals to self-help agencies made as needed; including American Cancer Society, Reach for Recovery, and other social service agencies
   g. patient verbalizes diet changes and modifies diet

II. UTERINE TUMORS: BENIGN

A. Assessment

1. Definition: abnormal growth within uterus; usually benign uterine myomas; also known as fibroids
2. Incidence: common between ages 24 and 40 years
3. Signs and symptoms
   a. bleeding most common
   b. as size increases, pressure may be felt
4. Diagnostic tests
   a. physical pelvic examination: emotional support of patient necessary
   b. nurse assists with preparing and labeling specimens
   c. proper draping of patient to preserve modesty
5. Usual treatments
   a. surgical excision, determined by age of patient
   b. conservative treatment if bleeding not excessive or if children still desired

III. CERVICAL CANCER

A. Assessment

1. Definition: abnormal growth in cervical area of uterus
2. Incidence: women over age 40 years
3. Predisposing factors
   a. first pregnancy at an early age
   b. frequent relations with numerous partners
   c. multiparity
   d. history of venereal disease

4. Signs and symptoms
   a. postmenopausal bleeding
   b. bleeding with intercourse
5. Diagnostic tests
   a. Pap smear (see Chapter 3)
   b. cervical biopsy
   c. colposcopy
   d. Schiller test
   e. cone biopsy
6. Complications: metastasizes (spreads) to other areas in the body
7. Usual treatments
   a. surgical excision
   b. radiation therapy—either internal implants or external
   c. chemotherapy

B. Planning, Goals/Expected Outcomes

1. Reduce emotional stress associated with diagnosis of cancer
2. Assist patient to recover fully from surgical procedure
3. Patient will comply with prescribed treatment plan

C. Implementation

1. Patient receives pre- and postoperative teaching as covered under "Perioperative Care." (pp. 187–190)
2. Offer support by allowing patient to verbalize fears and worries
3. Explain all procedures and activities to be performed

D. Evaluation

1. Patient recovers completely from surgical procedure
2. Patient verbalizes feelings and demonstrates an understanding of continued treatments
3. Family members aware of need for their assistance and social service agencies notified if needed

IV. ENDOMETRIOSIS

A. Assessment

1. Definition: endometrial tissue found outside uterus
2. Incidence: common disorder in women of childbearing age

3. Predisposing factors
   a. unknown
   b. could be related to family history
4. Signs and symptoms
   a. pain
   b. excessive menstrual flow
   c. bleeding between periods
   d. painful intercourse
5. Complications: infertility
6. Usual treatments
   a. conservative: administration of birth control pills
   b. surgical: excision of abnormal tissue outside uterus, possible hysterectomy

B. Planning, Goals/ Expected Outcomes

1. Patient will have a reduction of discomfort
2. Completely recovers from surgical procedure

C. Implementation

1. Administer medications and explain their schedule properly
2. Encourage patient to verbalize feelings concerning diagnosis
3. Provide appropriate pre- and postoperative care

D. Evaluation

1. Patient pain free
2. Patient takes medications correctly
3. Patient recovers completely from surgical procedure

V. MENOPAUSE

A. Assessment

1. Definition: end of woman's reproductive period; total cessation of menstruation
2. Incidence
   a. occurs between age 45 and 50 years; could occur between 35 and 58 years
   b. statistics
      (1) 25% by age 47 years
      (2) 50% by age 50 years
      (3) 75% by age 52 years
      (4) 95% by age 55 years
   c. artificial menopause occurs with surgical removal of ovaries
3. Signs and symptoms
   a. menstrual irregularity
   b. flushing of skin: "hot flashes"
   c. excessive perspiration
   d. fatigue
   e. emotional instability
   f. depression
4. Usual treatment: usually medical by administering estrogen replacement via oral medications—is controversial

B. Planning, Goals/ Expected Outcomes

1. Patient will adjust to menopause
2. Patient will maintain normal lifestyle and function
3. Patient will have decrease in symptoms of menopause
4. Patient will verbalize understanding of possible problems related to menopause

C. Implementation

1. Encourage good nutrition to maintain normal weight
   a. reduce the amount of fat in diet
   b. reduce amount of carbohydrates eaten
   c. reduce amount of red meat eaten
   d. encourage consumption of fish and poultry, fresh fruits, and vegetables
   e. encourage patient to exercise on daily basis
2. Encourage her to verbalize feelings related to this time in her life
3. Teach to report any unusual bleeding or spotting to physician

D. Evaluation

1. Patient adjusts to menopause and maintains normal activities
2. Symptoms of menopause reduced and made more tolerable
3. Patient verbalizes understanding of what is happening to her body
4. Patient verbalizes understanding of potential problems, such as bleeding after menses has stopped

■ Reproductive Disorders in Men

I. BENIGN PROSTATIC HYPERTROPHY (BPH)

A. Assessment

1. Definition/pathophysiology: enlargement of prostate not caused by inflammation or neoplasm; enlarged prostate pushes on urethra, causing difficulties in urination
2. Incidence: common in men over 45–50 years of age
3. Predisposing/precipitating factors
   a. aging process
   b. chronic urinary tract infections
4. Signs and symptoms
   a. decreased force of urine flow
   b. hesitancy in starting to void
   c. inability to empty bladder totally
   d. urgency and frequency
   e. nocturia
   f. dysuria
   g. overflow urinary incontinence
   h. hematuria
   i. enlarged prostate palpable on rectal examination
5. Diagnostic tests
   a. history and physical examination with rectal examination
   b. urine for culture and sensitivity, urinalysis
   c. cystoscopy
   d. intravenous pyelogram (IVP)
   e. complete blood count (CBC)
   f. blood urea nitrogen (BUN), serum acid phosphatase, alkaline phosphatase
6. Complications
   a. total blockage of urine output
   b. hydronephrosis
   c. pyelonephritis
   d. renal failure
7. Usual treatment
   a. urinary catheterization to drain bladder
   b. pharmacology
      (1) antibiotics
      (2) urinary tract antiseptics
      (3) antispasmodics
   c. suprapubic catheter possible for long-term drainage of bladder
   d. surgery
      (1) transurethral prostatectomy (TURP): performed with resectoscope inserted into penis, follows urethra to point of hypertrophy; electrocautery loop inserted, and excess tissue removed; only enlarged tissue removed, leaving normal tissue and prostatic capsule intact; treatment of choice for pa-tients with simple hyperplasia, for elderly, or poor risk patients; continuous bladder irrigation (CBI) set up with three-way Foley catheter afterwards
      (2) suprapubic prostatectomy: incision made into bladder through abdominal wall, and prostatic tissue removed; continuous bladder irrigation set up through cystotomy catheter from abdominal puncture site and Foley catheter inserted for drainage; may have CBI; causes sterility
      (3) retropubic prostatectomy: performed through low abdominal incision between pubic arch and prostatic capsule; prostatic capsule incised, and prostatic tissue removed; benefit—bladder not entered; causes sterility
      (4) perineal prostatectomy: approached through incision between scrotum and anus; prostatic capsule opened, and prostatic tissue removed; used only for prostatic cancer, causes impotence
   e. possibly, bilateral vasectomy may be performed at the time of prostatectomy to reduce risk of epididymitis

B. Planning, Goals/Expected Outcomes

1. Patient will understand need for medical and surgical regimen
2. Patient will be relieved of acute or chronic urinary retention
3. Patient will be free of pain
4. Patient will not develop complications of surgical procedure
5. Patient will have safe hospital stay

C. Implementation

1. Assist patient to understand surgical procedure
2. Provide emotional support for patient and significant others during diagnostic work-up and postoperative period
3. Explain to patient and significant others possibility of continuous bladder irrigation and hematuria; hematuria for 3–5 days
4. Monitor urinary drainage for blockage in drainage tubes, presence of clots, hematuria, oliguria, pyuria; report abnormal findings to team leader
5. Postoperative period
   a. monitor vital functions
      (1) particularly blood pressure if patient has

had spinal anesthesia: danger of hypotension

(2) intake and output: record each drainage tube separately

(3) continuous bladder irrigation at rate as ordered by physician

b. institute early ambulation as ordered; cough and deep breathe

c. perform catheter care using sterile technique

d. observe sterile technique for dressing changes

6. Administer pain medications per physician's order, watch for adverse effects in elderly population

7. Assist RN in assessment of geriatric patient in preoperative and postoperative periods for functions in sight, hearing, musculoskeletal function, steadiness on feet, vital signs, orientation

8. Provide safe environment, such as having bed in lowest position, call light easily available, side rails up at night; assist with activities of daily living and ambulation

9. Notify team leader immediately of any potential or actual problems in safety, such as confusion

D. Evaluation

1. Patient's voiding returned to normal
2. Patient complied with treatments
3. Patient's pain controlled
4. Patient recovered from surgery without complications

II. CANCER OF THE PROSTATE

A. Assessment

1. Definition/pathophysiology: malignant tumor of prostate gland
2. Incidence: in men over 60 years of age
3. Predisposing/precipitating factors
   a. cause unknown
   b. chronic urinary tract irritation
   c. cancer metastasized from other part of genitourinary tract
4. Signs and symptoms
   a. early stage, asymptomatic
   b. later stage, may be similar to prostatic hypertrophy
   c. symptoms of metastasis, such as back pain
5. Diagnostic tests
   a. similar to those for benign prostatic hypertrophy
   b. cystoscopy with biopsy
   c. serum acid and alkaline phosphatase; acid

phosphatase rises as cancer spreads outside prostatic capsule

6. Complications
   a. complete obstruction of urinary flow
   b. metastasis to other parts of genitourinary system
   c. metastasis to other parts of body
   d. perforation of bladder after surgery
7. Usual treatment
   a. early stages, probably transurethral approach (see "Benign Prostatic Hypertrophy")
   b. later stages, radical retropubic or perineal prostatectomy, in which prostate, capsule, seminal glands, bladder neck removed
   c. radiation therapy
   d. chemotherapy
   e. supportive measures, such as hydration and pain control

B. Planning, Goals/Expected Outcomes

1–5. Similar to planning under "Benign Prostatic Hypertrophy"
6. Patient will understand need, function, and side effects of radiation therapy
7. Patient will understand need, function, and side effects of chemotherapy
8. Patient will feel supported by nursing staff
9. Patient's spiritual needs will be met

C. Implementation

1–5. Similar to implementation under "Benign Prostatic Hypertrophy"
6. Assist patient to understand need, function, and adverse effects of radiation therapy (see "Cancer")
7. Assist patient to understand need, function, and adverse effects of chemotherapy (see "Cancer")
8. Provide environment so patient feels comfortable enough to express feelings and fears; use verbal and nonverbal supportive nursing care
9. If appropriate, assist patient to contact clergy of choice or meet needs on individual basis

D. Evaluation

1. Patient complied with radiation therapy
2. Patient complied with chemotherapy
3. Patient remained in stable emotional state
4. Patient received spiritual support

Questions

Margaret Simmons, age 62 years, calls her physician, by whom you are employed, to report that for the past 3 weeks she has been having episodes of vaginal bleeding.

1. Your most appropriate response would be to:

① Suggest she wait a few more weeks to see if the bleeding stops
② Tell her it probably doesn't mean anything, but you will arrange an appointment with the doctor
③ Suggest, jokingly, that she may need to resume taking birth control measures
④ Arrange an appointment with the physician as soon as possible

2. Mrs. Simmons makes an appointment to see the doctor for a pelvic examination and a Papanicolaou's smear. The nurse explains to Mrs. Simmons that:

① A vaginal douche is not to be taken before the examination
② A vaginal douche should be taken immediately before the appointment to assure clear visualization of the area
③ It is most important to be on time for the appointment so the doctor can spend sufficient time with her
④ If the bleeding stops, she is to cancel her appointment

3. Cancer of the cervix is one of the most treatable cancers if it is detected early. Women at the greatest risk for this cancer include women who had:

① Early onset of menstruation and malnutrition
② Children before the age of 20 or after 35 years
③ Frequent early sexual relations and multiple partners
④ Abstained from sexual intercourse and are obese

4. Breast self-examination is important for all women, but is especially important for those who:

① Are over age 50 years and had children before the age of 20

② Have very large breasts and breast-fed their children
③ Have a history of fibrocystic disease and are under age 40 years
④ Never had children and have an aunt with breast cancer

5. Which of the following explains the importance of assessing the patient's present functioning (growth and development) level?

① Assists staff to excuse current behaviors
② Assists staff to develop realistic goals for care
③ Assists client in understanding own behavior
④ Assists staff in determining admission status

Mrs. Simon is admitted for a modified radical mastectomy for a malignant breast tumor.

6. Preoperative teaching for Mrs. Simon should include:

① Preparation for a skin graft
② Beginning arm exercises
③ Use of an arm sling
④ Fitting of a prosthesis

7. Mrs. Simon returns from surgery with a Hemovac in place. Nursing interventions for a patient with a Hemovac include:

① Irrigating the tube as needed
② Not emptying the Hemovac
③ Avoiding kinks in the tubing
④ Pinning the Hemovac to the back of the patient's gown

8. In order to decrease the postoperative edema of the affected arm, the patient should:

① Elevate her arm on pillows above the heart
② Keep the arm fixed at her side
③ Apply a warm pad over the affected arm
④ Use only the unaffected arm for all activities

9. On the first postoperative day, the nurse recommends that Mrs. Simon begin arm exercises. The best exercise at this time is:

① Abducting the arm and flexing the elbow
② "Wall walking" every 4 hours
③ Using a rope pulley to extend her shoulder
④ Combing her hair with her affected arm

10. Mrs. Simon seems depressed about her loss at times and happy about the positive outcome of her surgery at other times. The nurse realizes that:

① Mrs. Simon is neurotic and should see the social worker
② Patients often have a difficult time adjusting to this
③ Mrs. Simon is simply vain and needs time to adjust
④ Patients often need some time alone after a loss like this

11. Mrs. Simon asks if she still has to do a monthly breast self-examination. Your best response would be:

① Yes, the cancer is likely to spread to the other breast
② No, there is no further risk of breast cancer
③ No, the doctor will do it every 3 months
④ Yes, there is an increased risk of a new cancer in the other breast

Mrs. Sands has been diagnosed with cervical cancer and is to have an internal radium implant in for the next 48 hours.

12. In caring for Mrs. Sands, you know that a problem during the time the implant is in place is often:

① Fear and isolation
② Nausea and vomiting
③ Vaginal bleeding
④ Pain from the implant

13. When caring for Mrs. Sands after the insertion of the implant, the nurse must protect herself from undue exposure to the radiation. To do this the nurse should:

① Care for the patient no more than 10 minutes per day
② Wear a lead apron and stand anywhere when giving direct care
③ Stand at the head of the bed whenever possible while giving care
④ Ask a family member to be present and to assist with patient care

14. In order to insure that no more radiation than the prescribed dose is received by Mrs. Sands's internal organs, the nurse should:

① Encourage the patient to turn side to side every 2 hours
② Elevate the head of the bed for meals

③ Administer laxatives as ordered to prevent constipation
④ Carefully maintain the patency of the urinary catheter

15. When it is time for the implant to be removed, the nurse has the responsibility of:

① Calling the radiology department to remind them
② Assisting the surgeon with the removal
③ Removing the implant and placing it in a lead container
④ Nothing—this is not a nursing responsibility

16. After removal of the implant, it is important to teach Mrs. Sands to:

① Avoid all pregnant women
② Limit her exposure to children to 30 minutes a day
③ Not sleep in the same bed as her husband for 1 month
④ Avoid sexual intercourse and douches for 6 weeks

17. Which of the following problems would not be normal following removal of the implant and would require that Mrs. Sands call the doctor?

① She experiences moderate constipation
② She notes brown, foul-smelling vaginal drainage
③ She develops urinary incontinence spontaneously
④ Her urine is slightly blood-tinged

Mike Dawson is a 70-year-old retired policeman who has been experiencing symptoms of frequency, urgency, and nocturia, which have been increasing over the last 2 months. He is diagnosed as having an enlarged prostate.

18. The doctor performed a rectal examination on Mr. Dawson. The purpose of this examination is to:

① Diagnose an enlarged prostate
② Check for the presence of blood
③ Definitively diagnose prostatic cancer
④ Diagnose the presence of an infection

19. Mr. Dawson is scheduled for a suprapubic prostatectomy. In doing preoperative teaching, the nurse should be sure to include:

① Information about his inevitable impotence

② The need for frequent postoperative dressing changes
③ That the patient will not have an external incision
④ That there is a chance cancer will be found

20. Postoperatively, Mr. Dawson is complaining of pain in the bladder and bladder spasms. The best medication the doctor would prescribe is:

① Demerol
② Morphine
③ Pro-Banthine
④ Aspirin

21. On the first postoperative day, Mr. Dawson is draining large amounts of urine through the dressing and little through the catheter. Your appropriate nursing intervention is to:

① Irrigate the catheter as ordered
② Change the dressing and record the approximate output
③ Call the doctor
④ Reinforce the dressing and irrigate the catheter

22. When the catheter is removed, Mr. Dawson is experiencing some dribbling and urinary incontinence. Which of the following should the nurse include in patient teaching?

① Recommending the use of an external catheter
② Advising his wife to purchase protective adult underpads
③ Instructing him to limit his intake
④ Instructing him to do perineal exercises to strengthen his urinary muscles

23. It is important for Mr. Dawson to avoid straining for a bowel movement, because this can increase the risk of bleeding. The medication most likely to be prescribed for this is:

① Metamucil
② Milk of magnesia
③ Colace
④ Dulcolax

24. Middle-aged persons should:

① Exercise less each decade after age 50 years
② Increase their sleep after age 50 years
③ Decrease their calories by 7.5% for each decade after age 25 years
④ Increase their diversional activities to prepare for retirement

25. The major cause of death in middle-aged men is:

① Heart disease
② Lung cancer
③ Cirrhosis
④ Stroke

26. Major physiologic changes that occur in middle age include:

① Increased peristalsis
② Increased metabolic rate
③ Increased rigidity of lung tissue
④ Increased visual accommodation

Martha Hayes is a 44-year-old mother of two who has been experiencing excessive vaginal bleeding for the past 2 months. She is in the gynecologist's office for her yearly Papanicolaou's smear.

27. Prior to the pelvic examination, the nurse should:

① Have the patient void
② Administer an enema
③ Catheterize the patient
④ Scrub the perineal area with antiseptic soap

28. The main reason for the above action is to:

① Obtain a stool specimen
② Obtain a sterile urine specimen
③ Decrease discomfort during the pelvic examination
④ Remove flatus and feces from the rectum

29. The doctor performed a Pap smear on Mrs. Hayes, which returned as a Class III smear. This means that the cells are:

① Normal
② Inflammatory
③ Malignant
④ Suggestive of malignancy

30. Mrs. Hayes is scheduled for a total abdominal hysterectomy. The night before surgery she receives a Betadine douche. The purpose of this is to:

① Minimize vaginal bleeding
② Cleanse the vaginal canal
③ Sterilize the vaginal canal
④ Decrease the number of malignant cells present

31. Mrs. Hayes is encouraged to ambulate frequently after surgery. The nurse knows that for this type of surgery, it is to prevent:

   ① Abdominal distention
   ② Wound infection
   ③ Diarrhea
   ④ Urinary retention

32. Mrs. Hayes asks if she will continue to have periods postoperatively. You would explain that because of the surgery she will:

① Experience surgical menopause
② Not have the uncontrolled bleeding she had preoperatively
③ Experience some changes associated with menses, but not have a period
④ Continue to have normal periods

Answers & Rationales

Guide to item identification (see pp. 3–5 for further details about each category)

I, II, III, or IV for the phase of the nursing process
1, 2, 3, or 4 for the category of client needs
A, B, C, D, E, F, or G for the category of human functioning
Specific content category by name; ie, cholecystectomy

1. (4) Bleeding at times other than normal menstrual periods may be abnormal. In this case, the bleeding is postmenopausal and has lasted longer than 2 weeks, which makes it a possible warning sign of cancer.
III, 4, A. Uterine Cancer.

2. (1) Douching can wash away material that can assist the physician in diagnosing the cause of any possibly abnormal bleeding or discharge.
III, 1 & 2, A. Pap Smear.

3. (3) One risk for cervical cancer is anything that causes chronic cervical irritation.
I, 2, A & F. Cervical Cancer.

4. (4) Family history is one of the greatest risk factors for breast cancer.
I & III, 2 & 4, A & F. Breast Cancer.

5. (2) "It is through an understanding of human development that the health provider can distinguish between the patient's chronological level and actual functioning level and, therefore, develop more realistic care plans." (Bauer & Hill, 1986:9). "Initially, it is impossible for the client to comply past his actual functioning age. The provider and the client will feel less frustrated if this is considered in the plan." (Bauer & Hill, 1986:39)
I & IV, 4, A. Adult Growth & Development.

6. (2) It is important that the patient be taught arm exercises preoperatively so that she can begin basic ones immediately after surgery.
III, 1, A & E. Breast Cancer.

7. (3) The tubing must remain patent for the Hemovac to function properly.
III, 2, D. Breast Cancer.

8. (1) Elevating the arm will help decrease the possible postoperative lymphedema.
III, 2, B & D. Breast Cancer.

9. (4) Combing the hair provides some movement without initiating vigorous exercises too early.
III, 2, A & D. Breast Cancer.

10. (2) It is common for the patient to experience this ambivalence over the loss of the breast combined with the positive removal of the cancer.
I, 2 & 4, A, F, & G. Breast Cancer.

11. (4) There is an increased risk of a second primary cancer in the opposite breast after a woman has cancer in one breast.
III, 1, A & D. Breast Cancer.

12. (1) While the implant is in place, she will be in a private room with staff and visitors allowed in for only limited periods. Also, the presence of an implant is usually very frightening for the patient.
I, 2, D, F, & G. Cervical Cancer.

13. (3) The important factors to remember when caring for a patient with an implant are time, distance and shielding. The nurse is most shielded, by the patient's body, when standing at the head of the bed.
III, 2, D. Cervical Cancer.

14. (4) Bladder distention would move the bladder closer to the source of radiation.
III & IV, 2, D & F. Cervical Cancer.

15. (1) It is the nurse's responsibility to note the time for the removal and to notify the radiologist if it is not done on time.
III, 2, D. Cervical Cancer.

16. (4) Because of the trauma to the vaginal and cervical mucosa caused by the radiation, all forms of irritation should be avoided for at least 6 weeks.
III, 4, A & D. Cervical Cancer.

17. (3) The sudden development of urinary incontinence could indicate the presence of a vesicovaginal fistula, which often occurs spontaneously after radiation therapy because of tissue breakdown between the bladder and vagina.
IV, 2, A & F. Cervical Cancer.

18. (1) The prostate is easily palpated rectally, and enlargement is easily detected.
IV, 2, A & F. BPH.

19. A suprapubic prostatectomy involves an incision into the bladder, which drains large amounts of urine postoperatively.
② III, 2 & 4, A & F. BPH/Prostatectomy.

20. Pro-Banthine is an antispasmodic and best treats the bladder spasms.
③ I & III, 2, B. BPH/Prostatectomy.

21. It is normal for the majority of the drainage to come out through the dressing in the early postoperative period until the edema around the urethra decreases.
② III, 2, F. Prostatectomy.

22. Perineal exercises will help the patient regain urinary control gradually.
④ III, 2, D & F. Prostatectomy.

23. Colace is a stool softener that decreases the amount of straining the patient will have to do.
③ I & III, 2, F. Prostatectomy.

24. The middle aged adult has a natural decrease in metabolism, requiring a 7.5% decrease in calories to maintain the same body weight.
③ III, 4, A & F. Adult Growth & Development.

25. Heart disease is the leading cause of death in middle aged men; therefore, the major health need in this group is centered on prevention of cardiovascular disease.
① I, 4, A & B. Adult Growth and Development.

26. The flexibility of lung tissue decreases during the middle age years.
③ IV, 4, A & B. Adult Growth and Development.

27. A full bladder can interfere with the pelvic exam.
① III, 1, A & F. Female Reproductive Disorders.

28. A full bladder can cause discomfort during the pelvic exam.
③ II, 1, A & C. Female Reproductive Disorders.

29. A Class III smear is merely suspicious for malignancy.
④ IV, 2, A & F. Female Reproductive Disorders.

30. Because the cervix will be removed, it is important to cleanse the vaginal canal prior to surgery.
② II, 2, D & F. Cervical Cancer.

31. Abdominal distention is one of the most common problems after a hysterectomy.
① II, 2, D & F. Cervical Cancer.

32. A total abdominal hysterectomy does not involve the removal of the ovaries, so the patient will still have some of the symptoms associated with menses but no actual menstruation.
③ III, 2, A & D. Cervical Cancer.

OXYGENATION

Cardiopulmonary Disorders. The need of every cell for oxygen requires balance in supply and demand; oxygenators are heart and lungs, and disorders associated with these organs are the greatest threat to life in the United States.

■ Cardiovascular Disorders

I. ARTERIOSCLEROSIS/ ATHEROSCLEROSIS

A. Assessment

1. Definitions/pathophysiology
   a. arteriosclerosis: condition in which arteries harden and narrow, causing them to lose their elasticity
   b. atherosclerosis: condition in which fatty deposits (plaques) form on inner lining of blood vessels.
2. Incidence
   a. most common condition in United States
   b. increasing risk with age
   c. more common in men; women's rate rises after menopause
3. Predisposing/precipitating factors
   a. high fat diet
   b. smoking
   c. familial tendency
   d. obesity
   e. sedentary lifestyle
4. Signs and symptoms (vary depending on degree and location of involved blood vessels)
   a. coronary involvement
      (1) chest pain
      (2) dyspnea
      (3) palpitations
      (4) fainting
      (5) fatigue
   b. cerebral involvement
      (1) transient ischemic attacks (TIAs)
      (2) loss of memory
      (3) headaches
      (4) deterioration of personality
   c. extremities
      (1) leg cramps
      (2) cool skin
      (3) color changes
      (4) numbness and tingling
      (5) reduced or absent peripheral pulses
      (6) skin ulcerations and gangrene
5. Diagnostic tests
   a. history and physical examination
   b. arteriograms
6. Usual treatment
   a. reduce cholesterol in blood with diet and drugs
   b. coronary, cerebral, and peripheral vasodilators (Table 7-1)
   c. reduce risk factors such as smoking, obesity, lifestyle, stress
   d. surgery to remove plaque or bypass obstructions

B. Planning, Goals/ Expected Outcomes

1. Patient will attain lower cholesterol level
2. Patient will avoid trauma of extremities
3. Pain of ischemia will be relieved
4. Patient will understand and comply with therapeutic restrictions

C. Implementation

1. Provide low fat, low calorie, low cholesterol diet and counseling (Tables 7-2, 5-5, 5-6, and 5-8)
2. Protect extremities from trauma
3. Provide skin care
4. Observe for and report any change in skin color,

TABLE 7–1. Antianginals (Vasodilators)

Class	Example	Action	Use	Common Side Effects	Nursing Implications
Vasodilators	Nitroglycerin, Persantine, Vasodilan, Isordil	Act on blood vessels to increase diameter, effective on coronary arteries	To treat angina, cerebral vasoconstriction and peripheral vascular disease	Excessive vasodilation, headache, orthostatic hypotension, tachycardia	Monitor blood pressure closely, teach how to take correctly, check for relief
Calcium channel blockers	verapamil (Calan)	Reduce oxygen demand, dilate coronary arteries	To treat vasospastic or stable angina	Hypotension, dizziness, CHF, peripheral edema, gastrointestinal upset	Monitor for signs of CHF, may also treat hypertension

CHF, congestive heart failure.

TABLE 7–2. Foods Low in Cholesterol

Skim milk	Sherbet	Fish
Buttermilk	Egg whites	Low fat cottage cheese
Coffee	Vegetable oils	Potatoes
Tea	Low fat margarine	Rice
Carbonated beverages	Oil and vinegar dressings	Spaghetti (nonegg noodles)
Whole grain breads	Lean meat	Noncream soups
Most cereals	Chicken with skin removed	Sugar
Fresh fruits	Turkey with skin removed	All vegetables

temperature, pain or numbness, pulse volume, or breaks in skin
5. Avoid tight clothing
6. Use protective devices such as bed cradles
7. Relieve or reduce pain
8. Administer appropriate prescribed vasodilators (Table 7-1)
   a. provide warmth for vasodilation with care, such as warm baths or hot water bottle to lower abdomen
   b. provide sufficient activity to increase blood flow without causing ischemia
   c. educate patient and family regarding diet, medication, activity, and risk factors

D. Evaluation

1. Patient's serum cholesterol reached normal level
2. Patient had no trauma to extremities
3. Patient's ischemic pain relieved
4. Patient understood and complied with therapeutic restrictions

II. HYPERTENSION

A. Assessment

1. Definition/pathophysiology: persistently high blood pressure greater than 140/90; must be consistently above this level to be classified as hypertension
   a. primary or essential
      (1) most common type
      (2) cause unknown
      (3) known risk factors
   b. secondary
      (1) follows other diseases such as renal disease, pregnancy, heart defects, or endocrine disorders
      (2) treated by treating primary disease
2. Incidence/predisposing factors
   a. age 30–70 years
   b. blacks are affected 2:1

   c. obesity
   d. smoking
   e. stress
   f. birth control pills and estrogen
   g. genetic factors, heredity
   h. males
3. Signs and symptoms (may be vague and usually late)
   a. headache
   b. fatigue
   c. irritability
   d. tachycardia
   e. blurred vision
   f. tinnitus
   g. nose bleeds
4. Diagnostic tests
   a. history of high blood pressure, treatments, family history
   b. postural blood pressure measurement (lying, sitting, standing)
   c. comparison of present with previous blood pressure readings (must go high on at least three separate occasions to be hypertension)
   d. chest radiograph
   f. fundoscopic eye examination
   g. laboratory examinations: blood urea nitrogen (BUN), hematocrit, urinalysis
5. Complications
   a. cardiac hypertrophy
   b. congestive heart failure
   c. transient ischemic attacks (TIAs)
   d. accelerated atherosclerosis, nephrosclerosis
   e. aneurysms and hemorrhages
   f. papilledema
6. Usual treatment
   a. antihypertensives (Table 7-3)
   b. reduce cholesterol in blood with diet and drugs
   c. reduce risk factors such as smoking, obesity, lifestyle, stress

B. Planning, Goals/ Expected Outcomes

1. Patient's blood pressure will be lowered through use of antihypertensives
2. Patient will follow low sodium, low cholesterol diet and lose weight (Tables 7-2, 7-4, and 5-3)
3. Patient's blood pressure will be maintained through stress management
4. Patient will understand and comply with therapeutic regimen

C. Implementation

1. Administer prescribed antihypertensives (Table 7-3)

TABLE 7–3. Antihypertensives

Class	Example	Action	Use	Common Side Effects	Nursing Implications
Thiazide diuretics	Hydrochlorothiazide (HydroDiuril)	Diuretic, K$^+$ wasting	To treat hypertension	Hypokalemia, hyponatremia, orthostatic hypotension, hyperglycemia	Teach high K$^+$, low Na$^+$ diet, check I&O, BP
Potassium-sparing diuretics	Spironolactone (Aldactone)	Diuretic, increase Na$^+$ and water excretion	To treat hypertension	Hyponatremia, hyperkalemia, GI upset, allergies	Monitor Na$^+$ and K$^+$, I&O, BP
Loop diuretics	Furosemide (Lasix)	Inhibit reabsorption of Na$^+$ and water	To treat hypertension	Orthostatic hypotension, hypovolemia, hyponatremia, hypokalemia	Watch for dehydration, monitor electrolytes, check BP, give high K$^+$ diet, store in light-resistant bottle
Sympathetic inhibitors	Methyldopa (Aldomet)	Lower BP by blocking of sympathetic impulses	To treat hypertension	Orthostatic hypotension, depression, impotence, bradycardia, Na$^+$ and water retention	Have patient change position slowly, use low Na$^+$ diet, avoid alcohol
Vasodilators	Hydralazine (Apresoline)	Lower BP by causing vasodilation	To treat hypertension	Excessive vasodilation, headache, tachycardia, Na$^+$ and water retention	Monitor I&O, BP, maintain low Na$^+$ diet

BP, blood pressure; GI, gastrointestinal; I&O, intake and output.

2. Assess and document symptoms and response to treatment
3. Provide and teach prescribed diet
4. Weigh daily
5. Monitor blood pressure
6. Assist in planning of exercise regimen
7. Educate patient and family about importance of blood pressure control

TABLE 7–4. High and Low Sodium Foods

Low Sodium Foods	High Sodium Foods
Chicken	Milk
Fish	Cheese
Lean meat	Tomato juice
Most fresh vegetables	Canned vegetables, soups
Most fresh fruits	Lunch meats
Bread	Salted foods, such as chips or nuts
No salt added foods	Condiments
Salt substitutes	Relish, pickles
Cereal	Peanut butter
Cooked rice	Processed foods
Fresh cooked beans	Butter
	Soft drinks
	Celery

D. Evaluation

1. Patient's blood pressure returned to and maintained at normal levels
2. Patient followed low sodium and cholesterol diet and attained normal weight
3. Patient followed stress reduction and exercise regimen
4. Patient understood and complied with therapeutic regimen

III. CORONARY ARTERY DISEASE (CAD)

A. Assessment

1. Definition/pathophysiology: coronary arteries provide the only blood supply to the myocardium, and any significant interference with flow through these vessels impairs the entire function of circulatory system; heart has vital function of pumping blood by its rhythmic contractions; very dangerous disorder of heart, heart muscle damaged by diminished oxygen supply or so weakened it can no longer function effectively as pump

2. Incidence
   a. leading cause of death in United States (myocardial infarction [MI])
   b. mortality rate declining
3. Predisposing/precipitating factors
   a. obesity
   b. hypertension
   c. smoking
   d. sedentary lifestyle
   e. age
   f. stress
   g. hereditary
   h. elevated lipids and blood pressure
4. Signs and symptoms
   a. chest pain
   b. fatigue
   c. palpitations
   d. dyspnea on exertion
   e. syncope
   f. edema
5. Diagnostic tests
   a. ECG: graph of electrical activity of heart
   b. exercise stress test: shows ECG during physical exercise, usually treadmill or stationary bike
   c. echocardiogram: uses ultrasonic beams to demonstrate shape, location, and size of heart
   d. angiography: using contrast media to demonstrate blood flow through coronary arteries and aorta
   e. chest radiograph: to demonstrate size, shape, and location of heart
   f. continuous cardiac monitoring
   g. Holter monitor: portable monitor that records heart activity during 24-hour period—patient keeps log of activity during this time; gives picture of ECG changes as patient goes through usual activities
   h. laboratory studies
      (1) complete blood count (CBC): to determine if anemia or infection is present
      (2) erythrocyte sedimentation rate (ESR): to check for inflammation
      (3) serum enzymes and isoenzymes: serum glutamic-oxaloacetic transaminase (SGOT), lactate dehydrogenase (LDH), creatine phosphokinase (CPK) taken soon after admission

      (4) lipids: elevation indicates risk of heart disease
      (5) BUN and creatinine: elevated with renal and/or liver damage
6. Usual treatment
   a. medications
      (1) cardiac glycosides slow and strengthen heart (Table 7-5)
      (2) antiarrhythmics restore and maintain rhythm of heart (Table 7-6)
      (3) vasodilators improve blood supply to myocardium (Table 7-1)
      (4) antianginals decrease pain in myocardium (Table 7-1)
      (5) anticoagulants treat abnormal clotting patterns or decrease risk of clot formation (Table 7–7)
      (6) diuretics reduce blood volume to correct hypertension and edema (Table 7-3)
      (7) analgesics control pain and relieve anxiety (Table 7-8)
      (8) calcium channel blockers relax muscles in coronary arteries (Table 7-1)
   b. diet (see Chapter 5)
      (1) low sodium (Table 7-4 and 5-3)
      (2) low fat and cholesterol (Table 7-7)
      (3) often high potassium if on thiazide diuretic (Table 7-9 and 5-4)
      (4) low calorie if weight reduction needed
   c. exercise
      (1) rest required in acute phase
      (2) exercise regimen to improve oxygenation, ordered by physician
      (3) oxygen therapy as needed based on blood gases
   d. surgery: coronary artery bypass, valve replacements
7. Complications
   a. angina pectoris
   b. myocardial infarction (MI)

B. Planning, Goals/ Expected Outcomes

1. Patient will have coronary artery disease controlled without surgery

TABLE 7–5. Cardiac Glycosides

Example	Action	Use	Common Side Effects	Nursing Implications
Digoxin (Lanoxin)	Acts on myocardium to increase force of contraction and cardiac output while slowing rate	To treat CHF, tachycardia	Arrhythmias, heart block, bradycardia, GI upset, muscle weakness, diplopia	Take apical pulse prior to giving, hold if >120 or <60, check K$^+$ if on diuretics, watch for toxicity

CHF, congestive heart failure; GI, gastrointestinal.

TABLE 7–6. Antiarrhythmics

Example	Action	Use	Common Side Effects	Nursing Implications
Procainamide hydrochloride (Procan)	Decreases cardiac irritability	To treat PVCs, tachycardia	Severe hypotension, bradycardia, GI upset, rash	Monitor BP, watch for side effects, use carefully in patients with CHF
Quinidine gluconate (Quinaglute)	Slows conduction through AV node	To treat atrial flutter or fibrillation	Vertigo, headache, PVCs, hypotension, tinnitus, CHF, GI upset	May increase digoxin toxicity, check apical rate, give with meals
Propranolol hydrochloride (Inderal)	Decreases impulses through AV node and increases refractory period	To treat supraventricular, ventricular and atrial arrhythmias	Fatigue, hypotension, CHF, bradycardia, GI upset, depression, bronchial constriction	Don't use with asthmatics, withdraw drug slowly, check pulse, monitor BP, watch for peripheral edema

AV, atrioventricular; BP, blood pressure; CHF, congestive heart failure; GI, gastrointestinal; PVCs, premature ventricular contractions.

2. Patient will comply with medical therapy
3. Patient will be prepared for surgery as needed

C. Implementation

1. Administer medications as ordered
2. Teach patient diet modifications
3. Monitor for any increase or change in pain
4. Provide preoperative teaching as needed with RN
5. Monitor postoperatively as directed

D. Evaluation

1. Patient complied with prescribed therapy
2. Patient had disease controlled without surgery
3. Patient recovered from surgery without complications

IV. ANGINA PECTORIS

A. Assessment

1. Definition/pathophysiology: chest pain caused by reduced blood flow from coronary arteries to myocardium

2. Predisposing/precipitating factors
   a. long-term result of atherosclerosis, hypertension, or diabetes mellitus
   b. immediate precipitating
      (1) emotional upset
      (2) exposure to cold
      (3) exertion
      (4) overeating
3. Signs and symptoms
   a. sudden severe chest pain, substernal, radiating to left arm, shoulder, and neck
   b. pallor
   c. cold clammy skin
   d. dyspnea
   e. anxiety
4. Diagnostic tests
   a. history and physical examination
   b. ECG and Holter monitoring
   c. exercise stress test
5. Usual treatment
   a. nitroglycerine, sublingually, to relieve acute pain (Table 7-1)
   b. vasodilators such as Nitro Bid or Isordil may prevent anginal attacks (Table 7-1)
   c. diet to reduce fat and cholesterol and maintain normal weight
   d. coronary bypass surgery

TABLE 7–7. Anticoagulants

Example	Action	Use	Common Side Effects	Nursing Implications
Heparin sodium	Acts to inhibit formation of prothrombin activator	To treat and prevent blood clots	Hemorrhage	Avoid use of other anticoagulants at same time, teach patient to avoid bleeding, monitor partial thromboplastin time (PTT), protamine sulfate antidote
Warfarin (Coumadin)	Acts to inhibit formation of prothrombin in liver	To treat and prevent blood clots	Hemorrhage	Avoid use of other anticoagulants at same time; vitamin K antidote.

TABLE 7–8. Analgesics

Class	Example	Action	Use	Common Side Effects	Nursing Implications
Nonnarcotics	Acetylsalicylic acid (aspirin)	Act to decrease pain as antiinflammatory	To treat less severe pain	Salicylism, allergic reactions, GI distress, ulcerogenic, anticoagulant, liver damage	Avoid use in patients with ulcers, on anticoagulants, don't overuse, keep away from children, monitor liver function
Narcotics	Morphine, meperidine (Demerol)	Act by inhibiting transmission of pain impulses, reduce cortical response, alter pain perception areas of brain	To treat and prevent pain	Drowsiness, dizziness, euphoria, respiratory depression, constipation, urinary retention, allergy, hypotension	Monitor effectiveness, watch for hypotension and respiratory depression, monitor I&O, bowel movements, tolerance

GI, gastrointestinal; I&O, intake and output.

B. Planning, Goals/ Expected Outcomes

1. Patient's pain will be relieved without progressing to myocardial infarction
2. Patient will learn to reduce or cope with physical and emotional stress
3. Patient will learn to avoid risk factors
4. Patient will reduce fat in diet and alter calories as needed to manage weight

C. Implementation

1. Assess and document symptoms of stress and pain
2. Teach patient to stop activity when pain appears
3. Ask patient to report chest pain promptly
4. Administer vasodilators and understand their actions, can be used as a preventative measure
5. Provide emotional support and assurance
6. Refer to dietician for diet therapy teaching and reinforce dietary instructions
7. Teach patient and family importance of drug therapy, dietary restrictions, and management of stress and activity

D. Evaluation

1. Patient's pain kept to minimum
2. Patient exercised according to ability and doctor's order

TABLE 7–9. Foods High in Potassium

Whole milk	Cantaloupes	Mustard greens
Coffee in quantity	Oranges	Baked potatoes
Bread	Peas	Salt substitutes
Bran cereals	Spinach	Peanuts
Dried apricots	Lima beans	Molasses
Dried prunes	Soybeans	Broiled beef
Bananas	White beans	
Watermelons	Squash	

3. Patient avoided exposure to cold, emotional stress, heavy meals, and overexertion
4. Patient maintained normal weight and followed ordered dietary modifications

V. MYOCARDIAL INFARCTION (MI)

A. Assessment

1. Definition/pathophysiology: obstruction of branch of coronary artery leading to areas of necrosis resulting from ischemia; heart's ability to recover depends on size and location of infarction
2. Incidence: Same as for CAD
3. Predisposing/precipitating factors
   a. emotional stress
   b. obesity
   c. smoking
   d. high fat diet
   e. familial tendency
   f. diabetes mellitus
   g. history of angina
   h. atherosclerosis
4. Signs and symptoms
   a. sudden, severe crushing chest pain, radiating down left arm or to jaw; may be mistaken for indigestion
   b. dyspnea
   c. symptoms of shock (anxiety, pallor, diaphoresis)
   d. leukocytosis
   e. elevated cardiac enzymes (CPK, LDH, SGOT)
   f. arrhythmias
5. Diagnostic tests
   a. history and physical examination
   b. ECG
   c. laboratory tests, serum cardiac enzymes, white blood count (WBC)
6. Complications
   a. cardiogenic shock

b. congestive heart failure
c. pulmonary edema
d. death
7. Usual treatment
   a. morphine, IV, for chest pain (Table 7-8)
   b. oxygen for respiratory distress
   c. cardiac monitoring
   d. drugs as required for arrhythmias (Table 7-6)
   e. bed rest
   f. cardiopulmonary resuscitation as needed

B. Planning, Goals/ Expected Outcomes

1. Patient will not experience life-threatening arrhythmias
2. Patient's pain will be relieved promptly
3. Patient will not experience oxygen deprivation
4. Patient will understand importance of and comply with exercise and dietary restrictions
5. Patient's anxiety will be reduced

C. Implementation

1. Record vital signs every hour during acute phase
2. Monitor pulse during activity
3. Provide prompt pain relief
4. Monitor oxygenation
5. Provide activity as permitted
6. Provide prescribed diet, sodium and caffeine restricted, and teach patient restrictions
7. Provide counseling as needed to reduce anxiety

D. Evaluation

1. Patient had no arrhythmias
2. Patient's pain relieved
3. Patient's oxygen levels maintained within normal range
4. Patient understood and followed exercise and dietary restrictions
5. Patient's anxiety reduced

VI. CONGESTIVE HEART FAILURE (CHF)

A. Assessment

1. Definition/pathophysiology: CHF occurs when heart fails to pump as it should, causing congestion when blood is not adequately circulated

2. Incidence
   a. may follow myocardial infarction
   b. increases with age
3. Predisposing/precipitating factors
   a. complication of other cardiovascular disorders
      (1) myocardial infarction
      (2) hypertension
      (3) arteriosclerosis
      (4) congenital and acquired heart defects
   b. hypervolemia
4. Signs and symptoms: vary according to degree of failure
   a. heart failure may be either right or left sided; however, either will lead to complete failure
   b. left-sided heart failure
      (1) dyspnea
      (2) orthopnea
      (3) productive cough with frothy, blood-tinged sputum
      (4) rales
      (5) fatigue
      (6) anxiety
   c. right-sided heart failure
      (1) dependent edema
      (2) distended neck veins
      (3) abdominal distension
      (4) liver enlargement
      (5) nausea and vomiting
      (6) anorexia
      (7) oliguria
      (8) weight gain
      (9) increased venous pressure
5. Diagnostic tests
   a. history and physical examination
   b. ECG
   c. arterial blood gases
   d. chest radiograph
6. Usual treatment
   a. limited activity or bed rest
   b. drug therapy
      (1) digitalis (Table 7-5)
      (2) diuretics (Table 7-3)
   c. oxygen therapy
   d. restricted sodium intake

B. Planning, Goals/ Expected Outcomes

1. Patient's cardiac workload will be reduced
2. Prescribed medications to reduce pulse rates, to reduce fluid volume, and to strengthen heart muscle will be taken
3. Oxygenation of tissues will be maintained
4. Patient and family will understand and comply with diet therapy, medication therapy, and activity

C. Implementation
(Will Vary According to Severity of Failure)

1. Monitor vital signs including apical pulse for 1 full minute before giving digitalizing drugs
2. Record intake and output (I&O)
3. Restrict fluids as ordered
4. Weigh daily
5. Monitor peripheral edema, elevate feet when sitting
6. Assess exercise tolerance
7. Provide low sodium diet (Table 7-4)
8. Explain expected outcomes of therapy
9. Listen to patient concerns
10. Teach patient and family importance of diet and exercise regimen

D. Evaluation

1. Patient's cardiac workload reduced
2. Prescribed medications taken as ordered
3. Oxygen concentration level is maintained to all tissues
4. Patient understood and complied with diet therapy, medication therapy, and activity

VII. PERIPHERAL VASCULAR DISORDERS

Chronic problems in blood vessels outside heart that cause cellular changes in these peripheral tissues, especially lower extremities

A. Arterial Vascular Disease
(Atherosclerosis Obliterans)

1. Assessment
   a. definition and pathophysiology: arterial insufficiency of lower extremities caused by atherosclerosis and usually affecting one extremity more than the other, although both are impaired.
   b. incidence: same as for arteriosclerosis
   c. predisposing/precipitating factors
      (1) atherosclerosis and all its risk factors
      (2) smoking
      (3) cold
      (4) anything causing arterial constriction
   d. signs and symptoms
      (1) all apparent below level of obstruction and dependent on extent, location, degree of occlusion, and amount of collateral circulation
      (2) pain
         (a) intermittent claudication: cramping pain brought on by exercise and relieved by rest
         (b) rest pain: burning, tingling, and numbness, noticeable at night and not associated with activity
      (3) cyanosis or pale color
      (4) skin temperature very cool to cold below level of obstruction, with potential areas of blue-black necrosis
      (5) trophic changes such as smooth, shiny, thin skin, little or no hair, and thick nails
      (6) impaired or absent peripheral pulses
   e. diagnostic tests
      (1) history and physical examination
      (2) arteriogram
      (3) Doppler studies
   f. usual treatment
      (1) disease not curable; treatment only done to relieve ischemic pain and improve blood flow
      (2) peripheral vasodilators such as Vasodilan (Table 7-1)
      (3) progressive structured exercise to increase collateral circulation
      (4) surgery
         (a) endarterectomy
         (b) femoral–popliteal bypass graft
         (c) sympathectomy
   g. complications
      (1) infection
      (2) amputation of affected part
2. Planning, goals/expected outcomes
   a. patient will have arterial blood flow maintained to lower extremities
   b. patient will not develop further injury to extremities
   c. patient will understand and comply with exercises to improve collateral circulation
3. Implementation
   a. teach patient proper vascular care (Chart 7-1)
   b. teach patient to avoid vasoconstrictors and promote vasodilatation
   c. teach patient Buerger-Allen exercises
      (1) lie with legs elevated to 45- to 90-degree angle until skin turns dead white
      (2) lower legs below level of rest of body without pressure behind knees
      (3) when legs become red, have patient lie flat for 3 to 5 minutes
4. Evaluation
   a. patient's arterial blood flow to lower extremities maintained
   b. no further tissue damage occurred
   c. patient understood and followed instructions to improve and maintain collateral circulation

CHART 7–1
INFORMATION FOR PATIENTS WITH PERIPHERAL
VASCULAR DISEASE

1. Keep warm without overheating.
2. Do not use tobacco in any form.
3. Take great care when foot is not injured. Avoid crowded places.
4. Wear wide toed shoes that cause no pressure and have adequate support for the arches.
5. Do not wear circular garters.
6. Do not sit with the knees crossed.
7. If the weight of the bedclothes is uncomfortable, use a pillow or bed cradle to hold the bedclothes off the feet.
8. Soak the feet in a basin of warm, soapy water for 5 minutes every day. Dry thoroughly, especially between the toes, by mopping, not rubbing.
9. Do not apply any medications to the feet without physician's directions.
10. If the feet are dry and scaly, rub with lanolin, olive oil, castor oil, or cold cream.
11. If feet are moist, use talcum powder.
12. Before filing nails, soak feet in warm (not hot) water for 5 minutes to soften nails. File straight across. Do not use a razor blade, knife, or scissors.
13. Proper first aid treatment is important. Consult your physician immediately for any redness, blistering, pain, or swelling.
14. Do not attempt to treat corns or calluses. Ask your physician what should be done.

Adapted from Keane, C.B. Essentials of Medical-Surgical Nursing. 2nd ed. Philadelphia, W.B. Saunders Company, 1986, p. 391.

B. Venous Disorders

1. Thrombophlebitis and embolism
   a. assessment
      (1) definition/pathophysiology:
         (a) thrombus: clump of platelet and fibrin that form clot; usually occurs as result of injury or sluggish venous blood flow, or an increase in number of platelet or red blood cells
         (b) embolus: clot that becomes dislodged and travels through circulation until it obstructs artery
      (2) predisposing/precipitating factors
         (a) venous stasis
         (b) irritation or inflammation of vein wall
         (c) long periods of standing or sitting
         (d) increased platelet or red blood cells
      (3) signs and symptoms of thrombophlebitis (embolus signs and symptoms depend on location)
         (a) positive Homan's sign
         (b) redness and heat over area
         (c) swelling and hardness over area
         (d) distension of surrounding veins
         (e) possible cyanosis
      (4) diagnostic tests
         (a) history and physical examination
         (b) arteriogram
         (c) nuclear scans
         (d) Doppler studies
      (5) usual treatment
         (a) complete bed rest
         (b) warm moist packs to affected area
         (c) anticoagulants
            (i) heparin, IV immediately for prevention of clot extension or further clot formation
            (ii) Coumadin, oral for long-term anticoagulant therapy to prevent recurrence (Table 7-7)
         (d) surgery
            (i) vein ligation to trap thrombus and prevent embolus
            (ii) plication of vena cava to filter out clots
            (iii) embolectomy to remove clot
      (6) complications
         (a) pulmonary embolus
         (b) stroke
         (c) death
   b. planning, goals/expected outcomes
      (1) patient will not develop thrombophlebitis or embolus
      (2) if patient develops thrombophlebitis, an embolus will not occur
      (3) patient will understand and comply with therapeutic regimen

c. implementation
  (1) preventative measures
    (a) avoid activities that promote venous stasis
    (b) use support stockings or antiembolic hose
    (c) exercise legs frequently when standing or sitting for long periods; do not cross legs
    (d) avoid constricting clothing
    (e) elevate legs when sitting
    (f) teach and promote all preventative measures
  (2) treatment
    (a) administer anticoagulants as ordered
    (b) apply warm moist packs to affected area
    (c) maintain bed rest
    (d) apply antiemboli stocking to unaffected leg
d. evaluation
  (1) patient did not develop thrombophlebitis or embolus due to preventative measures
  (2) if thrombophlebitis developed emboli did not result
  (3) patient followed therapeutic regimen to treat and prevent thrombophlebitis and emboli
2. Varicose veins
  a. assessment
    (1) definition/pathophysiology: enlarged, tortuous veins distended with pooled blood caused by stasis and incompetent valves
    (2) incidence: people with jobs requiring prolonged sitting or standing
    (3) predisposing/precipitating factors
      (a) obesity
      (b) prolonged sitting or standing
      (c) incompetent venous valves
      (d) multiple pregnancies
    (4) signs and symptoms
      (a) enlarged tortuous veins
      (b) fatigue and heaviness in legs after prolonged sitting or standing
      (c) dull or sharp leg pains
      (d) itching along course of vein
    (5) diagnostic tests: none common, except history and physical examination
    (6) usual treatment
      (a) external support with elastic bandages or support stockings
      (b) weight reduction
      (c) surgical therapy: vein ligation and stripping
  b. planning, goals/expected outcomes
    (1) patient will not develop varicose veins
    (2) patient will recover from surgery without complications

c. implementation
  (1) teach patient to avoid standing and sitting for prolonged periods of time
  (2) provide diet counseling for weight reduction
  (3) encourage use of support hose
d. evaluation
  (1) patient did not develop varicose veins
  (2) patient recovered from surgery without complications
3. Venous stasis ulcers
  a. assessment
    (1) definition/pathophysiology: ulcers, usually around ankles; result from venous stasis; heal slowly and often become chronic
    (2) incidence: result of chronic venous insufficiency
    (3) predisposing/precipitating factors
      (a) chronic venous stasis
      (b) prolonged sitting or standing
      (c) injury or trauma
    (4) signs and symptoms
      (a) ruddy red-brown coloration around ankles
      (b) edema
      (c) pink to reddish ulcer
    (5) usual treatment
      (a) warm, moist dressings
      (b) debridement
      (c) skin grafts to cover ulcer
  b. planning, goals/expected outcomes
    (1) patient's ulcer will heal without problems
    (2) patient will not develop further ulceration
  c. implementation
    (1) teach patient to prevent leg ulcer by wearing support hose, avoiding prolonged sitting or standing, and avoiding trauma
    (2) apply dressings and teach patient correct application technique
    (3) prevent infection
  d. evaluation
    (1) patient's ulcer healed without complications
    (2) patient's ulcer did not recur

C. Amputations

1. Assessment
  a. definitions/pathophysiology: traumatic or planned removal of upper or lower extremity
  b. predisposing/precipitating factors
    (1) peripheral vascular disease
    (2) crush injuries
    (3) malignancy
    (4) severe lacerations that disrupt circulation
    (5) any severe circulatory impairment

c. signs and symptoms
  (1) cold, cyanotic limb
  (2) with or without gangrene
  (3) decreased or absent pulses
  (4) ischemic pain
d. diagnostic tests
  (1) arteriogram
  (2) radiographs

2. Planning, goals/expected outcomes
  a. patient will be psychologically prepared for amputation
  b. patient will recover from surgery without complications
  c. patient will cope with amputation and participate in rehabilitation
  d. patient will be able to care for own stump and prosthesis

3. Implementation
  a. help patient prepare psychologically for amputation
  b. elevate stump for 24 hours postoperatively to decrease bleeding and swelling
  c. position stump to prevent flexion contractures after 24 hours
    (1) do not continue to elevate leg to prevent flexion contracture of hip and knee
    (2) position patient prone one hour out of four
  d. monitor dressing for bleeding
  e. begin rewrapping stump daily to shrink and prepare it for prosthetic fitting
  f. explain to patient about phantom limb pain
  g. offer patient emotional support
  h. begin range-of-motion exercises
  i. exercise upper extremities to increase strength
  j. support physical therapy exercises
  k. encourage patient to actively participate in rehabilitation

4. Evaluation
  a. patient adequately prepared for amputation
  b. patient recovered from surgery without complications
  c. patient coped with amputation and begins rehabilitation
  d. patient safely cares for stump and prosthesis

■ Diseases of the Blood

I. LEUKEMIA

A. Assessment

1. Definition/pathophysiology: malignant disorders of blood affecting white blood cells; classified by maturity of cells and origin of normal cells

  a. acute
    (1) preponderance of primitive cells called blasts
    (2) sudden onset with rapid progression
    (3) if remission is not achieved rapidly, death occurs
  b. chronic
    (1) predominant cells more mature
    (2) gradual onset and slow progression
    (3) more common in adults
    (4) longer survival time
  c. myeloid leukemias: arise from bone marrow
  d. lymphoid leukemias: arise from lymphatic system

2. Incidence
  a. acute more common in children
  b. most common cancer in children
  c. chronic more common in older adults

3. Predisposing/precipitating factors
  a. exposure to radiation in large doses
  b. exposure to certain chemicals such as benzene
  c. possibly viruses

4. Signs and symptoms
  a. anemia
  b. WBC may be above 50,000 with abnormal cells with certain types of leukemia
  c. severe neutropenia
  d. severe infections
  e. enlarged lymphatic tissue: liver, spleen, lymph nodes
  f. weakness and weight loss
  g. headache, confusion, central nervous system (CNS) symptoms as cells invade CNS
  h. bruising and bleeding due to low platelet counts

5. Diagnostic tests
  a. WBC, complete blood count (CBC)
  b. bone marrow aspiration
    (1) keep patient calm
    (2) apply pressure dressing to site
    (3) watch for excessive bruising or bleeding
  c. history and physical examination
  d. lymph node biopsy

6. Usual treatment
  a. chemotherapy to slow growth and produce remission of symptoms
  b. blood and platelet transfusions to maintain blood levels
  c. antibiotics to combat potential infections (Table 7-10)
  d. bone marrow transplant

7. Complications
  a. infection
  b. hemorrhage
  c. death

TABLE 7–10. Antibiotics

Class	Example	Action	Use	Common Side Effects	Nursing Implications
Penicillin	Ampicillin (Polycillin)	Bactericidal against sensitive organisms	To treat penicillin-sensitive organisms	Allergic reactions, GI upset, development of resistant organisms, anaphylaxis	Monitor for rash, check for allergy before administration, obtain C&S before starting
Aminoglycosides	Gentamicin (Garamycin), kanamycin (Kantrex)	Bactericidal	To treat gram-negative infections	Ototoxicity, nephrotoxicity, superinfections, small allergic potential	Monitor for hearing or renal changes, watch for superinfections
Cephalosporins	Cephalothin (Keflin), cephalexin (Keflex)	Bactericidal	To treat septicemia, penicillin-resistant organisms	Allergic reactions in many penicillin-sensitive patients, superinfections, nephrotoxicity, phlebitis (IV), diarrhea	Monitor for allergies, don't give with food, watch for superinfections
Tetracycline	Tetracycline (Achromycin)	Bactericidal	To treat pneumonia and bacterial diarrhea	Diarrhea, nausea, permanent discoloration of teeth and bones in children, superinfections, impaired bone growth	Monitor for allergies, don't give to children under 12 years of age or pregnant women, don't give with milk or antacids, give with enough water

C&S, culture and sensitivity; GI, gastrointestinal; IV, intravenous.

B. Planning, Goals/ Expected Outcomes

1. Patient will not suffer from life-threatening infections
2. Patient will not hemorrhage
3. Patient will have side effects of chemotherapy controlled
4. Patient will maintain ideal body weight
5. Patient and family will cope with diagnosis and possible terminal prognosis

C. Implementation

1. Protect from infection, using reverse isolation if necessary
2. Bleeding precautions, prevent trauma
   a. soft toothbrush
   b. no aspirin
   c. do not use safety razor
3. Encourage well balanced diet and teach patient nutritious foods (Chapter 5)
4. Monitor urinary function and maintain adequate hydration
5. Provide emotional support

D. Evaluation

1. Patient did not develop infection
2. Patient did not hemorrhage
3. Side effects of chemotherapy controlled
4. Patient's ideal body weight maintained
5. Patient and family coped with diagnosis

II. LYMPHOMA

A. Assessment

1. Definition/pathophysiology: cancers of cells of lymphoid system, lymphocytes and histiocytes; referred to as Hodgkin's disease or non-Hodgkin's lymphoma; tumors usually start in lymph nodes
2. Incidence
   a. more common in males
   b. peaks in early 20s and after age 50 years
3. Predisposing/precipitating factors
   a. unknown cause
   b. may be associated with virus
4. Signs and symptoms
   a. painless enlargement of lymph nodes, either in neck or groin, usually begin unilaterally and progress to bilateral
   b. generalized pruritus
   c. symptoms of pressure on organs as internal lymph nodes enlarge
   d. enlarged spleen and liver
   e. low-grade fever
   f. night sweats
   g. anemia
   h. increased WBCs
   i. weight loss
5. Diagnostic tests
   a. CBC
   b. lymph node biopsy
   c. bone marrow biopsy
   d. liver/spleen scan
   e. lymphangiogram
      (1) invasive test done by injecting radiopaque dye into lymph channels in feet and using

x-rays to visualize lymph nodes throughout abdomen
   (2) takes three or more hours to complete
   (3) top of feet remain blue from dye for up to 1 year
   (4) encourage coughing and deep breathing, because dye is excreted from body through lungs
   f. staging laparotomy to determine extent of disease
6. Usual treatment
   a. exploratory laparotomy with splenectomy and lymph node biopsy
   b. radiation therapy
   c. chemotherapy

B. Planning, Goals/ Expected Outcomes

1. Patient will have lymphoma diagnosed and treated early
2. Patient will understand diagnostic tests
3. Patient will recover from surgery without complications
4. Patient will have side effects of chemotherapy controlled
5. Patient will have side effects of radiation therapy controlled
6. Patient will maintain ideal body weight
7. Patient and family will cope with diagnosis

C. Implementation

1. Teach patient about diagnostic tests
2. Provide standard postoperative care
3. Encourage well-balanced diet and teach patient nutritious foods (see Chapter 5)
4. Provide emotional support
5. Prepare patient for radiation therapy as outpatient
6. Prepare patient for chemotherapy

D. Evaluation

1. Patient had lymphoma diagnosed and treated early
2. Patient understood diagnostic tests
3. Patient recovered from surgery without complications
4. Patient had side effects of chemotherapy controlled
5. Patient had side effects of radiation therapy controlled
6. Patient maintained ideal body weight
7. Patient and family coped with diagnosis

III. SICKLE-CELL DISEASE

A. Assessment

1. Definition/pathophysiology: hereditary disease, occurring mainly in blacks, in which hemoglobin takes on characteristic sickle shape, decreasing amount of oxygen it can carry
2. Predisposing/precipitating factors
   a. race/heredity: occurs mainly in blacks; nearly 10% of American blacks carriers of trait
   b. sometimes found in those of Mediterranean ancestry
3. Signs and symptoms
   a. anemia
   b. enlarged liver and spleen
   c. painful swollen fingers and toes (dactylitis)
   d. chronic leg ulcers
   e. cerebral infarcts, strokes
   f. aplastic anemia from overstress on bone marrow
   g. aseptic necrosis of bones
   h. vaso-occlusion
   i. renal infarcts, renal failure
   j. cholelithiasis
   k. pulmonary infarct and stasis
   l. cardiomegaly, congestive heart failure (CHF)
   m. infections
4. Diagnostic tests
   a. CBC
   b. sickle-cell prep
   c. genetic studies and history
5. Usual treatment
   a. treatment symptomatic and preventative
   b. drug therapy to combat sickling of red blood cells

B. Planning, Goals/ Expected Outcomes

1. Patient will remain in remission as long as possible
2. Patient will suffer from minimal complications
3. Patient will not develop life-threatening infections
4. Patient's pain will be controlled

C. Implementation

1. Educate patient and family about disease
2. Provide emotional support
3. Ensure adequate nutrition and hydration
4. Provide for genetic counseling
5. Prevent infections
6. Provide adequate pain medication as ordered

D. Evaluation

1. Patient remained in remission as long as possible
2. Patient developed minimal complications
3. No life-threatening infections occurred
4. Patient's pain was controlled

IV. SHOCK

A. Assessment

1. Definitions/pathophysiology: variety of causes—hemorrhagic, neurogenic, septic, vasogenic, anaphylactic, and cardiogenic—leading to cellular hypoxia and tissue necrosis
2. Predisposing/precipitating factors
   a. inadequate blood volume
   b. decreased cardiac output
   c. shift in body fluids from one compartment to another
   d. vascular collapse
   e. nervous system overstimulation
   f. exposure to allergens
3. Signs and symptoms
   a. hypotension
   b. tachycardia
   c. cold clammy skin
   d. pallor or cyanosis
   e. thirst
   f. restlessness
   g. oliguria
   h. decreasing level of consciousness
4. Usual treatment
   a. identify and reverse cause
   b. emergency situation that requires quick action to stop hemorrhage
   c. vasopressors (Table 7-11)
   d. replacement of lost volume and blood components

B. Planning, Goals/Expected Outcomes

1. Patient will not develop shock
2. Patient will have shock diagnosed and treated rapidly
3. Patient will recover from shock without long-term complications

C. Implementation

1. Assess patient frequently, monitor vital signs
2. Keep patient calm
3. Keep patient warm without overheating
4. Administer IV fluids, as ordered
5. Position patient with feet up to increase venous return if possible (modified Trendelenburg)
6. Give oxygen as ordered

D. Evaluation

1. Patient did not develop shock
2. Patient treated for shock immediately
3. Patient recovered from shock without complication

■ Pulmonary Disorders

I. PNEUMONIA

A. Assessment

1. Definition/pathophysiology: extensive inflammation of lung with consolidation of tissue as it fills with exudate
2. Predisposing/precipitating factors
   a. children or elderly
   b. weak, debilitated, chronically ill patients
   c. immobilized patients

TABLE 7–11. Vasopressors

Class	Example	Action	Use	Common Side Effects	Nursing Implications
Adrenergics	Dopamine	Cause vasoconstriction of peripheral vascular system while increasing blood flow to vital organs and kidneys	To treat shock	Hypertension, tachycardia, dizziness, headache, palpitations	Use with care in patients with hypertension, benign prostatic hypertrophy (BPH), chronic obstructive pulmonary disease (COPD), check I&O, BP

BP, blood pressure; I&O, intake and output.

d. after surgery
e. vomiting and aspiration
f. inhalation of toxins
g. trauma
h. immune suppressed patients
3. Signs and symptoms
   a. high fever, chills
   b. productive cough with rusty or blood-tinged sputum
   c. pleural pain
   d. general malaise and general weakness
   e. abnormal breath sounds
4. Diagnostic tests
   a. abnormal chest radiograph with areas of consolidation
   b. physical assessment of chest
   c. sputum culture and sensitivity
5. Usual treatment
   a. antiinfectives such as penicillin or erythromycin (Table 7-10)
   b. treatment specific to cause

B. Planning, Goals/ Expected Outcomes

1. High-risk patient will not develop pneumonia
2. Patient will recover without complications

C. Implementation

1. Control high temperatures with antipyretics
2. Maintain fluid and electrolyte balance; monitor I & O
3. Maintain good nutrition
4. Cough and deep breathe patient hourly
5. Monitor vital signs and respiratory status
6. Provide good oral hygiene
7. Preventive measures for high-risk patients
8. Suction as needed

D. Evaluation

1. High-risk patient did not develop pneumonia
2. Patient recovered without complications

II. TUBERCULOSIS (TB)

A. Assessment

1. Definition/pathophysiology
   a. infectious lung disease caused by *Mycobacterium tuberculosis*

b. characterized by encapsulated lesions containing bacilli
   c. lesions degenerate and become necrotic or heal with fibrosis and calcification
   d. disease never cured, just in remission
   e. can infect extra pulmonary sites, such as intestine, kidneys, and CNS
2. Incidence
   a. blacks, Native Americans
   b. increasing in recent years
3. Predisposing/precipitating factors
   a. not highly contagious
   b. poor living conditions, overcrowding with poor sanitation
   c. malnutrition
   d. highest rates among elderly, males, nonwhites, and immigrants
4. Signs and symptoms
   a. onset gradual
   b. cough
   c. low-grade fever in afternoon
   d. night sweats
   e. weight loss
   f. fatigue
   g. occasional hemoptysis
5. Diagnostic tests
   a. skin testing: positive test means only that person exposed to tubercle bacillus and has formed antibodies against it, not that they have active TB; further evaluation needed
   b. chest radiographs and tomograms
   c. positive sputum culture: only accurate mode of diagnosis
6. Usual treatment
   a. antitubercular agents effective almost always with combination therapy; must treat for 2 years (Table 7-12)

TABLE 7–12. Antitubercular Agents

Example	Common Side Effects	Nursing Implications
Isoniazid	Peripheral neuritis, hepatitis, hypersensitivity	Give pyridoxine, vitamin B_6 to prevent neuropathy, check liver enzymes, teach patient to take all medication for 2 years
Ethambutol	Optic neuritis, rash	Monitor color vision, monitor renal function
Rifampin	Hepatitis, febrile reaction	Turns urine red/orange, potentiates actions of other antibiotics
Streptomycin	Eighth cranial nerve damage, nephrotoxicity	Monitor hearing, use with caution in elderly, monitor renal function

b. prophylactic treatment for 1 year for those exposed and most susceptible
c. hospitalization only for diagnosis and early treatment then outpatient
d. *bacille Calmette-Guerin* (BCG) vaccine for high-risk, noninfected groups

B. Planning, Goals/Expected Outcomes

1. Patient will have diagnosis of TB made early
2. Patient will comply with drug therapy
3. TB will be in remission

C. Implementation

1. Control spread of infection through respiratory isolation until chemotherapy begun
2. Teach patient good hygiene
3. Administer medications as ordered
4. Immunize high-risk groups
5. Insure patient compliance for full course of drugs usually 1 year for prophylaxis and 2 years for treatment
6. Educate family of patient and other high-risk groups

D. Evaluation

1. Diagnosis of TB was made early
2. Patient complied with drug therapy
3. Patient experienced a remission

III. CHRONIC OBSTRUCTIVE PULMONARY DISEASE (COPD)

A. Assessment

1. Definition/pathophysiology
   a. term used to describe three diseases: asthma, bronchitis, and emphysema
   b. general pathology obstruction of small bronchioles and alveoli
   c. emphysema characterized by permanent distention of bronchioles and destruction of alveolar walls; air trapped after inhalation
2. Incidence
   a. among top ten leading causes of death in United States
   b. increasing morbidity and mortality rates directly attributable to cigarette smoking and air pollution
3. Predisposing/precipitating factors
   a. smoking
   b. air pollution
   c. genetic predisposition
   d. respiratory allergies
   e. chronic bronchitis
4. Signs and symptoms
   a. barrel chest
   b. pink skin color due to hypercapnia (high pCO_2)
   c. hypoxia (low O_2 concentration level)
   d. cough with thick, tenacious sputum or none
   e. shortness of breath and dyspnea on exertion
   f. severe activity intolerance
   g. abnormal breath sounds
5. Diagnostic tests
   a. pulmonary function tests show air trapping
   b. blood gas analysis shows CO_2 retention
   c. abnormal breath sounds and percussion of trapped air
6. Usual treatment
   a. antibiotics to prevent infections (Table 7-10)
   b. bronchodilators (Table 7-13)
   c. mucolytics and expectorants to aid in liquefying secretions
   d. oxygen in low levels for severe dyspnea; never more than 2 L/min of 20%–24% oxygen
7. Complications
   a. CHF
   b. cor pulmonale
   c. pneumonia

TABLE 7–13. Bronchodilators

Example	Action	Use	Common Side Effects	Nursing Implications
Aminophylline (Aminodur)	Relaxes bronchial smooth muscle and inhibits release of histamine, mild diuretics and cardiac stimulants	To treat asthma and bronchial spasms	GI upset, nervousness, frequency, diarrhea, insomnia, tachycardia, palpitations	Use with care in patients with hypertension, glaucoma, BPH and diabetes, monitor for CNS symptoms, give with food to decrease GI upset, avoid smoking

BPH, benign prostatic hypertrophy; CNS, central nervous system; GI, gastrointestinal.

B. Planning, Goals/ Expected Outcomes

1. Patient will maintain pO$_2$ of at least 60 mm Hg
2. Patient will maintain maximal activity level
3. Patient will remain free from infection
4. Patient will comply with therapy, especially avoiding respiratory irritants
5. Patient will stop smoking cigarettes

C. Implementation

1. Teach patient:
   a. to avoid respiratory irritants, especially cigarette smoking
   b. pursed lip and diaphragmatic breathing
   c. to drink plenty of fluids unless contradicted
   d. to eat multiple small meals a day rather than three large ones
   e. to avoid persons with infections
   f. to avoid over-the-counter drugs, especially antihistamines
2. Help patient to maintain optimal health status
3. Include family in educational programs
4. Achieve balance of rest and activity

D. Evaluation

1. Patient's pO$_2$ remained above 60 mm Hg
2. Patient remained active within limits of disease
3. Patient remained infection free
4. Patient complied with therapy and stopped cigarette smoking

IV. LUNG CANCER

A. Assessment

1. Definition/pathophysiology
   a. no early signs and symptoms
   b. less than 5% 5-year survival
   c. often widely metastatic at diagnosis
2. Incidence
   a. more common in men than women, although number of women is increasing dramatically
   b. most common cancer
   c. leading cause of cancer deaths
3. Predisposing/precipitating factors
   a. smoking
   b. air pollution
   c. usually over age 40 years
4. Signs and symptoms
   a. no early signs or symptoms
   b. cough, especially early morning
   c. late symptoms
      (1) chest pain
      (2) exertional dyspnea
      (3) hemoptysis
      (4) compression on surrounding areas
5. Diagnostic tests
   a. sputum cytology
   b. chest radiograph
   c. bronchoscopy: nursing responsibilities
      (1) patient NPO for 8 to 10 hours pretest
      (2) after test, NPO until gag reflex returns
      (3) check for gag reflex with tongue blade at back of throat before allowing food or fluids
      (4) monitor for bleeding or respiratory distress
   d. mediastinoscopy
   e. thoracentesis
   f. needle biopsy
   g. open biopsy
   h. lung scan
6. Usual treatment
   a. surgical resection
      (1) wedge resection
      (2) lobectomy
      (3) pneumonectomy
   b. chemotherapy
   c. radiation therapy
   d. immunotherapy

B. Planning, Goals/ Expected Outcomes

1. Patient will cope with diagnosis and potentially terminal nature of disease
2. Patient will understand diagnostic tests
3. Patient will recover from surgery without complications
4. Patient will have side effects of chemotherapy controlled
5. Patient will have side effects of radiation therapy controlled
6. Patient and family will cope with diagnosis

C. Implementation

1. Assist patient through diagnostic work-up
2. Provide emotional support
3. Request clergy or other counselors as needed
4. Monitor for postoperative complications (see "Chest Surgery," p.146)
5. Teach patient to avoid infections
6. Help patient cope with radiation or chemotherapy

D. Evaluation

accepted diagnosis and copes with poten-
rminal nature of disease
2. Patient recovered from surgery without complication
3. Patient had side effects of chemotherapy controlled
4. Patient had side effects of radiation therapy controlled
5. Patient and family coped with diagnosis

V. CHEST SURGERY

A. Preoperative Preparation

1. Assess respiratory status and function
2. Teach patient postoperative exercises, especially
breathing exercises
3. Teach patient special exercises to strengthen shoulder muscles and improve breathing efficiency

B. Postoperative Care

1. Position for maximum ventilation, drainage, and
comfort
   a. do not allow patient to lie on unaffected side
   after pneumonectomy
   b. position patient on unaffected side after all
   other chest surgery
   c. prevent tension pneumothorax and mediastinal
   shift by maintaining patency of chest tubes
   d. prevent rupture of bronchial stump
2. Monitor function of chest tubes (Fig. 7-1)
   a. do not allow tubing to become kinked
   b. do not empty bottle if it becomes full of drainage; notify doctor
   c. never raise drainage bottle above level of chest
   d. do not clamp tube unless specifically ordered
   for short periods of time; can cause tension
   pneumothorax
   e. do not dislodge tubes
   f. watch for fluctuation of water level with respiration or bubbling in water seal bottle until
   negative pressure is restored
   g. monitor rate of fluid drainage; no more than 100
   to 150 mL/hour is normal first few days
   h. monitor for occurrence of subcutaneous emphysema
   i. tape junctions of tubing to prevent leakage
   j. milk or strip only if specifically ordered
3. Apply occlusive dressing as tubes are removed
4. Monitor respiratory status, especially return of
breath sounds as lung reexpands
5. Check vital signs frequently

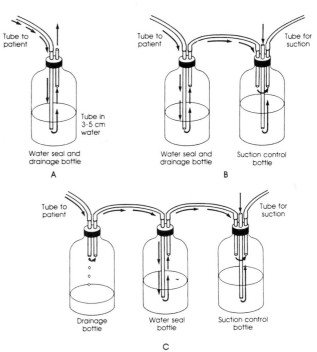

FIGURE 7–1. One-, two-, and three-bottle methods for providing a closed drainage system. *A,* In the one-bottle system, the drainage from the chest tube enters the bottle through the glass tube that has one end submerged under water to form a seal. This provides a one-way valve that prevents a backflow of air into the pleural cavity, which could collapse the lung. As fluid and air from the pleural cavity enter the drainage bottle, the air that is displaced in the bottle is vented through the short tube above water level. *B,* The second bottle in the two-bottle system acts as a trap to control and decrease the amount of suction within the chest tube. Otherwise, the suction might be too forceful and damage the pleural membrane. No drainage enters this bottle. Its only purpose is to control the force of suction applied. *C,* The third bottle in the three-bottle system also is used to regulate the amount of suction. This can be done by adjusting the length of the glass tube that is under water. (From Keane, C.B.: Essentials of Medical-Surgical Nursing. 2nd ed. Philadelphia, W.B. Saunders Company, 1986.)

VI. LARYNGEAL CANCER

A. Assessment

1. Definition/pathophysiology: common malignancy
of head and neck; may affect glottis, supra glottis,
or true cords
2. Incidence
   a. more common in men than women
   b. highest among smokers and drinkers
   c. increases after age 50 years
3. Predisposing/precipitating factors
   a. cigarette smoking and alcohol ingestion
   b. voice abuse
   c. may be associated with bronchiogenic cancer

4. Signs and symptoms
   a. hoarseness only early symptom
   b. late
      (1) pain
      (2) dysphagia
      (3) lymphadenopathy in throat
      (4) feeling of lump in throat
5. Diagnostic tests
   a. direct examination with laryngoscopy
   b. computed tomography (CT) scan of neck
   c. laryngogram
   d. biopsy
6. Usual treatment
   a. depends on stage of disease and spread
   b. radiation therapy: preoperatively, postoperatively, or instead of surgery in high-risk or elderly patients
   c. surgery
      (1) partial laryngectomy
      (2) hemilaryngectomy
      (3) total laryngectomy and tracheostomy with or without radical neck dissection
      (4) laryngoplasty after resection

B. Planning, Goals/ Expected Outcomes

1. Patient will understand diagnostic tests
2. Patient will be physically and psychologically prepared for surgery
3. Patient will recover from surgery without complications
4. Patient will learn acceptable, alternate form of communication
5. Patient will understand and tolerate radiation therapy without complications
6. Patient will cope with altered body image
7. Patient will maintain adequate nutritional status
8. Patient will be free from pain
9. Patient and significant others will cope with terminal prognosis

C. Implementation

1. Preoperative
   a. allow verbalization of fears
   b. establish alternate form of communication
   c. provide meticulous mouth care
   d. provide adequate nutritional intake
      (1) liquids
      (2) enteral nutrition
      (3) hyperalimentation
   e. prepare patient for preoperative radiation therapy
      (1) provide skin care as needed
      (2) provide artificial saliva for decreased salivation
2. Postoperative
   a. suction as needed through mouth or tracheostomy
   b. monitor for hemorrhage
   c. remove nasal crusts
   d. frequent mouth care
   e. maintain tube feedings or hyperalimentation as ordered
   f. monitor closely for tracheal-esophageal fistula formation
   g. medicate for pain frequently
   h. position in semi-Fowler's for maximal chest expansion
   i. ambulate early and encourage deep breathing to prevent pneumonia
   j. monitor wound drainage carefully
   k. offer support and encourage client to express grief
   l. teach patient stoma care
   m. suction as needed
   n. clean inner cannula as needed
   o. keep extra tracheostomy tube and obturator at bedside in case of emergency
   p. always use two people to change ties on tracheostomy tube
   q. teach patient to cover stoma when coughing
   r. suggest use of light, porous covering over healed stoma
   s. teach safety precautions
      (1) avoid showers
      (2) wear Medic Alert bracelet stating "Neck Breather"
   t. encourage patient to stop cigarette smoking and alcohol consumption
   u. encourage patient to work on alternate speech method

D. Evaluation

1. Patient recovered from surgery without complications
2. Patient learned alternate form of communication
3. Patient recovered from radiation therapy without complications
4. Patient coped with altered body image
5. Patient's nutritional status is adequate
6. Patient's pain is controlled
7. Patient and significant others cope with potentially terminal prognosis

■ Cardiopulmonary Resuscitation

I. ASSESSMENT: *A, B, C*

A. *Airway*

1. Look and listen for signs of distress
2. Check mouth and throat for obstruction

B. *Breathing*

1. Listen and feel for breathing
2. Look for chest movement
3. Note rate and quality of respirations

C. *Circulation*

1. Check for presence and strength of carotid pulse
2. Monitor rate and quality of pulse

D. Level of Consciousness

1. Degree of orientation
2. Responsiveness

E. Pupils

1. Check for size and shape
2. Monitor for response to light

II. IMPLEMENTATION

A. Restore Airway

1. Clear mouth and throat
2. Head tilt–chin lift maneuver if no sign of spinal injury: if neck injury suspected, use jaw-thrust maneuver
3. Two full breaths
4. Monitor chest for movement

B. Restore Circulation

1. Compress heart by pressing over lower sternum
2. If single rescuer, compression 15 times at first, then at rate of two breaths to 15 compressions
3. If two rescuers, rate of one breath to five compressions

III. EVALUATION

A. Stop When Patient Returns to Spontaneous Respiration and Heart Beat

B. Stop When Another Rescuer Takes Over

C. Stop When You Are Exhausted

D. Stop When Patient Pronounced Dead

■ Fluid and Electrolyte Balance

I. NORMAL FLUID BALANCE

Fluid intake and output should be equal, homeostasis (average intake and output is about 2500 mL/day)

A. Fluid Intake

1. Water in food and beverages makes up about 90% of total intake
   a. drinking water and beverages account for about 60% of intake or 1500 cc
   b. fluids in moist foods accounts for about 1000 cc or 30% of intake
2. Water metabolism makes up about 10% of intake or 250 mL; result of byproducts of oxidative metabolism of various nutrients

B. Fluid Output

Environmental factors, such as temperature and relative humidity and amount of physical exercise, will influence output

1. Fluid loss in urine about 1500 mL/day
2. Fluid loss in water vapor from exhaled air via lungs about 700 mL
3. Fluid loss by perspiration about 150 mL
4. Fluid loss via feces 150 mL

C. Regulation of Fluid Intake

1. Thirst primary regulator of water intake
2. Thirst center located in hypothalamus
3. Receptors in thirst center sensitive to water loss

and cause person to feel thirsty and seek water; with water loss, osmotic pressure of extracellular fluid increases and osmoreceptors in hypothalamus stimulated

D. Regulation of Fluid Output

1. Some water loss is related to body functions and largely unavoidable
   a. water loss via perspiration is a necessary part of body's temperature control mechanism
   b. water lost in feces via undigested food wastes
   c. water lost via evaporation from lungs and diffusion through skin not easily controlled
2. Urine production primary regulator of fluid output
   a. antidiuretic hormone (ADH) from the pituitary controls water loss through urine
   b. ADH secretion is inhibited with increased fluid intake, leading to increased urine output
   c. ADH secretion is stimulated when fluid intake is low, leading to decreased urine output
   d. diuretics may be prescribed to increase urine output
   e. natural diuretics include coffee, tea, and alcohol

E. Distribution of Body Water

1. Intracellular: fluid contained within all cells; represents 75% of total body water; contains large amounts of potassium, phosphate, and protein
2. Extracellular: fluid not contained inside cell; represents 25% of total body water; contains large amounts of sodium, chloride, and bicarbonate ions

F. Fluid Dynamics

Movement of fluid from one compartment to another via the following dynamics

1. Diffusion: movement of substance from area of high concentration to one of low concentration
2. Active transport: transport of substances across membrane from area of low concentration to one of high concentration; requires energy expenditure
3. Osmosis: movement of water across semipermeable membrane into solution with high solute concentration
4. Filtration: passage of fluid through semipermeable membrane as result of difference in hydrostatic pressure

G. Additional Concepts

1. Sodium attracts water; a concentration of sodium anywhere in the body attracts water until sodium is diluted to "normal" concentration
2. If there is a high level of sodium in plasma, blood volume increases because water is drawn into capillaries to dilute sodium
3. If there is a high level of sodium in interstitial fluid, water is attracted to dilute sodium, resulting in edema
4. If concentration of ions in either intracellular or extracellular spaces changes, water will shift from an area of low concentration to an area of high concentration until concentrations are equal; shift shrinks or expands respective spaces

■ Fluid Imbalances

I. EDEMA

A. Assessment

1. Definition/pathophysiology: abnormal accumulation of fluid in interstitial spaces of tissues; third space
2. Incidence: occurs whenever there is shift of fluids to third space
3. Predisposing/precipitating factors: multiple medical/surgical conditions may cause edema, including
   a. renal failure
   b. congestive heart failure
   c. cirrhosis
   d. corticosteroid therapy
   e. excessive salt intake
   f. hypertension
4. Types of edema
   a. pitting edema: tissues hold indentation made by pressure of fingertips for as long as 10 minutes (volume of interstitial fluid increased)
   b. localized edema: fluid drawn to site of injury, insect bite, burn, or other trauma
   c. generalized or dependent edema: affected by gravity
      (1) facial edema develops if patient is in a prone position
      (2) sacral and shoulder edema occurs when patient is on bed rest in a supine position
      (3) dependent edema of lower extremities occurs when patient has been sitting or standing for long periods of time
5. Signs and symptoms
   a. full bounding pulse
   b. tachycardia

c. jugular vein distention
d. increased arterial and central venous blood pressure (CVP)
e. rapid weight gain
f. peripheral, dependent edema
g. tachypnea, dyspnea, or cyanosis
h. if severe, pulmonary edema
6. Diagnostic tests
   a. CBC
   b. serum electrolytes
   c. daily weights
7. Usual treatment
   a. correction of underlying problem if possible
   b. diuretics (Table 7-3)
   c. low sodium diet (Table 5-3)

B. Planning, Goals/ Expected Outcomes

1. Patient will comply with treatment plan
2. Patient will identify and avoid high sodium foods
3. Patient will be free of edema

C. Implementation

1. Monitor intake and output
2. Observe and record signs and symptoms of edema
3. Weigh patient daily: same time, same scale, same clothes, and same nurse if possible
4. Instruct patient to avoid high sodium foods
5. Administer diuretics as prescribed, such as Lasix and hydrochlorothiazide (Table 7-3)
6. Elevate extremities when sitting to decrease edema
7. Assess breath sounds for presence of fluid rales

D. Evaluation

1. Patient complied with treatment plan
2. Patient identified and avoided high sodium foods
3. Patient free of edema

II. DEHYDRATION

A. Assessment

1. Definition/pathophysiology: excessive loss of water from body tissues
2. Predisposing/precipitating factors
   a. decreased intake of water and electrolytes
   b. loss of water and electrolytes via severe vomiting or diarrhea
   c. hemorrhage
   d. severe burns

3. Signs and symptoms
   a. thirst
   b. loss of skin turgor
   c. cracked lips and dry mucous membranes
   d. decreased urine output (normal output 30 mL/ hour)
   e. concentrated urine: dark amber color and odorous
   f. low central venous pressure
   g. orthostatic hypotension
   h. severe dehydration may result in hypotension, stupor, and marked oliguria
4. Diagnostic tests
   a. CBC
   b. serum electrolytes
   c. 24-hour urine output
5. Usual treatment
   a. oral fluid replacement if dehydration is mild
   b. isotonic IV fluids, such as Ringer's lactate, if dehydration is severe

B. Planning, Goals/ Expected Outcomes

1. Patient will recognize symptoms of dehydration
2. Patient will maintain adequate oral intake
3. Patient will remain well hydrated

C. Implementation

1. Administer IV fluids as ordered
2. Encourage adequate oral fluid intake
3. Closely monitor intake and output
4. Observe, record, and report signs and symptoms of dehydration
5. Attempt to identify cause of dehydration

D. Evaluation

1. Patient recognized symptoms of dehydration
2. Patient maintained adequate oral intake
3. Patient remained well hydrated

■ Electrolyte Imbalances

I. HYPERNATREMIA

Normal serum sodium 135 to 145 mEq/L

A. Assessment

1. Definition/pathophysiology: serum sodium elevated above 145 mEq/L

2. Predisposing/precipitating factors
   a. increased salt intake without increase in water intake
   b. loss of water without loss of sodium
   c. profuse, watery diarrhea
   d. severe burns
   e. dehydration
3. Signs and symptoms
   a. pitting edema
   b. excessive weight gain; more than 2 lb/day
   c. dyspnea
   d. increased blood pressure
   e. symptoms of dehydration
4. Diagnostic tests
   a. CBC
   b. serum electrolytes
   c. urinary electrolytes
5. Usual treatment
   a. correct cause of imbalance
   b. limit sodium intake
   c. limit water intake

B. Planning, Goals/ Expected Outcomes

1. Patient's serum sodium will return to normal
2. Patient will not have further problems with excessive sodium

C. Implementation

1. Record intake and output
2. Help identify cause of imbalance
3. Restrict sodium intake (Tables 7-4 and 5-3)
4. Restrict fluids

D. Evaluation

1. Patient's serum sodium returned to normal
2. Patient had no further problems with excessive sodium

II. HYPONATREMIA

A. Assessment

1. Definition/pathophysiology: serum sodium less than 135 mEq/L
2. Predisposing/precipitating factors
   a. diuretics, sodium wasting
   b. profuse diaphoresis
   c. excessive water intake without sodium
   d. excessive gastrointestinal losses

3. Signs and symptoms
   a. mental confusion
   b. restlessness
   c. weakness
   d. muscle twitching
   e. abdominal cramping
   f. if severe: convulsions, coma, and death
4. Diagnostic tests
   a. CBC
   b. serum electrolytes
   c. urine electrolytes
5. Usual treatment
   a. correct cause of imbalance
   b. oral administration of sodium (salt water, salt tablets, or foods high in sodium) with great care
   c. IV administration of isotonic (0.9%) sodium chloride or Ringer's lactate

B. Planning, Goals/ Expected Outcomes

1. Patient's serum sodium will return to normal
2. Patient will not develop further problems with low sodium

C. Implementation

1. Administer oral sodium as ordered
2. Maintain accurate intake and output
3. Monitor IV fluids carefully
4. Monitor patient's vital signs and fluid balance when replacing sodium

D. Evaluation

1. Patient's serum sodium returned to normal
2. Patient had no further problems with low sodium

III. HYPERKALEMIA

Normal serum potassium 3.5 to 5.0 mEq/L

A. Assessment

1. Definition/pathophysiology: serum potassium more than 5.0 mEq/L
2. Predisposing/precipitating factors
   a. renal failure (unable to excrete potassium)
   b. severe burns or crush injuries (cell destruction releases intracellular potassium)
   c. adrenal insufficiency

d. overuse of salt substitutes containing potassium
e. increased intake of potassium orally through foods or medication
3. Signs and symptoms
   a. diarrhea/nausea
   b. muscle weakness/flaccid paralysis
   c. cardiac arrhythmias
   d. if severe and uncorrected, cardiac arrest may occur
4. Diagnostic tests
   a. CBC
   b. serum electrolytes
   c. urinary electrolytes
5. Usual treatment
   a. correct cause of imbalance
   b. decreased potassium intake if mild (Tables 7-9 and 5-4)
   c. if severe: Kayexalate orally or enemas (cation-exchange resin) or dialysis

B. Planning, Goals/ Expected Outcomes

1. Patient's serum potassium will return to normal
2. Patient will not have further problems with excessive potassium

C. Implementation

1. Monitor intake and output
2. Maintain cardiac monitoring
3. Check pulse carefully for arrhythmias
4. Observe character and rate of respirations
5. Administer Kayexalate orally or per enema as ordered

D. Evaluation

1. Patient's serum potassium level returned to normal
2. Patient had no further problems with excessive potassium

IV. HYPOKALEMIA

A. Assessment

1. Definition/pathophysiology: serum potassium less than 3.5 mEq/L
2. Predisposing/precipitating factors
   a. diuretics, potassium wasting
   b. loss of fluid from gastrointestinal tract

(1) vomiting
(2) diarrhea
(3) nasogastric (NG) tubes
3. Signs and symptoms
   a. fatigue, weakness
   b. anorexia leading to nausea/vomiting
   c. cardiac arrhythmias
   d. severe hypokalemia may result in hypotension, flaccid paralysis, and death due to cardiac arrest
4. Diagnostic tests
   a. CBC
   b. serum electrolytes
   c. urinary electrolytes
5. Usual treatment
   a. correct cause of imbalance
   b. increase oral potassium intake: potassium rich foods or oral potassium salts (Tables 7-9 and 5-4)
   c. IV administration of potassium salt, such as potassium chloride (KCl); IV potassium always given in diluted solution because undiluted injection of KCl would always be fatal

B. Planning, Goals/ Expected Outcomes

1. Patient's serum potassium will return to normal
2. Patient will not have further problems with low potassium

C. Implementation

1. Administer oral potassium as ordered
2. Maintain accurate intake and output
3. Monitor IV fluids carefully
4. Monitor patient vital signs and fluid balance when replacing potassium
5. Monitor pulse carefully for arrhythmias

D. Evaluation

1. Patient's serum potassium returned to normal
2. Patient had no further problems with low potassium

V. HYPERCALCEMIA

Normal serum calcium, 9 to 11 mg/dL

A. Assessment

1. Definition/pathophysiology: serum calcium greater than 11 mg/dL

2. Predisposing/precipitating factors
   a. excess doses of vitamin D
   b. prolonged immobilization
   c. hyperparathyroidism
   d. excessive calcium intake
   e. many types of cancer
3. Signs and symptoms
   a. deep bone pain
   b. anorexia, nausea, vomiting
   c. polyuria, polydypsia
   d. mental changes, lethargy
   e. if chronic, may result in kidney stones
4. Diagnostic tests
   a. CBC
   b. serum electrolytes
   c. urine electrolytes
5. Usual treatment
   a. correct cause of imbalance
   b. mild hypercalcemia treated by forcing fluids and limiting oral calcium intake
   c. acute or severe hypercalcemia treated by administering IV sodium chloride plus diuretics, such as furosemide, to increase calcium excretion in urine

B. Planning, Goals/ Expected Outcomes

1. Patient's serum calcium will return to normal
2. Patient will not have further problems with high calcium

C. Implementation

1. Limit oral calcium intake
2. Monitor intake and output
3. Observe and report mental changes or lethargy
4. Monitor for signs and symptoms of kidney stones

D. Evaluation

1. Patient's serum calcium returned to normal
2. Patient had no further problems with high calcium

VI. HYPOCALCEMIA

A. Assessment

1. Definition/pathophysiology: serum calcium less than 9 mg/dL
2. Predisposing/precipitating factors
   a. burns

b. acute pancreatitis
   c. surgical removal of parathyroid glands
   d. hypoparathyroidism
3. Signs and symptoms
   a. numbness and tingling of fingers and toes and area around mouth (circumoral paresthesia)
   b. muscle and abdominal cramping
   c. carpopedal spasms, tetany
   d. convulsions
4. Diagnostic tests
   a. CBC
   b. serum electrolytes
   c. urinary electrolytes
5. Usual treatment
   a. correct cause of imbalance
   b. administer calcium orally
   c. administer IV calcium salts, such as calcium gluconate

B. Planning, Goals/ Expected Outcomes

1. Patient's serum calcium will return to normal
2. Patient will not have further problems with low calcium

C. Implementation

1. Administer oral or IV calcium as ordered
2. Maintain accurate intake and output
3. Observe seizure precautions (padded side rails up, padded tongue blade at bedside) until calcium deficit corrected
4. Check for early signs of tetany

D. Evaluation

1. Patient's serum calcium returned to normal
2. Patient had no further problems with low calcium

■ Acid–Base Imbalances

Decreased arterial pH indicates state of acidosis that may be of either metabolic or respiratory origin; in metabolic acidosis, serum bicarbonate level below normal; in respiratory acidosis, pCO_2 elevated; increased arterial pH indicates state of alkalosis that may be either metabolic or respiratory; in metabolic alkalosis, serum bicarbonate level above normal; in respiratory alkalosis, pCO_2 decreased

I. RESPIRATORY ACIDOSIS

A. Assessment

1. Definition/pathophysiology: condition in which arterial blood pH below 7.35 caused by retention of CO_2 that combines with H_2O to form carbonic acid (H_2CO_3)
2. Predisposing/precipitating factors
   a. hypoventilation
   b. acute pulmonary edema
   c. aspiration
   d. pneumonia
   e. pneumothorax
   f. oversedation
   g. COPD
   h. ascites
3. Signs and symptoms
   a. headache
   b. increased pulse, blood pressure, respirations
   c. mental cloudiness
   d. weakness
   e. symptoms of increased intracranial pressure
   f. cardiac arrhythmias
4. Diagnostic tests
   a. history and physical examination to determine underlying cause
   b. blood gas, pH, and electrolyte levels
5. Usual treatment
   a. reversal of cause
   b. improvement of ventilation
   c. bronchodilators (Table 7-13)
   d. pulmonary hygiene
   e. oxygen and mechanical ventilation if acute
6. Complications
   a. cardiac arrhythmias from elevated serum potassium
   b. hypotension
   c. congestive heart failure
   d. shock
   e. increased intracranial pressure from vasodilatory effect of CO_2 on cerebral blood vessels

B. Planning, Goals/Expected Outcomes

1. Patient will have adequate ventilation
2. Patient will not develop complications from respiratory acidosis
3. Patient will not develop complications from oxygen therapy

C. Implementation

1. Specific implementations depend on cause of ventilatory impairment; the following are general measures to increase ventilation
   a. establish patent airway
   b. administer mechanical ventilatory aids as prescribed
   c. facilitate removal of tracheobronchial secretions by teaching and encouraging patient to cough and deep breathe, taking in adequate fluids
   d. prevent respiratory infections
2. Administer antibiotics or bronchodilators
3. Monitor patient's blood gases and signs and symptoms of worsening hypoventilation and acidosis
4. administer prescribed drugs, such as sodium bicarbonate, if necessary to neutralize excess acid
5. Administer oxygen cautiously, especially to patients with COPD, in order to increase tissue oxygenation without causing respiratory depression
   a. monitor for signs of CO_2 narcosis, such as respiratory depression, decreasing level of sensorium, cardiac arrhythmias
   b. monitor for signs of oxygen toxicity, such as pulmonary edema, presence of blood in tracheobronchial secretions

D. Evaluation

1. Patient effectively coughed and deep breathed
2. Blood gases normal
3. Patient showed no signs of respiratory distress
4. Patient had no evidence of CO_2 narcosis, O_2 toxicity, or rebound respiratory alkalosis

II. RESPIRATORY ALKALOSIS

A. Assessment

1. Definition/pathophysiology: condition in which arterial blood pH greater than 7.45 caused by a decrease in pCO_2 secondary to increased alveolar ventilation
2. Predisposing/precipitating factors
   a. anxiety
   b. hysteria
   c. early salicylate intoxication
   d. gram-negative septicemia
   e. mechanical ventilators
3. Signs and symptoms
   a. lightheadedness
   b. inability to concentrate

c. numbness and tingling of fingertips and around mouth
d. tinnitus
e. fainting
4. Diagnostic tests
  a. history and physical to determine underlying cause
  b. blood gas, pH, and electrolyte levels
5. Usual treatment
  a. rebreather bag
  b. sedation
6. Complications
  a. tetany, convulsions
  b. hypokalemia
  c. dizziness and fainting

B. Planning, Goals/ Expected Outcomes

1. Underlying cause of respiratory alkalosis will be identified and eliminated
2. Patient's acid–base balance will be restored
3. Patient will be free from complications of treatment for respiratory alkalosis

C. Implementation

1. Specific interventions dependent on cause
  a. salicylate abuse: instruct patient regarding appropriate use of aspirin
  b. anxiety reaction: assist patient to recognize and cope with situations that provoke anxiety; teach patient to take slow deep breaths or temporarily hold breath in situations that precipitate hyperventilation; breathe into paper bag
  c. mechanical ventilation: monitor ventilatory settings and patient's blood gases and electrolytes
2. Administer rebreathing mask, prescribed sedatives, or 5% CO_2 for inhalation
3. Maintain seizure precautions
4. Monitor blood gases and electrolytes during treatment to detect overshoot metabolic acidosis

D. Evaluation

1. Underlying cause of patient's respiratory alkalosis identified and corrected
2. Patient's blood pH, HCO_3^-/H_2CO_3, and electrolytes within normal limits; no signs or symptoms of alkalosis
3. Patient did not sustain injuries
4. Patient showed no evidence of overshoot metabolic acidosis

III. METABOLIC ACIDOSIS

A. Assessment

1. Definition/pathophysiology: condition in which arterial blood pH below 7.35; caused by either accumulation of fixed (nonvolatile) acid or base deficit
2. Predisposing/precipitating factors
  a. diabetic ketoacidosis
  b. lactic acidosis
  c. late salicylate poisoning
  d. uremia
  e. starvation
  f. diarrhea from intestinal fistula
  g. administration of large quantities of isotonic saline or ammonium chloride
3. Signs and symptoms
  a. headache
  b. confusion
  c. drowsiness
  d. Kussmaul's respiration: rapid and deep breathing
  e. nausea/vomiting
4. Diagnostic tests
  a. history and physical examination to determine underlying cause
  b. blood gas, pH, and electrolyte levels
5. Usual treatment: dependent on cause
6. Complications
  a. fluid and electrolyte loss from vomiting and diarrhea
  b. cardiac arrhythmias from elevated serum potassium
  c. hypotension
  d. congestive heart failure

B. Planning, Goals/ Expected Outcomes

1. Underlying cause of the patient's metabolic acidosis will be identified
2. Patient's acid–base balance will be restored
3. Patient will not develop complications from metabolic acidosis
4. Patient will not develop complications from the therapy for metabolic acidosis

C. Implementation

1. Specific implementations depend on underlying cause
  a. diabetic ketoacidosis: administer prescribed insulin, fluids, and potassium; instruct patient on insulin and diet therapy

b. renal tubular disease: replace bicarbonate kidneys unable to reabsorb
c. lactic acidosis: improve tissue perfusion via cardiovascular support
2. If therapy of underlying cause will not reverse acidosis rapidly enough, administer prescribed drugs, such as sodium bicarbonate or sodium lactate, to neutralize acid
3. Monitor I & O; replace fluid and electrolytes lost from vomiting, diarrhea, or osmotic diuresis
4. Monitor patient for manifestations of overshoot metabolic alkalosis; monitor for manifestations of hypokalemia, because as acidosis is corrected, potassium reenters cells; administer prescribed potassium supplements

D. Evaluation

1. Underlying cause of metabolic acidosis identified
2. Patient's blood pH and HCO_3^-/H_2CO_3 and urine pH normal; no signs or symptoms of metabolic acidosis
3. Patient had no evidence of fluid or electrolyte imbalance
4. Patient had not sustained injuries

IV. METABOLIC ALKALOSIS

A. Assessment

1. Definition/pathophysiology: condition in which arterial blood pH greater than 7.45 caused by either loss of acid or gain of base
2. Predisposing/precipitating factors
   a. vomiting or gastric suctioning
   b. potassium loss
   c. hyperaldosteronism and Cushing's syndrome
   d. excessive ingestion of alkali
3. Signs and symptoms
   a. tingling in fingers and toes
   b. dizziness
   c. hypertonic muscles
   d. depressed respirations
4. Diagnostic tests
   a. history and physical to determine underlying causes
   b. blood gas, pH, and electrolyte levels

5. Usual treatment
   a. reverse underlying disorder
   b. administer sodium chloride IV
6. Complications
   a. respiratory depression from blunting of respiratory drive caused by H^+ deficiency
   b. tetany, convulsions
   c. hypokalemia

B. Planning, Goals/ Expected Outcomes

1. Underlying cause of metabolic alkalosis will be identified
2. Patient's acid–base balance will be restored
3. Patient will be free from complications from therapy for metabolic alkalosis

C. Implementation

1. Specific implementations depend on the underlying cause
   a. excessive ingestion of sodium bicarbonate: instruct patient regarding appropriate use of sodium bicarbonate-containing drugs
   b. chloride loss: administer prescribed chloride replacements
   c. potassium deficit: administer prescribed potassium supplements, encourage foods high in potassium
2. If treatment of underlying cause will not reverse alkalosis rapidly enough, administer prescribed acidifying drugs, such as ammonium chloride or Diamox
3. Observe seizure precautions
4. Monitor blood gases and electrolytes during therapy to detect overshoot metabolic acidosis

D. Evaluation

1. Underlying cause of metabolic alkalosis identified
2. Patient's blood pH, HCO_3^-/H_2CO_3 normal
3. No evidence of overshoot metabolic acidosis
4. Patient's serum potassium within normal limits

Questions

1. Fatty materials deposited within the arteries is termed:

① Hypercholesterolemia
② Ankylosis
③ Atherosclerosis
④ Hyperuricemia

Mr. Anthony is 60 years old with a 5-year history of emphysema. He is admitted to the hospital for pneumonia, with a chief complaint of shortness of breath and congestion.

2. Using Maslow's Hierarchy of Needs, the most basic need of Mr. Anthony at this point in time would be:

① Safety
② Air
③ Self-esteem
④ Food

3. An important problem at this point in Mr. Anthony's care would be:

① Altered nutritional status due to inability to swallow
② Potential for depression secondary to chronic illness
③ Inadequate oxygenation due to chronic lung disease
④ Impaired circulation secondary to congestive heart failure

4. His wife reports that he usually sleeps on two or three pillows at home. Which of the following nursing interventions is most appropriate based on this information?

① Have him assume the semi-Fowler's position for sleep
② Allow him to sit in a chair to sleep
③ Ambulate TID with breathing exercises
④ Apply oxygen as needed for dyspnea

5. Because of his current breathing problem, Mr. Anthony is most likely to have problems with:

① Loss of consciousness
② Dehydration
③ Fatigue
④ Dementia

6. Which of the following would indicate that Mr. Anthony's problems are resolving?

① He is able to sleep through the night without nocturia
② He sits up at the bedside for meals without distress
③ He has resumed normal bowel habits
④ He ambulates the length of the hall without dyspnea

7. Based on Mr. Anthony's diagnosis of both pneumonia and emphysema, the medications most likely to have been ordered by the physician include:

① Digoxin and Lasix
② Penicillin and aminophylline
③ Digoxin and streptomycin
④ Lasix and theophylline

Ann Clark is a 65-year-old mother of three, admitted with a diagnosis of chronic leukemia. She is admitted in acute distress and seriously ill.

8. Most leukemias involve changes in the:

① Erythrocytes
② Platelets
③ Monocytes
④ Lymphocytes

9. Because of the changes in the white blood cells of a leukemic, the nurse knows to expect Mrs. Clark to demonstrate:

① Enlargement of the lymph nodes
② A lower resistance to infections
③ A greater risk of phlebitis
④ An increase in clotting activity

10. Thrombocytopenia frequently occurs in leukemia. Nursing interventions to prevent excessive bleeding include:

① Using swabs for mouth care
② Encouraging dry meals
③ Maintaining strict bed rest
④ Avoiding people with infections

11. It seems to the nurse that Mrs. Clark is often irritable and difficult to please. This is probably an indication that:

① She is very neurotic
② This is typical behavior for women of her age when hospitalized
③ This is a symptom of her illness and outside her control
④ She has not accepted her illness and needs spiritual help

Mr. Hammer was brought in through the emergency room complaining of sudden, severe chest pain while at work. He is now anxious, short of breath, and diaphoretic.

12. The doctor orders morphine sulfate to be given intravenously. The nurse knows that the purpose of this is to:

① Relieve any nausea and vomiting
② Increase the respiratory rate
③ Increase the blood circulation
④ Relieve the severe pain

13. When Mr. Hammer is stabilized 2 days later, he continues to be very apprehensive and states that he feels like he is going to die. His wife asks the nurse why he is this way and if he is going to die. The nurse should explain that:

① People who are dying often feel this way
② He is not going to die now, so she can stop worrying
③ This is usual after heart attacks and will resolve with proper reassurance
④ This is an indication that he may have suffered cerebral hypoxia during the attack

14. The doctor has ordered Coumadin to help prevent further occlusions. Nursing care should include:

① Increasing intake of iron-rich foods
② Monitoring stools for blood
③ Having protamine sulfate on hand
④ Monitoring WBCs

15. In order to prevent problems from Coumadin, Mr. Hammer should be taught to:

① Take his apical pulse daily
② Avoid sexual intercourse
③ Avoid any products containing aspirin
④ Increase his intake of potassium

16. Your patient is suffering from peripheral arterial disease. Appropriate teaching would include:

① Elevating the legs whenever possible
② Wearing support stockings
③ Applying a warm water bottle to the lower abdomen
④ Avoiding standing for any length of time

Mr. Martin is admitted with a diagnosis of congestive heart failure for the last 5 years with increasing symptoms over the last 2 days.

17. Mr. Martin has been experiencing increased edema of the ankles and lower extremities. On the basis of this, the nurse knows that his heart failure is probably:

① Right sided
② Left sided
③ Complete
④ Cor pulmonale

18. He is placed on a low sodium diet to help control the edema. Foods allowed on this diet would include:

① Fresh fruits
② Canned soups
③ Milk and cheese
④ Lunch meat

19. Mr. Martin is to be placed on medication to strengthen his heart and decrease his edema. The most likely combination of drugs would be:

① Lasix and Pronestyl
② Isuprel and digoxin
③ Digoxin and Diuril
④ Lasix and Diuril

20. Based on the above combination of drugs, what problem would predispose Mr. Martin to drug toxicity?

① Hyponatremia
② Hypercalcemia
③ Hypophosphatemia
④ Hypokalemia

21. In order to prevent drug toxicity, the nurse should teach Mr. Martin to increase his intake of:

① Milk
② Oranges
③ Fresh vegetables
④ Cheeses

22. Daily weights are ordered for Mr. Martin to monitor:

① Fluid balance
② Body fat
③ Blood volume
④ Appetite

23. Mr. Martin suddenly exhibits respiratory distress with frothy sputum. The nurse realizes that he has probably developed:

① A pulmonary embolus
② Right-sided heart failure

③ Pulmonary edema
④ Cor pulmonale

24. The nurse is ordered to apply rotating tourniquets. The most dangerous practice would involve:

① Leaving the tourniquets on for 15 minutes at a time
② Applying less pressure than needed to occlude the arteries
③ Using a blood pressure cuff to apply the pressure
④ Discontinuing the tourniquets at the same time

Mr. Wilson is an elderly gentleman brought to the hospital by his son for increasing respiratory difficulties. Mr. Wilson tells you that he has been treating himself for years and doesn't really need any of this "fancy" medicine.

25. Mr. Wilson's first test was a chest radiograph. Preparation for this test includes:

① Wearing only a hospital gown
② Nothing by mouth for 8 hours
③ A cleansing enema prior to the test
④ Injection of a dye into the trachea

26. The doctor performs a bronchoscopy on Mr. Wilson. When he returns from the test, the nurse must:

① Realize that he will not be able to speak for several hours
② Suction him frequently for the next 24 hours
③ Provide cool gargles to prevent bleeding
④ Withhold food and fluids until the gag reflex returns

27. Which of the following should be promptly reported if it occurs after the bronchoscopy?

① Blood-streaked sputum
② Swelling of the neck
③ Hoarseness
④ Discomfort when swallowing

28. The doctor orders that Mr. Wilson receive oxygen. The nurse's primary responsibility for this includes:

① Explaining the dangers of it to Mr. Wilson
② Preventing him from becoming dependent on the oxygen
③ Administering it with the same care as any medication
④ Adjusting the flow as needed based on assessments of cyanosis

29. The most accurate way to determine the need for oxygen in a patient with COPD is by:

① Observing the skin color
② Noting changes in the vital signs
③ Asking the patient how he or she feels
④ Blood gas analysis

30. Mr. Wilson has been diagnosed as having COPD. The doctor orders postural drainage. The purpose of this is to:

① Increase the blood supply to the lungs
② Strengthen the respiratory drive
③ Remove fluid from the pleural cavity
④ Remove mucus from the bronchial tree and lungs

31. The best time for the postural drainage to be done is:

① Before breakfast and dinner
② Right before visiting hours
③ Only during the night shift
④ After breakfast and lunch

32. You are teaching Mr. Wilson to cough and deep breathe effectively. You would include all of the following in your instructions *except*:

① Assume a sitting position, leaning forward slightly
② Feel the breaths distend your abdomen
③ Exhale quickly and cough forcefully
④ Splint the chest and abdomen with a pillow

33. Mr. Wilson's sputum will be:

① Thick and tenacious
② Thin and watery
③ Blood tinged and frothy
④ Highly contagious

34. Mr. Wilson is now ready for discharge and is apologizing to all the nurses about how stubborn he was when he came in. His original reluctance to enter the hospital was probably a result of:

① A bad past experience in the hospital
② His distrust of people in the medical profession
③ A fear of the unknown and anxiety about a new environment
④ His fear of dying in the hospital

35. A thoracentesis is done to remove fluids from the:

① Spaces around the alveoli
② Bronchioles and main bronchi
③ Pleural space
④ Area between the skin and the pleura

36. The most common symptom of thrombophlebitis in the lower leg is:

① Cyanosis of the affected limb
② Positive Homans' sign in the affected leg
③ Severe ankle edema in the affected leg
④ Distention of the affected vessels

37. A nursing intervention contraindicated in thrombophlebitis would be:

① Maintaining strict bedrest
② Turning the patient from side to side
③ Applying warm packs to the affected leg
④ Massaging the affected leg

38. Hypertension can be described as a disease that:

① Can be controlled with treatment
② Can be cured
③ Often disappears without treatment
④ Is usually fatal

39. The treatment for hypertension is usually directed at:

① Lowering the blood pressure to below normal levels
② Repairing the damaged blood vessels
③ Increasing the urine output
④ Preventing further damage to the blood vessels

40. Your patient has just returned from an above the knee amputation. Immediate postoperative care includes:

① Elevating the stump on several pillows
② Positioning the patient on the unaffected side
③ Leaving the stump flat on the bed with the head of the bed elevated
④ Having the patient lie in a prone position

41. The day after surgery, the best position for your patient to assume for at least one hour out of four is:

① Prone with the stump straight
② Supine with the stump elevated
③ Sitting with the stump dependent
④ Semi-Fowler's with the stump on pillows

Mr. Carter has returned from surgery for a left lobectomy for cancer of the lung.

42. The surgeon wrote an order to turn the patient to the left side and back only. This was done to:

① Facilitate expansion of the left lung
② Prevent hemorrhage
③ Reduce pain
④ Facilitate drainage from the operative area

43. Mr. Carter had a chest tube inserted. When transferring him from the cart to his bed, the nurse must be careful to:

① Disconnect the tube from the drainage bottle
② Keep the drainage bottle below the level of the chest
③ Clamp the chest tube until the patient is stable
④ Wait until the doctor is present to prevent displacement

44. If the closed chest drainage is disrupted:

① Air will enter the thoracic cavity and collapse the lung
② Air will escape the thoracic cavity and expand the lung
③ Water in the drainage bottle will flow into the pleural cavity
④ Hemorrhage will result

45. Postoperatively, frequent coughing and deep-breathing exercises are:

① Prohibited because of the severe pain
② Supervised by the surgeon only
③ Needed for adequate ventilation in the unaffected lung
④ Done only if the patient is not in too much pain

Answers & Rationales

Guide to item identification (see pp. 3–5 for further details about each category)

I, II, III, or IV for the phase of the nursing process
1, 2, 3, or 4 for the category of client needs
A, B, C, D, E, F, or G for the category of human functioning
Specific content category by name; ie, cholecystectomy

1. ③ Atherosclerosis is caused by fatty deposits in the lining of the coronary vessels.
IV, 2, B. Coronary Artery Disease.

2. ② Oxygen is one of the most basic needs for life.
I & IV, 4, B. Pneumonia.

3. ③ Oxygenation is always a priority in the basic health needs.
II, 4, B. Pneumonia.

4. ① Semi-Fowler's position allows for the best expansion of the lungs and best approximates his sleeping position at home.
III, 2, B. Pneumonia & COPD.

5. ③ Decreased oxygenation leads to fatigue.
I & IV, 2, B. Pneumonia & COPD.

6. ④ One way to assess improvement in oxygenation is through increased ability to perform activities without increasing fatigue.
IV, 2, B. Pneumonia.

7. ② Antibiotics are used to treat pneumonia, and bronchodilators are used to treat emphysema.
I & IV, 2, B & D. Pneumonia & COPD.

8. ④ Most leukemias (about 70%) involve changes in the lymphocytes.
I, 2, B. Leukemia.

9. ② The increase in the white blood cells, the leukocytes, in leukemia is misleading, because most of them are immature and therefore ineffective. The patient, therefore, has a lower resistance to infection.
I, 2, B. Leukemia.

10. ① A low platelet count is common. Using soft swabs for mouth care decreases the risk of bleeding from the mucous membranes.
III, 2, B. Leukemia.

11. ③ It is not unusual for the leukemic to seem irritable and short tempered. The nurse should accept that this behavior is a part of the disease process.
I, 2, B & G. Leukemia.

12. ④ Morphine sulfate is the drug of choice for the pain of a myocardial infarction.
IV, 2, B. MI & Medications.

13. ③ It is common for patients to fear death after a near death experience, especially after a heart attack. These fears usually resolve with honest reassurance.
III, 2 & 3, B & G. MI.

14. ② An adverse effect of Coumadin is abnormal bleeding.
III, 2, B. MI & Medications.

15. ③ Aspirin is also an anticoagulant, plus it is an irritant to the stomach. A combination of the two can lead to increased anticoagulant effects plus GI bleeding.
III, 4, B. MI & Medications.

16. ③ Warmth to the lower abdomen can safely cause the pelvic vessels to dilate, thereby increasing the blood flow to the extremities.
III, 4, B. Peripheral Arterial Disease.

17. ① Right-sided heart failure is characterized by a back-up of pressure in the venous return, the periphery.
I, 2, B. CHF.

18. ① Fresh fruits are very low in sodium, as are most fresh foods.
III, 2, B & F. CHF.

19. ③ In order to strengthen his heart and to decrease his edema, he will need a cardiac glycoside, digoxin, and a diuretic, Diuril.
IV, 2, B & F. CHF.

20. ④ Thiazide diuretics cause the loss of potassium.
IV, 2, B & F. CHF.

21. ② Oranges are high in potassium.
II, 2, B & G. CHF.

22. ① An indirect way to measure a patient's fluid balance is to weigh him or her at the same time, on the same scale, and in the same clothes daily.
III, 1 & 2, B. CHF.

23.
③   Left-sided heart failure is characterized by an increased pressure in the pulmonary vasculature leading to pulmonary edema.
IV, 2, B. CHF.

24.
④   Discontinuing all tourniquets at the same time could instantly increase the circulating volume by almost 3 L, resulting in severe hypervolemia. The tourniquets are released slowly in sequence.
IV, 1 & 2, B. CHF.

25.
①   Preparation for a chest radiograph requires only that no metal be above the waist.
III, 1, B. COPD.

26.
④   Xylocaine is sprayed into the back of the throat to inhibit the gag reflex. Food and fluid must be withheld until the gag reflex returns to prevent aspiration.
III, 1 & 2, B & D. COPD.

27.
②   Swelling of the neck might represent subcutaneous emphysema, which would mean that the integrity of the lung had been interrupted.
III, 2, B. COPD.

28.
③   Oxygen has all the same dangers and entails the same responsibilities as any other medication.
II, 1 & 2, B. COPD.

29.
④   With a chronic lung disease patient, the only accurate way to determine hypoxia is through blood gases.
I, 2, B. COPD.

30.
④   Postural drainage is designed to drain excessive secretions from throughout the bronchial tree.
IV, 1, B. COPD.

31.
①   The coughing following postural drainage is excessive and could trigger vomiting if done after meals.
III, 1, B. COPD.

32.
③   Forceful coughing is unnecessary and exhausting. Slow exhalation is the objective for the chronic lung disease patient.
III, 2, B. COPD.

33.
①   The sputum of a patient with COPD is always thick and tenacious.
III, 2, B. COPD.

34.
③   Fear of the unknown is one of the greatest fears patients exhibit.
I, 2, G. COPD.

35.
③   Fluid is not normal in the pleural space. A thoracentesis is done to remove this abnormal collection of fluid.
III, 2, B. Thoracentesis.

36.
②   Homans' sign is pain in the calf when the foot is dorsiflexed. It is a characteristic sign of lower leg thrombophlebitis.
I, 2, B. Thrombophlebitis.

37.
④   Massaging the leg can dislodge the clot, leading to an embolus.
III, 2, B. Thrombophlebitis.

38.
①   Hypertension is a lifelong problem that can be controlled with diet, medication, and other therapies.
I, 2, A & C. Hypertension.

39.
④   The purpose of the treatment in hypertension is to minimize the damage to the blood vessels. Since the disease has no early warning symptoms, some damage is often found at the time of diagnosis.
IV, 2, B. Hypertension.

40.
①   Elevating the stump for 24 hours postoperatively helps to decrease edema.
III, 2, B & F. PVD/Amputation.

41.
①   Flexion contractures occur easily in lower leg amputations if the leg is not extended regularly for stretching.
II, 2, D & E. PVD/Amputations.

42.
④   Gravity will help facilitate drainage from the operative site.
IV, 2, B. Lung Cancer.

43.
②   The drainage bottle in closed water seal drainage should always be kept below the level of the lungs.
III, 2, B & D. Chest Tubes.

44.
①   If the closed drainage system is disrupted, the pleura loses the negative pressure and the lung collapses.
I, 2, B & D. Chest Tubes.

45.
③   The unaffected lung is very prone to underinflation, atelectasis, and infection. Coughing and deep-breathing exercises are vital to a normal return of respiratory function.
III, 2, B. Thoracotomy.

SENSORY/PERCEPTUAL ALTERATIONS

Normal Function

I. Communication system in body

II. Coordinates sensory and motor activites

III. Receives, interprets and relays messages

IV. Composed of nerve cells, which have two properties in common; excitability and conductivity

■ Disorders of the Cerebral/ Central Nervous System

I. INCREASED INTRACRANIAL PRESSURE (IICP)

A. Assessment

1. Definition/pathophysiology
   a. normal pressure of brain matter, intracranial blood volume, and cerebrospinal fluid (CSF) within skull normally is 15 mm Hg.
   b. because the cranium is rigid, an increase in any substance causes an increase in intracranial pressure
2. Predisposing/precipitating factors
   a. head injury with swelling
   b. stroke
   c. brain tumors
   d. infections
   e. intracranial bleeding
3. Signs and symptoms
   a. level of consciousness—varies from:
      (1) alert and oriented to person, place, and time
      (2) confused or disoriented
      (3) lethargic and obtund
      (4) comatose, various levels
   b. pupillary response—response on affected side ranges from:
      (1) unilateral dilatation
      (2) sluggish reaction to light
      (3) nonreactive
      (4) fixed
   c. papilledema
   d. blurred vision
   e. vital signs
      (1) increased systolic blood pressure with widened pulse pressure
      (2) decreased pulse
      (3) decreased, irregular respirations
      (4) elevated temperature
   f. motor function
      (1) weakness: flaccid, paresis
      (2) paralysis of limbs, extremities
   g. sensory function
      (1) paraesthesia
      (2) absence of feeling
      (3) reflex activity
         (a) corneal: decreased, absent
         (b) gag: decreased, absent
         (c) Babinski: positive, present
         (d) deep tendon (DTR): hyper-hypoactive
   h. headache
   i. nausea/vomiting
   j. seizure activity
4. Diagnostic test: presence of signs and symptoms and physical examination
5. Usual treatment
   a. dexamethasone (Decadron) to reduce cerebral edema
   b. osmotic diuretics such as mannitol to decrease cerebral edema
   c. treatment of cause of increased pressure

B. Planning, Goals/ Expected Outcomes

1. Patient will not develop increased intracranial pressure
2. Patient will not develop complications of increased intracranial pressure
3. Patient will recover from increased intracranial pressure without permanent damage

C. Implementation

1. Observe for signs and symptoms of intracranial pressure
2. Administer medications to decrease pressure as ordered
3. Avoid activities that would increase pressure (Table 7-14)
   a. monitor intracranial pressure (ICP) lines (4–15 mm Hg if client has one)
   b. position properly, with head of bed elevated 30 degrees
   c. prevent flexion and hyperextension of neck
   d. avoid coughing, straining, Valsalva maneuver
   e. monitor fluid and electrolyte balance
   f. fluid intake limited (1500–1800 mL/24 hours)
4. Control environment
   a. quiet atmosphere
   b. reassuring touch without startling
5. Administer treatments appropriate to cause as ordered

TABLE 7–14. Some Do's and Don'ts in Care of Patients with Increased Intracranial Pressure

Do:
1. Conduct neurologic checks at least once every hour unless more frequent monitoring indicated.
2. Report changes immediately.
3. Maintain a patent airway and adequate ventilation to ensure proper oxygen and carbon dioxide exchange.
4. Elevate the head of the bed 15 to 30 degrees to facilitate return of blood from the cerebral veins.
5. Use measures to maintain normal body temperature. Elevations of temperature raise blood pressure and cerebral blood flow. Shivering also can increase ICP.
6. Monitor intake and output.
7. Give passive range of motion exercises.

Don't:
1. Allow patient to become constipated or have any reason to perform Valsalva maneuver.
2. Hyperextend, flex, or rotate the patient's head.
3. Flex the patient's hips (as in female catheterization).
4. Place patient in Trendelenburg position for any reason.
5. Allow patient to perform isometric exercises.

From Keane, C.B. Essentials of Medical-Surgical Nursing. 2nd ed. Philadelphia, W.B. Saunders Company, 1986.
ICP, intracranial pressure.

D. Evaluation

1. Patient does not develop increased intracranial pressure
2. Patient does not develop complications of increased intracranial pressure
3. Patient recovered from increased intracranial pressure without permanent damage

II. INFECTIOUS CONDITIONS

A. Meningitis

1. Assessment
   a. definition: inflammation of membrane covering brain and spinal cord
   b. incidence: occurs at any age
   c. predisposing/precipitating factors
      (1) complication of another bacterial disease
      (2) could follow penetrating head wound
      (3) could result from exposure to virus
   d. signs and symptoms
      (1) severe, persistent headache
      (2) neck pain and stiffness: nuchal rigidity
      (3) photophobia
      (4) irritability
      (5) nausea, vomiting
      (6) signs of upper respiratory infection
      (7) seizures
   e. diagnostic tests
      (1) spinal tap (lumbar puncture)
         (a) needle inserted into arachnoid space between L3 and L4

         (b) sterile technique must be used
         (c) nurse responsible for:
            (i) positioning
            (ii) obtaining materials
            (iii) labeling specimens
            (iv) reassuring patient
            (v) bed rest for 8 hours to reduce headache
      (2) neurologic check
   f. usual treatments
      (1) specific antibiotics for causative organism
      (2) anticonvulsants
      (3) supportive care
2. Planning, goals/expected outcomes
   a. patient will have relief of headache pain
   b. patient will not have increased seizure activity
   c. patient will not develop problems of immobility
   d. patient and family will be supported emotionally
3. Implementation
   a. room darkened and noise-free
   b. anticonvulsants administered on time
   c. patient turned frequently
   d. deep breathing encouraged, no coughing
   e. adequate hydration maintained
   f. all procedures explained to patient and family
4. Evaluation
   a. patient obtained relief from headaches and discomfort
   b. patient did not develop increased seizure activity
   c. patient did not develop problems of immobility
   d. patient and family verbalized understanding of procedures and treatment plan

B. Encephalitis

1. Assessment
   a. definition: infection and inflammation of brain tissue
   b. incidence: anyone
   c. predisposing/precipitating factors
      (1) exposure to virus
      (2) bite of mosquito or tick
   d. signs and symptoms
      (1) sudden or slow onset
      (2) headache
      (3) fever
      (4) restlessness
      (5) lethargy
      (6) muscular weakness
      (7) coma
      (8) mental confusion
      (9) disorientation
   e. diagnostic tests
      (1) lumbar puncture

(2) electroencephalogram (EEG)
(3) good history and physical examination
f. complications: death
g. usual treatment
(1) supportive care
(2) anticonvulsants
(3) IV therapy
(4) sedative for rest
(5) steroids (Decadron) to reduce cerebral edema
(6) medication to relieve headache pain, non-narcotics
2. Planning, goals/expected outcomes
a. patient will be made comfortable
b. seizures will be decreased
c. patient will receive supportive care to prevent complications of immobility
d. emotional support will be given to patient and family
3. Implementation
a. room noise free and darkened
b. anticonvulsants administered
c. patient turned frequently
d. adequate hydration maintained
e. procedures and patient activities explained to family and patient
4. Evaluation
a. patient's comfort was maintained
b. patient's seizure activity was decreased
c. patient and family were supported emotionally

III. ACUTE DISORDERS

A. Trauma: Head Injury

1. Assessment
a. definitions
(1) concussion: closed head injury
(2) contusion: brain tissue bruised
(3) subdural hematoma: venous bleeding; blood filled swelling between arachnoid membrane and dura mater
(4) epidural hematoma: bleeding from large artery, medical emergency
b. incidence: most frequent cause of death between age 1 and 35 years
c. predisposing/precipitating factor: trauma
d. signs and symptoms
(1) outward signs
(a) bruising
(b) swelling
(c) laceration
(d) bleeding
(2) signs of increasing intracranial pressure (Chart 7-2)
e. diagnostic tests
(1) radiograph of skull; no special preparation
(2) cerebral angiography
(a) injection of radiopaque dye into carotid artery to visualize arterial system
(b) series of pictures taken
(c) client usually NPO
(d) check for allergies to iodine
(e) post test: check injection site, level of consciousness, and vital signs
(3) electroencephalography
(a) records electrical impulses from brain
(b) wash hair prior to test
(c) usually no stimulants: coffee, tea, or certain medications prior to test
(4) brain scan, computed tomographic (CT) scan
(a) use of computer to get three-dimensional picture
(b) no special preparation
(c) no pain
(5) magnetic resonance imaging (MRI): similar to CT scan
f. complications
(1) exacerbation of symptoms
(2) death
g. usual treatment
(1) conservative first
(a) maintain open airway

CHART 7–2
SIGNS OF INCREASING INTRACRANIAL PRESSURE

Sign	Nursing Assessment
Change in level of consciousness	Note change in awareness, whether increasing or decreasing; orientation; decreasing response to stimulation
Change in vital signs	Slowing pulse rate; elevated systolic blood pressure with decreased diastolic blood pressure leading to increased pulse pressure; labored breathing; rising body temperature
Change in limb movement	Extreme restlessness; muscle weakness or paralysis
Change in pupil size	Bilateral or unilateral dilation; unilateral dilation may be sign of cerebral hemorrhage with rapid deterioration

(b) observe for signs of increased intra-cranial pressure
(c) check for leakage of cerebrospinal fluid
    (i) check ears, nose
    (ii) fluid will test positive for glucose on Chemstix; mucus will not
(2) surgical intervention if necessary, usually to drain hematoma

2. Planning, goals/expected outcomes
  a. patient will be aware of possible complications of head injury
  b. patient will understand diagnostic tests to be performed
  c. patient will be observed for changes in neurologic status

3. Implementation
  a. head injury instructions will be given to patient and family if not admitted to hospital (Chart 7-3)
  b. full explanation of diagnostic tests will be given
  c. neurologic check will be performed
    (1) level of consciousness
    (2) neuromuscular responses
    (3) pupillary reactions
    (4) vital signs

4. Evaluation
  a. patient and family aware of potential complications and understand need to return to hospital
  b. patient verbalizes understanding of diagnostic tests
  c. patient's neurologic checks within normal range

B. Cerebral Vascular Accident (CVA, Stroke)

1. Assessment
  a. definition
    (1) interruption in blood flow to area of brain
    (2) may be caused by:
      (i) cerebral thrombosis
      (ii) cerebral hemorrhage
      (iii) an embolism
      (iv) pressure on blood vessel
  b. incidence: third most common cause of death in United States; most common cause of neurologic disability
  c. predisposing/precipitating factors
    (1) hypertension
    (2) atherosclerosis
    (3) heart disease
    (4) obesity
    (5) smoking
    (6) diabetes mellitus
  d. signs and symptoms vary with area of brain affected
    (1) aphasia
    (2) weakness or paralysis
    (3) visual disturbances
    (4) dizziness, ataxia
    (5) confusion
    (6) slurred speech
    (7) headache, loss of consciousness
  e. diagnostic tests
    (1) CT scans, brain scans show areas of ischemia

CHART 7–3
INSTRUCTIONS FOR HOME CARE AFTER HEAD INJURY

1. Avoid strenuous physical activities for at least 24 hours after injury
2. Apply icebag to areas of swelling; continue for at least 24 hours after injury
3. Give light diet for 24 hours after injury
4. Arouse patient every 2 hours day and night for at least 24 hours

CALL DOCTOR IMMEDIATELY OR RETURN TO EMERGENCY ROOM IF
1. Patient becomes confused, irrational, disoriented, "talks out of head," doesn't know where he or she is
2. Unable to arouse patient
3. Patient continues to be nauseated or vomits more than once
4. Patient has trouble with balance
5. Patient complains of double or blurred vision
6. Headache persists or becomes more intense 12 hours after injury

(2) lumbar puncture
(3) angiography
(4) EEG
f. complications
(1) paralysis
(2) aphasia: all types; eg, receptive, expressive
(3) visual disturbances
(4) death
g. usual treatments
(1) maintain open airway
(2) surgical intervention if stroke caused by thrombus or embolus; procedure is endarterectomy (removal of plaques from inner wall of artery)
(3) medical
(a) anticonvulsant to prevent seizures
(b) stool softeners to prevent constipation
(c) corticosteroids to reduce inflammation
(d) analgesics to reduce pain and headache
2. Planning, goals/expected outcomes
a. maintain patent airway and oxygen supply
b. assess vital signs and neurologic status
c. maintain fluid and electrolyte balance
d. insure adequate nutrition
e. maintain proper gastrointestinal function
f. maintain good mouth care
g. prevent problems of immobility
h. support patient and family emotionally
3. Implementation
a. loosen clothing and position to maintain open airway
b. assess vital signs and perform neurologic check; notify physician of any changes
c. monitor IV and oral fluids
d. offer diet as tolerated; check gag reflex prior to feeding
e. adjust diet to needs of patient, to prevent either constipation or diarrhea; include fruits, fluids, and fiber as tolerated
f. cleanse mouth prior to each meal to enable patient to taste food
g. turn every 2 hours to prevent decubiti
h. encourage active range of motion to unaffected limbs, passive range of motion to affected areas
i. encourage deep breathing and coughing
j. encouarge emotional health by:
(1) explaining activities and procedures to patient and family
(2) assist patient to communicate, avoiding frustration
(3) anticipate needs of patient
(4) place materials patient may need near unaffected extremity
(5) keep family informed of all progress and procedures

4. Evaluation
a. patient returned to optimum health for condition
b. patient performed basic activities of daily living alone or with assistance, as dictated by extent of disability
c. patient and family able to verbalize feelings related to diagnosis
d. used social service agencies as needed

C. Spinal Cord Injuries

1. Assessment
a. definition
(1) injury to spinal cord in which cord severed or compressed, causing decreased function
(2) classified according to location
(a) cervical
(b) thoracic
(c) lumbar
b. incidence: occurs most frequently in men between age 20 and 40 years
c. predisposing/precipitating factors
(1) most result from trauma
(2) accidents: auto, diving, gunshot wounds, falls
(3) spinal cord tumors
d. signs and symptoms
(1) symptoms occur below level of cord affected
(2) paralysis
(3) decreased perspiration in paralyzed area
(4) bowel and bladder dysfunction
(5) if cervical, would see:
(a) hypotension
(b) decreased body temperature
(c) bradycardia
(d) respiratory complications
e. diagnostic tests
(1) complete physical and neurologic examination
(2) radiographs
f. complications
(1) infections: bladder, lung, decubiti
(2) mental depression
(3) death
g. usual treatments
(1) immediate care
(a) handle with extreme care at scene of accident
(b) head and spine stabilized before transfer
(2) supportive treatment
(a) prevent shock
(b) control hemorrhage
(3) traction

(a) Crutchfield tongs
(b) halo ring and fixation pins
(4) begin rehabilitation to assist patient's return to a productive life
2. Planning, goals/expected outcomes
a. proper anatomic alignment will be maintained
b. infection will be prevented
c. proper fluid intake and output will be maintained
d. constipation will be prevented
e. likelihood of development of decubiti will be reduced
f. patient and family will deal with emotional aspects of accident and injury
3. Implementation
a. patient maintained in proper traction and correct positions
b. provide sterile wound and catheter care to prevent infection
c. encourage deep breathing and coughing
d. monitor intake and output; force fluids to prevent bladder problems
e. encourage diet high in fiber and bulk
f. encourage high protein diet
g. begin bowel retraining program
(1) establish regular time for elimination
(2) give laxative, stool softeners, suppositories as ordered
h. change patient's position frequently to prevent pressure
i. encourage patient and family to verbalize feelings
j. refer to psychiatrist, social workers, and other members of support team
4. Evaluation
a. patient recovers physically to highest level of functioning possible
b. patient and family adjust emotionally to condition
c. complications of immobility decreased or prevented
d. patient maintains adequate food and fluid intake

D. Brain Tumors

1. Assessment
a. definition: new growth of tissue (benign or malignant) within brain; space-occupying lesion
b. incidence: dependent on type of tumor
(1) cause unknown
(2) 2% of yearly cancer deaths
c. predisposing/precipitating factors
(1) heredity
(2) congenital
(3) radiation
(4) secondary to cerebral trauma
(5) metastases from other sites
d. signs and symptoms: dependent on location and rate of growth
(1) headache*
(2) nausea and vomiting*
(3) papilledema*
(4) signs of ICP (see section I)
(5) dizziness
(6) personality changes
(7) localized clinical manifestations
(a) seizure activity
(b) motor deficits
(c) sensory deficits
(d) speech deficits
e. diagnostic tests
(1) history and physical examination
(2) visual and fundoscopic examination
(3) skull radiograph
(4) EEG
(5) angiogram
(6) nuclear magnetic resonance imaging (NMRI)
(7) CT scan
f. complications
(1) shock
(2) uncontrolled ICP
(3) seizures
(4) residual paralysis, paraesthesia
g. usual treatment: alone or in combination
(1) surgery
(2) radiation
(3) chemotherapy
2. Planning, goals/expected outcomes
a. patient will have stable vital and neurologic signs
b. patient will not develop signs of ICP
c. patient will not develop complications of immobility
d. patient will recover from craniotomy without complications
3. Implementation
a. establish and maintain patent airway
b. assess vital signs
c. prevent neck flexion
d. turn every 2 hours
e. body position: dependent on type of craniotomy
(1) supratentorial: elevate head of bed 30 degrees
(2) infratentorial: position from side to side, not on back
f. establish baseline neurologic assessment
g. monitor, assess, and evaluate neurologic status in terms of baseline data
h. check level of consciousness

* Classic triad of symptoms for brain tumor.

i. vital signs
j. monitor and control ICP
  (1) position properly with head of bed elevated 30 degrees, unaffected side
  (2) prevent flexion and hyperextension of neck
  (3) avoid coughing, straining, Valsalva maneuver
  (4) monitor fluid and electrolyte balance
  (5) fluid intake limited (1500–1800 mL/24 hours)
k. administer appropriate medications as ordered
  (1) Decadron
  (2) osmotic diuretics, IV mannitol
  (3) Dilantin to prevent seizures
  (4) cimetadine (Tagamet)
l. assess for pain and administer analgesic
  (1) codeine as needed
  (2) Tylenol as needed
  (3) narcotic analgesics (morphine and Demerol) *contraindicated;* mask symptoms of ICP
m. log rolling (if necessary)
n. eye care: patches to prevent corneal ulcerations if blink reflex absent
o. range of motion (ROM), passive exercises
p. let family participate in care, activities
q. teach patient/family ADL, diet, activity, medication, safety measures
4. Evaluation
  a. patient's vital and neurologic signs stable
  b. patient did not develop signs of ICP
  c. patient did not develop complications of immobility
  d. patient recovered from craniotomy without complications

IV. CHRONIC DISORDERS

A. Epilepsy

1. Assessment
  a. definition
    (1) abnormal electrical activity of brain resulting in seizure activity
    (2) excessive firing at times, other times normal
    (3) classification on basis of origin
      (a) idiopathic: cause unknown
      (b) cause known; eg, blow on head, endocrine disorder
  b. incidence: affects 1% to 2% of population, occurs in families with history of disease
  c. predisposing/precipitating factors
    (1) unknown problem in brain chemistry
    (2) trauma at birth
    (3) infectious diseases
    (4) inherited disorder

(5) head injury
(6) metabolic disorders
(7) cerebral vascular accident
d. classification of seizures
  (1) generalized seizures
    (a) absence seizure (petit mal): brief loss of consciousness, "staring" expression with immediate return to alert state; usually affects children
    (b) tonic–clonic seizure (grand mal): tonic (stiffening) and clonic (twitching) phases; may be accompanied by aura, loss of consciousness, incontinence; drowsy after seizure; can progress to status epilepticus, a prolonged seizure with no periods of consciousness; a medical emergency
    (c) myoclonic seizure: single or repetitive muscle flexion spasms
    (d) atonic seizure: brief loss of posture or muscle tone; person conscious during attack
  (2) partial seizures: involves a localized area of cerebral cortex
    (a) simple partial: localized motor or sensory disturbance usually without loss of consciousness
    (b) complex partial: psychomotor, temporal lobe seizures; often involves tongue, hands, feet, and/or trunk; may or may not involve loss of consciousness
e. diagnostic exams
  (1) initially based on symptoms present
  (2) EEG
  (3) skull radiograph
  (4) lumbar puncture
  (5) brain scan
  (6) cerebral angiography
f. complications
  (1) death from status epilepticus
  (2) school failures related to loss of attention
  (3) emotional disorders related to public's intolerance
g. usual treatments
  (1) drug therapy
    (a) phenytoin (Dilantin)
      (i) action: stabilize neuronal membranes, limit seizure activity by controlling passage of sodium ions across cell membrane
      (ii) use: grand mal and psychomotor seizures
      (iii) side effects: ataxia, slurred speech; gingival hyperplasia, thrombocytopenia, nausea and vomiting
      (iv) nursing implications: do not stop drug suddenly, call doctor if side

effects develop, stress importance of good oral hygiene
- (b) phenobarbital
  - (i) action: depress monosynaptic and polysynaptic transmission in CNS
  - (ii) use: all forms of epilepsy
  - (iii) side effects: drowsiness, lethargy, nausea and vomiting, rash
  - (iv) nursing implications; do not stop abruptly
2. Planning, goals/expected outcomes
   a. patient and family will understand condition and ways to keep it under control
   b. patient and family will become aware of medications, side effects, and responsibilities
   c. patient and family will become aware of first aid treatment for seizures
3. Implementation
   a. encourage patient and family to discuss feelings related to diagnosis
   b. stress need to comply with medication plan
   c. instruct in side effects of medications
   d. warn not to drink alcohol
   e. refer to social agencies that deal with epilepsy
   f. instructions for emergency care
      (1) do not restrain during seizure
      (2) remove harmful objects
      (3) maintain airway
      (4) protect from environmental dangers

B. Parkinson's Disease

1. Assessment
   a. definition/pathophysiology: group of neurologic symptoms, progressive and debilitating, probably related to absolute lack of dopamine in brain
   b. predisposing/precipitating factors
      (1) idiopathic: primary cause unknown
      (2) atherosclerosis
      (3) drug induced, especially phenothiazine and Rauwolfia tranquilizers
      (4) toxic reaction to substances such as carbon dioxide and mercury poisoning
      (5) trauma
   c. signs and symptoms
      (1) tremors at rest that decrease with movement and are absent while asleep
      (2) tremors more pronounced with stress
      (3) muscle rigidity
      (4) poor balance
      (5) shuffling gait
      (6) decreased salivation and sweating
      (7) constipation
   d. diagnostic tests
      (1) history and physical examination
      (2) presence of symptoms
      (3) no laboratory or diagnostic abnormalities
   e. usual treatment
      (1) drug therapy: dopamine derivatives to control symptoms (Table 7-15) along with anticholinergics (Table 7-16)
      (2) physical therapy: to maintain mobility and function
2. Planning, goals/expected outcomes
   a. patient will cope with physical changes
   b. patient will remain as active as possible
   c. patient will understand and comply with therapeutic regimen
3. Implementation
   a. support patient emotionally
   b. assess patient closely after medication started to ensure optimum dose
   c. encourage patient independence
4. Evaluation
   a. patient adjusts to physical changes
   b. patient remains independent
   c. patient follows therapeutic regimen

C. Multiple Sclerosis

1. Assessment
   a. definition/pathophysiology: progressive demyelinating disease of central nervous system characterized by periods of remission and exacerbation; inflammation and resultant demyelination means that no impulses transmitted to affected muscles
   b. predisposing/precipitating factors
      (1) young white women

TABLE 7–15. Antiparkinsonian Drugs

Example	Action	Use	Common Side Effects	Nursing Implications
Levodopa and carbidopa (Sinemet)	Increases level of dopamine in CNS	To control symptoms of Parkinson's disease	Nausea/vomiting, anorexia, orthostatic hypotension, dry mouth, ataxia, headache, dysphagia, anxiety, insomnia, urinary retention, hypertension	Use with caution in patients with cardiovascular, respiratory, endocrine, hepatic disease or with ulcers, glaucoma, diabetes or psychosis

CNS, central nervous system.

TABLE 7–16. Anticholinergics

Example	Action	Use	Common Side Effects	Nursing Implications
Atropine sulfate	Inhibits the effect of acetylcholine as transmitter for impulses in parasympathetic nervous system at synapses	To treat Parkinson's disease, to decrease saliva and respiratory secretions preoperatively	Dry mouth, blurred vision, acute glaucoma, constipation, dilated pupils, urinary retention, tachycardia	Avoid use in patients with glaucoma, BPH, myasthenia gravis, CHF and hypertension; monitor vital signs; check for side effects; monitor I&O

BPH, benign prostatic hypertrophy; CHF, congestive heart failure; I&O, intake and output.

(2) possible viral origin
(3) currently unknown cause
c. signs and symptoms
(1) early symptoms vague
(2) motor dysfunctions
   (a) diplopia
   (b) muscle weakness and eventual paralysis
   (c) muscle spasticity
(3) sensory dysfunctions
   (a) patchy or total blindness
   (b) paresthesias
   (c) neuropathies with pain and burning
   (d) tinnitus and deafness
(4) coordination
   (a) ataxia
   (b) scissors gait
   (c) intention tremors, absent at rest
   (d) nystagmus
   (e) dysphagia
   (f) scanning speech
(5) mentation
   (a) depression
   (b) labile emotions with inappropriate euphoria

(6) other
   (a) urinary and bowel incontinence
   (b) sexual dysfunction
   (c) extreme fatigue
d. diagnostic tests
(1) no easily available tests
(2) diagnosis made through analysis of symptoms
(3) nerve biopsy shows demyelination
e. usual treatment
(1) symptomatic supportive therapy mainly
(2) adrenocorticotrophic hormone (ACTH) injections to increase patient's own cortisol level and induce remissions (Table 7-17)
2. Planning, goals/expected outcomes
a. patient will maintain independence and function as long as possible
b. patient will cope with progressive disability
c. patient will understand and comply with therapeutic regimen
d. patient and family will cope with terminal prognosis of disease
3. Implementation
a. maintain independence
b. provide emotional support

TABLE 7–17. Anti-Inflammatories

Class	Example	Action	Use	Common Side Effects	Nursing Implications
Steroids	Cortisone acetate	Block inflammatory, allergic and immune responses similar to glucocorticoids	To treat a wide variety of inflammatory, autoimmune, allergic disorders, to replace natural glucocorticoids	Na^+ and water retention, GI ulceration, hypertension, CHF, delayed wound healing, protein breakdown, osteoporosis, cataracts, leukopenia, diabetes, hypokalemia	Warn patient to avoid infections; increased needs during stress and illness; monitor for Addison's disease; give with antacids; use low salt, high potassium diet; teach patient not to stop taking drug without doctor's approval
Nonsteroidal drugs	Ibuprofen (Motrin)	Act by inhibiting prostaglandin synthesis	To reduce inflammation of arthritis and other disorders	Prolonged bleeding time, edema, tinnitus, GI distress, rash	Avoid in patients with ulcers or asthma; teach that it takes weeks to reach full effect; give with food or milk; watch for side effects

CHF, congestive heart failure; GI, gastrointestinal.

c. prevent potential complications associated with decrease mobility
d. monitor ability to swallow and prevent choking
e. encourage patient to join multiple sclerosis (MS) support group
f. plan with patient for discharge and home care
g. encourage good health practices to keep disease in remission
h. help patient cope with terminal prognosis
4. Evaluation
   a. patient maintains independence within limitations of disease
   b. patient copes with disability and prognosis
   c. patient follows therapeutic regimen

D. Myasthenia Gravis

1. Assessment
   a. definition/pathophysiology: progressive disorder of acetylcholine that inhibits transmission across myoneural junction and produces severe muscle weakness
   b. predisposing/precipitating factors
      (1) probably autoimmune
      (2) no specific risk factors
   c. signs and symptoms
      (1) ptosis
      (2) difficulty chewing and swallowing
      (3) severe muscle weakness, gradual at first then increasing
      (4) fatigue
      (5) eventually, inability to walk
      (6) all skeletal muscles weaken, with eventual loss of ability to breathe
   d. diagnostic tests
      (1) Tensilon test: injection of edrophonium (Tensilon), producing immediate increase in muscle strength
      (2) inject neostigmine with return of muscle strength
   e. usual treatment
      (1) if disease is mild, symptomatic treatment with potassium chloride, ephedrine, and guanidine
      (2) plasmapheresis
      (3) anticholinesterase therapy, neostigmine (Prostigmin) or pyridostigmine (Mestinon), to inactivate acetylcholinesterase and improve muscle strength (Table 7-18)
      (4) ACTH and prednisone as immunosuppressive therapy (Table 7-17)
2. Planning, goals/expected outcomes
   a. patient will maintain independence as long as possible
   b. patient will cope with physical disability
   c. patient will understand and comply with therapeutic regimen
   d. patient and family will cope with terminal diagnosis
3. Implementation
   a. monitor for cholinergic crisis from drugs
      (1) symptoms of cholinergic crisis
         (a) nausea and vomiting
         (b) abdominal cramps
         (c) diarrhea
         (d) blurred vision
         (e) pallor
         (f) facial muscle twitching
         (g) hypotension
      (2) have atropine on hand as antidote
   b. observe for myasthenic crisis from undermedication with cholinergic drugs
      (1) symptoms of myasthenic crisis
         (a) increased pulse and respiration
         (b) increased blood pressure
         (c) anoxia, cyanosis
         (d) incontinence
         (e) decreased urine output
         (f) absent cough and swallow reflex
   c. provide emotional support
   d. teach patient to avoid stress
   e. educate patient about nature of disease
   f. teach patient correct medication administration and symptoms and treatment of cholinergic crisis
   g. avoid drugs that cause dangerous effects such as CNS depressants, thyroid drugs, "mycin" antibiotics, phenothiazines, and cardiac drugs
   h. help patient adjust to terminal diagnosis

TABLE 7-18. Cholinergics

Example	Action	Use	Common Side Effects	Nursing Implications
Pyridostigmine bromide (Mestinon)	Inhibits destruction of acetylcholine, promoting stimulation of receptors	To treat myasthenia gravis	Headache, weakness, miosis, bradycardia, abdominal cramps, diarrhea, nausea/vomiting, excess saliva, bronchospasms, hypotension, muscle cramps	Avoid in patients with obstructions, asthma, epilepsy or ulcers; watch closely for side effects; check vital signs; give before meals

4. Evaluation
   a. patient remains independent within physical limitations
   b. patient accepts diagnosis and nature of disease
   c. patient follows therapeutic regimen

■ Eye: Normal Function

I. LOCATION

In protective bony orbit in skull

II. COMPOSITION

Three layers of tissue

A. Sclera

1. Thick, white fibrous tissue
2. Cornea: transparent section over front of eyeball that permits light rays to enter

B. Choroid

1. Middle vascular area
2. Extends to ciliary body, which helps control shape of lens
3. Brings nutrients and oxygen to the eye
4. Front pigment section (iris) that gives eye color
5. Pupil lies in center of iris

C. Retina

1. Physiology of vision occurs
2. Contains receptors of the optic nerve
3. Neurons shaped like rods and cones
4. Cones permit perception of color, and rods permit perception of light and shade

III. CHAMBERS

A. Anterior

Contains aqueous humor; maintains slight forward curve in cornea

B. Posterior

Contains vitreous humor; keeps eyeball in its spherical shape

IV. CONJUNCTIVA

Mucous membrane that covers eyeball and eyelid; keeps eyeball moist

V. LENS

Transparent structure behind iris that focuses light rays on retina

VI. LACRIMAL APPARATUS

Glands that produce tears to lubricate and cleanse

■ Visual Disorders

I. CONJUNCTIVITIS

A. Assessment

1. Definition: inflammation of the conjunctiva
2. Predisposing factors: bacteria and allergens
3. Signs and symptoms
   a. purulent drainage
   b. itching
   c. eyes erythematous
4. treatment: ophthalmic antibiotics

B. Planning, Goals/ Expected Outcomes

1. Patient will administer ophthalmic ointment as prescribed
2. Infection will diminish

C. Implementation

1. Encourage frequent hand washing to prevent transmission to others
2. Cleanse eyelids and remove crusts before administering ophthalmic medications
3. Instruct client how to administer ophthalmic ointment

D. Evaluation

1. No evidence of infection
2. Absence of drainage and itching

II. CATARACT

A. Assessment

1. Definition: transparent crystalline lens becomes clouded and opaque
2. Incidence
   a. higher in patients with diabetes or on steroids
   b. more common in seventh through ninth decades of life
3. Predisposing factors
   a. congenital
   b. result of diabetes, steroids
   c. senile cataracts as result of aging process
   d. infections or trauma
   e. radiation therapy to head
4. Signs and symptoms
   a. gradual loss of vision
   b. progressive blurring
5. Diagnostic examinations
   a. examination with ophthalmoscope (absence of red reflex)
   b. patient history
6. Usual treatments
   a. surgical removal of completely opaque (ripe) lens with or without lens implant
   b. corrective lenses are necessary after surgery unless an artificial lens is implanted at time of surgery

B. Planning, Goals/ Expected Outcomes

1. Patient will verbalize understanding of usual preoperative and postoperative care and routines
2. Patient will verbalize understanding of precautions necessary to prevent infection and dislodgement of implanted lens
3. Patient will verbalize understanding of expected results on vision of cataract extraction and of implantation of lens

C. Implementation

1. Instruct patient to avoid coughing, bending, or rapid head movements
2. Provide bed rest for amount of time prescribed by physician, if at all
3. Maintain patient flat in low Fowler's position
4. Have patient deep breathe (avoid coughing)
5. Have patient avoid straining (give stool softener)
6. Help patient avoid vomiting (an antiemetic will usually be ordered)
7. Observe and report pain or bleeding
8. Position patient on unoperated side

D. Evaluation

1. Patient is free of infection
2. Patient's implanted lens is not dislodged

III. GLAUCOMA

A. Assessment

1. Definition: Intraocular pressure increases because of imbalance between production and drainage of aqueous humor as angle of drainage closes
   a. acute (closed-angle) glaucoma: dramatic onset of symptoms; immediate treatment is required, usually surgery
   b. chronic (open-angle) glaucoma: symptoms develop slowly and may be ignored; if condition is not diagnosed early, there may be permanent loss of vision
2. Incidence
   a. increases over 40 years of age
   b. family history increases risk
3. Signs and symptoms
   a. painless loss of peripheral vision
   b. halos around lights
   c. permanent loss of vision
   d. pain, malaise, nausea and vomiting (late symptoms)
4. Diagnostic examinations
   a. measurement of intraocular pressure
   b. measurement of visual fields
   c. history of symptoms
5. Usual treatments
   a. miotics used to decrease intraocular pressure by constricting pupil and increasing outflow of humor
   b. iridectomy: surgical incision through cornea to remove part of iris to allow for drainage of humor

B. Planning, Goals/ Expected Outcomes

1. Patient will be free from pain
2. Patient will not suffer permanent loss of vision

C. Implementation

1. Administer eye medications on schedule
2. Inform patient that drugs containing atropine should be avoided
3. Inform patient that straining and lifting are discouraged

D. Evaluation

1. Patient does not experience pain
2. Patient's vision loss does not progress

IV. DETACHED RETINA

A. Assessment

1. Definition: sensory layer separates and unable to receive visual stimuli
2. Incidence: more common among those over age 40 years
3. Predisposing factors
   a. penetrating injury
   b. sudden blow
   c. tumors or eye hemorrhage
   d. cause frequently unknown
4. Signs and symptoms
   a. spots and flashes of light
   b. floating spots
   c. loss of vision in affected area
5. Preoperative care
   a. patient should be on bed rest
   b. cover both eyes with patches to prevent further detachment
6. Surgical treatments
   a. immediate surgery with drainage of fluid from subretinal space so that retina returns to normal position
   b. retinal breaks are sealed by various methods that produce inflammatory reactions
      (1) cryosurgery
      (2) electrodiathermy
      (3) photocoagulation (use of a laser beam)

B. Planning, Goals/ Expected Outcomes

1. Patient will not develop further loss of vision
2. Patient will have improved vision after surgery

C. Implementation

1. Postoperative nursing care
   a. physician's orders will be specific; provide care individually
   b. patient may be kept on complete bed rest for 1 day or longer; sandbags may be ordered on both sides of the head for immobilization
   c. patient should not be turned or moved unless movement ordered
   d. both eyes may be covered; patient should always have call light within reach
   e. prior to discharge, patient instructed to avoid jarring or bumping head and not to do any heavy lifting
2. Maintain bed rest pre- and postoperatively as ordered
3. Maintain eye patches to prevent further detachment
4. Instructions given to avoid sudden, jarring movements

D. Evaluation

1. Patient's vision loss does not progress
2. Patient's vision improves following surgery

■ Hearing: Normal Auditory Function

I. OUTER EAR

Picks up sound waves from environment and takes to eardrum (tympanic membrane)

II. MIDDLE EAR

Contains malleus, incus, and stapes bones, which transmit sound waves from eardrum to inner ear

III. INNER EAR

Contains cochlea, which has duct filled with fluid that vibrates when sound waves from stirrup bone strikes against it; hair-like cells (organ of Corti) pick up sound waves and transmit them through auditory nerve to hearing center of brain (sense of balance also located in inner ear)

■ Auditory Disorders

I. OTOSCLEROSIS

A. Assessment

1. Definition: results from bony ankylosis of stapes, which interferes with vibration of stapes and transmission of sound to inner ear
2. Incidence
   a. more common among women
   b. hearing loss usually becomes apparent to patient during second and third decades of life
3. Predisposing factors: cause unknown, but majority of patients have family history of disease

4. Signs and symptoms
   a. progressive loss of hearing
   b. tinnitus (ringing or buzzing in the ears)
5. Diagnosis: hearing test
6. Usual treatments
   a. hearing aid
   b. surgery; stapedectomy (removal of diseased bone and replacement with prosthetic implant)

B. Planning, Goals/ Expected Outcomes

1. Patient will verbalize understanding of usual preoperative and postoperative care and routines
2. Patient will verbalize understanding of major precautions necessary to prevent infection and dislodgement of prosthesis
3. Patient verbalizes understanding of expected effects of surgery on hearing

C. Implementation

1. Preoperative instructions should include information that movement may cause dizziness for 48 to 96 hours after surgery
2. Bedrest for 24 hours after surgery will be expected in order to prevent dislodgement of the prosthesis
3. Precautions to avoid dislodgement of prosthesis include
   a. avoid blowing nose
   b. avoid coughing and sneezing
   c. if nauseated, request antiemetic so that vomiting avoided
4. reinforce physician's explanation of effects of surgery and explain that edema and accumulation of blood in ear may diminish hearing in operative ear until resolved
5. postoperative
   a. keep in supine position or as ordered by physician
   b. do not turn patient
   c. deep breathe every 2 hours, but do not allow coughing
   d. check for drainage; report excessive bleeding
   e. may have vertigo when ambulatory; stay with patient and avoid quick movements

D. Evaluation

1. Patient is free of infection
   a. afebrile
   b. negative cultures of ear drainage

2. Patient's prosthesis does not dislodge
   a. improvement in hearing
   b. absence of dizziness and tinnitus

II. ACUTE OTITIS MEDIA

A. Assessment

1. Definition: acute infection of middle ear usually resulting from spread of microorganisms to middle ear through eustachian tube during upper respiratory infections
2. Incidence: more common in young children
3. Signs and symptoms
   a. fever
   b. severe earache
   c. diminished hearing
   d. pus present in auditory canal (if eardrum has perforated)
4. Diagnosis
   a. using otoscope, physician notes that eardrum red and bulging
   b. culture of ear drainage
5. Usual treatments
   a. myringotomy: incision in eardrum that may prevent spontaneous rupture and allow purulent material to escape
   b. antibiotics given to control infection
   c. fluids encouraged
6. Complications
   a. usually occur when otitis media goes untreated
   b. mastoiditis: middle ear connects with mastoid process by complex passages through which infection can travel
   c. scarring or permanent perforation of the eardrum
   d. hearing loss
   e. meningitis
   f. chronic otitis media: chronic discharge from ear, reduction of hearing, and sometimes slight fever

B. Planning, Goals/ Expected Outcomes

1. Patient will be free from earache
2. Patient will not experience hearing loss

C. Implementation

1. Patient takes medications as prescribed by physician

2. Importance of follow-up ear examination after course of antibiotic therapy stressed
3. Patient instructed in symptoms of recurrence of acute otitis media

D. Evaluation

1. Patient does not experience earache
2. Patient experiences no permanent hearing loss

Questions

Mr. Daniels is admitted for a neurologic work-up. The first test to be performed is a lumbar puncture.

1. Mr. Daniels tells you that he does not understand the procedure and doesn't really know what to expect. Your best response to him would be to:

   ① Tell him that you will call the doctor to come explain the procedure to him
   ② Explain the proper position for the procedure, tell him to relax and breathe normally, and say that local anesthetic is used to prevent pain
   ③ Explain that the doctor will be inserting a large needle into the spinal column and withdrawing some of the fluid from around his spinal cord and brain to test for an infection
   ④ Tell him that someone will explain the procedure when it is time and that there is no need to worry about being hurt or paralyzed by the test

2. The most effective way to help Mr. Daniels relieve his anxiety over the test is to:

   ① Give him a brief explanation of the exact procedure
   ② Reassure him that his doctor is experienced in this procedure
   ③ Ask him exactly what he is anxious about and listen to him
   ④ Ask him to write down his questions to give to the doctor before the test

3. After the lumbar puncture is completed, Mr. Daniels should be:

   ① Encouraged to ambulate
   ② Placed in Trendelenburg for 2 hours to equalize the pressure
   ③ Encouraged to lie flat on his back for 6–12 hours
   ④ Placed on strict bed rest for at least 48 hours

4. Mr. Daniels is also scheduled for an electroencephalogram (EEG). The main reason for an EEG is to:

   ① Identify the location of a brain tumor
   ② Diagnose epilepsy
   ③ Administer small shocks and record brain response
   ④ Record the normal electrical activity of brain cells

5. In preparing him for the EEG, the nurse should:

   ① Sedate him with phenobarbital
   ② Withhold all medications
   ③ Keep him awake for 48 hours before the test
   ④ Shampoo his hair

6. The nurse is trying to determine a patient's level of consciousness. The nurse can best describe the patient as:

   ① Alert and able to state name and time
   ② Seems to be comatose
   ③ Remains unable to respond
   ④ Somewhat stuporous and doesn't know location

7. Which of the following could the nurse chart to give the most objective observation concerning neuromuscular status?

   ① Paralysis of lower extremities
   ② Unable to grip nurse's hand with left hand but strong grip with right
   ③ Weak and lethargic most of the time; confused at frequent intervals
   ④ Poor response to painful stimuli

8. You are to check the patient's pupillary response. This is best done:

   ① In a well-lighted room with a flashlight
   ② In a darkened room with a penlight
   ③ After the patient has received a mydriatic
   ④ After the patient has received a miotic

9. When caring for a patient who suffers from dysarthria, it is important for the nurse to:

   ① Administer tube feedings accurately
   ② Maintain adequate fluid intake
   ③ Face the patient when speaking so they can lip read
   ④ Speak slowly and clearly and allow time for response

10. Which of the following statements regarding meningitis is true? It:

    ① Is an inflammation of brain tissue
    ② Can be caused by a tick bite
    ③ Occasionally follows a CVA
    ④ Can be caused by a bacteria or viral infection

11. When a patient has meningitis, it is important that the nurse:

① Provide a quiet, dimly lit environment for the patient
② Ventilate the room properly and provide sufficient sunlight
③ Eliminate strong odors and unpleasant sights to prevent vomiting
④ Allow frequent visits from family to prevent depression from isolation

12. Your patient is scheduled for a cerebral computed tomography (CT scan). You can best prepare the patient by:

① Premedicating the patient for pain
② Keeping the patient NPO for at least 12 hours prior to the test
③ Protecting the patient from overexposure to radiation
④ Assuring the patient that this is a safe and painless test

13. After which of the following operations must vomiting be absolutely prevented?

① A prostatectomy
② A cholecystectomy
③ A colon resection
④ A cataract extraction

14. A high fever often accompanies meningitis. A nursing intervention most helpful in relieving the febrile delirium would be:

① Restraining the patient to prevent self-injury
② Applying a warm water bottle to the back of the neck
③ Increasing fluid intake to prevent dehydration
④ Application of cool compresses or an icebag to the head

15. When a patient is admitted with a head injury, one of the most important aspects of nursing care would be:

① Restraining the patient to prevent self-injury
② Administering phenobarbital to prevent convulsions
③ Carefully monitoring the patient's vital signs
④ Turning the patient frequently to prevent paralysis

16. Patients with head injuries are not given sedatives because these drugs may:

① Produce coma
② Mask the patient's symptoms
③ Increase the patient's blood pressure
④ Lead to cerebral hemorrhage

17. If the patient has suffered a head injury, there is a risk that cerebrospinal fluid leakage may occur. It should be suspected in head injured patients with:

① Bleeding from the nose or mouth
② Purulent, thick drainage from the nose or ears
③ Clear yellow or pink tinged fluid from the nose or ears
④ Watering of the eyes and drainage of mucus from the nose

18. In order to confirm the presence of cerebrospinal fluid drainage, the nurse should:

① Test the fluid for the presence of glucose
② Send a specimen to the laboratory for diagnosis
③ Test for the presence of albumin
④ Send a culture for sensitivity

19. If there is confirmed leakage of cerebrospinal fluid, the patient should be:

① Cautioned against blowing or picking the nose
② Positioned with the head lower than the rest of the body
③ Cautioned against moving the head at all
④ Encouraged to blow the nose to remove secretions

20. Which of the following is not considered a cause of stroke?

① Cerebral thrombosis
② Cerebral hemorrhage
③ Cerebral encephalitis
④ Cerebral atherosclerosis

21. A patient who has had a stroke should have range of motion exercises done regularly. This is an important nursing intervention because the:

① Muscles have been damaged by the interruption of blood flow
② Bone and joints have been affected and contractures may occur
③ Part of the brain controlling muscles has been destroyed and will never function normally
④ Use of the muscles may return if compli-

cations involving the musculoskeletal system have been prevented

22. When a stroke has been caused by a hemorrhage, the nurse should:

① Position the patient flat in bed
② Have the patient cough and deep breathe hourly
③ Position the patient in semi-Fowler's
④ Administer Coumadin as ordered

23. Approximately half of epileptics who experience grand mal seizures experience a warning sign referred to as a(n):

① Prodromal symptom
② Aura
③ Sequela
④ Icteric

24. If the nurse comes upon a patient having a seizure, the nurse should:

① Protect the head from injury and turn the patient to the side if possible
② Restrain the patient to prevent injury
③ Place an object between the teeth and move the patient to an upright position
④ Move the patient to the floor and hold the patient down

25. When "log rolling" a patient to the side, it is important for the nurse to:

① Elevate the head of the bed slightly to avoid pressure on the back
② Raise the knees slightly to avoid pressure on the hips
③ Support the back with pillows and place a pillow between the legs to avoid back strain
④ Remove the pillow from under the patient's head and place it under the shoulders

Answers & Rationales

Guide to item identification (see pp. 3–5 for further details about each category)

I, II, III, or IV for the phase of the nursing process
1, 2, 3, or 4 for the category of client needs
A, B, C, D, E, F, or G for the category of human functioning
Specific content category by name; ie, cholecystectomy

1.
② The nurse should explain the procedure in broad terms without interjecting information that will needlessly frighten the patient.
III, 1, A & C. Lumbar Puncture.

2.
③ The best way to reassure a patient is first to find out exactly what that patient is anxious about.
III, 1, A & C. Lumbar Puncture.

3.
③ Lying flat for 6–12 hours will allow the pressure to return to normal and decrease the risk of spinal headache.
III, 1, C. Lumbar Puncture.

4.
④ An EEG simply records the electrical activity of the brain.
I, 1, C. EEG.

5.
④ The electrodes need to make good contact with oil free skin.
III, 1, C. EEG.

6.
① When collecting and recording data, the most objective description should always be used.
I & II, 2, C. Neurologic Assessment.

7.
② The statements charted should be as objective and descriptive as possible.
I & II, 2, C. Neurologic Assessment.

8.
② To see the change in the pupils, the room should be dimly lit and a focused light source used to test the pupils.
I & II, 2, C. Neurologic Assessment.

9.
④ Dysarthria means that the patient has difficulty speaking, so the nurse should speak slowly and clearly and allow time for response.
III, 2, C. Neurologic Assessment.

10.
④ Meningitis is an inflammation of the membranes covering the brain and spinal cord caused by a virus or bacteria.
I, 2, C & D. Meningitis.

11.
① With the photosensitivity and irritability exhibited in patients with meningitis, the environment should be as calm and controlled as possible.
III, 2, C & D. Meningitis.

12.
④ The CT scan is a simple, painless test with a variety of uses.
III, I, C. CT Scan.

13.
④ The patient with a cataract extraction must avoid any activity that would increase intra-ocular pressure and precipitate acute glaucoma.
II, 2, C. Cataract.

14.
④ Cool compresses or icebags applied to the forehead help relieve the febrile delirium.
II, 2, C & F. Meningitis.

15.
③ Patients with head injuries may develop increased intracranial pressure and a widening pulse pressure (the difference between the systolic and diastolic blood pressures) is an early sign of this.
III, 2, A & C. Head Injury.

16.
② Decrease in the level of consciousness is an important sign in patients with head injuries, and sedatives will themselves alter the consciousness.
IV, 2, C. Head Injury.

17.
③ Cerebrospinal fluid is clear, yellowish fluid and often leaks from the nose or ears with severe head injuries.
I, 2, C. Head Injury.

18.
① Cerebrospinal fluid contains glucose, whereas normal nasal drainage does not.
III, 2, C & D. Head Injury.

19.
① If the integrity of the skull is disrupted in the nasal region, bacteria from the nose can easily migrate into the cerebrospinal fluid.
II, 2, C & D. Head Injury.

20.
③ Encephalitis does not cause a stroke.
I, 2, C. CVA.

21. A stroke may cause only temporary loss of
④ function, so it is important to prevent contractures so that the patient has the opportunity to regain maximal function.
III, 2, C & E. CVA.

22. Positioning in semi-Fowler's allows for in-
③ creased venous return. Also, intracranial pressure is lessened.
III, 2, C. CVA.

23. An aura is the set of symptoms that precede a
② grand mal seizure.
IV, 2, C. Seizures.

24. Protecting the head from trauma and decreas-
① ing the risk of aspiration are the priorities for patient safety.
III, 2, O, Seizures.

25. Supporting the back and body as an immove-
③ able whole is the principle of "log rolling."
III, 1, C & E. Laminectomy.

PROTECTIVE FUNCTIONS

■ Sexually Transmitted Diseases

I. GONORRHEA

A. Assessment

1. Definition/pathophysiology: most common type of sexually transmitted disease and major public health problem, caused by *Neisseria gonorrhoeae*, and easily transmitted from one person to another
2. Predisposing/precipitating factors
   a. sexually active individuals with multiple partners at greater risk
   b. exposure to microorganism
   c. newborns can contract from infected mothers
3. Signs and symptoms
   a. women
      (1) 80% without symptoms
      (2) vaginal discharge
      (3) pain in lower abdomen
      (4) burning in urination
      (5) may involve ovaries and tubes, causing sterility
   b. men
      (1) dysuria
      (2) whitish or yellowish pus discharge from penis
      (3) inflammation of prostate and testes, leading to sterility
   c. both
      (1) septic arthritis
      (2) meningitis
      (3) peritonitis
      (4) endocarditis
4. Diagnostic test: culture of organisms from discharge
5. Usual treatment
   a. penicillin and other antibacterials such as sulfa drugs (Table 7-19)
   b. penicillin given by injection in long-acting form to give high blood level and prolonged action
   c. tetracycline or streptomycin can be used if patient is penicillin sensitive
   d. avoid further sexual contact until cultures are negative

B. Planning, Goals/Expected Outcomes

1. Patient will not contract gonorrhea
2. Patient will understand and comply with therapy
3. Patient will recover without permanent complications

C. Implementation

1. Teach patient about risk to others until infection is cured
2. Ask patient about sexual contacts, because they all must receive treatment
3. Teach patient that successful treatment does not bring immunity

TABLE 7-19. Pharmacologic Treatment of Syphilis, Gonorrhea, Herpes Genitalis

Disease	Drugs	Action	Side Effects	Nursing Implications
Syphilis	Penicillin such as penicillin G benzathine	Bactericidal	Pain and sterile abscess at injection site Neuropathy	Ask patient about allergy to penicillins or other antibiotics
	Tetracycline	Bacteriostatic	Anorexia Nausea Eosinophilia Dysphagia	Inactivated by milk and milk products
Gonorrhea	Penicillin such as ampicillin	Bactericidal semisynthetic broad spectrum	Nausea Vomiting Pain at injection site (see above)	Danger of hypersensitivity reaction as with all antibiotics
	Tetracycline Spectinomycin	Inhibits protein synthesis in pathogen	Insomnia Dizziness Pain at injection site Nausea	Danger of hypersensitivity reaction
	Erythromycin	Inhibits bacterial cell protein synthesis	Gastritis Abdominal pain Cholestatic jaundice	Inactivated by high acid medium Avoid taking with fruit juices
Herpes genitalis	Acyclovir (Zovirax) for cutaneous use only	Inhibits herpesvirus DNA synthesis	Transient burning Stinging	Not a cure, symptomatic treatment only Apply ointment with gloves or finger cot

4. Avoid self-contamination through use of gloves and good hand-washing
5. Administer medications as ordered

D. Evaluation

1. Patient did not develop gonorrhea
2. Patient compiled with therapy and gonorrhea cured
3. Patient recovered without permanent complications

II. SYPHILIS

A. Assessment

1. Definition/pathophysiology: generalized infection caused by spirochete, *Treponema pallidum*, and transmitted mainly through sexual contact, but also through any contact with body fluids
2. Predisposing/precipitating factors
   a. sexual contact with infected persons
   b. multiple sexual contacts increases risk
   c. infants born of infected mothers
   d. contact with infected bodily fluids
3. Signs and symptoms
   a. primary stage
      (1) chancre, hard sore on mucous membranes of mouth or genitalia
      (2) often unnoticed in women because it is in vagina
      (3) sore highly infectious in this stage
      (4) enters bloodstream within 3 days
      (5) headache
      (6) enlarged lymph nodes near chancre
      (7) symptoms disappear in 3 to 8 weeks
   b. secondary stage
      (1) slight malaise and headache
      (2) some patients asymptomatic
      (3) skin rash or sore throat
      (4) loss of patches of hair
      (5) arthritis, neuritis, retinitis
      (6) symptoms eventually subside when disease enters latent period
   c. tertiary stage
      (1) begins 1 year after infection, but serious symptoms may not occur for 4 to 5 years
      (2) invasion of all body tissues by spirochetes
      (3) nervous system involvement common
4. Diagnostic tests
   a. Veneral Disease Research Laboratory (VDRL) blood serum test for primary and secondary stages
   b. examination of cerebrospinal fluid from lumbar puncture for tertiary stage

c. fluorescent treponema antibody absorption test (FTA-ABS) for all stages
5. Usual treatment
   a. penicillin antibiotic of choice, in one massive, injectable long-acting dose
   b. if patient is penicillin sensitive, use tetracycline or erythromycin (Table 7-19)
   c. contacting and treatment of sexual contacts

B. Planning, Goals/Expected Outcomes

1. Patient will not contract syphilis
2. Patient will comply with therapy to treat disease
3. Patient will recover without long-term or life-threatening complications

C. Implementation

1. Teach patient to avoid casual sexual contact to avoid exposure to disease
2. Encourage compliance with therapy
3. Be nonjudgmental
4. Teach patient that treatment offers no immunity to further disease

D. Evaluation

1. Patient did not contact disease
2. Patient complied with therapy and disease successfully treated
3. No permanent complications occurred

■ Skin Disorders

I. BURNS

A. Assessment

1. Definition/pathophysiology: burns are injuries to skin caused by agents such as heat, electricity, chemicals, or radiation
2. Classification
   a. amount of body surface
      (1) rule of nines, a way of expressing portions of body surface burned
         (a) head and neck: 9%
         (b) anterior trunk: 18%
         (c) posterior trunk: 18%
         (d) each arm: 9%
         (e) each leg: 18%
         (f) genitalia and perineum: 1%
   b. depth of burn, old method

(1) first degree: involves epidural layer only

(2) second degree: involves superficial to deep dermis

(3) third degree: involves all layers of dermis, extends into subcutaneous tissues

(4) fourth degree: includes muscle and bone

   c. depth of burn, new method

(1) partial thickness: epidermal appendages (sweat and oil glands and hair follicles) intact and wound will heal itself if no further injury occurs

(2) full thickness: involves all layers of skin and destruction of epidermal appendages and requires grafting for healing to occur

3. Signs and symptoms

   a. first degree: red dry skin and pain

   b. second degree: mottled white to cherry red, skin moist with or without blisters, and extreme pain

   c. third degree: white and leathery to charred, skin dry without elasticity, and little or no pain

   d. fourth degree: skin charred to dead white, without pain

4. Usual treatment

   a. depth of wound assessed

   b. IV Ringer's lactate to maintain fluid balance and prevent shock

   c. pain medication: often IV morphine for severe pain

   d. continuous replacement of lost fluids with care to prevent fluid overload

   e. monitor respiratory status if upper respiratory tract burned

   f. open method

     a. wounds left open to air in sterile settings

     b. wet compresses or soaks used to debride burn

   g. closed method

(1) occlusive dressings with silver sulfadiazine antibiotic cream to control infection

(2) debridement of wound

   h. skin grafting

B. Planning, Goals/Expected Outcomes

1. Patient will recover from burns without permanent impairment
2. Patient will not develop infection
3. Patient will maintain positive nitrogen balance and fluid balance so healing can occur
4. Patient will not develop contractures
5. Patient will cope with emotional aspects of burn injury
6. Patient will understand and comply with therapy for burns after discharge

C. Implementation

1. Emergency treatment

   a. minor burns treated with immersion in ice water and application of cold compresses

   b. never apply salves or any greasy substance

   c. for severe burns, simply cover area with clean occlusive bandage and transfer patient to hospital immediately; never try to remove clothes stuck to burn

2. Nursing interventions

   a. prevention of infection a top priority

   b. application of topical medications

   c. strict aseptic technique when caring for burns

   d. assess scar tissue and prevent contractures

   e. encourage prescribed exercises to prevent contractures and maintain function

   f. maintain adequate fluid intake

   g. encourage diet high protein, high vitamin C, iron, and calcium (see Chapter 5)

   h. provide emotional support to patient and family, especially if burns are disfiguring

   i. teach patient and family home care for discharge

D. Evaluation

1. Patient recovered without complications
2. Patient did not develop infection
3. Patient maintained positive nitrogen balance and good fluid balance
4. Patient did not develop contractures
5. Patient coped with disfigurement caused by burns
6. Patient able to care for burns at home

■ PERIOPERATIVE CARE

I. PREOPERATIVE PERIOD

A. Assessment

1. Laboratory data

   a. ECG

   b. CBC, make sure hemoglobin at least 10 g/mL and no elevated WBCs

   c. urinalysis

   d. liver function studies for clotting factors, albumin, and function

   e. chest radiograph

2. Vital signs for baseline normal
3. Allergies
4. Nutritional status

   a. obesity increases risk in many ways

(1) venipuncture and intubation harder

(2) effect of general anesthesia prolonged

(3) more respiratory complications

(4) time of surgery prolonged

(5) slowed healing time and more risk of wound disruption

(6) more easily dehydrated

b. malnourishment

(1) protein depletion means poorer healing

(2) fewer defensive cells to fight infections

(3) postoperatively, always in catabolic state

5. Chronic health problems that increase risk of surgical problems

a. heart disease

b. diabetes

c. circulatory impairment

d. respiratory problems such as COPD and asthma

e. circulatory problems

f. smoking

g. liver disease

6. Psychologic readiness

a. fear of unknown greatest fear

b. need adequate explanation of procedures and what to expect

c. assess specific fears of patient

7. Spiritual needs

a. fear of not waking up

b. often need to speak to clergy

c. use available resources to meet spiritual needs, such as anointment for Catholics

8. Learning needs

a. postoperative exercises

b. knowledge of surgery and outcome

B. Planning, Goals/ Expected Outcomes

1. Patient will be adequately physically prepared for surgery

2. Patient will be adequately psychologically prepared for surgery

C. Implementation

1. Patient teaching

a. general information about surgery

b. coughing and deep breathing

c. leg exercises

d. turning

2. Preparation of skin per hospital policy

3. Restriction of oral intake

a. NPO after midnight

b. sometimes have IV started for hydration

4. Elimination

a. enemas until clear often given prior to surgery of lower intestine

b. occasionally catheterized before surgery

5. Rest

a. need good night's sleep, so sedative often given night before surgery

b. need to remain quiet and rested day of surgery

6. Consent for surgery signed and on chart before any narcotics or sedatives given

7. Immediate preoperative care

a. surgical gown and cap

b. all hairpins and metal objects removed

c. wedding ring may be taped on

d. all valuables off and safely stored

e. dentures out

f. identification bracelet on and correct

g. have patient void before surgery

h. medication given about 30 minutes before surgery to:

(1) reduce anxiety and promote rest

(a) Nembutal sodium or Seconal sodium: sedatives

(b) Vistaril hydrochloride: mild tranquilizer

(c) Demerol or morphine sulfate: narcotics

(2) decrease secretion of mucus and other body fluids: atropine sulfate or Robinul

(3) reduce nausea and vomiting with Vistaril

(4) enhance effects of anesthesia, sedatives, narcotics, and tranquilizers

D. Evaluation

1. Patient physically prepared for surgery

2. Patient psychologically prepared for surgery

II. INTRAOPERATIVE PERIOD

A. Anesthesia

1. Inhalation or general anesthesia

2. Intravenous agents

3. Regional

a. topical

b. rectal

c. spinal

B. Safety

1. Verify patient identity

2. Position so no pressure on bony prominences

3. Hypothermia

a. slows metabolic rate

b. slows oxygen consumption

c. slows bleeding

4. Sponge and instrument counts

III. POSTOPERATIVE PERIOD

A. Immediate Postoperative Period

1. Assessment
   a. level of consciousness
   b. patent airway
   c. vital signs
   d. IV fluids
   e. operative site
2. Planning, goals/expected outcomes
   a. patient will recover from anesthesia without difficulty
   b. patient airway will remain patent
   c. patient will not develop postoperative complications
3. Implementation
   a. position for safety and to maintain patent airway
   b. administer oxygen as ordered
   c. maintain IV flow rate
   d. assist in patient comfort
   e. provide warm blankets
   f. have emesis basin available if nausea and vomiting occur
   g. monitor urine output; at least 30 mL/hour
   h. provide emotional support
4. Evaluation
   a. patient recovered from anesthesia without difficulty
   b. patient airway remained patent
   c. patient did not develop postoperative complications

B. General Postoperative Period

1. Assessment
   a. vital signs
   b. symptoms of shock or hemorrhage
   c. dressings
   d. respiratory status
   e. tubes and drains
   f. wound
      (1) infection: presence of any redness or purulent drainage
      (2) dehiscence: any wound separation
      (3) evisceration: protrusion of abdominal contents
   g. elimination
      (1) adequate urinary output; at least 30 mL/hour
      (2) return of peristalsis
      (3) hiccoughs
   h. pain
   i. emotional reaction to surgery
2. Planning, goals/expected outcomes
   a. patient will not develop any complications
   b. patient will recover from surgery
3. Implementation
   a. vital signs: compare with preoperative levels
   b. dressings
      (1) check hourly first day
      (2) reinforce as needed
      (3) change using sterile technique as ordered
      (4) accurately describe wound and amount, color, and consistency of drainage
   c. respiratory status
      (1) cough and deep breathe hourly; use incentive spirometer
      (2) ambulate
      (3) auscultate breath sounds for abnormalities
   d. wound care (Tables 7-20 and 7-21)
      (1) clean wound as ordered using sterile technique
      (2) monitor for wound infection, usually 5 to 7 days after surgery
      (3) teach patient home care of wound
      (4) prevent dehiscence with binder
      (5) treat dehiscence with bed rest in (semi-Fowler's position with knees gatched), clean dressing, and notification of physician

TABLE 7–20. Phases of Wound Healing

Wounding Phase	1. Tissue integrity is disrupted; bleeding occurs; clots form; site is contaminated by bacteria and foreign bodies.
Inflammatory Phase	2. Capillary permeability and vasodilation increase; fluid (transudate) leaks into the wound; swelling occurs.
	3. WBCs and macrophages migrate to the site.
	4. Shreds of fibrin are laid down to fill the wound base.
Proliferative Phase	5. Dried proteins form a scab.
	6. Epithelial and endothelial cells and fibroblasts migrate to the wound, multiply, and follow the fibrin network. Fibroblasts synthesize collagen.
	7. Capillary vessels bud.
	8. Granulation continues. If wound cavity is large and the wound edges are not approximated, excessive amounts of granulation tissue (*proud flesh*) fill the defect.
Scarring Phase	9. Epithelial covering becomes multilayered.
	10. Collagen is synthesized to form connective tissue and scar tissue.
	11. Collagen production becomes balanced by collagen degradation and absorption.
	12. Scar tissue shrinks and contracts.

From Miller, B.F. & Keane, C.B. Encyclopedia and Dictionary of Medicine, Nursing and Allied Health. 3rd ed. Philadelphia, W.B. Saunders Company 1983. WBCs, white blood cells.

TABLE 7–21. Nutrients Affecting Wound Healing

Nutrient	Specific Component	Contribution to Wound Healing
Proteins	Amino acids	Needed for neovascularization, lymphocyte formation, fibroblast proliferation, collagen synthesis, and wound remodelling.
		Required for certain cell-mediated responses including phagocytosis and intracellular killing of bacteria.
	Albumin	Prevents wound edema secondary to low serum oncotic pressure.
Carbohydrates	Glucose	Needed for energy requirement of leukocytes and fibroblasts to function in inhibiting activities of wound infection
Fats	Essential unsaturated fatty acids	Serve as building blocks for prostaglandins that regulate cellular metabolism, inflammation, and circulation.
	a. Linoleic	
	b. Linolenic	Constituents of triglycerides and fatty acids contained in cellular and subcellular
	c. Arachidonic	membranes.
Vitamins	Ascorbic acid	Hydroxylates proline and lysine in collagen synthesis.
		Enhances capillary formation and decreases capillary fragility.
		A necessary component of complement that functions in immune reactions and increases defenses to infection.
	B complex	Serve as cofactors of enzyme systems.
	Pyridoxine, pantothenic and	Required for antibody formation and white blood cell function.
	folic acid A	Enhances epithelialization of cell membranes.
		Enhances rate of collagen synthesis and cross-linking of newly formed collagen.
		Antagonizes the inhibitory effects of glucocorticoids on cell membranes.
	D	Necessary for absorption, transport, and metabolism of calcium.
		Indirectly affects phosphorus metabolism.
	E	No special role known; may be important if there is a fatty acid deficiency.
	K	Needed for synthesis of prothrombin and clotting factors VII, IX, and X.
		Required for synthesis of calcium-binding protein.
Minerals	Zinc	Stabilizes cell membranes.
		Needed for cell mitosis and cell proliferation in wound repair.
	Iron	Needed for hydroxylation of proline and lysine in collagen synthesis.
		Enhances bactericidal activity of leukocytes.
		Secondarily, deficiency may cause decrease in oxygen transport to wound.
	Copper	An integral part of the enzyme, lysyloxidase, that catalyzes formation of stable collagen crosslinks.

From Miller, B.F. & Keane, C.B. Encyclopedia and Dictionary of Medicine, Nursing and Allied Health. 3rd ed. Philadelphia, W.B. Saunders Company, 1983. Originally from Schumann, D. (1979). Preoperative measures to promote wound healing. *Nurs. Clin. North Am.* 14:683.

(6) treat evisceration with bed rest, moist sterile dressing, and preparation of patient for return to surgery for reclosure of wound; medical emergency

e. elimination
  (1) encourage ambulation
  (2) use nasogastric tube to treat nausea, vomiting, and severe distension
  (3) increase diet as peristalsis returns (see Chapter 5)
    (a) clear liquid
    (b) full liquid
    (c) soft diet
    (d) regular diet
  (4) ensure that patient voids at least 30 mL/ hour, and within 8 to 12 hours after surgery
f. pain
  (1) medicate patient with narcotics
  (2) promote comfort through backrubs, repositioning, and other nursing measures
g. provide emotional support as needed
h. discharge teaching
  (1) teach normal restrictions such as no lifting, driving, or intercourse, usually for 4 to 6 weeks
  (2) teach care specific to surgery

  (3) arrange for visiting nurses or other help as needed after discharge
4. Evaluation
  a. patient recovered from surgery
  b. patient did not develop postoperative complications

■ Immune/Autoimmune Disorders

I. ACQUIRED IMMUNE DEFICIENCY SYNDROME (AIDS)

A. Assessment

1. Definition/pathophysiology: viral disorder caused by human T-lymphotrophic virus, type III, or HIV, which destroys T lymphocytes and renders the individual unable to fight off disease
2. Predisposing/precipitating factors
  a. homosexual men
  b. IV drug users
  c. hemophiliacs
  d. Haitians

3. Signs and symptoms
   a. presence of specific opportunistic infections or cancer
      (1) *Pneumocystis carinii* pneumonia
      (2) Kaposi's sarcoma
   b. swollen glands in neck, armpits, and groin
   c. rapid weight loss
   d. unexplained fever
   e. chronic diarrhea
   f. skin changes
   g. fatigue
   h. cough and shortness of breath
   i. 75% mortality rate within 3 to 4 years of diagnosis
4. Diagnostic tests
   a. presence of HIV virus
   b. presence of *Pneumocystis carinii* parasite or Kaposi's sarcoma
5. Usual treatment: AZT and experimental, mainly supportive therapy

B. Planning, Goals/ Expected Outcomes

1. Patient will not develop opportunistic infections
2. Patient and family will cope with emotional aspects of disease
3. Patient will understand and comply with precautions to prevent spread of disease
4. Patient will cope with terminal prognosis

C. Implementation

1. Educate patient on modes of spread
2. Avoid contamination of blood or serum
3. Use good hand-washing
4. Provide emotional support
5. Follow hospital isolation procedures

D. Evaluation

1. Patient did not develop opportunistic infection
2. Patient and family coped with diagnosis of AIDS
3. Patient understood and complied with precautions to limit spread of disease
4. Patient coped with impending death

II. CANCER

A. Assessment

1. Definition
   a. abnormal growth of cells, with alteration in cell's DNA that causes cell to multiply rapidly

and spread (metastasize) to other parts of body
   b. cancer cells take over normal cells' nourishment and space
2. Incidence
   a. occurs at any age; some age-specific cancers
   b. incidence increases with age
   c. often associated with exposure to "carcinogens" (substances in environment that can add to likelihood of cancer development)
3. Predisposing/precipitating factors
   a. major risk factors for cancer (Table 7-22)
   b. age
   c. exposure to chemical carcinogens
   d. obesity
   e. cigarette smoking
4. Signs and symptoms
   a. seven warning signals of cancer (*caution*)
      (1) *C*hange in bowel or bladder habits
      (2) *A* sore that does not heal
      (3) *U*nusual bleeding or discharge
      (4) *T*hickening or lump in breast or elsewhere

TABLE 7–22. Major Risk Factors for Cancer

Lung	Heavy smoker over age 50 years
	Smoked a pack a day for 20 years
	Cigarette cough
	Started smoking at age 15 years or before
Breast	Lump or nipple discharge
	History of breast cancer
	Close relatives with history of breast cancer
	Age over 35 years; especially over 50 years
	Never had children; first child after age 30 years
Colon rectal	History of rectal polyps
	Rectal polyps run in family
	History of ulcerative colitis
	Blood in stool
	Over age 40 years
Uterine cervical	Unusual bleeding or discharge
	Frequent sex in early teens or with many partners
	Low income background
	Poor care during or following pregnancy
	Age 40 to 49 years
Uterine endometrial	Unusual bleeding or discharge
	Late menopause (after age 55 years)
	Diabetes, high blood pressure and obesity
	Age 50 to 64 years
Skin	Excessive exposure to sun
	Fair complexion
	Work with coal tar, pitch, or creosote
Oral	Heavy smoker and drinker
	Poor oral hygiene
	Chewing tobacco
Ovary	History of ovarian cancer among close relatives
	Age 50 to 59 years
Prostate	Over age 65 years
Stomach	History of stomach cancer among close relatives
	Diet heavy in smoked, pickled, or salted foods
	Some link with blood group A

(5) *Indigestion or difficulty swallowing*
(6) *Obvious change in wart or mole*
(7) *Nagging cough or hoarseness*
  b. others specific to site of cancer
5. Diagnostic tests
  a. biopsy: surgically taking piece of tissue to examine microscopically
  b. radiographs
    (1) use of radiopaque liquids; eg, barium for gastrointestinal (GI) tract
      (a) nurse needs to be sure ordered prep given prior to examination; usually cleansing enemas or nothing by mouth, or clear liquid diet only
      (b) after examination, nurse needs to check for laxative order to aid in elimination of barium
    (2) use of radioactive materials to "scan" body; radioactive material concentrates in tumor areas, creating "hot spots"; no special preparation; patient not radioactive
    (3) CT scan
      (a) uses computer and low radiation to obtain three-dimensional picture
      (b) possibly enemas for abdominal scan; explain procedure to patient
    (4) MRI
      (a) uses magnetic fields, no radiation
      (b) some patients experience claustrophobia during test
      (c) no prep except explanation
  c. endoscopy: use of fiberoptic flexible scope to examine internal GI system
6. Usual treatment
  a. surgical excision of tumor and surrounding tissues
  b. chemotherapy: use of drugs that interfere with cell metabolism and inhibit tumor growth and spread (Tables 7-23, and 7-24)
  c. radiation therapy: use of radiation from x-rays, radium, and other sources to destroy tumor with minimal damage to normal tissue; can be internal or external

B. Planning, Goals/ Expected Outcomes

1. Patient will identify risk factors related to cancer
2. Patient will know seven warning signals of cancer
3. Patient will follow prescribed treatment plan
4. Patient will be assisted in dealing with side effects of treatment
5. Patient will participate in continued check-ups for cancer recurrence or prevention

TABLE 7–23. Chemotherapeutic Agents (Antineoplastics)

Alkylating agents	Inhibit cell growth and division by reacting with DNA
Antimetabolites	Prevent cell growth by competing with metabolites in the production of nucleic acid
Anticancer antibiotics	Block cell growth by binding with DNA
Plant alkaloids	Prevent cellular reproduction by altering protein synthesis and nucleic acids through some still unknown mechanism
Steroid hormones	Inhibit the growth of hormone susceptible tumors by changing their chemical environment

6. Patient will be assisted to deal with emotional aspects of diagnosis

C. Implementation

1. Assist patient to learn side effects of carcinogens such as sun, chemicals, and smoking
2. Modify diet by reducing fat intake and increasing fiber intake (see Chapter 5)
3. Identify seven warning signs of cancer
4. Encourage patient to participate in treatment process
  a. identify social support system
  b. refer to social service agencies such as American Cancer Society (ACS), Ostomy Association, I Can Cope, for assistance
5. Assist patient to take measures to reduce side effects of treatments (Table 7-25)
6. Make outpatient appointments, arrange follow-up visits, and for continued monitoring
7. Help patient verbalize feelings concerning diagnosis
8. Make referrals to appropriate resources and people as needed such as ACS, Reach for Recovery, psychiatrist, social worker

D. Evaluation

1. Patient recovered from treatment of primary cancer
2. Patient avoided sun, smoking, and other carcinogens
3. Patient modified diet
4. Patient kept follow-up appointments
5. Side effects of cancer treatments reduced or coped with
6. Patient discussed feelings concerning diagnosis and learned ways to cope
7. Support systems identified and utilized effectively by patient

TABLE 7–24. Pharmacologic Treatment of Cancer

Class	Example	Action	Use	Adverse Effects	Nursing Implications
Alkylating agents	Cyclophosphamide (Cytoxan) Chlorambucil	Interfere with rapidly proliferating tissues; the DNA molecule is damaged	Hodgkin's disease and other lymphomas Leukemia	Anorexia Nausea Vomiting Reversible alopecia Bone marrow suppression Hemorrhagic cystitis	Given by IV or oral route Push fluids to increase output to try to prevent hemorrhage Cystitis Hematuria or dysuria needs to be immediately reported to team leader
Antimetabolites	Methotrexate Fluorouracil (5FU)	Prevent the reduction of folic acid to tetrahydrofolate; folic acid is critical to metabolism of the proliferating cell	Lymphatic leukemia Lymphosarcoma Lymphoblastic leukemia Choriocarcinoma	Bone marrow suppression Stomatitis Hemorrhagic enteritis Hepatic dysfunction Gastrointestinal system disorders	Hemorrhagic enteritis could lead to perforation Watch for blood in stools Increase in abdominal pain
Natural products	Vinblastine Vincristine Dactinomycin	Block cell division	Choriocarcinoma Hodgkin's lymphomas Melanomas Sarcomas	Anemia Pancytopenia Nausea Vomiting Diarrhea Stomatitis Reversible alopecia Phlebitis	Given by IV route Monitor for bone marrow, hepatic or renal impairment Monitor for bronchospasm
Hormones	Adrenocorticosteroids	Suppress cell reproduction	Acute lymphocytic leukemia	Cushingoid symptoms	Monitor for cushingoid symptoms, such as diabetes mellitus symptoms
	Estrogens Androgens	Change hormone environment	Male hormones for female reproductive organ cancers; female hormones for male reproductive cancers	Nausea Vomiting Water retention Impotence in men, decreased libido in women Menstrual irregularities Opposite sex characteristics	Monitor for signs and symptoms of hypercalcemia, such as renal calculi Monitor for symptoms of cholestatic jaundice
Miscellaneous agents	Hydroxyurea	Suppress DNA synthesis	Melanoma	Bone marrow suppression Anorexia Nausea Vomiting Stomatitis Elevated blood urea nitrogen (BUN)	Monitor for renal toxicity

III. SYSTEMIC LUPUS ERYTHEMATOSUS (SLE)

A. Assessment

1. Definition/pathophysiology: chronic, systemic, inflammatory disease involving connective tissue and multiple body systems; probably autoimmune in nature; characterized by remissions and exacerbations; variable course of disease
2. Incidence
   a. women more than men
   b. nonwhite women more than white
   c. women most often during childbearing years

TABLE 7–25. Radiation Treatment of Cancer

Area Irradiated	Effect	Nursing Management
Abdomen/pelvis	Cramps, diarrhea	Opium tincture, camphorated diphenoxylate with atropine (Lomotil), low residue diet, maintain fluid and electrolyte balance
Head	Alopecia	Encourage patient to wear wig or head covering
	Mucositis	Mouthwash with viscous lidocaine, cool carbonated drinks, ice pops, soft, nonirritating diet
	Monilial infection	Nystatin mouthwash, avoidance of commercial mouthwash
	Dental caries	Fluoride applied to teeth prophylactically, provide gingival care
Chest	Lung tissue devitalization	No smoking, avoidance of people with upper respiratory infections, provide humidifier if necessary
	Pericarditis	Control arrhythmias with appropriate agents (procainamide, disopyramide phosphate), monitor for heart failure
Kidneys	Nephritis, lassitude, headache, edema, dyspnea on exertion, hypertensive nephropathy, azotemia, secondary anemia	Maintain fluid and electrolyte balance, watch for signs of renal failure

3. Predisposing/precipitating factors
   a. drug-induced syndrome: hydralazine (Apresoline) and procainamide (Pronestyl)
   b. stress
   c. genetic predisposition
4. Signs and symptoms
   a. joint inflammation, arthritis like
   b. insidious onset
   c. extreme fatigue, generalized weakness and anorexia
   d. weight loss
   e. fever
   f. "butterfly rash": raised rash across cheeks and bridge of nose
   g. generalized rash
   h. polymyositis
   i. vasculitis: often direct cause of death
      (1) renal
      (2) central nervous system
      (3) cardiac
   j. hypertension
   k. peripheral vascular disease
   l. gastrointestinal problems
      (1) pain
      (2) cramping
      (3) nausea and vomiting
   m. pneumonitis
   n. Raynaud's phenomenon
5. Diagnostic tests
   a. CBC
   b. lupus erythematosus (LE) prep
   c. assessments of affected organ systems
6. Complications
   a. peripheral vascular disease, loss of limbs
   b. hypertension
   c. stroke
   d. renal failure
   e. congestive heart failure
   f. chronic obstructive pulmonary disease
7. Usual treatments
   a. antiinflammatories
      (1) steroids (Table 7-17)
      (2) nonsteroidal (Table 7-17)
   b. Plaquenil, antimalarial for skin lesions
   c. topical steroids
   d. symptomatic treatment to each affected body system; ie, antihypertensives

B. Planning, Goals/ Expected Outcomes

1. Patient's skin integrity will be maintained
2. Patient's pain and discomfort will be decreased
3. Patient's symptoms will be controlled
4. Patient will cope with altered body image
5. Patient will not suffer from excessive complications

6. Patient will maintain maximal level of independence
7. Patient will understand and comply with medical regimen

C. Implementation

1. Maintain skin integrity
   a. use cool baths
   b. avoid soaps and powders
   c. apply topical steroids as ordered
2. Administer medication as ordered
3. Avoid things that exacerbate disease
   a. sunlight
   b. stress
   c. pregnancy
4. Provide frequent rest periods

5. Encourage maximal independence
6. Provide high protein (unless renal involvement), high vitamin and iron diet
7. Monitor for easy bruising and injury
8. Allow grieving over potential terminal nature of disease

D. Evaluation

1. Patient's skin remained intact
2. Patient stated relief or control of pain and discomfort
3. Patient coped with altered body image
4. Patient's symptoms were controlled
5. Patient understood and complied with medical regimen
6. Patient maintained maximal independence

Questions

1. A malignant tumor differs from a benign tumor in that the malignant tumor:

① Grows more slowly
② Spreads more easily
③ Is easily removed by surgery
④ Is encapsulated

2. The term metastasis is best defined as:

① The spread of malignant cells to another part of the body
② A second primary tumor in a new location
③ The presence of malignant cells in a tumor
④ Contamination of the tumor with bacteria

3. Cancer is spread in many ways. One way it is *not* spread is:

① Through the circulatory system
② On surgical instruments and gloves during surgery
③ Through sexual intercourse with a cancer patient
④ Through the lymphatic system

4. Risk factors for the development of cancer include all the following except:

① Smoking
② Asbestos
③ Testosterone
④ Sunlight

5. Which of the following is no longer recommended by the American Cancer Society as a test for early detection of cancer?

① Monthly breast self-examination and a mammogram for women over age 50 years
② Yearly stools tested for guaiac on all people over age 50 years
③ Digital rectal examination for men over age 40 years
④ Annual sputum analysis and yearly chest radiograph for smokers

6. In order to prevent cancer and to screen for its early detection, the nurse must know:

① Those at greatest risk for each cancer
② The cause of all cancers
③ The prognosis for the treatment of all cancers
④ The current treatment protocol for each cancer

7. If a person is a heavy smoker and a heavy drinker for years, he or she is at greatest risk for:

① Lung cancer
② Laryngeal cancer
③ Stomach cancer
④ Oral cancer

8. A cancer patient is often described as being in remission. This means that the patient is:

① Cured of the cancer permanently
② Free of the cancer for at least 5 years
③ Free of the cancer for an undetermined time
④ Currently having active disease and in need of treatment

9. Cancer in general is most correctly diagnosed by:

① A culture
② A biopsy
③ Laboratory analysis of blood
④ Diagnostic radiographs

10. Side effects of external radiation are usually:

① Generalized to all body systems
② Localized to the area tested
③ Minimal if the dose is given all at once
④ Serious and potentially life threatening

11. When caring for the patient receiving external radiation, the nurse should take extra precautions with the skin over the site of the therapy. Care of this area should include:

① Daily cleansing with soap and water
② Application of lotion to prevent drying
③ Avoidance of tight clothing over the site
④ Avoiding any contact with the area

12. When radiation therapy is given to the mouth and upper neck, which of the following side effects is likely to develop?

① Stomatitis
② Alopecia
③ Thrombocytopenia
④ Leukopenia

13. If the above side effect does develop, the most appropriate nursing intervention to treat it is:

① Avoid intramuscular injections
② Place the patient in reverse isolation
③ Encourage the patient to wear a wig or scarf
④ Administer Xylocaine gargle before meals as ordered

14. Before caring for the patient with cancer, it is very important for the nurse to know:

① The usual treatment for that cancer
② The patient's social support system
③ Whether the patient knows the diagnosis
④ The most recent experimental therapy available

15. Gonorrhea is a venereal disease that:

① Is incurable in women
② Can be contracted only once, then the person has immunity
③ Is not highly infectious
④ Can be cured with antibiotics like penicillin

16. It is difficult to control the spread of gonorrhea because:

① Women with the disease are often misdiagnosed
② Few women have symptoms severe enough to seek treatment
③ The symptoms are very similar to those of syphilis
④ Men have so few symptoms of the disease

17. The patient receiving chemotherapeutic agents in the treatment of cancer may suffer from numerous side effects, including leukopenia, thrombocytopenia, anemia, and gastrointestinal distress and bleeding. The nurse knows that these side effects occur because:

① Chemotherapeutic agents are toxins
② Both normal and abnormal rapidly dividing cells are destroyed
③ The dosages of chemotherapy are usually higher than they should be to insure cure
④ Chemotherapeutic agents are lethal to all cells

18. Nursing interventions for the patient suffering from leukopenia secondary to chemotherapy would include:

① Protecting the patient from infections
② Avoiding venipunctures for blood work
③ Providing for periods of rest
④ Administering antiemetics before meals

19. Nursing interventions for the patient with thrombocytopenia secondary to chemotherapy would include:

① Protecting the patient from infections
② Avoiding venipunctures for blood work
③ Providing for periods of rest
④ Administering antiemetics before meals

20. Nursing interventions for the patient with anemia secondary to chemotherapy would include:

① Protecting the patient from infections
② Avoiding venipunctures for blood work
③ Providing for periods of rest
④ Administering antiemetics before meals

21. Nursing interventions for the patient suffering from gastrointestinal distress secondary to chemotherapy would include:

① Protecting the patient from infections
② Avoiding venipunctures for blood work
③ Providing for periods of rest
④ Administering antiemetics before meals

22. If the patient is suspected of suffering from gastrointestinal bleeding secondary to chemotherapy, the nurse should:

① Test all stools and urine for blood
② Administer only cold liquids
③ Avoid venipunctures that could increase blood loss
④ Place the patient on complete bed rest

Answers & Rationales

Guide to item identification (see pp. 3–5 for further details about each category)

I, II, III, or IV for the phase of the nursing process
1, 2, 3, or 4 for the category of client needs
A, B, C, D, E, F, or G for the category of human functioning
Specific content category by name; ie, cholecystectomy

1. ② The major characteristic of a malignant tumor is its ability to spread beyond the limits of normal cells.
I, 2, D & F. Cancer.

2. ① Metastasis involves the spread of a malignant cell from its point of origin to another part of the body.
I, 2, D & F. Cancer.

3. ③ Cancer cannot be spread through personal contact.
I, 2, D & F. Cancer.

4. ③ All are risk factors except the male hormone testosterone. The nurse should be aware of risk factors to teach and protect patients.
I, 2, D & F. Cancer.

5. ④ All are routine screening examinations except the sputum analysis and chest radiograph, which were dropped because they did nothing to improve the early detection of cancer.
I & III, 2 & 4, D & F. Cancer.

6. ① Knowing the risk factors for each type of cancer allows the nurse to screen and do health promotion with the correct populations.
I & III, 2 & 4, D. Cancer.

7. ② The combination increases a person's risk for cancer of the larynx.
I, 2, D & F. Cancer.

8. ③ Remission means that the disease is temporarily under control, but the time it lasts is undetermined.
I, 2, D & F. Cancer.

9. ② A biopsy is the only absolute way to diagnose cancer.
I, 2, D. Cancer.

10. ② Side effects from radiation are more likely to be localized to the area exposed, although some systemic effects may occur.
I, 2, D. Cancer/Radiation Therapy.

11. ③ The nurse should teach the patient to avoid any irritation of the irradiated skin, which may increase the breakdown of the skin.
III, 2, D. Cancer/Radiation Therapy.

12. ① Stomatitis is the irritation of the mucous membranes caused by either radiation or chemotherapy.
III, 2, D. Cancer/Radiation Therapy.

13. ④ The mouth is very sore with stomatitis, and local anesthesia must be administered before meals or mouth care.
III, 2, D. Cancer/Radiation Therapy.

14. ③ Before the nurse cares for the cancer patient, it is important to determine exactly what the patient has been told about the condition.
III, 2, D & G. Cancer.

15. ④ Gonorrhea can be treated with antibiotics.
IV, 4, A & D. STDs.

16. ② Only about 10% of women exhibit symptoms of gonorrhea, making it very difficult to diagnose because most women don't know they have it.
IV, 4, A. STDs.

17. ② The side effects of chemotherapy and radiation therapy occur because both malignant and normal rapidly dividing cells are destroyed. The cells of the bone marrow and the mucous lining of the gastrointestinal tract are some of the most rapidly dividing cells in the body.
I, 2, D. Cancer/Chemotherapy.

18. ① A lowered white blood cell count increases the patient's risk of contracting an infection.
III, 2, D. Cancer/Chemotherapy.

19. ② A low platelet count predisposes the patient to bleeding.
III, 2, D. Cancer/Chemotherapy.

20. ③ Red blood cells are also destroyed by chemotherapy, leaving the patient anemic and fatigued.
III, 2, C & D. Cancer/Chemotherapy.

21. Gastrointestinal distress occurs because of destruction of the mucous membrane lining of the
④ tract, which often leads to nausea, vomiting, diarrhea and anorexia. Antiemetics before meals may help the patient to eat.
III, 2, D & F. Cancer/Chemotherapy.

22. Testing the urine and stools for blood will confirm the presence of gastrointestinal and uri-
① nary tract bleeding.
III, 2, D. Cancer/Chemotherapy.

MOBILITY/ ACTIVITY/ COMFORT

■ Hazards of Immobility

I. GENERALIZED

A. Survival

Adults need mobility to survive

B. Duration

Many and varied problems arise if patient is immobilized for even 24 hours, and problems increase with length of immobilization

C. Avoidance

Most problems can be avoided with proper nursing care

D. Extent

Immobility affects all body systems

II. CARDIOVASCULAR SYSTEM

A. Assessment

1. Blood vessels
   a. muscular activity aids in movement of blood
   b. with no activity, blood flow sluggish
   c. inadequate nourishment to all cells
   d. decreased flow predisposes clot formation
2. Workload of heart
   a. heart works harder when body at rest and supine
   b. more frequent use of Valsalva maneuver every time patient moves up in bed
3. Blood pressure
   a. orthostatic changes occur within hours
   b. patient at risk for fainting or falling

B. Nursing Interventions

1. Exercises to maintain adequate circulation, within limits of patient's condition
   a. passive range of motion
   b. active range of motion
   c. isometric exercises

2. Positioning
   a. teach patient to change position without using Valsalva maneuver
   b. change position, minimally at least every hour and completely every 2 hours
   c. elevate head of bed at intervals
   d. encourage patient to move extremities, even a little, as much as possible

III. RESPIRATORY SYSTEM

A. Assessment

1. Pulmonary stasis and accumulation of secretions
   a. wheezing
   b. productive cough
   c. altered respiratory depth and rate
2. Inadequate aeration of lungs
   a. shortness of breath
   b. pain
   c. feeling of tightness in chest

B. Nursing Interventions

1. Have patient cough and deep breathe
2. Frequent turning
3. Adequate hydration
4. Change position to include semi-Fowler's to Fowler's
5. Support incision or painful area during coughing
6. Medicate as needed to encourage coughing
7. Avoid codeine and other cough suppressants
8. Provide rest periods
9. Give frequent mouth care

IV. GASTROINTESTINAL SYSTEM

A. Assessment

1. Ingestion
   a. decreased appetite
   b. emotions often low so less willing to eat
   c. usually low protein intake
2. Elimination
   a. constipation related to:
      (1) decreased peristalsis
      (2) physical inactivity
      (3) inability to use bedpan
      (4) decreased muscle tone
      (5) embarrassment over using bedpan and asking for help
      (6) amount and type of food eaten
      (7) fluid intake

b. impaction
   (1) absence of stools for 3 days
   (2) may have diarrhea as liquid seeps around impaction

B. Nursing Interventions

1. Check patient's dietary intake
   a. provide adequate liquids
   b. increase bulk and roughage in diet (see Chapter 5)
2. Provide privacy for defecation
3. Use bedside commode if at all possible
4. Position patient sitting on bedpan if patient must remain in bed
5. Encourage patient to follow normal bowel habits
6. Administer stool softeners (Colace) or bulk laxatives (Metamucil) as ordered
7. Institute bowel training program

8. Avoid cathartics or enemas unless absolutely necessary

V. MUSCULOSKELETAL SYSTEM

A. Assessment

1. Range of motion (see Chapter 3 and Fig. 7-2)
   a. muscle activity maintains range of motion
   b. without joint motion, muscles lose elasticity and shorten
   c. fibrous tissue develops
   d. contractures may occur and cause permanent damage
2. Osteoporosis
   a. new bone formed because of stress and strain placed on bones by walking and standing
   b. inactivity causes depletion of calcium, phosphorus, and nitrogen in bone
   c. demineralization causes increased bone porosity and increased risk factors

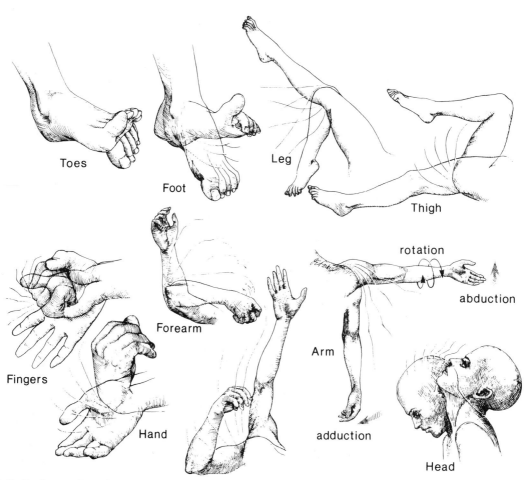

FIGURE 7–2. Bed exercises for postoperative patients. (From Watson, J.E.: Medical-Surgical Nursing and Related Physiology. 2nd ed. Philadelphia, W.B. Saunders Company, 1979.)

B. Nursing Interventions

1. Prevent foot drop with foot board
2. Use supportive devices to prevent contractures and deformities
3. Active and passive range of motion exercises (see Figure 7-2)
4. Stand and allow weight bearing if possible
5. Increase calcium in diet through foods such as yogurt, sardines, greens, milk, or cheese (see Table 5-7)

VI. INTEGUMENTARY SYSTEM

A. Assessment

1. Decubitus ulcers: lesions produced by sloughing of inflamed and necrosed tissue
   a. caused by pressure, especially over bony prominence (Fig. 7-3)
   b. caused by shearing force
2. Erythema begins within 1 to 2 hours of pressure and congestion because of impaired blood flow
3. Breakdown most likely to occur if individual is malnourished, obese, elderly, or has circulatory impairment
4. Other risk factors include warm, moist skin subjected to irritating substances such as urine, feces, sweat, or other discharges
5. Classification
   a. Stage I
      (1) skin is deep pink, red, or mottled
      (2) skin is warm and firm or tightly stretched
      (3) reversible; no permanent skin damage
   b. Stage II
      (1) skin blistered, cracked, or abraded
      (2) skin integrity disrupted
      (3) skin around area red and warm
   c. Stage III
      (1) skin ulcerated with crater-like sore
      (2) underlying tissues involved
      (3) usually infected
      (4) infection causes continued erosion and copious secretions
   d. Stage IV
      (1) deep ulceration and necrosis involving deep underlying muscle and maybe bone
      (2) extensively infected
      (3) ulcer either dry and covered with thick necrotic tissue or wet and oozing

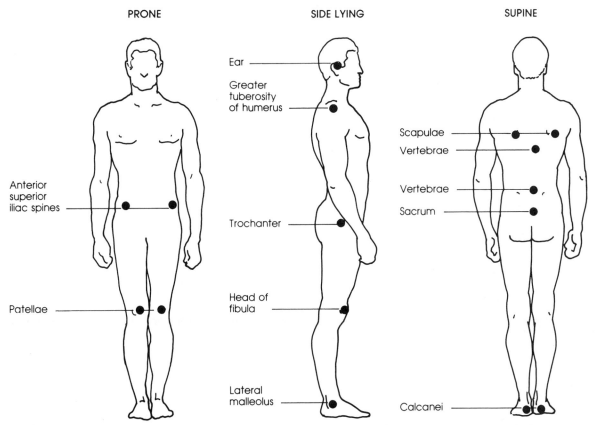

FIGURE 7–3. Bony prominences most susceptible to skin breakdown, according to position. (From Keane, C.B.: Essentials of Medical-Surgical Nursing. 2nd ed. Philadelphia, W.B. Saunders Company, 1986.)

B. Nursing Interventions

1. Prevention of ulcers is much easier than treatment
   a. frequent position changes
   b. pad all bony prominences
   c. support extremities
   d. turn at least every 2 hours or more frequently
   e. use special devices such as egg crate mattress, foam pads, flotation pad, sheepskin, Clinitron bed, or other therapeutic devices to distribute pressure and help prevent breakdown
   f. keep patient and all linens clean and dry
   g. use lotion to moisturize skin
   h. massage all potential breakdown areas
   i. maintain adequate nutrition and hydration
   j. reposition to avoid shearing force of sliding patients
2. Treatment of pressure sores varies by institution
   a. keep ulcer clean and dry
   b. care required constantly to prevent further damage
   c. use protocol established by institution for treatment

VII. URINARY SYSTEM

A. Assessment

1. Stasis common when patient is not in upright position
2. When patient is supine, urine flow is sluggish and pooling occurs
3. Calculi and infections are common with stasis
4. Loss of bladder tone from distention
5. Lose control of urinary sphincters because of excessive pressure
6. Retention with overflow and incontinence is common

B. Nursing Interventions

1. Encourage adequate fluid intake, at least 2 to 3 L/day
2. Have patient void regularly
3. Restrict calcium intake
4. Encourage acid-ash foods such as cranberry juice, cereals, fish, meats, and vitamin C to acidify urine
5. Have women sit and men stand to void to facilitate bladder emptying
6. Use appropriate methods to encourage voiding (see Chapter 3)
7. Catheterize as a last resort; physician's order necessary

VIII. PSYCHOLOGIC ASPECTS

A. Assessment

1. Loss of independence
2. Sense of hopelessness is common
3. Feelings of isolation and depression
4. Worry over family and financial matters

B. Nursing Interventions

1. Allow maximum independence and decision making on part of patient
2. Help patient set realistic goals
3. Help patient see own worth and maintain dignity
4. Arrange consults with social services as needed

■ Musculoskeletal Disorders

I. TRAUMATIC DISORDERS

A. Casts

1. Assessment
   a. types of casts
      (1) long or short leg casts
      (2) walking casts with extra support for weight bearing
      (3) spica casts cover trunk and one or two extremities
   b. observe closely for pressure on nerves or blood vessels
   c. observe for numbness, tingling, or increased pain
   d. observe distal tissues for impaired circulation; assess color and warmth by checking blanching
   e. monitor for signs of infection: elevated temperature, presence of foul odor
   f. check for warmth or "hot spots" under cast, which could signal inflammation
2. Nursing interventions
   a. allow cast to dry completely before moving it
   b. if moving wet cast, use palms, not fingertips
   c. support cast on pillows
   d. leave cast exposed to air until dry
   e. do not use hair drier or heat source on cast
   f. cast takes at least 24 hours to dry or longer in higher humidity
   g. keep cast clean, dry, and free from bodily secretions
   h. tape edges of cast to prevent irritation
   i. continually monitor circulation and sensation under cast
   j. monitor for complications

k. teach patient home cast care, especially not to stick objects under cast

l. elevate casted extremities to decrease normal swelling

B. Traction

1. Assessment
   a. traction: application of mechanical pull to a body part to
      (a) reduce and set a fracture
      (b) immobilize a part
      (c) relieve pain
   b. types of traction (Fig. 7-4)
      (1) skeletal: traction applied directly to bone
      (2) skin: traction applied directly to skin
         (a) Buck's extension: lower extremity, usually to treat fractured hip
         (b) Russell's: for fractured hip or knee
         (c) cervical or pelvic: for cervical or lumbar strain
   c. be sure weights hang free
   d. observe all skin areas for possible pressure sores
   e. monitor pin sites for possible infection
   f. assess for impaired circulation or undue pressure on nerves
2. Nursing interventions
   a. maintain proper body alignment for traction and countertraction
   b. turn and position patient as allowed by type of traction
   c. clean pin sites daily and dress per institutional policy
   d. provide diversional activities
   e. use fracture bedpan

C. Fractures

1. Assessment
   a. types of fractures (Fig. 7-5)
      (1) complete: bone broken in two parts with complete separation of parts
      (2) incomplete: bone broken into two parts that do not separate
      (3) comminuted: bone shattered into more than two fragments
      (4) closed or simple: skin not broken
      (5) open or compound: break in skin with protrusion of bone fragments
      (6) greenstick: common in children when bone is partially bent and partially broken
      (7) other types include pathologic, longitudinal, spiral, transverse, oblique

   b. predisposing/precipitating factors
      (1) old age
      (2) osteoporosis; greatest in postmenopausal women
      (3) trauma
      (4) cancer
   c. signs and symptoms
      (1) pain
      (2) swelling
      (3) deformities
      (4) of fractured hip: leg shortened, abducted, and externally rotated
   d. diagnostic tests
      (1) history of injury
      (2) radiographic examination
      (3) physical examination
   e. usual treatment
      (1) goal is to reunite bone fragments in as close to normal alignment as possible, so that bone can heal normally; healing occurs in 4 stages:
         (a) blood from trauma clots and forms hematoma between broken ends of bone
         (b) granulation tissue forms that becomes firm and becomes link between pieces of broken bone
         (c) new bone tissue enters area, forming woven bone; ends have begun to knit
         (d) immature cells replaced by mature cells, callus formed, tissue resembles normal bone
      (2) closed reduction
         (a) bones realigned without surgery
         (b) once bones are in alignment, cast is usually applied to hold bones in alignment
      (3) open reduction
         (a) surgical realignment of bone fragments
         (b) cast or traction usually applied postoperatively
      (4) internal fixation
         (a) follows open reduction
         (b) application of screws, plates, pins, nails, and so on to hold fragments in alignment
         (c) may also involve removal of damaged bone and replacement with prosthesis
         (d) used for the elderly, because it provides immediate bone strength
         (e) increased risk of infection
      (5) external fixation
         (a) sturdy external frame with multiple pins through bone
         (b) used with extensive open fractures with soft tissue damage
         (c) if infected, fractures do not heal properly
         (d) with multiple traumas

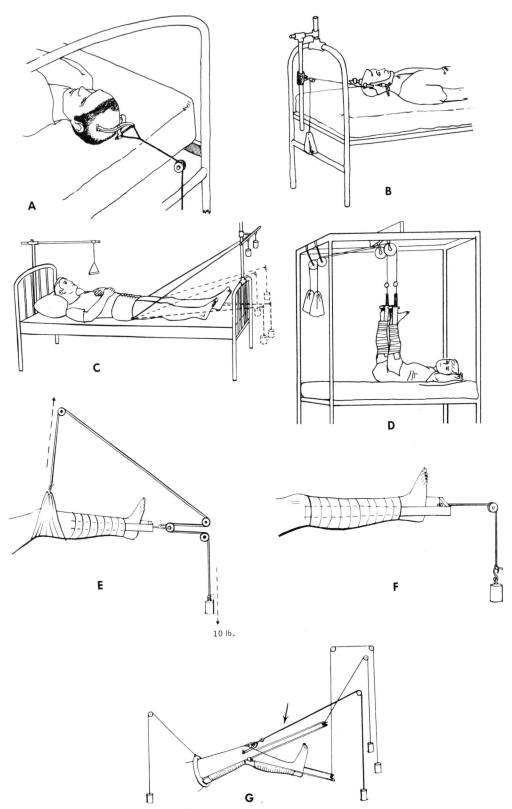

FIGURE 7–4. Types of traction. *A,* Cervical traction using tongs. *B,* Cervical traction using a halter. *C,* Pelvic traction. *D,* Balanced suspension traction using a Thomas splint with a Pearson attachment. *E,* Russell traction, which may be used in the treatment of the shaft of the femur. *F,* Buch's extension. *G,* Balanced suspension traction using a Thomas splint with a Pearson attachment. (*A* through *D* from Weibe, A.M.: Orthopedics in Nursing. Philadelphia, W.B. Saunders Company, 1961. *E* through *G* from Sutton, A.L.: Bedside Nursing Techniques. 2nd ed. Philadelphia, W.B. Saunders Company, 1969.)

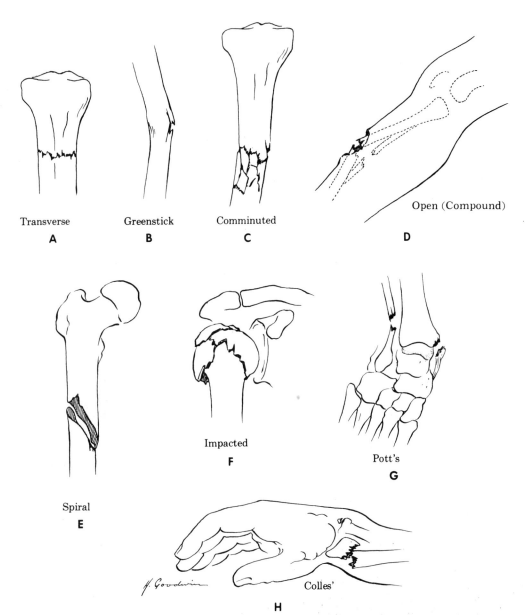

Transverse
A

Greenstick
B

Comminuted
C

Open (Compound)
D

Spiral
E

Impacted
F

Pott's
G

Colles'
H

FIGURE 7–5. Types of fractures. *A*, Simple complete transverse. *B*, Incomplete (greenstick). *C*, Comminuted. *D*, Compound (open), *E*, Spiral. *F*, Impacted. *G*, Pott's. *H*, Colles'. (From Watson, J.E.: Medical-Surgical Nursing and Related Physiology. 2nd ed. Philadelphia, W.B. Saunders Company, 1979.)

    (e) more freedom of movement than with traction

    (f) greater risk of infection with multiple open pin sites

2. Planning, goals/expected outcomes
  a. patient will have fracture treated and heal without complications
  b. patient will not develop problems of immobility
  c. patient will understand and comply with home care instructions

3. Implementation
  a. monitor circulation and sensation distal to fracture
  b. usual postoperative care
  c. meticulous care of pin site and incision to prevent infection

  d. monitor for pulmonary embolus or with fractures of long bones, fat embolus
  e. prevent complications of immobility
  f. teach patient and family home care for discharge
  g. for hip pinning
    (1) turn patient to unaffected side
    (2) partial weight bearing for affected hip 3 to 6 months
    (3) out of bed day after surgery
    (4) keep leg abducted with pillows

4. Evaluation
  a. fracture healed without complications
  b. no complications of immobility occurred
  c. patient and family understood and followed discharge instructions

II. CHRONIC DISORDERS

A. Arthritis

Rheumatoid and osteoarthritis (Chart 7-4)

1. Assessment
   a. definition/pathophysiology
      (1) rheumatoid arthritis
         (a) systemic inflammatory collagen disease causing pathologic changes within joint, leading to permanent deformity
         (b) pathology, chronic inflammation of synovial membranes and formation of pannus
      (2) osteoarthritis
         (a) nonsystemic, progressive degenerative joint disease
         (b) degeneration of cartilage with wear and tear with formation of bony buildup, Heberden's nodes
   b. predisposing/precipitating factors
      (1) rheumatoid
         (a) unknown; probably autoimmune in nature
         (b) onset age 30–40 years; some instances of juvenile arthritis
      (2) osteoarthritis
         (a) joints of wear and tear
         (b) highly stressed joints
         (c) obesity
         (d) onset rare before age 40 years
   c. signs and symptoms
      (1) rheumatoid
         (a) redness and swelling of joints

CHART 7–4
COMPARISON OF RHEUMATOID ARTHRITIS AND OSTEOARTHRITIS

Characteristic	Rheumatoid arthritis	Osteoarthritis
Definition	A systemic disease, but pathologic changes and disability result from chronic inflammation of the joints.	A progressive degenerative joint disease.
Pathology	Chronic inflammation of synovial membranes and formation of chronic granulation tissue (pannus) in the joint. Pannus capable of eroding cartilage in joints, and spreading to bone, ligaments, and tendons.	Microscopic changes in the cartilage in the joint. Eventually there is loss of cartilage, bony enlargement, and malalignment of joints.
Etiology	Unknown. Evidence that the pathologic changes are immunologic.	Unknown. May be due to "wear and tear" of aging.
Rheumatoid factors (autoantibodies)	Usually present.	Usually absent.
Age at onset	30 to 40 years.	50 to 60 years; rarely before 40.
Weight	Normal or underweight.	Usually overweight.
General state of health	Usually anemic, "chronically ill." Low-grade fever and slight leukocytosis.	Well nourished.
Appearance of joints	Early: soft tissue swelling. Late: ankylosis: extreme deformity. Joint involvement usually symmetric and generalized.	Early: slight joint enlargement. Late: enlargement more pronounced, slight limitation of motion. Joints usually involved are weight bearing; spine, hips, and knees.
Muscles	Pronounced muscular atrophy, particularly in later stages.	Usually not affected.
Other	Morning stiffness, pain on motion, swelling and tenderness of joints. Subcutaneous nodules. Typical rheumatoid changes seen on radiograph.	Stiffness, relieved by moderate motion; joint malalignment. Symptoms increase in cold, wet weather.

From Keane, C.B. Essentials of Medical-Surgical Nursing. 2nd ed. Philadelphia, W.B. Saunders Company, 1986, p. 561.

(b) deformity and displacement of proximal joints

(c) pain on motion

(d) underweight

(e) anemia

(f) chronic low-grade fever, slight leukocytosis

(g) presence of rheumatoid factors

(h) muscle atrophy

(i) morning stiffness

(2) osteoarthritis

(a) pain and stiffness on movement

(b) distal joint enlargement

(c) presence of Heberden's nodes

(d) symptoms aggravated by humidity and temperature changes

(e) weight-bearing joint involvement

(f) localized, nonsystemic symptoms

d. diagnostic tests

(1) CBC

(2) rheumatoid factor

(3) radiographs

e. usual treatment

(1) antiinflammatory agents (Table 7-17)

(a) nonsteroidal

(b) steroids

(2) remissive agents

(a) gold

(b) D-penicillamine

(c) Plaquenil

(3) orthopedic splints during acute inflammation to prevent deformity

(4) total joint replacement

2. Planning, goals/expected outcomes

a. patient will maintain functional abilities as long as possible

b. patient will cope with diagnosis of chronic disease

c. patient will understand and comply with therapy

d. patient will recover from surgery without complications

3. Implementation

a. balance rest and activity

b. exercise only to point of pain

c. apply heat and cold to control pain

d. administer medications as ordered

e. encourage well-balanced diet

f. assist with discharge planning including need for home assistance

g. after total hip replacement

(1) monitor immediately for shock and hemorrhage

(2) keep leg widely abducted (four pillows) and prevent flexion or external or internal rotation

(3) prevent infection

(4) teach patient home care

(5) do not lie on operative side

(6) do not adduct legs, including crossing legs for 1 year

(7) do not bend or flex hip more than 90 degrees for 1 year

(8) partial weight bearing for 3 months

4. Evaluation

a. patient remained functional

b. patient coped with diagnosis of chronic disease

c. patient understood and followed therapeutic regimen

d. patient recovered from total joint surgery without complications

B. Ruptured Intervertebral Disc

1. Assessment

a. definition/pathophysiology: protrusion of disc outside of normal intervertebral space causing pressure on adjacent nerves and nerve roots

b. predisposing/precipitating factors

(1) poor body mechanics

(2) heavy lifting

(3) prolonged sitting such as long distance truck drivers

(4) sudden strenuous exercise

c. signs and symptoms

(1) 95% occur in lumbar spine

(2) pain in lower back radiating down back of leg to foot

(3) pain increases with walking, sneezing, coughing, or straining

(4) pain in arm and hand if cervical injury

d. diagnostic tests

(1) myelogram: radiopaque dye injected into spinal column to visualize patency of column

(a) patient assumes side-lying, knee-chest position for lumbar puncture

(b) force fluids after test to decrease risk of spinal headache

(c) keep patient flat for 6 to 12 hours after test

(2) radiographs

(3) electromyogram (EMG)

(4) CT scan or MRI of spine

e. usual treatment

(1) conservative therapy

(a) bed rest

(b) cervical or pelvic traction

(c) hot packs

(d) medication: muscle relaxants such as Robaxin or Valium (Table 7-26)

(e) back braces

(f) special exercises after acute episode

(2) laminectomy: removal of a portion of vertebra to decrease pressure

TABLE 7–26. Muscle Relaxants

Example	Action	Use	Common Side Effects	Nursing Implications
Methocarbamol (Robaxin)	Reduces transmission of impulses from spinal cord to skeletal muscles	To treat painful skeletal muscle spasms or other disorders	Drowsiness, lightheadedness, headache, hypotension, GI distress, rash	Watch for sensitivity, warn patient about impaired mental functioning, avoid alcohol or other depressants, give with food or milk, watch for hypotension

    (3) spinal fusion: fusion of two or more vertebra when multiple vertebra involved
    (4) chemolysis: chymopapain injections to dissolve affected disc
2. Planning, goals/expected outcomes
  a. patient will not develop ruptured intervertebral disc
  b. patient will recover without surgery
  c. patient will recover from surgery without complications
  d. patient will understand and comply with therapeutic regimen and exercises to prevent recurrence
3. Implementation
  a. maintain bed rest with patient in semi-Fowler's with knees slightly raised to decrease pressure on spine
  b. administer medications and treatments as ordered
  c. postoperative care
    (1) log-roll patient
    (2) use fracture bedpan
    (3) allow men to stand to void
    (4) encourage patient to avoid sitting
    (5) prevent constipation
  d. teach patient discharge care
  e. encourage patient to follow exercises and other instructions
  f. teach patient good body mechanics
4. Evaluation
  a. ruptured disc did not occur
  b. patient recovered without surgery
  c. patient recovered from surgery without complications
  d. patient understood and followed therapeutic regimen

Questions

Mrs. Masters is an elderly woman admitted for a fractured left hip. She had a pinning done yesterday. You know that because of her age and diagnosis, she is at risk for developing decubitus ulcers.

1. Which of the following would *not* be a risk factor for skin breakdown?

   ① Emaciation or obesity
   ② Adequate hydration
   ③ Wrinkles in the sheets
   ④ Urinary incontinence

2. When bathing Mrs. Masters, you notice a reddened area around her right shoulder. To prevent any further skin impairment, the nurse should:

   ① Place a rubber ring under her shoulder
   ② Rub the area vigorously with her fingertips
   ③ Gently massage around the area and report your findings to the nurse
   ④ Keep her positioned only on her left side to decrease the pressure on the right

3. Another problem Mrs. Masters is likely to develop because of her age and her diagnosis would be constipation. The most appropriate nursing measure to treat this would be:

   ① Get her up to the bathroom three times daily
   ② Give her milk of magnesia TID
   ③ Administer enemas till clear
   ④ Add prune juice and fiber to her diet

Andy, age 20 years, fractured his leg while skiing. He is placed in skeletal traction.

4. The primary purpose of skeletal traction is to:

   ① Maintain the patient on bed rest
   ② Prevent shifting of the bone fragments
   ③ Reduce and set the fracture
   ④ Relieve the painful muscle spasms

5. Nursing care for Andy while he is in skeletal traction must include:

   ① Inspecting and cleaning of pin sites each shift
   ② Turning him to the unaffected side each shift
   ③ Getting him up in the chair for meals
   ④ Encouraging him to exercise both legs

6. After the fracture has begun to heal, a long leg cast is applied. Andy complains that he is now having pain. The most appropriate initial action would be to:

   ① Call the doctor
   ② Medicate with the ordered analgesics
   ③ Elevate the casted leg
   ④ Check the circulation of the toes on the casted leg

7. Andy is complaining that the skin under the cast is itching. Your best intervention to relieve the itching would be to:

   ① Tell him not to put anything down the cast to scratch it
   ② Ask the doctor to order an antipruritic
   ③ Pour some alcohol down the cast
   ④ Tell him this means that the leg is healing and the cast will be removed soon

Betty Olson, age 40 years, is admitted with severe rheumatoid arthritis.

8. The treatment regimen prescribed for Mrs. Olson would most likely be:

   ① Bed rest until all symptoms subside
   ② Daily bicycle riding
   ③ A balance between rest and exercise
   ④ Vigorous exercise followed by complete rest

9. The drug of choice to treat rheumatoid arthritis is:

   ① Aspirin
   ② Acetaminophen
   ③ Codeine
   ④ Copper

10. Side effects of the above drug can be avoided if the patient takes the drug:

    ① Only at bedtime
    ② With food
    ③ Before arising in the morning
    ④ With at least three glasses of water

11. The type of arthritis seen most commonly in the elderly is:

    ① Acute rheumatoid arthritis
    ② Gouty arthritis
    ③ Osteoarthritis
    ④ Traumatic arthritis

Answers & Rationales

Guide to item identification (see pp. 3–5 for further details about each category)

I, II, III, or IV for the phase of the nursing process
1, 2, 3, or 4 for the category of client needs
A, B, C, D, E, F, or G for the category of human functioning
Specific content category by name; ie, cholecystectomy

1. Adequate hydration helps to prevent tissue breakdown.
② I, 2, E. Immobility.

2. Gentle massage will help to restore circulation without causing tissue trauma. Potential breakdown should always be reported and charted.
③ III, 2, E. Immobility.

3. Constipation is associated with decreased mobility and with the decreased peristalsis of age. It is preferable to treat it with dietary measures rather than medications.
④ III, 2, E. Immobility.

4. Skeletal traction actually reduces and sets fractures by direct pull on the bone.
③ IV, 2, E. Traction.

5. When a patient is in skeletal traction, the pin sites must be cleaned and inspected each shift.
① III, 2, D & E. Traction.

6. The first action is to check the circulation in the toes and, if it is impaired, then to call the doctor.
④ III, 2, E. Fracture/Cast.

7. Never put anything down a cast. Antipruritics such as Benadryl or Atarax will help the itching.
② III, 2, B. Fracture/Cast.

8. It is important for the arthritic patient to balance rest and activity to maintain function and reduce deformity.
③ II, 2, E. Rheumatoid Arthritis.

9. Aspirin, a nonsteroidal antiinflammatory, is the drug of choice for arthritis.
① III, 2, F. Rheumatoid Arthritis.

10. Aspirin causes gastrointestinal distress and possible gastrointestinal bleeding if taken on an empty stomach. Food helps to decrease this side effect.
② III, 2, E. Rheumatoid Arthritis.

11. Osteoarthritis is a result of the degeneration of the bones that occurs with aging.
③ I, 2, E. Osteoarthritis.

METABOLISM/ELIMINATION

■ Endocrine Disorders

Normal endocrine function is shown in Chart 7-5

I. THYROID

A. Hyperthyroidism

1. Assessment
   a. definition/pathophysiology: disease in which thyroid secretes excessive amounts of various thyroid hormones
   b. predisposing/precipitating factors
      (1) women between age 30 and 50 years
      (2) family history of hyperthyroidism
      (3) may be autoimmune
   c. signs and symptoms
      (1) hypermetabolic symptoms
      (2) weakness and fatigue
      (3) weight loss with increased appetite
      (4) insomnia
      (5) tachycardia and palpitations
      (6) dyspnea
      (7) exophthalmus (protrusion of eyeballs), not reversible with treatment of disease
      (8) goiter
   d. diagnostic tests
      (1) T_3 and T_4
      (2) elevated thyroid-stimulating hormone (TSH) if secondary hyperthyroidism
   e. usual treatments
      (1) radioactive I^{131}
      (2) antithyroid drugs (Table 7-27): drugs must be given several months before surgery to produce euthyroid state
      (3) subtotal thyroidectomy
2. Planning, goals/expected outcomes
   a. patient will have hyperthyroidism diagnosed and treated before permanent damage occurs
   b. patient will understand and comply with therapeutic regimen
   c. patient will recover from partial thyroidectomy without complications
3. Implementation
   a. preoperative care
      (1) keep patient calm and quiet to decrease metabolic rate
      (2) prepare patient adequately for tests
      (3) maintain weight through high calorie diet: 3000–4000 cal/day
      (4) maintain cool environment
      (5) check vital signs regularly
      (6) administer medications as ordered
      (7) prepare patient emotionally for surgery
   b. postoperative care
      (1) place patient in Fowler's position to facilitate breathing
      (2) have calcium gluconate on hand in case symptoms of hypoparathyroidism occur
      (3) have tracheostomy set at bedside and monitor for respiratory distress due to possible laryngeal nerve damage
      (4) monitor for symptoms of thyroid storm, a condition of severe hypermetabolism with severe tachycardia, fever, tachypnea, and possible death from heart failure
      (5) check dressing frequently for tightness and drainage, especially sides and underneath neck
      (6) report difficulty swallowing or talking
      (7) make sure patient understands medication usage on discharge; may need lifelong thyroid replacement
4. Evaluation
   a. patient diagnosed and treated for hyperthyroidism without permanent complications
   b. patient followed therapeutic regimen pre- and postoperatively
   c. patient recovered from thyroidectomy without complications

B. Hypothyroidism

1. Assessment
   a. definition/pathophysiology: inadequate production of thyroid hormones leading to hypometabolic state; cretinism is hypothyroidism in childhood; myxedema is hypothyroidism in adulthood
   b. predisposing/precipitating factors
      (1) thyroidectomy
      (2) thyroid treatment
      (3) prenatal thyroid treatment
   c. signs and symptoms
      (1) goiter
      (2) symptoms of hypometabolism
      (3) decreased appetite with increased weight gain
      (4) constipation
      (5) slowed mentation
      (6) excessive sleep
      (7) dry, scaly skin, and dry hair
      (8) depression
      (9) edema
      (10) accelerated cardiovascular disease
   d. diagnostic tests
      (1) high serum cholesterol
      (2) low levels of thyroid hormones
      (3) low TSH secondary to pituitary disease

CHART 7–5
FUNCTIONS OF ENDOCRINE GLANDS

Gland	Hormone	Action on Target Tissue
PITUITARY		
anterior lobe	thyroid-stimulating hormone (TSH); also called thyrotropin	controls all known activities of thyroid glandular cells; influences body's metabolic processes
	growth hormone (GH); also called somatotropic hormone (SH) and somatotropin	causes growth of all tissues capable of growing; enhances protein synthesis, increases utilization of fats, and conserves carbohydrate by decreasing use of glucose
	follicle-stimulating hormone (FSH)	stimulates development of ovarian follicles and estrogen secretion; stimulates production of sperm
	luteinizing hormone (LH)	affects maturation of ovarian follicles, ovulation, and progesterone secretion; stimulates Leydig cells of testes and testosterone secretion;
	prolactin (PRL)	maintains corpus luteum and secretion of progesterone; promotes lactation
	adrenocorticotropic hormone (ACTH); also called adrenocorticotropin and corticotropin	controls secretion of some of the hormones of the adrenal cortex; eg, the glucocorticoids (chiefly cortisol and, to some extent, aldosterone and adrenal sex hormones)
posterior lobe	vasopressin (VP); also called antidiuretic hormone (ADH)	elevates blood pressure in relatively high doses; conserves water by decreasing urinary output
	oxytocin (OT)	activates uterine contraction and, in response to sexual stimulation, transports sperm during coitus; increases secretion of milk
intermediate part	melanocyte-stimulating hormone (MSH)	increases pigmentation of skin
THYROID	thyroxine (T_4); also called tetraiodothyronine and levothyroxine triiodothyronine (T_3); also called liothyronine	stimulate metabolism (catabolic phase); eg, increase respiratory rate and utilization of oxygen, production of body heat, gluconeogenesis, strength and force of heart rate, and enhance muscle tone
	calcitonin	decreases serum calcium
PARATHYROID	parathyroid hormone (PTH); also called parathormone	maintains constant serum level of calcium
ADRENAL		
cortex	glucocorticoids (chiefly cortisol)	increase protein breakdown, impair utilization of glucose, and increase hepatic output of glucose, hence are called diabetogenic hormones; essential for survival under stress
	mineralocorticoids (chiefly aldosterone)	promote retention of sodium and loss of potassium and hydrogen in urine

Chart continued on following page

CHART 7–5 *CONTINUED*

Gland	Hormone	Action on Target Tissue
	androgens and estrogens	(see under testes and ovaries)
medulla	epinephrine, norepinephrine (to a much smaller extent)	increase cardiac output, elevate blood glucose and blood lipids, raise blood pressure
OVARIES	estrogens: beta-estradiol, estrone, and estriol	cause proliferation and growth of sexual organs and other reproductive tissues; induce proliferative phase of the menstrual cycle
	progesterone	prepares endometrium for implantation of the fertilized ovum, decreases frequency of uterine contractions, promotes secretory changes in mucosal lining of uterine tubes for nutrition of fertilized ovum, prepares mammary tissue for lactation
PLACENTA	human chorionic gonadotropin (hCG)	maintains the corpus luteum and stimulates progesterone secretion
	human placental lactogen (hPL)	acts in combination with prolactin to induce lactation; also promotes growth and acts as an insulin antagonist
TESTES	androgens: testosterone, dihydrotestosterone, androstenedione	promote development of male sex characteristics in fetus, stimulate descent of testes into scrotum, stimulate protein production, responsible for masculinization
ISLETS OF LANGERHANS OF PANCREAS		
beta cells	insulin	promotes uptake, storage, and use of glucose, particularly by liver, muscles, and fat tissue, increases transport of glucose into cells and their usage of glucose, causes active transport of many amino acids into cells, promotes protein synthesis and inhibits catabolism of proteins, depresses rate of gluconeogenesis, and has synergistic effect with GH
alpha cells	glucagon	causes glycogenolysis in liver and release of glucose, which raises blood glucose level, increases rate of gluconeogenesis, which causes continued hyperglycemia
delta cells	somatostatin	inhibits secretion of both insulin and glucagon; also secreted by hypothalamus as growth hormone inhibiting hormone
THYMUS	thymosin	induces differentiation of T-lymphocytes involved in cell-mediated immunity

From Miller, B.F. & Keane, C.B. Encyclopedia and Dictionary of Medicine, Nursing and Allied Health. 3rd ed. Philadelphia, W.B. Saunders Company, 1983, pp. 377–378.

TABLE 7–27. Antithyroid Agents

Example	Action	Use	Common Side Effects	Nursing Implications
Iodine (SSKI, saturated solution of potassium iodide)	Inhibits thyroid hormone formation, blocks thyroid hormone release	To treat hyperthyroidism	Nausea, metallic taste, rash, hyperemia, fever, headache	Dilute in water or juice, give after meals, store in light-resistant bottles, give with other antithyroid agents
Propylthiouracil (PTU)	Inhibits oxygenation of iodine, blocking iodine's ability to bind with thyroid to form thyroxine	To treat hyperthyroidism	Agranulocytosis, headache, vertigo, nausea/vomiting, rash, arthralgia, loss of taste	Use carefully in pregnancy, watch for signs of hypothyroidism, monitor complete blood count (CBC), avoid use of iodine, store in light-resistant container, give with meals

e. usual treatment
    (1) thyroid medication: Synthroid, thyroid
    (2) partial thyroidectomy if goiter does not decrease with medications
2. Planning, goals/expected outcomes
  a. patient will have hypothyroidism diagnosed and treated before irreversible damage occurs
  b. patient will understand and comply with therapeutic regimen
3. Implementations
  a. keep patient comfortable
  b. provide protection for skin
  c. provide emotional support
  d. treat constipation with fluids and diet
  e. provide extra warmth for patient
  f. teach patient life-long medication regimen
4. Evaluation
  a. patient did not develop complications of hypothyroidism
  b. patient followed therapeutic regimen

II. PARATHYROID

A. Hypoparathyroidism

1. Assessment
  a. definition/pathophysiology: drop in parathormone that results in drop in serum calcium level by increasing its excretion in renal tubules
  b. predisposing/precipitating factors
    (1) accidental removal with thyroidectomy
    (2) irradiation of thyroid
    (3) idiopathic atrophy
  c. signs and symptoms
    (1) numbness and tingling around mouth and fingertips
    (2) muscle tetany
    (3) convulsions

    (4) cardiac arrhythmias
    (5) laryngeal spasms
  d. diagnostic tests
    (1) serum calcium, decreased
    (2) serum parathormone, decreased
    (3) serum phosphorus, increased
  e. usual treatments
    (1) calcium gluconate IV; immediate treatment
    (2) with chronic disease, calcium and vitamin D along with parathormone replacement
2. Planning, goals/expected outcomes
  a. patient will be diagnosed and treated for disease before life-threatening complications occur
  b. patient will understand and comply with therapeutic regimen
3. Implementation
  a. monitor for early signs of tetany
  b. monitor calcium levels
  c. teach patient correct medication regimen for discharge
4. Evaluation
  a. patient did not develop complications of hypoparathyroidism
  b. patient followed therapeutic regimen

B. Hyperparathyroidism (von Recklinghausen's Disease)

1. Assessment
  a. definition/pathophysiology: excessive synthesis and excretion of parathormone leading to excessively high levels of calcium in blood
  b. predisposing/precipitating factors
    (1) postmenopausal women
    (2) renal failure
  c. signs and symptoms
    (1) osteoporosis
    (2) pathologic fractures

(3) anorexia

(4) constipation

(5) renal stones

(6) renal failure

(7) increased myocardial contractility and sensitivity to digitalis

(8) decreased reflexes

(9) muscle flaccidity

(10) depression

(11) decreased mentation

d. diagnostic tests

(1) serum calcium, increased

(2) serum parathormone, increased

(3) serum phosphorus, decreased

e. usual treatments

(1) infusion of isotonic saline plus large dose of diuretic such as Lasix to promote diuresis of calcium (Table 7-3)

(2) administration of oral phosphorus

(3) administration of mithramycin to inhibit skeletal release of calcium

(4) administration of calcitonin to decrease rate of skeletal breakdown

(5) surgical removal of all but small portion of tissue

2. Planning, goals/expected outcomes

a. patient will be diagnosed and treated for condition before life-threatening complications occur

b. patient will understand and comply with therapeutic regimen

c. patient will recover from surgery without complications

3. Implementation

a. monitor vital signs

b. monitor for life-threatening complications

c. monitor output carefully

d. monitor electrolytes

e. care for patient postoperatively as for thyroidectomy patient

4. Evaluations

a. patient received prompt treatment

b. patient followed therapeutic regimen

c. patient recovered from surgery without complications

III. ADRENALS

A. Cushing's Syndrome

Excess adrenocortical hormone

1. Assessment

a. definition/pathophysiology: group of symptoms caused by excessive amounts of cortisol; caused by:

(1) excessive secretion of adrenocorticotropic hormone (ACTH)

(2) functional tumor of adrenal cortex

(3) ectopic production of ACTH by tumor commonly associated with lung cancer

(4) iatrogenic due to steroid therapy most common cause

b. predisposing/precipitating factors

(1) lung cancer

(2) adrenal cortical tumors

(3) steroid therapy

c. signs and symptoms

(1) altered metabolism

(a) protein catabolism and muscle wasting

(b) increased fat deposits around shoulders, face, and trunk

(c) increased blood glucose levels and increased resistance to insulin

(d) calcium release from bones and osteoporosis

(2) fluid and electrolyte imbalances

(a) sodium retention

(b) fluid retention

(c) potassium loss

(3) immunosuppression and increased susceptibility to infection

(4) decreased collagen tissue formation

(a) striae

(b) increased bruising

(c) decreased wound healing

(5) hypertension

(6) gastric hyperacidity and decrease of gastric mucosa

(7) hirsutism

(8) inability to withstand stress

(9) altered libido

d. diagnostic tests

(1) serum cortisol level: normally diurnal secretion pattern, constant level with Cushing's

(2) serum electrolytes

(3) vital signs

(4) blood sugar

(5) CBC

(6) serum protein levels

e. usual treatments

(1) regulate cortisone therapy carefully

(2) administer diuretics to control edema and hypertension (see Table 7-3)

(3) bilateral adrenalectomy for adrenal tumors

2. Planning, goals/expected outcomes

a. patient will have symptoms of Cushing's syndrome controlled as much as possible

b. patient will recover from surgery for adrenal tumor without complications

c. patient will understand and comply with therapeutic regimen

3. Implementation

a. monitor vital signs

b. monitor intake and output
c. daily weights
d. protect from infections
e. maintain low calorie, low sodium, high potassium, high protein, high calcium, low fat diet (see Chapter 5)
f. administer antacids to control hyperacidity
g. administer medications as ordered
h. teach patient symptoms of hyperglycemia
i. warn patient not to vary medication dosage without specific physician's orders
j. teach patient to avoid stress
k. teach patient to avoid trauma
l. provide emotional support
m. teach patient self-care for discharge
4. Evaluation
a. patient develops minimal side effects
b. patient recovers from surgery without complications
c. patient follows therapeutic regimen

B. Addison's Disease: Adrenocortical Insufficiency

1. Assessment
a. definition/pathophysiology: deficiency of adrenocortical hormones, glucocorticoids, and mineralocorticoids, which leads to death if not treated promptly; caused by:
(1) nonfunctioning adrenal tumor
(2) pituitary malfunction
(3) atrophy of adrenals secondary to cortisone therapy
b. predisposing/precipitating factors
(1) adrenal tumor
(2) pituitary tumor
(3) steroid therapy
c. signs and symptoms
(1) vague symptoms early in disease
(2) electrolyte imbalance
(a) hyponatremia
(b) hyperkalemia
(c) hypovolemia and hypotension
(3) hypoglycemia
(4) inability to withstand stress
(5) bronzing of skin
(6) cardiac arrhythmias
(7) anorexia
(8) decreased mentation
(9) depression
(10) coma and death
d. diagnostic tests
(1) plasma cortisol levels
(2) serum electrolytes
e. usual treatment
(1) removal of tumor

(2) replacement of hormones with steroid therapy
2. Planning, goals/expected outcomes
a. patient will not develop life-threatening complications of Addison's disease
b. patient will understand and comply with life-long steroid therapy
3. Implementation
a. monitor vital signs
b. protect from stress
c. observe for hypoglycemia
d. monitor for signs of shock
e. teach patient about life-long steroid therapy
4. Evaluation
a. patient did not develop life-threatening complications
b. patient understood and followed life-long steroid therapy

IV. DIABETES MELLITUS

A. Assessment

1. Definition/pathophysiology: absolute deficiency of insulin leading to problems in oxidation and metabolism of glucose and complex syndrome of disorders
a. categories
(1) Type I, insulin-dependent diabetes mellitus (IDDM)
(a) little or no insulin produced
(b) requires insulin daily
(c) must follow prescribed diet therapy and exercise program
(d) potential renal, retinal, cardiovascular, and neurologic problems
(e) potential for hyper- and hypoglycemia
(2) Type II, noninsulin-dependent diabetes mellitus (NIDDM)
(a) controlled by diet or oral hypoglycemic agents
(b) most patients obese
(c) rarely develop ketosis or hypoglycemia
2. Predisposing/precipitating factors
a. genetic predisposition
b. obesity
c. possibly viral origin
d. possibly immunologic, autoimmune factors
e. incidence increasing; over 10 million in United States
3. Signs and symptoms
a. polyuria
b. polyphagia
c. polydypsia
d. weight loss with IDDM
e. fatigue and lack of energy

f. weight gain with NIDDM
g. infections
h. symptoms of complications in renal, retinal, cardiovascular, and neurologic systems
4. Diagnostic tests
   a. fasting blood sugar
   b. glucose tolerance tests
   c. urinalysis
   d. urinary function studies
5. Usual treatments
   a. insulin or oral hypoglycemic agents (Table 7-28) and insulin (Table 7-29)
   b. diet modification, diabetic exchange list (see Chapter 5)
   c. prescribe regular exercise regimen

B. Planning, Goals/ Expected Outcomes

1. Patient will be diagnosed with diabetes before permanent complications occur
2. Patient will not develop complications of diabetes
3. Patient will maintain blood sugar within specified limits
4. Patient will understand and comply with therapeutic regimen of insulin administration, foot care, home glucose monitoring, diet modification, exercise, and regular health care
5. Patient and family will cope with diagnosis of chronic disease

C. Implementation

1. Patient education
   a. insulin administration
      (1) injection techniques
      (2) sites (Fig. 7-6)
      (3) types of insulin
      (4) storage of insulin
      (5) mixing of insulins

b. pathophysiology of diabetes
c. complications of diabetes
   (1) neuropathy: death of peripheral nerves, leading to paresthesias and eventually anesthesia
   (2) retinopathy: vascular leakage in retina and eventual loss of vision
   (3) nephropathy: renal vascular damage eventually leading to renal failure
   (4) vascular damage: peripheral vascular degeneration, accelerated atherosclerosis, coronary heart disease
d. home glucose testing
   (1) urine testing for glucose (sugar) and ketone bodies (acetone)
   (2) home glucose monitor of blood from finger stick
e. exercise regimen
f. diet teaching
   (1) six food exchanges (Table 5-9)
   (2) do not skip meals
   (3) follow prescribed meal plan
   (4) do not eat foods other than those in meal plan
   (5) check with physician before altering diet
g. foot care
   (1) do not go barefoot
   (2) wash and dry feet daily and carefully
   (3) wear white cotton socks to absorb perspiration
   (4) examine feet daily for sores
   (5) wear well-fitting shoes
   (6) do not cut nails or corns; see a podiatrist
   (7) do not burn feet with hot bath water
   (8) see doctor immediately for any foot trauma
h. teach patient signs of hyper- and hypoglycemia and what to do if either occurs (Chart 7-6)
i. encourage patient to express feelings
j. encourage patient to seek other resources, such as dieticians and social service, as needed
k. help patient achieve self-care competency

TABLE 7–28. Oral Hypoglycemic Agents

Name	Dosage	Metabolism	Duration of Effect
Tolbutamide (Orinase)	500–3000 mg daily total, taken BID or TID Available in 250- and 500-mg tablets	Metabolized by liver Excreted in urine	6–12 hours
Acetohexamide (Dymelor)	250–1500 mg daily total, taken once a day or BID Available in 250- and 500-mg tablets	Metabolized by liver Excreted in urine	12–24 hours
Chlorpropamide (Diabinese)	100–500 mg daily total, taken once daily Available in 100- and 250-mg tablets	Very little metabolized by liver 99% excreted in urine	Up to 60 hours
Tolazamide (Tolinase)	100–500 mg daily total, taken once daily or BID Available in 100-, 250-, and 500-mg tablets	Metabolized by liver Excreted in urine	12–24 hours

From Keane, C.B. Essentials of Medical-Surgical Nursing. 2nd ed. Philadelphia, W.B. Saunders Company, 1986.

TABLE 7–29. Insulin Regimens

Regimen	Type Insulin Used	Time Administered with Expected Time-Action Curve*	Advantages	Disadvantages
a) Single-dose	Intermediate insulin (I)	7 A.M. (I) — Noon — 6 P.M. — Midnight — 7 A.M.	1 injection should cover noon and PM meal; hypoglycemia during sleep is not a problem	No fasting, breakfast, or nighttime coverage of hyperglycemia
b) Split-mixed dose	Intermediate and regular insulin (I) + (R)	7 A.M. (I) + (R) — Noon — 6 P.M. — Midnight — 7 A.M.	2 injections provide coverage over 24-hour period	2 injections required; "locks" patient into set meal pattern
c) Split-mixed dose	Intermediate and regular insulin (I) + (R)	7 A.M. (I) + (R) — Noon — 7 P.M. (R) — 9 P.M. (I) — Midnight — 7 A.M.	3 injections provide coverage over 24 hours, particularly over early AM hours	3 injections required; evening intermediate insulin dose may potentiate early morning hypoglycemia
d) Multiple dose	Regular insulin and intermediate insulin (R) + (I)	7 A.M. (R) — Noon (R) — 7 P.M. (R) — 9 P.M. (I) — Midnight — 7 A.M.	Allows more flexibility in meal times and amount of food intake	4 injections required; requires premeal blood glucose checks; establishing and following individualized algorithm; tighter control may predispose to hypoglycemia
e) Multiple dose (insulin delivery via the pump is similar to this regimen)	Regular insulin and longest-acting insulin (R) + (LA)	7 A.M. (R) + (LA) — Noon (R) — 7 P.M. (R) — Midnight — 7 A.M.	Provides insulin delivery pattern that more closely simulates normal endogenous insulin pattern; allows for some flexibility in food-intake pattern	Requires 3 or 4 injections plus premeal and blood glucose check on retiring; requires establishing and following individualized algorithm; tight control may predispose to hypoglycemia

* Short-acting insulin —————. Long-acting insulin -------.
From Price, M.J. Insulin and oral hypoglycemic agents. Nurs. Clin. North Am. Dec.:695, 1983.

D. Evaluation

1. Patient diagnosed with diabetes early
2. Patient did not develop complications
3. Patient's blood sugar remained within specified limits
4. Patient followed diabetic therapeutic regimen
5. Patient and family accepted diagnosis of chronic disease

■ Digestive Disorders

I. PEPTIC ULCER DISEASE

A. Assessment

1. Definition/pathophysiology: ulceration of mucous lining of lower esophagus, stomach and duodenum that may involve submucosal and muscular layers (Fig. 7-7)
2. Incidence
   a. gastric
      (1) two times more common in men
      (2) age over 50 years
      (3) often malnourished
      (4) familial tendency
      (5) lower socioeconomic class
   b. duodenal
      (1) four times more common in men
      (2) between ages 25 and 50 years
      (3) highly stressed individuals
      (4) over 80% of all ulcers
      (5) blood type O
3. Predisposing/precipitating factors
   a. smoking
   b. diet not clearly documented
   c. economic and social status
   d. stress
   e. ulcerogenic drugs, such as aspirin, corticosteroids, and nonsteroidal antiinflammatories
   f. high alcohol consumption
   g. chronic stress
   h. physiologic stress; eg, burns, major trauma
4. Signs and symptoms
   a. epigastric pain that may be burning, gnawing, or aching
   b. nausea and vomiting more often in gastric ulcers
   c. weight loss
   d. anorexia
   e. eructations
   f. pain less in early morning and just after eating

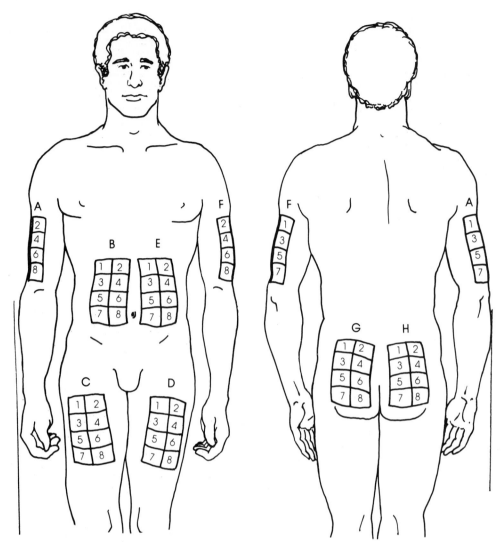

FIGURE 7–6. Rotation sites for injection of insulin. (From Keane, C.B.: Essentials of Medical-Surgical Nursing. 2nd ed. Philadelphia, W.B. Saunders Company, 1986.)

with duodenal; greater at those times with gastric

  g. pain worse on empty stomach and 2–3 hours after eating, when gastric acid level high with duodenal ulcer

  h. pain better on empty stomach for gastric

  i. melena with duodenal

  j. hematemesis with gastric

5. Diagnostic tests

  a. history and physical exam

  b. CBC

  c. upper gastrointestinal radiographic series (barium swallow); PN responsibilities:

   (1) patient education: explain procedure

   (2) administer cathartics and enemas as ordered night before

   (3) keep patient NPO after midnight

   (4) administer cathartics or enemas after procedures as ordered

  d. endoscopic examination of esophagus, stomach, duodenum; direct visualization with a flexible scope; PN responsibilities:

   (1) patient education

   (2) administer cathartics and enemas as ordered

   (3) keep patient NPO after midnight

   (4) administer preprocedure medications as ordered

   (5) monitor for return of swallowing reflex in postprocedure period; NPO until then

   (6) monitor vital signs in postprocedure period

  e. observe stools for occult blood

CHART 7–6
COMPARISON OF HYPOGLYCEMIC (INSULIN) REACTION AND HYPERGLYCEMIA (DIABETIC KETOACIDOSIS)

Hypoglycemic Reaction	Hyperglycemia
Causes	
Overdosage of insulin	Failure to take insulin
Skipped or delayed meal	Illness or infection
Unplanned strenuous exercise	Overeating or eating sweets
	Severe stress (surgery, trauma, emotional upset)
Symptoms	
Early stage: tremor, dizziness, numbness in mouth, cool wet skin, fluttering in chest, hunger	Polyuria, polydipsia, polyphagia, blurred vision, dizziness
Middle stage: headache, mental confusion, combative behavior	Loss of appetite, stomach cramps, nausea and vomiting, dehydration, fatigue
	Deep, rapid breathing
	Loss of consciousness
Treatment	
Early stage: If patient can swallow, give orange juice, 6–7 Life Saver mints, glucose tablets or gel	Physician may prescribe insulin
Late stage: If patient cannot swallow, give glucagon, 2-mg kit (home or hospital); give IV glucose	Hospital admission for severe cases
Prevention	
Eat meals 4–5 hours apart, plus prescribed snack	Take correct dose of insulin
Take correct dose of insulin. Test urine or blood for sugar, especially during illness	See physician for illnesses
Eat extra food for extra exercise; ie, activity other than regular exercise	Follow diet; don't overeat or eat sweets

From Keane, C.B. Essentials of Medical-Surgical Nursing. 2nd ed. Philadelphia, W.B. Saunders Company, 1986, p. 525.

---

    f. gastric analysis
    g. observe vomitus for "coffee ground" appearance or bright red blood; test for occult blood
6. Complications
    a. hemorrhage
    b. perforation
    c. obstruction
    d. after surgery: "dumping syndrome," which is nausea, weakness, palpitations, sweating, syncope, diarrhea about 30 minutes after ingestion of food
7. Usual treatments
    a. pharmacologic (Table 7-30); primary treatment
       (1) histamine receptor antagonists
       (2) antacids
       (3) anticholinergics
       (4) analgesics, sedatives

    b. dietary modification possible, particularly reduction in caffeine, alcohol (Table 7-31)
    c. reduction of stress
    d. stop smoking
    e. surgical intervention; done only if medication fails or for complications
       (1) subtotal gastrectomy: removal of ulcerated portion of stomach (Fig. 7-8)
       (2) vagotomy: division of branch of tenth cranial nerve, vagus, that sends cerebral stimuli to stomach muscles and glands, thereby reducing gastric motility and secretions
       (3) total gastrectomy: removal of stomach (see "Cancer of the Stomach," further on)
       (4) closure if perforation has occurred
       (5) pyloroplasty for obstruction of duodenum:

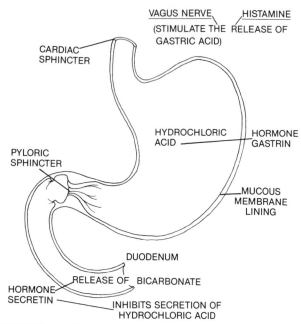

FIGURE 7–7. The stomach.

plastic surgery of pylorus to provide larger opening; done with vagotomy

f. nasogastric tube to decompress the gastrointestinal tract and remove gastric acid

B. Planning, Goals/Expected Outcomes

1. Patient will identify and alleviate risk factors
2. Patient will be free from pain
3. Patient will not develop complications from peptic ulcer
4. Patient will maintain adequate nutrition

C. Implementation

1. Assist patient to identify presence of risk or precipitating factors in life
2. Modify diet to eliminate ulcerogenic substances, such as caffeine, alcohol, and medications
3. Modify time frame of diet to include regular meals or possibly six small meals a day

TABLE 7–30. Pharmacologic Treatment of Peptic Ulcer

Class	Example	Action	Use	Common Side Effects	Nursing Implications
Histamine receptor antagonists	Cimetidine (Tagamet)	Inhibit histamine at receptor sites on parietal cells	Decrease gastric acid secretion	Agranulocytosis Mental confusion Dizziness Bradycardia Mild diarrhea Impotence Interstitial nephritis Lower sperm count	Monitor BUN; antacids should not be given at same time (1 hour before or 2 hours after)
Antacids: nonsystemic systemic	Nonsystemic: Mylanta Systemic: bicarbonate of soda (baking soda)	Elevate gastric acid pH	Weaken gastric acidity	Anorexia Constipation (aluminum) or diarrhea (magnesium)	Can interfere with absorption of certain medications, such as tetracycline; do not give together Systemic antacids can cause alkalosis
Anticholinergics	Clidinium bromide (Quarzan)	Block acetylcholine	Decrease GI motility and inhibit gastric acid secretion	Headache Confusion Excitability Palpitations Blurred vision Urinary retention	Contraindicated in narrow-angle glaucoma Obstructive uropathy; obstruction of GI tract Paralytic ileus Monitor vital signs, intake and output
Analgesics	Oxycodone hydrochloride (Percodan)	Binds with opiate receptors in CNS	Control moderate to severe pain	Sedation Clouded sensorium Hypotension Bradycardia Depressed respirations Nausea Vomiting Constipation	Monitor vital signs, particularly respirations

BUN, blood urea nitrogen; CNS, central nervous system; GI, gastrointestinal.

TABLE 7–31. Bland Diet

Foods Allowed	Foods Prohibited
Milk	Preserved meats
Cheeses	Smoked fish
Butter or margarine	Raw vegetables
Beef and lamb, roasted or broiled	Raw fruits
Chicken, roasted or broiled	Pastries
Fish, broiled or poached	Preserves
Cream soups	Candies
Cooked vegetables	Alcoholic beverages
Bananas	Caffeine
Baked apples without skins	Carbonated beverages
Stewed fruits	High fiber foods
Applesauce	Spices or condiments
Bread	Acidic foods
Custard	Fried foods
Ice cream	Fatty foods
Pudding	Smoked meats
Plain cakes	

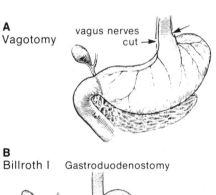

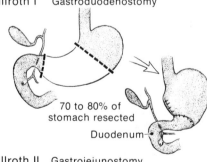

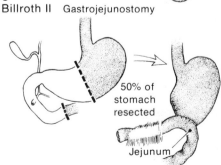

FIGURE 7–8. Subtotal gastric resection. *A*, Vagotomy. *B*, Billroth I (gastroduodenostomy). *C*, Billroth II (gastrojejunostomy). (From Watson, J.E.: Medical-Surgical Nursing and Related Physiology. 2nd ed. Philadelphia, W.B. Saunders Company, 1979.)

4. Stop smoking
5. Administer medications as ordered (Table 7-30)
6. Help patient understand and comply with surgical intervention
7. Assist RN to educate patient in preoperative phase regarding:
   a. surgical procedure
   b. need to cough and deep breathe
   c. early ambulation
   d. possible presence of drainage tubes
8. Assist RN in postoperative period to monitor
   a. vital functions
   b. intake and output; list each drainage tube separately
   c. early ambulation, cough and deep breathe
   d. medicate for pain as ordered
9. Help patient to identify signs and symptoms of complications and to notify nurse and doctor
10. Monitor patient for signs and symptoms of perforation, hemorrhage, obstruction; notify team leader immediately
11. Ensure intake of adequate fluids and nutrients
12. Help patient comply with pharmacologic treatment of nausea, vomiting, diarrhea, constipation (Table 7-32)
13. Prevent/treat "dumping syndrome"
    a. small, frequent meals
    b. low carbohydrate, high protein, moderate fat diet to slow gastric emptying
    c. drink liquids only between meals, not with meals
    d. lie down on left side for 1 hour after meals

D. Evaluation

1. Peptic ulcer healed
2. Patient had no pain
3. Patient recovered from ulcer or surgery without complications
4. Patient achieved adequate nutrition

II. HIATAL HERNIA

A. Assessment

1. Definition/pathophysiology: protrusion of part of stomach, often proximal area, through esophageal hiatus in diaphragm upward into mediastinal cavity; reflux of acid gastric contents, often, causing gastritis in herniated portion and causing bleeding and anemia
2. Incidence: small, asymptomatic hiatal hernias appear in many people, as shown by upper gastrointestinal series

TABLE 7–32. Pharmacologic Treatment of Nausea, Vomiting, Diarrhea, Constipation

Class	Example	Action	Use	Common Side Effects	Nursing Implications
Antiemetics: phenothiazines anticholinergics antihistamines	Phenothiazine: prochlorperazine maleate (Compazine)	Act on the chemoreceptor trigger zone in the medulla	Inhibit nausea and vomiting	Agranulocytosis Orthostatic hypotension Blurred vision Urinary retention Cholestatic jaundice	Do not give with antacids Monitor for CNS depression Moniter vital signs Moniter for alkalosis from loss of acidity
Laxatives: irritant saline bulk forming lubricant stool softeners	Irritant: castor oil	Stimulate intestinal mucosa	Increase motility and secretion	Abdominal cramps Fluid depletion Hypokalemia Hypotension	May interfere with absorption of food and medication
Antidiarrheals: demulcents protectants adsorbents astringents opiates	Opiate: diphenoxylate (Lomotil)	Inhibit motility and propulsion, diminish digestive secretions	Slow down or stop diarrheal stool	Sedation Lethargy Tachycardia Paralytic ileus Dry mouth	Treat the cause as well as the symptom; if diarrhea caused by a poison, do not treat diarrhea until poison is eliminated Monitor for hypovolemia and hypokalemia Monitor for acidosis Contains atropine, so contraindicated in glaucoma

CNS, central nervous system.

3. Predisposing/precipitating factors
   a. congenital weakness
   b. trauma
   c. increased intraabdominal pressure
   d. relaxation of gastric sphincter and musculature
   e. obesity
   f. anorexia nervosa, bulimia
4. Signs and symptoms
   a. heartburn
   b. regurgitation
   c. dysphagia
   d. sternal pain; may mimic angina after a heavy meal
   e. difficulty in breathing
   f. esophagitis from acid gastric contents pushed up on esophageal mucous membrane
5. Diagnostic tests
   a. history and physical examination
   b. chest and abdominal radiograph
   c. upper gastrointestinal radiographic examination
   d. esophagoscopy
6. Complications
   a. esophageal ulcer
   b. stenosis of distal portion of esophagus
   c. esophagitis
   d. occult bleeding, melena
   e. anemia
   f. gastritis

7. Usual treatments
   a. weight reduction
   b. positioning
      (1) avoid lying down after meals for 1 hour
      (2) sleep with head of bed elevated
   c. antacids
   d. small, frequent meals
   e. surgical repair

B. Planning, Goals/Expected Outcomes

1. Patient will identify and alleviate risk factors
2. Patient will be free from pain
3. Patient will not develop complications of hiatal hernia
4. Patient will understand and comply with therapeutic regimen

C. Implementation

1. Assist patient to identify presence of risk and precipitating factors
2. Assist patient to increase exercise and decrease calorie intake to decrease obesity
3. Administer antacids to weaken gastric acidity

4. Teach to use positioning to prevent increase in herniation
5. Teach to use positioning to prevent gastric reflux
6. Encourage patient to avoid heavy meals
7. Prepare patient for surgery
8. Provide postoperative care for patient as per ulcer surgery

A. Evaluation

1. Patient will remain asymptomatic
2. Patient had no pain
3. Patient recovered from surgical repair without complications

III. GASTRIC CANCER

A. Assessment

1. Defintion/pathophysiology: cancerous growth in stomach usually carcinoma; cause unknown; most start in lesser curvature, causing no symptoms until it spreads to sphincters
2. Incidence: declining in United States but still accounts for about 15,000 deaths/year
3. Predisposing/precipitating factors
   a. chronic gastric ulcers
   b. chronic gastritis
   c. familial tendency
4. Signs and symptoms
   a. early, usually vague
   b. late in disease, decrease in gastric motility
   c. anorexia
   d. weight loss
   e. weakness
   f. anemia
   g. pain
   h. melena
   i. hematemesis
   j. dysphagia
   k. constipation
   l. vomiting, possibly "coffee ground" material from old blood
5. Diagnostic tests
   a. history and physical exam
   b. CBC and electrolytes
   c. upper and lower gastrointestinal radiographic studies
   d. gastroscopy with biopsy: PN responsibilities (see "Peptic Ulcer Disease")
   e. gastric analysis: NG tube passed, stimulant such as histamine given, then stomach contents removed; contents analyzed for free and total acid, occult blood, and lactic acid; patient NPO after midnight
6. Complications
   a. metastasis, often to liver
   b. obstruction of pyloric or cardiac sphincter
   c. malnutrition
   d. malabsorption
   e. hemorrhage
   f. perforation with peritonitis
   g. shock
   h. after surgery: "dumping syndrome" (see "Peptic Ulcer Disease")
   i. vitamin B_{12} deficiency: pernicious anemia
7. Usual treatments
   a. surgical treatment
      (1) radical subtotal gastrectomy: resection of tumor plus ridge of healthy tissue, with anastomosis of stump of stomach to jejunum
      (2) total gastrectomy with removal of stomach; anastomosis between ends of esophagus and jejunum
      (3) less radical subtotal gastrectomy if tumor metastasized
   b. radiation and chemotherapy if patient not surgical candidate
   c. radiation and chemotherapy after surgery if metastasis known or suspected; radiation and chemotherapy in combination for cancer of stomach to slow down growth of tumor

B. Planning, Goals/Expected Outcomes

1. Patient will be prepared for surgery
2. Patient will be free of pain
3. Patient will have no complications of surgery
4. Patient will maintain adequate nutrition
5. Patient will have controlled side effects from usage of radiation and chemotherapy
6. Patient will cope with diagnosis and prognosis

C. Implementation

1. Assist RN to provide preoperative care
   a. explain diagnostic procedures
   b. explain surgical procedure
   c. explain radiation and chemotherapy
   d. monitor intravenous therapy; intake and output
   e. monitor NG tube for contents, pressure, output, placement; keep nares lubricated with water soluble lubricant
   f. provide support for patient and significant others
2. Assist RN to provide postoperative care
   a. monitor vital functions

b. monitor intake and output, including NG tube output
c. monitor intravenous therapy and blood
d. monitor hyperalimentation feeding if appropriate
e. turn, cough, and deep breathe hourly
f. administer pain medication as ordered
g. give nose and mouth care
h. when ordered, provide multiple small, dry meals
i. administer vitamin B_{12} intramuscularly to treat pernicious anemia every 2 weeks
3. Administer pain medication as ordered
4. Monitor or assist RN to assess for postoperative complications
a. monitor vital signs
b. monitor for blood in nasogastric drainage; some old blood normal first few days
c. monitor for increased abdominal pain and distention
d. auscultate for bowel sounds
e. monitor intake and output for overhydration or dehydration
f. monitor for signs and symptoms of infections, especially respiratory
g. if patient on parenteral hyperalimentation, check for glucosuria
5. Assist RN to monitor hyperalimentation feeding, blood administration, intravenous therapy, or enteral tube feeding as appropriate
6. Assist patient to eat frequent, small, bland, dry meals with vitamin supplements
7. Assist patient to understand and comply with the function of radiation and chemotherapy (Tables 7-23 and 7-24)
8. Monitor for bone marrow suppression, radiation burns on skin; be sure radiation markings on skin not removed
9. Assist patient to comply with pharmacologic treatment for nausea, vomiting, diarrhea, or constipation (Table 7-32)
10. Assist patient and significant others with feelings about malignant disease and altered body image
11. Assist patient to contact clergy as appropriate

D. Evaluation

1. Patient was adequately prepared for surgery
2. Patient free from pain
3. Patient had no complications from surgery
4. Patient maintained adequate nutrition
5. Cancer growth slowed
6. Patient is stable emotionally and spiritually

■ Lower Intestinal Disorders

I. DIVERTICULOSIS/ DIVERTICULITIS

A. Assessment

1. Definition/pathophysiology
   a. diverticulosis: presence of one or many pouches formed by herniation of mucous membrane through defect in muscular coat of intestine
   b. diverticulitis: inflammation of one or multiple diverticula of colon; caused by bacteria or other irritating substances collected in blind pouches of diverticula
2. Incidence: approximately 10% of population over 50 years of age, 40% over 70 years of age
3. Predisposing/precipitating factors
   a. chronic constipation from stress and low fiber diet
   b. congenital weakness of colon
   c. constipation from spastic colon syndrome
4. Signs and symptoms
   a. crampy pain in left lower quadrant of abdomen
   b. bowel irregularity with diarrhea
   c. generalized abdominal cramps
   d. narrow stools from fibrotic strictures
   e. melena possible
   f. occult bleeding
   g. low-grade fever
   h. elevated WBC
5. Diagnostic tests
   a. history and physical examination
   b. sigmoidoscopy: direct visualization of sigmoid colon
   c. barium enema: lower gastrointestinal radiographic series
   d. colonoscopy: endoscopic examination of entire colon by means of colonoscope admitted transanally; PN responsibilities:
      (1) patient education concerning examination
      (2) administer cathartics and enemas as ordered night before examination
      (3) keep patient NPO after midnight
      (4) monitor for rectal bleeding after examination
      (5) monitor for signs and symptoms of bowel perforation after examination
      (6) monitor vital signs
6. Complications
   a. anemia
   b. abscess
   c. peritonitis
   d. hemorrhage through erosion of arterial blood vessel
7. Usual treatments

a. pharmacologic treatment to reduce bacterial flora and soften fecal mass (Table 7-33)
   (1) antispasmodics
   (2) tranquilizers
   (3) sedatives
   (4) bowel antimicrobials such as neomycin
   (5) stool softeners
   (6) evacuant suppositories
b. intravenous fluids
c. surgical treatment if untreatable medically
   (1) primary resection with end to end anastomosis: removal of area of disease and inflammation and reconnection of both ends of colon
   (2) "double barrel" colostomy if complications such as perforation, fistula, obstruction; this is two-stage procedure; in first stage, diseased part of colon resected, but two ends of colon brought out to abdominal wall as stomas; allows inflammation process to subside while fecal flow diverted to proximal stoma; after 6–8 weeks, second stage involves closure of colostomy and anastomosis of two ends of colon for normal fecal flow
d. soft, high residue, low roughage, low carbohydrate diet

B. Planning, Goals/ Expected Outcomes

1. Assist patient to identify and alleviate risk factors
2. Patient will be free of pain
3. Patient will maintain normal bowel elimination
4. Patient will be prepared for surgery
5. Patient will develop no complications of surgery
6. Patient will maintain integrity of the skin
7. Patient will adjust to altered body image
8. Patient will be able to care for colostomy if appropriate
9. Patient and significant others will cope with disease and surgery

D. Implementation

1. Identify presence of risk or precipitating factors in life
2. Assist patient to identify and use high-residue foods such as bran and fruits (Table 7-34)
3. Assist patient to understand and comply with pharmacologic regimen
4. Assist RN to prepare patient for surgery as appropriate

TABLE 7–33. Pharmacologic Treatment of Diverticulitis

Class	Example	Action	Use	Common Side Effects	Nursing Implications
Antispasmodics	Dicyclomine hydrochloride (Bentyl)	Direct spasmolytic action on smooth muscle	Spastic colon	Headache Dizziness Palpitations Urinary retention Paralytic ileus	Monitor intake and output Monitor vital signs
Tranquilizers, sedatives	Diazepam (Valium)	Depress the CNS in the limbic system	Antianxiety	Drowsiness Hypotension Cardiovascular collapse Abdominal discomfort	Possible addiction Dosage should be reduced in elderly patients Do not withdraw abruptly
Bowel antimicrobials	Neomycin sulfate	Inhibit protein synthesis in bacterial cell	"Sterilize colon" for surgery	Headache Ototoxity Nephrotoxicity	Ask patient about drug allergies Monitor intake and output Hydrate well to avoid renal toxicity
Stool softeners	Docusate sodium (Colace)	Reduce surface tension of liquid content of the bowel	Incorporate more liquid in stool	Bitter taste Mild abdominal cramping Diarrhea	—
Evacuant suppositories	Bisacodyl (Dulcolax)	Direct action on smooth muscle at the colon	Increase peristalsis	Nausea Vomiting Abdominal cramps Diarrhea	Monitor for laxative dependence, particularly in elderly

CNS, central nervous system.

TABLE 7–34. High-Residue Foods

Milk	Raw vegetables	Fried foods
Whole grains	Nuts	Cheese
Bran	Tough meats	Cooked corn
Fruits with seeds or skin	Pork	Popcorn
Raw fruits except bananas		

    a. patient education about procedure
    b. let patient express fears and anxieties
    c. teach to turn, cough, and deep breathe
    d. explain possibility of drainage tubes
    e. explain possibility, appearance, and care of stoma as appropriate
    f. monitor intravenous therapy
    g. monitor intake and output
5. Monitor patient and assist RN in postoperative care
    a. turn, cough, and deep breathe hourly
    b. monitor vital functions
    c. measure intake and output; record each drainage tube separately
    d. provide stoma care with skin care
    e. auscultate for bowel sounds
    f. monitor for signs and symptoms of hemorrhage, perforation, or peritonitis
6. Provide pouch to fit snugly around stoma to prevent leakage of intestinal contents onto skin, which can cause chemical burn; use skin barrier
7. wash skin well, and dry well
8. Administer enemas into proximal stoma as ordered by physician
9. Administer enemas to distal stoma and rectum as ordered by physician prior to closure of colostomy and reanastomosis
10. Assist client to watch stoma care, then gradually to become involved in self-care or involve family member in care
11. Allow patient to express feelings concerning altered body image
12. Encourage use of "ostomy" visitor

D. Evaluation

1. Patient's diverticulitis healed without complications
2. Patient's diverticulitis did not recur
3. Patient had pain controlled
4. Patient recovered from surgery without complications
5. Patient learned ostomy self-care
6. Patient went through reanastomosis without complications

II. ULCERATIVE COLITIS

A. Assessment

1. Definition/pathophysiology: inflammation of large intestine that contains ulcerations of mucosa of colon; disease tends to begin in rectum and sigmoid colon, then ascend upward possibly to include entire colon
2. Incidence: associated with persons under high stress; young adults, genetic predisposition
3. Predisposing/precipitating factors
    a. cause unknown
    b. stress
    c. autoimmune factors
    d. repeated intestinal infections
    e. family tendency
4. Signs and symptoms
    a. diarrhea, can be bloody
    b. abdominal pain
    c. rectal bleeding
    d. nausea
    e. weight loss
    f. dehydration
    g. anemia
    h. body wasting, cachexia
5. Diagnostic tests
    a. history and physical examination
    b. stool examination for ova and parasites
    c. sigmoidoscopy
    d. barium enema
    e. colonoscopy
    f. CBC and electrolytes
6. Complications
    a. carcinoma of colon
    b. megacolon with perforation of colon
    c. peritonitis
    d. hemorrhage
    e. hypokalemia, hypocalcemia, iron deficiency
    f. volume depletion
    g. malabsorption
    h. stricture formation
    i. arthritis
    j. nephrolithiasis
7. Usual treatments
    a. pharmacologic (Table 7-35)
       (1) antidiarrheal medication
       (2) sedation
       (3) antibiotics, particularly sulfonamides (Table 7-10)
       (4) steroids (Table 7-17)
       (5) anticholinergics (Table 7-16)
       (6) analgesics (Table 7-8)
    b. rest, particularly after meals
    c. hydration: intravenous, oral

TABLE 7–35. Pharmacologic Treatment of Ulcerative Colitis

Class	Example	Action	Use	Common Side Effects	Nursing Implications
Corticotropic hormones	ACTH (corticotropin)	Stimulate adrenal gland	Stimulate whole endocrine system	Sodium and fluid retention Convulsions Dizziness Hemorrhage Euphoria	Watch for overstimulation of endocrine system Side effects of Cushing's syndrome
Corticosteroids	Prednisone	Suppress immune response	Decrease inflammation	Euphoria Congestive heart failure Hypertension Edema	Medication must be stepped down Monitor for glucosuria
Antibiotics	Sulfasalazine	Decrease bacterial folic acid synthesis	Treat infectious process in colon or secondary infection	Leukopenia Nausea Vomiting Diarrhea Toxic nephrosis	Check for allergies Push fluids to prevent crystallization in renal tubules
Antidiarrheals Anticholinergics	Atropine sulfate	Inhibit acetylcholine	(see Table 7-32) Slow diarrhea	Headache Restlessness Ataxia Hallucinations	Watch for tachycardia and urinary retention Contraindicated in acute glaucoma
Analgesics			(see Table 7-30)		

d. intake and output
e. psychotherapy
f. diet: well balanced, low residue, high protein (Table 7-36 and Chapter 5)
g. vitamin and mineral supplements
h. avoidance of milk and milk products if lactose intolerance present
i. surgical (less than 20% require this): total colectomy with ileostomy
j. parenteral hyperalimentation possible

TABLE 7–36. High Calorie, High Protein, Low Residue, Bland Diet for Inflammatory Bowel Disease

Type	Reason	Examples	Foods to avoid
High protein	Healing of mucosal tissue Replacement for malabsorbed protein in diet	Eggs Meat Cheese	Milk in early stages or if patient is sensitive to milk
High calorie	Spare protein Energy production Restore nutritional deficits	Pastas Desserts Meat Poultry Bread products Sugar Honey Hard candy	Ice cream Very cold foods High fat foods
Low residue, bland	Avoid irritation of mucosal lining	Eggs, except fried Small amounts of cheese Tender meat, not fried Small amounts of margarine, butter Cooked or canned vegetables and fruits Strained fruit juice Cooked, nonwhole grain cereals Gelatin desserts Sponge cake Plain custard Ices Hard candy Gum drops Plain gravy Salt	Heavy roughage Alcohol Raw vegetables Highly spiced foods Raw fruits Whole grain breads and cereals Fried foods Nuts Popcorn Milk Pepper

B. Planning, Goals/Expected Outcomes

1. Patient will identify and alleviate risk factors
2. Patient will maintain fluid and electrolyte balance
3. Patient will maintain normal nutrition
4. Patient will maintain integrity of skin

C. Implementation

1. Assist patient to reduce stress, avoid intestinal infections
2. Assist patient to understand and comply with pharmacologic treatment to decrease diarrhea and pain (Table 7-35)
3. Assist patient to understand and comply with need to increase fluids and electrolytes through oral route or intravenous route
4. Assist patient to understand and comply with dietary modification to decrease intestinal irritation (see "Regional Enteritis [Crohn's Disease]")
5. Maintain medical asepsis by cleaning perianal area after each diarrheal stool
6. Prepare patient for surgery if appropriate
7. Assist patient to have uncomplicated surgical recovery (see "Regional Enteritis [Crohn's Disease]")
8. Assist patient to not develop complications of colectomy with ileostomy (see "Regional Enteritis [Crohn's Disease]")

D. Evaluation

1. Patient's ulcerative colitis will be in remission
2. Patient had no recurrence
3. Patient had pain controlled
4. Patient's fluid and electrolyte balance maintained
5. Patient maintained adequate nutrition
6. Patient's skin integrity maintained

III. REGIONAL ENTERITIS (CROHN'S DISEASE)

A. Assessment

1. Definition/pathophysiology: inflammatory process of unknown etiology; affects primarily terminal portion of ileum but can affect any portion of small or large intestine; inflammatory segments can be separated by normal intestine; chronic disease with relapses of acute inflammatory symptomatology
2. Incidence
   a. occurs in both sexes about equally
   b. higher occurrence in persons of Jewish origin
   c. highest occurrence in persons age 15–35 years
3. Predisposing/precipitating factors
   a. familial tendency
   b. abnormal immune response
4. Signs and symptoms
   a. early signs are insidious
   b. abdominal cramping and pain unrelieved by defecation
   c. diarrhea
   d. scar tissue with constriction of intestinal lumen
   e. crampy abdominal pain particularly after meals
   f. anorexia, anemia
   g. weight loss, malnutrition
   h. constant irritating discharge, causing chronic diarrhea
   i. fever if abscess present
   j. abdominal tenderness
   k. constriction of parts of intestine, particularly distal ileum on gastrointestinal radiographic examinations
   l. melena
5. Diagnostic tests
   a. history and physical examination
   b. proctosigmoidoscopic examination with biopsy to rule out ulcerative colitis (colitis ruled out if rectosigmoid are normal)
   c. upper gastrointestinal radiographic examination (barium swallow)
   d. lower gastrointestinal radiographic examination (barium enema)
   e. endoscopic examination
   f. colonoscopy; PN responsibilities:
      (1) educate patient about procedures
      (2) give laxatives and enemas as ordered
      (3) keep patient NPO
      (4) monitor for bleeding or signs and symptoms of perforation
      (5) monitor vital signs
   g. CBC, electrolytes, clotting time
6. Complications
   a. strictures of the intestinal lumen
   b. malabsorption syndrome
   c. abscesses
   d. fistulas
   e. perianal ulcerations
   f. transmural penetration with perforation
   g. hemorrhage
   h. peritonitis
7. Usual treatments
   a. pharmacologic (Table 7-35)
   b. high calorie, high protein, low residue, bland diet with vitamin and iron supplements (Table 7-36 and Chapter 5)
   c. hydration by intravenous route
   d. blood transfusion possible
   e. surgical interventions

(1) resection of colon with end to end anastomosis if limited to particular area

(2) permanent colostomy depending on area of inflammation: removal of diseased portion of large intestine, with remaining end of colon brought to surface of abdomen through artificial opening called a stoma; anus sutured closed

(3) permanent ileostomy: removal of diseased portion of colon and ileum, with remaining end of ileum brought to surface of abdomen through artifical opening called stoma; anus sutured closed

f. total parenteral hyperalimentation nutrition may be required

B. Planning, Goals/ Expected Outcomes

Same as for ulcerative colitis

C. Implementation

1, 2, 3. Same as ulcerative colitis

4. Assist patient to understand and comply with dietary modifications to decrease intestinal irritation (Table 7-36)

5. Maintain medical asepsis by cleaning perianal area after each diarrheal stool

6. Assist RN to prepare patient for surgery as appropriate (see "Diverticulosis/Diverticulitis")

7. Monitor patient and assist RN in postoperative care

a. similar to diverticulosis/diverticulitis except stoma permanent

b. ileostomy drains diarrheal stool frequently, about 1200 mL/day; report to doctor if over 1500 mL/day

c. drainage pouch must be emptied frequently

d. drainage pouch must fit snugly around stoma to avoid spilling ileal contents onto skin, causing chemical burn

e. pouch must be changed immediately if leakage occurs: use skin barrier such as Stomahesive or karaya

f. monitor vital signs: intake and output; record each drainage bag separately

g. monitor for growth of yeast or fungus around stoma; use Mycostatin powder to treat

h. assist patient to look at surgical site and slowly begin to involve patient in care of appliance

i. provide much emotional support for patient and significant others

j. allow patient to express feelings, anxieties, and fears about surgical procedure

k. encourage "ostomy" visitor

8. Assist client to understand dietary restrictions and comply with avoiding foods that produce gas or malodors, such as asparagus, beans, and nuts

D. Evaluation

1. Patient's regional enteritis in remission
2. Patient's disease did not recur
3. Patient's pain was controlled
4. Patient's fluid and electrolyte balance maintained
5. Patient maintained adequate nutrition
6. Patient's skin integrity maintained
7. Patient learned and practiced self-care of ileostomy

IV. HERNIA

A. Assessment

1. Definition/pathophysiology: protrusion of intestine contained in hernial sac occurring in groin where abdominal area meets thighs; increased abdominal pressure from lifting, coughing, sneezing, or an accident often cause

a. direct: hernia sac pushes directly outward through weakest point in abdomen

b. indirect: hernia sac pushes downward into inguinal canal

c. femoral: protrusion of loop of intestine into femoral canal

d. incisional: protrusion of an organ at the site of the incision

2. Incidence: direct and indirect more common in males, femoral more common in females

3. Predisposing/precipitating factors

a. congenital weakness of abdominal wall

b. acquired weakness of abdominal wall related to straining or the aging process

c. trauma

d. obesity

e. pregnancy

4. Types

a. reducible: the hernial sac can be placed back into abdominal cavity

b. irreducible: hernia cannot be reduced

c. strangulated: irreducible plus obstruction of blood and intestinal flow

5. Signs and symptoms

a. outpouching of the hernia sac when patient is upright or straining

b. pain may be present in certain circumstances

c. if the herniation becomes obstructed, there is:

(1) colicky abdominal pain

(2) vomiting

(3) distention of the hernial sac

d. auscultation of bowel sounds from outpouching
6. Diagnostic tests: history and physical examination
7. Complications
   a. strangulation
   b. peritonitis
8. Usual treatments
   a. surgery
      (1) herniorrhaphy: removal of hernial sac
      (2) hernioplasty: reinforcement of suture line with overlay of synthetic sutures or mesh
   b. manual reduction with or without truss

B. Planning, Goals/ Expected Outcomes

1. Patient will identify and alleviate risk factors
2. Patient will be prepared for surgery
3. Patient will have no complications of surgery
4. Patient will be free of pain

C. Implementation

1. Teach patient dangers of poor body mechanics, obesity, and prolonged coughing from allergies or heavy smoking
2. Encourage patient to lose weight, practice good body mechanics, stop smoking, and treat allergies as appropriate
3. Give preoperative explanations and teaching similar to that for other surgeries of abdominal area
4. Monitor in the postoperative period in manner similar to that for other surgeries of abdomen
5. Medicate for pain as ordered by physician
6. Teach patient to support incisional area with hands or pillow while coughing, sneezing, or performing other activities that increase abdominal pressure

D. Evaluation

1. Patient verbalizes knowledge of risk factors
2. Patient's hernia did not recur
3. Patient recovered from surgery without complications
4. Patient's pain controlled

V. HEMORRHOIDS

A. Assessment

1. Definition/pathophysiology: enlarged varicose veins in rectal and anal area; may be internal or external; caused by prolonged, increased abdominal pressure and prolonged pressure on rectal, anal area
2. Incidence: fairly common; more common in women than in men
3. Predisposing/precipitating factors
   a. pregnancy
   b. prolonged sitting
   c. chronic constipation
   d. hard, dry stools
   e. obesity
4. Signs and symptoms
   a. may be asymptomatic
   b. pain
   c. burning
   d. itching
   e. bright red blood on stool
   f. visible or palpable mass in anal area
5. Diagnostic tests
   a. history and physical examination
   b. digital examination (rectal examination)
   c. proctoscopic examination to rule out tumors
6. Complications
   a. anal fissure
   b. thrombosis of hemorrhoid
   c. strangulation of varicosity
7. Usual treatments
   a. symptomatic
      (1) maintain cleanliness of area
      (2) astringent topical medication to shrink mucous membrane
      (3) stool softeners and laxatives
      (4) high residue diet to keep stool soft
      (5) sitz baths
   b. surgical
      (1) hemorrhoidectomy: removal of hemorrhoids by excision, clamp, cautery, or cryosurgery
      (2) conservative surgical treatment, Barron's ligation (rubber band ligation): hemorrhoids bound with rubber ligatures to produce necrosis, then sloughing of ligated portion

B. Planning, Goals/ Expected Outcomes

1. Patient will identify and alleviate risk factors
2. Patient will be free of pain
3. Patient will not develop complications of hemorrhoids
4. Patient will be prepared for surgery
5. Patient will not develop complications of hemorrhoidectomy

C. Implementation

1. Assist patient to identify presence of risk or precipitating factors
2. Teach patient to use symptomatic treatments
3. Teach patient signs and symptoms of complications and notify nurse or doctor
4. Give preoperative explanations and teachings
5. Monitor postoperatively for vital functions, intake and output
6. Turn, cough, deep breathe, early ambulation
7. Medicate for pain as ordered by physician
8. Monitor for signs and symptoms of complications, such as hemorrhage, perforation of colon

D. Evaluation

1. Patient's hemorrhoids remained asymptomatic
2. Patient did not develop complications of hemorrhoids
3. Patient's surgery was uneventful and without complications

VI. COLON/RECTAL CANCER

A. Assessment

1. Definition/pathophysiology: cancerous process in intestine that is relatively rare in small intestine and relatively common in large intestine; most colorectal cancers arise from preexisting polyps; polyp is growth, protruding from mucous membrane; polyps can be benign or malignant, but all need to be removed from colon; polyps may be attached by stalk or have broad base
2. Incidence: colorectal cancer most common intestinal cancer in United States; age of affected persons usually over 40 years
3. Predisposing/precipitating factors
   a. cause unknown
   b. polyps in colon and rectum
   c. chronic inflammation, such as ulcerative colitis
   d. diverticula
   e. lesions; pathologic discontinuity of tissue-like mucous membrane
   f. familial history
4. Signs and symptoms
   a. blood in feces
   b. anemia, weakness, and fatigue
   c. changes in bowel patterns; constipation alternating with diarrhea
   d. changes in stool shape due to strictures
   e. obstruction in colon due to polyps or tumorous growth
   f. weight loss, anorexia
   g. abdominal pain, rectal pain
   h. abdominal distention
5. Diagnostic tests
   a. history and physical examination
   b. proctosigmoidoscopy with biopsy
   c. upper gastrointestinal radiographic examination (barium swallow)
   d. lower gastrointestinal radiographic examination (barium enema)
   e. colonoscopy with biopsy
   f. CBC and electrolytes
   g. stool for occult blood
6. Complications
   a. obstruction of the colon
   b. hemorrhage
   c. metastasis within digestive system
   d. metastasis beyond digestive system
   e. malnutrition
   f. malabsorption
7. Usual treatments
   a. cancer chemotherapy (see "Cancer")
   b. radiation therapy (see "Cancer")
   c. surgery: depends on location and presence of metastasis
      (1) colon resection with end to end anastomosis for localized tumor polyp with no metastasis
      (2) colon resection with end to end anastomosis may be done as palliative treatment for metastatic cancer
      (3) abdominal perineal resection for cancer of rectum: involves cutting of colon above tumor, removal of affected portion of colon through perineal incision; remaining end of colon brought out to abdomen through opening called stoma
      (4) colostomy may be performed for inoperable tumors or in presence of partial or complete obstruction to allow emptying of colon through stoma
      (5) NPO and NG tube prior to surgery to decompress and rest the gastrointestinal tract
      (6) cathartics and enemas prior to surgery
      (7) intestinal anti-infectives like Neomycin prior to surgery to kill intestinal bacteria
      (8) drainage tubes in surgical area postoperatively to remove excess body fluids that collect in areas of inflammation
      (9) indwelling catheter possible
      (10) intravenous therapy
      (11) blood transfusion possible
      (12) total parenteral hyperalimentation nutrition possible
      (13) pain medication

B. Planning, Goals/ Expected Outcomes

1. Patient will identify and alleviate risk factors
2. Patient will not develop complications
3. Patient will understand and comply with cancer chemotherapy or radiation
4. Patient will be prepared for surgery
5. Patient will have uncomplicated recovery from surgery
6. Patient will maintain skin integrity
7. Patient will adjust to altered body image
8. Patient will be able to perform self-care with ostomy appliances
9. Patient will cope with diagnosis and prognosis

C. Implementation

1. Assist patient to understand and comply with early detection through rectal examination, proctoscopic examination, stool guaiac examination after age 40 years
2. Assist patient to comply with need for removal of rectal and colon polyps
3. Teach patient signs of complications, such as increased abdominal pain and bleeding, and to report these to physician or nurse immediately
4. Teach patient action, adverse effects, and treatment of adverse effects of cancer chemotherapy and radiation therapy (Tables 7-23 and 7-24)
5. Assist patient to comply with protocol for cancer chemotherapy or radiation therapy
6. Assist RN to prepare patient for surgery (see "Diverticulosis/Diverticulitis")
7. Monitor patient and assist RN in postoperative care of patient (similar to diverticulosis/diverticulitis, except there is only one stoma; because colostomy is permanent, anus sutured closed)
   a. auscultate for bowel sounds
   b. monitor for type and consistency of stool; closer colostomy to ileum, more watery the stool; closer the colostomy to rectum, more normal the consistency of stool due to normal reabsorption of fluid in large intestine
   c. assist patient to understand, if appropriate, means to help control regularity of bowel movements through diet and colonic irrigations; closer colostomy to rectum, greater the chance of bowel regularity through bowel training regimen
   d. monitor drainage tubes, including perineal drain, if present after abdominal perineal resection
   e. notify physician of signs and symptoms of complications, such as frank blood draining

from or around stoma, paralytic ileus, melena, changes in bowel pattern, extensive skin excoriation, hypotension, fluid and electrolyte abnormalities, acid–base abnormalities
8. Have enterostomal therapist assist patient; contact ostomy club
9. Assist patient to look at surgical site and gradually assist in own care
10. Educate patient and significant others in care of stoma and ostomy appliances
11. Allow patient to ventilate fears, anxieties, anger, depression
12. Provide emotional and spiritual support to patient and significant others
13. Assist patient to contact clergy as appropriate

D. Evaluation

1. Patient's tumor successfully treated with no recurrence
2. Patient recovered from treatment without complications
3. Patient received successful palliative treatment
4. Patient's skin remained intact
5. Patient adjusted to altered body image
6. Patient assumed self-care
7. Patient's spiritual needs met; patient coped with diagnosis and prognosis

■ Liver and Biliary Disorders

I. HEPATITIS

A. Assessment

1. Definition/pathophysiology: inflammation of liver; inflammation causes necrosis of hepatocytes; if liver heals with no scar tissue, it is termed acute; if scar tissue and nodules occur, it is termed chronic; liver has immense capability for regeneration, thereby producing resistance to permanent damage
2. Incidence: 85% of viral hepatitis attributed to hepatitis A virus or hepatitis B virus
3. Predisposing/precipitating factors
   a. amebiasis of *Entamoeba histolytica* type, leading to amebic abscess; results from ingestion of contaminated food and water
   b. anicteric, viral hepatitis primarily of infants and children that produces no jaundice
   c. viral type called cholangiolitic or cholestatic, associated with obstructive jaundice in biliary tract
   d. hepatitis A virus (HAV), infectious, usually

transmitted by oral–fecal route; especially prevalent in environments with overcrowding and poor sanitation; higher incidence among children and young adults; when HAV antibody detected in serum, it usually coincides with disappearance of HAV in stool, usually 1–2 months after onset of disease; HAV antibody seems to confer long-term, even life-long, immunity to HAV

  e. hepatitis B virus (HBV), transmitted in blood, blood products, contaminated needles and body fluids like tears, saliva, and semen; infant can be infected by its mother during pregnancy; great risk exists in commercially prepared clotting concentrates obtained from commercial donors, because testing for hepatitis B surface antigen (HB$_5$Ag) concentrates not as reliable in commercial clotting concentrates as in whole blood; six different antigens detectable in serum; onset and progression of HBV differs from HAV in that HBV has more insidious onset and longer course, because it is more difficult to rid body of HBV than HAV

  f. non-type A and non-type B, cluster category of remaining types of virus-induced hepatitis; similar to hepatitis B, but not caused by HAV or HBV; highly associated with blood transfusions from paid donors rather than volunteers

  g. fulminant, acute hepatitis in which patient lapses into coma as result of extensive necrosis to liver by poisonous chemicals, medication overdosages, and virus

  h. hepatitis C, newly found variety; little known about it

4. Signs and symptoms
  a. amebic: severe diarrhea, gastrointestinal upset; anorexia, abdominal pain
  b. anicteric: gastrointestinal upset, anorexia, low-grade fever, absence of jaundice
  c. cholestatic or cholangiolitic: jaundice, fatigue, hepatomegaly, bilious vomit, pruritus
  d. hepatitis A virus: symptoms usually occur 2–7 weeks after ingestion of contaminated food; includes gastrointestinal and respiratory disturbances with sudden onset jaundice, hepatomegaly, tenderness of liver, pruritus, muscular aches and pains, weight loss
  e. hepatitis B virus: may be asymptomatic or more usually has an insidious onset 6 weeks to 6 months after contact with contaminated product; includes sudden onset of fever, chills, severe headache, gastrointestinal upset, jaundice, pruritus, hepatomegaly, tenderness of liver, splenomegaly
  f. non-type A or non-type B: incubation time, 6–9 weeks

  g. fulminant: sudden onset of high fever, gastrointestinal upset, convulsions, coma, death, usually within 10–14 days

5. Diagnostic tests
  a. history and physical examination
  b. blood work
    (1) CBC
    (2) prothrombin time
    (3) liver enzymes, including SGOT, serum glutamic-pyruvic transaminase (SGPT), to indicate amount of liver damage
    (4) serum bilirubin
    (5) serum for antigens for HAV or HBV
  c. urinalysis
    (1) color: dark yellow to brown could indicate presence of bilirubin
    (2) urobilirubin: indicator of abnormal levels of bilirubin waste
    (3) presence of red blood cells (RBC), WBC, protein, indicating poor renal filtration
  d. stool examination
    (1) presence of HAV
    (2) clay color: too little bilirubin
    (3) dark color: too much bilirubin
    (4) melena: blood in stool
  e. liver biopsy: cells to assist with diagnosis, indicator of extent of liver damage
    (1) explain procedure
    (2) position patient on right side
    (3) instruct patient to remain on bed rest
    (4) obtain baseline vital signs prior to procedure and frequent vital signs after procedure
    (5) observe for bleeding at puncture site
    (6) maintain blood and body fluid precautions
    (7) maintain pressure on biopsy site

7. Complications
  a. acute becomes chronic with extensive necrosis of hepatocytes
  b. opportunistic pathogenic organism invasion
  c. impaired clotting ability, increased bleeding time due to impaired metabolism or splenomegaly
  d. hepatic encephalopathy
  e. hepatic coma
  f. altered metabolism of digestion
  g. altered detoxification of medications

8. Usual treatments
  a. bed rest with bathroom privileges as needed
  b. diet depends on patient's needs and metabolism; may range from diet as tolerated to diet high in protein, carbohydrate, and calories and low in fat for tissue repair with little need of fat metabolism (protein restricted only if blood ammonia level increased)

c. isolation precautions; serum, needle, or enteric
d. passive immunity such as human gamma globulin

B. Planning, Goals/ Expected Outcomes

1. Patient will understand and comply with need for bed rest
2. Patient will comply with dietary regimen
3. Patient will not develop complications for hepatitis
4. Patient's skin will remain intact
5. Patient will comply with isolation regulations
6. Patient will comply with medication regimen

C. Implementation

1. Explain to patient that reason for fatigue is decreased metabolism by the liver
2. Assist patient with activities of daily living
3. Assist patient in finding and using acceptable diversional activities
4. Explain reason for prescribed diet and assist patient to make choices that are acceptable

5. Monitor vital signs, intake and output, hematuria, melena, changes in neurologic signs, such as decreased state of consciousness
6. Assist patient to change position every 2 hours; watch for reddened areas, particularly over bony prominences; clean skin with nonirritants, particularly if pruritus present owing to bile salt accumulation
7. Explain disease process and need for isolation techniques; assist patient with compliance
8. Assist patient to comply with pharmacologic treatment (Table 7-37)
9. Avoid all drugs that are detoxified in liver
10. Increase fluid levels by intravenous, oral routes
11. Vitamin K preparations as ordered
12. Monitor laboratory values for liver function
13. Use warm water, baking soda, and lotion for bath for pruritus; avoid soap
14. Maintain bleeding precautions

D. Evaluation

1. Patient's energy levels returned to normal
2. Adequate nutrition achieved
3. Patient recovers without complications
4. Patient's skin remained intact

TABLE 7–37. Pharmacologic Treatment of Hepatitis

Drug	Action	Use	Side Effects	Nursing Implications
Human immune globulin	Antiviral drug that contains antibodies against various diseases	Bolsters immune system	Urticaria Local pain Headache Malaise Anaphylaxis	Obtain history of allergy or reaction to immunization
Hepatitis B immune globulin	Antiviral drug that contains antibodies against hepatitis B virus	Bolsters immune system	Anaphylaxis	Obtain history of allergy or reaction to immunization
Hepatitis B vaccine	Causes body to produce antibodies against hepatitis B	Immunization of high risk populations	Pain at injection site Slight fever Malaise	The vaccine will *not* prevent hepatitis B in patients who are incubating the virus prior to vaccination
Vitamin K	Improved clotting ability in the presence of depressed prothrombin time	Replacement of vitamin K in liver disease	Transient hypotension Nausea Vomiting Dizziness Sweating Flushing Bronchospasms Anaphylaxis	Monitor prothrombin time
Antiemetics such as Emete-con (benzquinamide hydrochloride)	Prevent or treat nausea due to impaired metabolism	May be given ½ hour prior to meals or to treat nausea	May cause drowsiness	Avoid phenothiazines, such as Compazine, which is detoxified in liver
Antacids such as Mylanta	Counteract gastric acidity	After meals to help neutralize gastric acidity	Diarrhea	Systemic antacids should be avoided to prevent alkalosis

5. Disease not transmitted to others
6. Patient's liver healed
7. Patient's pain controlled

II. CIRRHOSIS

A. Assessment

1. Definition/pathophysiology: chronic inflammatory disease of liver, characterized by abnormal formation of fibrous connective tissue (scar tissue), which causes abnormal partitioning of liver into irregular nodules, degenerative changes of parenchymal cells, and fatty infiltration
2. Incidence: approximately 20% of chronic alcoholics develop cirrhosis
3. Predisposing/precipitating factors: disease has long latency period; can be due to multiple factors which include:
   a. alcoholism (Laennec's cirrhosis) with progressive destruction of hepatocytes, fatty infiltration, and resultant portal hypertension
   b. nutritional deficiencies, particularly of protein, kwashiorkor; alcoholics often have nutritional deficiencies
   c. biliary disorders from chronic inflammation of bile ducts and retention of bile from obstructive pathology
   d. toxic results from chemical poisons, such as carbon tetrachloride, or overdosage of certain medications, such as chlorpromazine
   e. metabolic disorders, such as those of amino acid metabolism
4. Signs and symptoms: lengthy latency period tends to be followed by rapid onset of abdominal pain, abdominal swelling, hematemesis, edema, and possibly jaundice; signs and symptoms related to failure of liver's normal functions
   a. fluid retention from abnormal fluid and electrolyte balance, leading in advanced stages to ascites
   b. bleeding from abnormal clotting factors
   c. malnutrition from abnormal metabolism
   d. toxic effects from many medications due to abnormal detoxification
   e. fever and dehydration from poor nutrition and inadequate fluid intake
   f. spider angiomas from abnormal clotting factors and capillary fragility
   g. delirium tremens from withdrawal of alcohol
   h. hypoglycemia and hypoproteinemia due to poor nutrition and abnormal metabolism
   i. hypertension from congestion in the portal system
   j. abnormal neurologic symptoms from poor metabolism of chemicals, particularly ammonia (NH_3), which is formed from nitrogen in protein joined to hydrogen
   k. fatigue and weight loss from abnormal metabolism
   l. esophageal varices from portal hypertension
5. Diagnostic tests
   a. history and physical examination
   b. liver biopsy: PN responsibilities:
      (1) explain procedure
      (2) obtain baseline vital signs prior to procedure, frequent vital signs after procedure
      (3) position patient on right side after biopsy
      (4) monitor for bleeding at puncture site
      (5) keep patient on bed rest per physician's order with pressure on puncture site
   c. liver enzymes
   d. CBC
   e. liver scan
6. Complications
   a. ascites: late symptom, abnormal accumulation of serous fluid in peritoneal cavity secondary to portal hypertension and hypoproteinemia
   b. portal hypertension: abnormally increased pressure in portal system due to scar tissue obstruction in portal venous system
   c. esophageal varices: varicosities in esophagus secondary to prolonged portal hypertension; varices large, fragile, and bleed easily
   d. hepatic encephalopathy (coma): changes in neurologic status secondary to abnormal detoxification and retention of chemicals in blood; marked changes in state of consciousness, progressing to coma, flapping tremors (asterixis)
   e. hemorrhage from abnormal clotting factors
7. Usual treatments: supportive in nature; includes:
   a. rest to decrease energy expenditure
   b. restriction of alcohol—absolutely no alcohol
   c. diet
      (1) early in disease, can be diet as tolerated to high protein, high calorie for tissue repair, with supplemental vitamins and minerals
      (2) late in the disease, restricted proteins to limit hepatic encephalopathy, high calorie to use carbohydrates and fats as tolerated, plus supplemental vitamins and minerals (see Table 5-10)
   d. assessment for signs of bleeding, such as spider angioma, hematemesis, guaiac positive stool and urine, vital signs
   e. neurologic signs to monitor for abnormalities
   f. paracentesis to relieve symptoms of ascites
   g. monitor laboratory values for liver status
   h. fluid restriction to decrease edema
   i. pharmacologic treatment
      (1) antibiotics (Table 7-10)

(2) vitamin K
(3) diuretics

B. Planning, Goals/ Expected Outcomes

1. Patient will identify and alleviate risk factors
2. Patient will improve nutritional status
3. Patient will decrease energy expenditure
4. Early signs of complications will not be undetected
5. Patient will have decreased anxiety

C. Implementation

1. Assist patient to identify presence of risk or precipitating factors, such as alcoholism
2. Administer medications as ordered (Table 7-38)
3. Assist patient to understand reason for restrictions in diet, such as for salt and protein, and assist patient in selection of choices acceptable to patient (Tables 7-39 and 5-10)
4. Assist patient to rest; assist with and provide diversional activities
5. Monitor patient's vital signs, intake and output, neurologic signs, signs of bleeding, weight
6. Provide emotional support to patient and significant others; assist with spiritual needs as appropriate

D. Evaluation

1. Progression of patient's disease slowed
2. Adequate nutrition achieved as tolerated by patient
3. Patient's energy levels increased

4. Complications in patient's condition prevented or detected and treated
5. Patient's anxiety decreased, spiritual needs met

III. CHOLELITHIASIS/ CHOLECYSTITIS

A. Assessment

1. Definition/pathophysiology
   a. cholelithiasis: presence of gallstones in the gallbladder
   b. cholecystitis: inflammation of the gallbladder
2. Incidence: more common in women than in men; more common in obese patients
3. Predisposing/precipitating factors
   a. most frequently caused by presence of gallstones
   b. other factors include: chemical irritants, medications such as Ilosone, bacteria such as Staphylococcus or Streptococcus and obstruction in biliary tract from stones or tumor
   c. phrase "fair, fat, forty, fertile, and female" used in reference to high-risk group
   d. increasingly documented after pregnancy and delivery
4. Signs and symptoms
   a. acute cholecystitis
      (1) may be gradual onset or sudden; moderate amount of pain and tenderness in abdomen, particularly in right upper quadrant
      (2) nausea and vomiting, malaise, and low-grade fever
      (3) abdominal pain may radiate to back and right shoulder area
      (4) if complete obstruction occurs, pain becomes excruciating with high-grade fever and more pronounced nausea and vomiting

TABLE 7–38. Medications Used in Cirrhosis

Drug	Action	Use	Common Side Effects	Nursing Implications
Broad-spectrum antibiotics, eg, neomycin	Disinfect the bowel	Decrease the production of ammonia in the colon	Headache Lethargy Ototoxicity Nephrotoxicity	Watch for oliguria, elevation of BUN
Vitamin K	Improve clotting ability	Replacement of vitamin K	Transient hypotension Nausea Vomiting Dizziness Sweating Bronchospasms Anaphylaxis	Monitor prothrombin time
Diuretics such as Lasix (furosemide)	Reduce blood volume	Decrease edema	Fluid and electrolyte depletion	Monitor intake and output, vital signs, K^+ level

BUN, blood urea nitrogen.

TABLE 7–39. High and Low Protein Foods

Low Protein Foods	High Protein Foods
Fruits, fresh or canned	Meats
Green vegetables	Eggs
Carrots	Fish
Potatoes	Milk
Margarine	Soybeans
Prepared low protein items such as breads	Gelatin
	Protein supplements
Farina	Yogurt
Sherbet	Peanut butter
Corn starch	Cheeses
Wheat starch	Legumes
	Protein fortified cereals

Low Protein Diet

RESTRICTIONS	REASON
Milk	Restrict the exogenous source
Milk products	of nitrogen in amino acids;
Eggs	NH_3 = ammonia; ammonia
Cheese	build-up = hepatic
Meat	encephalopathy
Fish	
Fowl	
Legumes	
Meat extracts, such as gravies, soups	

(5) visible jaundice present in about 25% of patients; patients with obstruction
(6) may have clay-colored stools and dark urine if obstruction present

b. chronic cholecystitis
  (1) symptoms less pronounced and progress more slowly than in acute
  (2) most common symptoms: discomfort after eating, nausea, and flatulence
  (3) if particularly large meal or high fat meal has been ingested, symptoms become more pronounced and include regurgitation, eructation and vomiting
  (4) may be mild right upper quadrant pain
  (5) untreated chronic cholecystitis can lead to damage of gallbladder and liver

5. Diagnostic tests
  a. history and physical examination
  b. CBC, watching for elevated WBC
  c. liver enzymes as indicators of inflammation
  d. cholecystography: radiopaque dye in form of tablets administered night before test; examination done to evaluate capacity of gallbladder to fill, concentrate bile, and empty; PN responsibilities:
    (1) explain procedure to patient
    (2) administer cathartics and enemas as ordered night before
    (3) administer tablets as ordered after fat free supper
    (4) keep patient NPO as ordered by physician
  e. intravenous cholangiography: radiopaque dye as contrast medium, administered IV by physi-

cian, to determine patency of hepatic and common bile ducts
  f. CT scan; PN responsibilities:
    (a) explain test to patient
    (b) restriction of fluids per physician's order to concentrate dye
    (c) administer cathartics and enemas per physician's order

6. Complications
  a. cholelithiasis becomes cholecystitis by stones moving into bile ducts
  b. rupture of gallbladder
  c. tear in bile ducts
  d. hepatitis secondary to obstruction in biliary tract
  e. jaundice

7. Usual treatments
  a. preferred treatment in acute cholecystitis is cholecystectomy after acute episode subsides
  b. if cholecystectomy not possible, then cholecystotomy, which is draining of gallbladder with removal of stones, followed by cholecystectomy at future time
  c. in chronic cholecystitis preferred treatment is cholecystectomy if stones present
  d. if stones not present, preferred treatment rest, antibiotics, antispasmodics, analgesics, low-fat diet, and hydration by intravenous or oral route

B. Planning, Goals/ Expected Outcomes

1. In acute cholecystitis
  a. patient will be free from pain
  b. patient will have an uncomplicated recovery from surgery
2. In chronic cholecystitis
  a. patient will identify the presence of risk or precipitating factors in life
  b. patient will comply with diet modification to low-fat diet, avoidance of heavy meals
  c. patient will be free of complications

C. Implementation

1. In acute cholecystitis
  a. assist patient to understand pathology of cholecystitis and reason cholecystectomy preferred treatment
  b. assist patient in preoperative period by:
    (1) explaining diagnostic tests
    (2) explaining surgical procedure
    (3) teaching coughing and deep breathing procedure, possible presence and care of drain-

age tubes, pain medication, early ambulation

    (4) maintaining fluid balance
    (5) monitoring for signs and symptoms of complications
    (6) reporting abnormalities to RN
  c. assist patient in the postoperative period by:
    (1) monitoring vital functions
    (2) monitoring for bleeding
    (3) monitoring drainage of tubes
    (4) helping patient cough and deep breathe, ambulate frequently
    (5) medicating for pain per physician's orders
    (6) reporting abnormalities to RN
2. In chronic cholecystitis
  a. assist patient to identify risk factors and precipitating factors in life
  b. assist patient to comply with low fat diet (Tables 7-40 and 5-6)
  c. assist patient to comply with pharmacologic regime (Table 7-41)
  d. assist patient to identify signs and symptoms of complications and report them to physician

D. Evaluation

1. Patient's pain alleviated
2. Patient recovered from surgery without complications
3. Acute cholecystitis prevented
4. Patient complied with diet modification
5. Patient recovered without complication

TABLE 7–40. Low Fat Diet

Contents	Reason
Foods are prepared with the avoidance of added fat *Foods avoided include:* 1. meats, particularly fatty cuts 2. meat gravies, creams 3. lard 4. oils 5. dairy products of cream, butter, eggs 6. nuts 7. avocados *Food substitutions include:* 1. lean meats, such as veal, liver, lamb 2. lean meats that are broiled, baked or roasted 3. dairy products of skim milk cottage cheese, margarine 4. all kinds of breads and cereals 5. all kinds of vegetables 6. three eggs per week, not fried	Fat is the main stimulator of the gallbladder to contract in order to release bile; the contractions cause pain in the inflamed gallbladder, particularly in the presence of stones; during contraction, small stones can be expelled into the bile ducts, blocking them and causing acute pain

IV. PANCREATITIS

A. Assessment

1. Definition/pathophysiology: inflammatory condition of pancreas that can be acute or chronic; primarily exogenous functions of pancreas diminished, with endogenous functions of islets of Langerhans possibly affected in later stages; digestive enzymes of pancreas released into pancreatic tissue, producing autodigestion
2. Incidence: higher in alcoholics (men) and persons with cholelithiasis (women)
3. Predisposing/precipitating factors
  a. alcoholism
  b. drug toxicity, such as acetaminophen overdose
  c. obstruction in biliary tract
  d. viral infection
  e. nutritional deficiencies
  f. etiology often unknown
4. Signs and symptoms
  a. in acute pancreatitis: signs and symptoms related to rapid onset of necrosis, suppuration, gangrene, and hemorrhage in the pancreas
    (1) moderate to severe epigastric pain
    (2) nausea and vomiting
    (3) malaise and fever
    (4) eructation, hiccoughing
    (5) collapse from pain, fluid and electrolyte loss
    (6) rigid abdomen over umbilicus
    (7) jaundice if due to biliary obstruction
  b. in chronic pancreatitis: signs and symptoms related to loss of exogenous functions with diminished production of pancreatic enzymes; in long-standing chronic pancreatitis, symptoms of deficiency of endogenous islets of Langerhans may be present
    (1) bulky, fatty, foul-smelling stool due to malabsorption of protein, carbohydrate, fats
    (2) weight loss
    (3) malaise
    (4) nausea and vomiting
    (5) fever
    (6) wasting of muscle tissue
    (7) easy bruising due to malabsorption of fat soluble vitamins A, D, E, and K
    (8) signs and symptoms of diabetes mellitus
5. Diagnostic tests
  a. history and physical examination
  b. CT scan of pancreas
  c. abdominal radiographs
  d. fiberoptic endoscopy to visualize head of the pancreas
  e. pancreatography: radiographic examination performed during surgery in which contrast medium is injected into pancreatic duct

TABLE 7–41. Medications Used in Cholelithiasis/Cholecystitis

Drug	Action	Use	Common Side Effects	Nursing Implications
Antibiotics such as ampicillin	Bactericidal agent	Kill pathogenic organisms, causing or contributing to cholecystitis	Nausea Vomiting Diarrhea Stomatitis Yeast infection Anemia Thrombocytopenia Leukopenia	Question patient about allergy to penicillin or any antibiotics prior to administration
Antispasmodics such as Pro-Banthine (propantheline bromide)	Smooth muscle relaxants	Treat spasms in bile ducts	Headache Insomnia Palpitations Blurred vision Constipation	Overdose can cause curarelike symptoms
Analgesics such as meperidine	Central-acting analgesic	Treat pain of cholecystitis	Sedation Euphoria Hypotension Nausea Vomiting Constipation Urinary retention	Controlled substance, watch for respiratory depression Morphine not used, since it increases spasms of the duct
Chenodiol	Suppressor of hepatic synthesis of cholesterol	Gradual dissolution of gallstones through biliary cholesterol desaturation	Diarrhea Cramps Nausea Vomiting Liver toxicity	Watch for hepatic enzyme elevations

    f. liver enzymes, amylase, lipase
    g. CBC
6. Complications
    a. acute hemorrhagic pancreatitis
    b. malabsorption with malnutrition
    c. diabetes mellitus
7. Usual treatments
    a. in acute pancreatitis
      (1) maintain bed rest with bathroom privileges
      (2) analgesics for pain
      (3) maintain hydration with intravenous fluids
      (4) keep patient NPO
      (5) possible gastrointestinal decompression with NG tube to intermittent suction
      (6) administer antibiotics if appropriate
      (7) administer steroids if appropriate
      (8) when eating, may require supplemental pancreatic extracts
    b. in chronic pancreatitis
      (1) encourage rest
      (2) give supplemental pancreatic enzymes with each meal
      (3) give analgesics
      (4) ensure adequate nutrition

B. Planning, Goals/Expected Outcomes

1. Patient will identify and alleviate risk factors, especially alcohol
2. Patient will be free of pain
3. Patient will maintain adequate hydration
4. Patient will maintain adequate nutrition
5. Patient will not develop complications

C. Implementation

1. Assist patient to identify presence of risk or precipitating factors in life, such as alcoholism
2. Assist patient in compliance with bed rest with bathroom privileges; assist patient with diversional activities
3. Educate patient about the pharmacologic regimen; administer medications as ordered (Table 7-42)
4. Monitor intake and output; administer intravenous hydration as appropriate; monitor for signs and symptoms of overhydration or dehydration
5. Educate patient to need for pancreatic enzymes with meals and patterns of adequate nutrition
6. Monitor patient's vital functions; report abnormalities to team leader
7. Monitor for signs and symptoms of diabetes mellitus

D. Evaluation

1. Pain free or pain controlled
2. Patient's hydration and nutrition was maintained
3. Patient did not develop complications or received early treatment of complications

TABLE 7–42. Medications Used in Pancreatitis

Drug	Action	Use	Common Side Effects	Nursing Implications
Analgesics such as meperidine		(see Table 7-8)		
Antibiotics such as ampicillin		(see Table 7-10)		
Steroids such as prednisone	Decrease inflammation	Treat inflammatory symptoms	Euphoria Hypertension Edema Gastrointestinal irritation Peptic ulcer	Can produce symptoms of diabetes mellitus Can cause pancreatitis Drug dosage must be reduced slowly
Pancreatic extract such as pancreatin (Viokase)	Supplemental replacement of pancreatic enzymes	(also see Table 7-17) Aids digestion of starches, fats, proteins	Nausea Vomiting	Antacids may negate the effect

■ Renal/Urinary Disorders

I. URINARY TRACT DISORDERS

A. Cystitis

1. Assessment
   a. definition/pathophysiology: inflammation of urinary bladder; may be primary or secondary to ascending urethritis or secondary to descending nephritis or ureteritis; pathogenic organism usually bacteria, often *E. coli* in women
   b. incidence: more common in women than in men
   c. predisposing/precipitating factors
      (1) infection in another part of urinary system
      (2) poor perineal hygiene
      (3) dehydration
      (4) urinary catheterization
      (5) tight clothing around groin
      (6) obstruction in urethra or bladder, such as prostatic hypertrophy or urethritis
      (7) vaginal infections
      (8) sexual intercourse (women)
   d. signs and symptoms
      (1) dysuria
      (2) hematuria
      (3) frequency and urgency of urination
      (4) chills and fever if infection in other parts of urinary system as well as bladder
   e. diagnostic tests
      (1) history and physical examination
      (2) urine culture and sensitivity
      (3) urinalysis
      (4) CBC
      (5) cystoscopy
   f. complications
      (1) acute cystitis becomes chronic
      (2) involvement in other parts of urinary tract, such as ureteritis and pyelonephritis

   g. usual treatment
      (1) pharmacologic (Table 7-43)
         (a) antibiotics
         (b) urinary antiseptics
         (c) urinary analgesics
         (d) analgesics (antispasmodics)
      (2) treat obstruction if present
         (a) removal of hypertrophy of prostate (see "Benign Prostastic Hypertrophy [BPH]")
         (b) dilation of urethra
2. Planning, goals/expected outcomes
   a. patient will identify and alleviate risk factors in life
   b. patient will be free of pain
   c. patient will be free of infection
   d. patient will not have complications
3. Implementation
   a. assist patient in carrying out good personal hygiene, selecting clothes not binding in groin area, avoiding irritant soaps, avoiding physical irritations such as prolonged bike riding
   b. assist patient to understand and comply with pharmacologic regimen; push fluids, particularly acid-ash fruit juices, such as cranberry juice
   c. administer smooth muscle antispasmotics, such as dicyclomine hydrochloride
   d. obtain culture and sensitivity specimens, sterile technique with catheters
   e. monitor patient for signs and symptoms of extending infection; notify team leader
   f. force fluids
   g. monitor intake and output
   h. ensure patient takes full course of antibiotics
4. Evaluation
   a. patient's cystitis cured, bladder mucosa healed
   b. patient complied with pharmacologic regimen
   c. patient's pain controlled
   d. patient's urine culture grew no bacteria
   e. patient recovered without complications

TABLE 7–43. Medications Used in Urinary Tract Infections

Drug	Action	Use	Common Side Effects	Nursing Implications
Antibiotics, particularly penicillin-like, oxacillin	Inhibit pathogenic cell wall synthesis	Treat systemic infections	Anaphylaxis Thrombocytopenia Neuropathy Hepatitis Interstitial nephritis	Resists penicillinase Ask patient about medication allergy, particularly to penicillin prior to administration
Urinary tract antibiotics such as co-trimoxazole (sulfamethoxazole trimethoprim)	A sulfonamide bacteriostatic agent	Decrease bacterial folic acid synthesis	Aplastic anemia Nausea Vomiting Headache Toxic nephrosis	Must push fluids to prevent crystalluria Check for sulfa allergy
Urinary tract antiseptics such as nalidixic acid (NegGram)	Inhibit microbial DNA synthesis	In acute and chronic urinary tract infections caused by gram negative pathogens	Drowsiness Weakness Headache Abdominal pain Diarrhea Photosensitivity	Needs renal and liver function studies for long-term therapy Resistant bacteria may develop early
Urinary tract analgesics such as phenazopyridine hydrochloride (Pyridium)	Local anesthetic	Anesthetic effect on urinary mucosa	Headache Nausea	Urine turns reddish orange May alter Clinistix; use Clinitest for accuracy
Analgesics such as Demerol	Narcotic analgesic	Central pain reliever	Nausea Vomiting Hypotension	May cause urinary retention, constipation
Steroids such as prednisone	Antiinflammatory	Treat inflammation; try to limit autoimmune response	Euphoria Fluid retention Congestive heart failure	Dose must be tapered when stopping treatment to prevent addisonian crisis

B. Urethritis

1. Assessment
   a. definition/pathophysiology: inflammation of urethra, causing mucous membrane to swell; can impede flow of urine
   b. incidence: high in cases of gonorrhea, particularly in males
   c. predisposing/precipitating factors
      (1) gonorrhea
      (2) prostatitis
      (3) catheterization
      (4) sexually transmitted nonspecific pathogen
   d. signs and symptoms
      (1) frequency and urgency
      (2) burning on urination, dysuria
      (3) purulent discharge
   e. diagnostic tests
      (1) history and physical examination
      (2) urine culture and sensitivity
      (3) culture and sensitivity of discharge
      (4) cystoscopy
   f. complications
      (1) cystitis
      (2) hydronephrosis
      (3) pyelonephritis
      (4) uremia
      (5) renal failure
   g. usual treatment
      (1) antibiotics
      (2) analgesics
      (3) dilation of stricture of urethra

2. Planning, goals/expected outcomes
   a. patient will identify and alleviate risk factors in life
   b. patient will understand and comply with treatment
   c. patient will be free of pain
   d. patient will experience no recurrence
3. Implementation
   a. assist patient to identify personal risk factors and accept treatment for causes such as gonorrhea, nonspecific sexually transmitted pathogen, or stricture
   b. assist patient to comply with pharmacologic therapy or dilation
   c. provide pain medication as ordered
   d. instruct patient to avoid recurrence, such as being careful with selection of sexual partners and having early signs of gonorrhea treated quickly
4. Evaluation
   a. patient's urethritis healed
   b. patient complied with treatment
   c. patient's pain controlled
   d. patient recovered without complications
   e. patient's condition did not recur

C. Pyelonephritis

1. Assessment
   a. definition/pathophysiology: inflammation of kidney and renal pelvis; can be acute or chronic; can involve glomerulus, tubules or interstitial

renal tissue; damage to glomeruli results in impairment of filtration process; kidney becomes enlarged, inflammation in mucosa present, abscesses can form

b. incidence: occurs most frequently in children and young people, persons with recent sore throat, scarlet fever, or streptococcal infections, and persons with previous infection in lower urinary tract

c. predisposing/precipitating factors
    (1) previous sore throat, scarlet fever
    (2) previous streptococcal infection that may cause autoimmune response
    (3) infection in lower genitourinary tract that ascends to kidney
    (4) presence of indwelling urinary catheter
    (5) pregnancy with vesicoureteral reflux

d. signs and symptoms
    (1) in acute pyelonephritis
        (a) dull pain in flank, costovertebral angle (CVA) tenderness
        (b) chills and fever
        (c) headache
        (d) malaise
        (e) hematuria, pyuria
        (f) wine-colored urine
        (g) frequency and urgency
        (h) cloudy urine from albuminuria, WBCs
        (i) edema secondary to protein loss
        (j) hypertension
    (2) in chronic nephritis (nephrosis)
        (a) may occur right after acute attack or appear after long interval that was asymptomatic
        (b) may occur with no history of acute attack
        (c) in early stages:
            (i) malaise
            (ii) albuminuria
            (iii) hematuria
            (iv) possibly anemia
        (d) in second stage (follows latent stage that is usually asymptomatic): edema, particularly in face, legs, and arms
        (e) in final stage:
            (i) uremia
            (ii) kidney failure

e. diagnostic tests
    (1) history and physical examination
    (2) urinalysis
    (3) urine for culture and sensitivity
    (4) intravenous pyelogram (IVP)
    (5) kidney, ureter, and bladder (KUB) radiograph
    (6) cystoscopy
    (7) CT scan
    (8) BUN and creatinine levels

f. complications
    (1) uremia
    (2) renal failure
    (3) septicemia
    (4) hypertension
    (5) opportunistic secondary infections

g. usual treatment
    (1) bed rest
    (2) antibiotics
    (3) urinary antiseptics
    (4) analgesics
    (5) high protein, low sodium diet (Table 7-44 and Chapter 5)
    (6) hydration by intravenous method and orally as long as output maintained
    (7) steroid hormones possible
    (8) hemodialysis possible
    (9) kidney transplant drastic method

2. Planning, goals/expected outcomes
  a. patient will be free of infection
  b. patient will be free of pain
  c. patient will not develop secondary infection
  d. patient will not develop recurrence
  e. patient will maintain adequate nutrition and hydration

3. Implementation
  a. assist patient to understand and comply with pharmacologic regimen (Table 7-43)
  b. assist patient to comply with bed rest; provide diversional activities
  c. administer pain medication as ordered
  d. assist patient to understand need to avoid per-

TABLE 7–44. High Protein, Low Sodium Diet*

High Protein Foods	Reason
Milk	Replace protein lost in urine
Eggs	Protein needed for tissue repair
Lean meat, fish, poultry	
Vegetables	Provide adequate calories for energy
Fruits	
Whole grain, enriched bread and cereal	
Butter, margarine	

Foods High in Sodium to Be Avoided	Reason
(may be 500–1000 mg/day)	Prevent or limit edema, thereby decrease hypertension
Salt at the table	
Salted, preserved foods like hot dogs, cold cuts	Less sodium causes less fluid retention, therefore increased urinary output
Kosher meats	
Salted snack foods like chips, peanuts, popcorn	
Spices and condiments such as bouillon cubes, meat tenderizers, pickles, soy sauce	
Cheeses	
Peanut butter	

* Used in presence of edema, hypertension, oliguria.

sons with infections, avoid becoming overly fatigued and undernourished
   e. assist patient to take full regimen of antibiotics and steroids as appropriate
   f. assist patient to understand and comply with high protein, low sodium diet plus hydration at levels prescribed by physician (Table 7-44)
4. Evaluation
   a. patient's infection cleared
   b. patient did not develop secondary infection
   c. patient did not suffer recurrence
   d. patient maintained adequate nutrition and hydration

II. URINARY CALCULI (NEPHROLITHIASIS)

A. Assessment

1. Definition/pathophysiology: presence of calculi in kidney and urinary tract; caused by abnormal precipitation of chemicals out of urine; majority of kidney stones composed of calcium and magnesium in combination with phosphate or oxalate; calculi range from very large to as small as grains of sand; smaller stones can be passed from kidney into ureters to bladder and down urethra; some stones mainly composed of uric acid (urate)
2. Incidence: occurrence higher in males than females, particularly in those between ages of 30 and 50 years, with sedentary occupations
3. Predisposing/precipitating factors
   a. persistent urinary tract infections
   b. obstruction of flow of urine, such as with benign prostatic hypertrophy
   c. stasis of urine due to immobility
   d. abnormalities in metabolism of certain chemicals
   e. diet high in calcium, phosphates, purines, oxalates
   f. insufficient fluid intake
   g. overusage of sodium bicarbonate (alkaline urine leads to increased precipitation of calcium)
4. Signs and symptoms
   a. may produce no symptoms unless dislodged from renal pelvis into ureter
   b. colicky pain in flank region of the costovertebral angle (CVA tenderness)
   c. pain may radiate around to abdomen and down to genitalia
   d. colicky pain may not be controllable by medication or position change
   e. nausea and vomiting
   f. hematuria

   g. fever
   h. pain on urination
   i. frequency and urgency
   j. pyuria
   k. diaphoresis
   l. pain may stop spontaneously once stone passes either into bladder or out urethra
5. Diagnostic tests
   a. history and physical examination
   b. urinalysis
   c. CBC
   d. cystoscopy: surgical placement of scope through urethra into bladder for direct visualization: PN responsibilities
      (1) teach patient what to expect from procedure, depending on whether performed under local anesthesia or general anesthesia
      (2) intake and output
      (3) vital signs
      (4) strain urine for stones
      (5) monitor for voiding after procedure
   e. urine culture and sensitivity
   f. KUB radiographs
   g. intravenous pyelogram
6. Complications
   a. stone lodged in ureter or urethra
   b. hydronephrosis secondary to obstruction
   c. pyelonephritis
   d. perforation of ureter, with development of septic shock
   e. peritonitis from perforation
   f. stone moved to bladder, blocks urethra
   g. cystitis, urethritis
7. Usual treatment
   a. antibiotics
   b. analgesics
   c. hydration, intravenous or oral
   d. cytoscopy with passage of ureteral catheter and stone basket to remove stone
   e. cystoscopy with passage of instrumentation to crush stone in ureter or bladder and remove (litholapaxy)
   f. nephrolithotomy: surgical removal of stone from kidney
   g. pyelolithotomy: surgical removal of stone from renal pelvis
   h. ureterolithotomy: surgical removal of stone from ureter

B. Planning, Goals/ Expected Outcomes

1. Patient will identify and alleviate risk factors
2. Patient will be free from pain
3. Patient will not develop complications

C. Implementation

1. Assist patient to identify foods high in calcium and phosphorus to be avoided (Table 7-45)
2. Assist patient during diagnostic studies, surgical procedures
   a. PN responsibilities: preoperative
      (1) patient education about procedures
      (2) teach patient to cough and deep breathe
      (3) teach patient about early ambulation and pain medication
      (4) strain urine for stones
   b. PN responsibilities: postoperative
      (1) monitor vital functions
      (2) intake and output
      (3) cough and deep breathe
      (4) early ambulation
      (5) pain medication as ordered
3. Monitor intake and output; monitor vital signs
4. Monitor for signs and symptoms of infection
5. Monitor for signs and symptoms of peritonitis

D. Evaluation

1. Patient's stones removed
2. Patient's infection cleared
3. Patient's pain was controlled
4. Patient's stones did not recur
5. Patient recovered without complications

III. HYDRONEPHROSIS

A. Assessment

1. Definition/pathophysiology: renal pelvis and calices of kidney distend with urine as outflow obstructed; as disease progresses, nephrons destroyed; as distention progresses and pressure builds, muscular walls of renal pelvis and calices stretch; replaced by fibrous tissue progressing to functionless sac
2. Incidence: higher in males than females

TABLE 7–45. Foods to be Avoided in Renal Calculi

Foods High in Calcium	Foods High in Phosphorus
Milk	Milk
Milk products	Milk products
Leafy vegetables	Whole grain cereals
Whole grains	Rye and whole grain breads
	Dried fruits
	Fish, shellfish
	Chocolate, nuts
	Cream sauces

3. Predisposing/precipitating factors
   a. obstruction of urinary tract, such as
      (1) ureteral tumors
      (2) calculi
      (3) benign or malignant prostatic hypertrophy
      (4) cancer of bladder and urethra
      (5) edema from urinary tract infections affecting ureters or urethra
   b. atrophy of urinary tract
4. Signs and symptoms
   a. dull and nagging pain in kidney area (CVA tenderness)
   b. sharp pain in kidney area
   c. hematuria
   d. pyuria
   e. elevated WBC if infection develops
   f. fever
5. Diagnostic tests
   a. history and physical examinations
   b. urinalysis
   c. culture and sensitivity of urine
   d. pyelography
   e. cystoscopy
   f. intravenous pyelogram (IVP)
   g. CT scan
6. Complications
   a. uremia if both kidneys involved
   b. renal failure
   c. pyelonephritis
7. Usual treatment
   a. treat cause
   b. bladder catheterization to drain urine
   c. prostatectomy
   d. nephrostomy tube to drain pelvis of kidney
   e. antibiotics (Table 7-10)
   f. analgesics (Table 7-8)
   g. antipyretics

B. Planning, Goals/ Expected Outcomes

1. Patient will understand and comply with treatment
2. Patient will have adequate intake and output
3. Patient will be free of pain
4. Patient will not develop complications

C. Implementation

1. Assist patient to understand need for treatments and comply with treatments
   a. urinary antiseptics and antibiotics: to reduce edema by decreasing infection in urinary tract (see Table 7-43)
   b. IVP

c. nephrostomy with placement of drainage tubes: PN responsibilities
   (1) teach patient about procedure
   (2) usual preoperative teaching
   (3) postoperative care with coughing and deep breathing, monitoring vital functions, using sterile technique for tube care, recording intake and output
d. urinary catheter: PN responsibilities
   (1) urinary catheter care
   (2) intake and output
   (3) assess for blood, pus
e. prostatectomy (see "Benign Prostatic Hypertrophy [BPH]")
2. Monitor intake and output
3. Hydration by intravenous route or oral route
4. Administer pain medications as ordered
5. Use sterile technique to prevent further infection
6. Monitor vital functions for signs of infections; administer antibiotics as ordered

D. Evaluation

1. Patient's hydronephrosis reversed
2. Patient's infection cleared
3. Patient maintained adequate fluid levels and adequate output
4. Patient's pain controlled
5. Patient recovered without complications

IV. RENAL FAILURE: ACUTE AND CHRONIC

A. Assessment

1. Definition/pathophysiology: inability of kidney to carry on normal function; can be caused by multiple factors; kidney failure affects multiple body functions, including fluid and electrolyte balance, acid–base balance, excretion of waste products, control of blood pressure; renal failure can be acute with recovery or can become chronic
2. Incidence: higher in males than females
3. Predisposing/precipitating factors
   a. prerenal causes
      (1) circulatory collapse with decreased blood flow to kidney
      (2) severe dehydration
      (3) prolonged hypotension
      (4) physical trauma
   b. renal causes
      (1) infection/inflammation
      (2) toxic chemicals, such as mercury

(3) nephrotoxic medications, such as multiple antibiotics
(4) electrolyte imbalances, such as hyperkalemia
(5) diabetes mellitus
(6) blood transfusion reaction
(7) lupus erythematosus
(8) polycystic kidneys
   c. postrenal causes
      (1) benign prostatic hypertrophy
      (2) urinary calculi
      (3) lower urinary tract obstruction
4. Signs and symptoms
   a. of acute renal failure
      (1) nausea, vomiting
      (2) diarrhea
      (3) oliguria (decreased output), which may progress to anuria (no output)
      (4) headache, drowsiness, lethargy from retained waste products (urea)
      (5) possibly hypertension from retained fluids
      (6) possibly hypertension secondary to circulatory collapse or severe dehydration
      (7) signs and symptoms of electrolyte imbalances
      (8) elevated BUN, creatinine levels
   b. of chronic renal failure (end-stage) (Fig. 7-9)
      (1) very high serum BUN and creatinine levels due to tubular necrosis
      (2) hyperkalemia
      (3) cardiac arrest from hyperkalemia
      (4) hypertension may become malignant
      (5) susceptibility to infection
      (6) gastrointestinal problems
      (7) anorexia with nausea and vomiting
      (8) uremic breath
      (9) anemia with weakness
      (10) bleeding tendencies
      (11) oliguria to anuria
      (12) pruritus from uremic frost
      (13) fluid and electrolyte imbalances
      (14) acid–base imbalances
      (15) anasarca (severe generalized edema)
      (16) neurologic signs and symptoms progressing to convulsions, coma, and death
5. Diagnostic tests
   a. history and physical examination
   b. BUN and creatinine levels
   c. kidney function tests
   d. CT scan
   e. intravenous pyelogram (IVP): PN responsibilities
      (1) teach patient about procedure
      (2) keep patient NPO prior to examination
      (3) administer cathartics or enemas night before as ordered

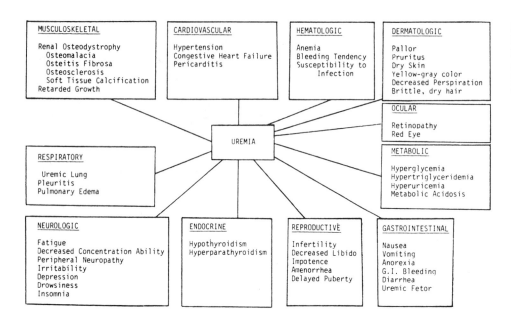

MUSCULOSKELETAL	CARDIOVASCULAR	HEMATOLOGIC	DERMATOLOGIC

Renal Osteodystrophy
  Osteomalacia
  Osteitis Fibrosa
  Osteosclerosis
  Soft Tissue Calcification
Retarded Growth
	Hypertension
	Congestive Heart Failure
	Pericarditis
		Anemia
		Bleeding Tendency
		Susceptibility to
		  Infection
			Pallor
			Pruritus
			Dry Skin
			Yellow-gray color
			Decreased Perspiration
			Brittle, dry hair

OCULAR

Retinopathy
Red Eye

METABOLIC

Hyperglycemia
Hypertriglyceridemia
Hyperuricemia
Metabolic Acidosis

RESPIRATORY

Uremic Lung
Pleuritis
Pulmonary Edema

UREMIA

NEUROLOGIC	ENDOCRINE	REPRODUCTIVE	GASTROINTESTINAL
Fatigue Decreased Concentration Ability Peripheral Neuropathy Irritability Depression Drowsiness Insomnia	Hypothyroidism Hyperparathyroidism	Infertility Decreased Libido Impotence Amenorrhea Delayed Puberty	Nausea Vomiting Anorexia G.I. Bleeding Diarrhea Uremic Fetor

FIGURE 7–9. Systemic effects of uremia. (From Lewis, S.M.: Pathophysiology of chronic renal failure. Nurs. Clin. North Am., 16:501, 1981.)

    (4) ask patient if allergic to any iodine dyes
    (5) vital signs before and after procedure
    (6) monitor intake and output
    (7) watch for allergic reaction
  f. urinalysis for presence of blood, protein, WBC, sugar
  g. radiograph of kidney to assess for size, urinary tract obstruction: kidney, ureter, and bladder (KUB)
6. Complications
  a. hypertension
  b. fluid and electrolyte abnormalities
  c. acid–base imbalances
  d. hemorrhage
  e. anasarca
  f. convulsions
  g. coma
  h. death
7. Usual treatment
  a. treat cause if possible
  b. peritoneal dialysis: sterile catheter placed in peritoneal space to allow input of dialysate solution; solution left in for prescribed period of time, then drained out; principle involves diffusion of fluid through semipermeable membrane, in this case, peritoneal membrane; fluid toxins and waste products pulled into hypertonic dialysate solution and then drained out; output should be more than input (Fig. 7-10)
  c. hemodialysis: surgical arteriovenous shunt created to allow arterial blood to be tapped and then channeled to hemodialysis machine, which uses external physical semipermeable membranes for diffusion; blood that has had fluids and chemicals removed then returned to venous circulation

  d. renal transplant: if appropriate, diseased kidney removed and donor kidney surgically implanted; danger of rejection present

B. Planning, Goals/ Expected Outcomes

1. Patient will identify reason for and comply with fluid restrictions
2. Patient will maintain fluid, electrolyte, and acid–base balance
3. Patient will identify need for alternate form of removal of waste products normally performed by kidney
4. Patient will comply with needs of alternate form of removal of waste products
5. Patient will be free of complications for renal failure
6. Patient will be free of pain

C. Implementation

1. Assist patient to understand and comply with fluid restrictions; maintain intake and output
2. Monitor for signs and symptoms of fluid, electrolyte, or acid–base balance; report abnormalities to team leader
3. Assist patient to understand need for alternative form of removal of wastes
4. In peritoneal dialysis: monitor intake and output, vital signs, signs of peritonitis, infection, fluid overload
5. In hemodialysis: monitor intake and output, vital signs, signs of infection at site of shunt or systemic;

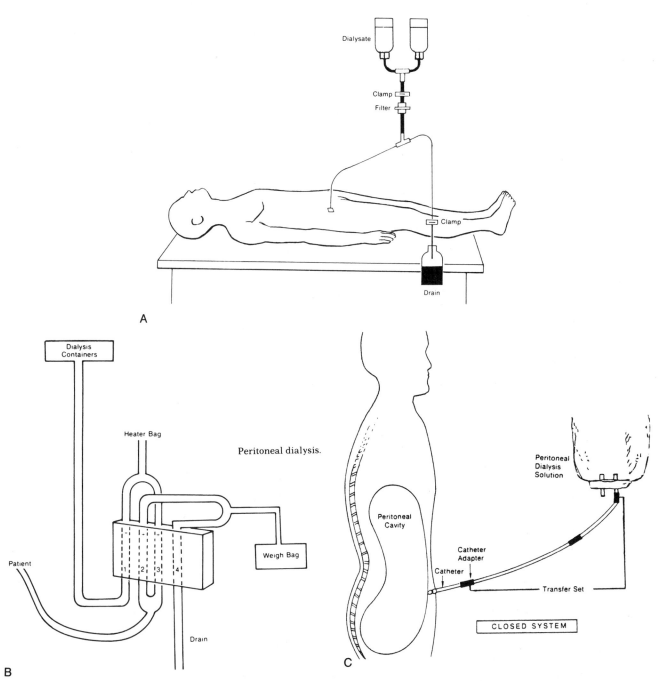

FIGURE 7–10. Peritoneal dialysis. *A,* Manual, three-way method. *B,* Cycler dialysis. During fluid instillation, tube allows warm solution to flow into the peritoneal cavity; tube 4 allows drainage from the weighing bag into the floor drain; and tubes 1 and 2 are closed. At the end of the "drain" cycle, tubes 3 and 4 are closed, and tube 1 is opened to allow flow from the containers into the heater bag. Tube 2 then allows drainage from the patient to flow into the weighing bag. *C,* Method for continuous ambulatory peritoneal dialysis. (From Sorrells, A.J.: Peritoneal dialysis: A rediscovery. Nurs. Clin. North Am., 16:515, 1981.)

monitor for circulation through shunt by listening with stethoscope for "whooshing" sound at shunt site

6. In renal transplant: monitor intake and output, vital signs, signs of transplant rejection, fever, malaise, increased WBC, hypertension; report abnormalities to team leader

7. Teach patient signs and symptoms of complications and to report them to nurse and doctor; monitor for signs and symptoms of complications and report to team leader

8. Administer pain medications as ordered; monitor for complications; provide symptomatic treatment as needed

D. Evaluation

1. Patient maintained adequate fluid balance
2. Patient maintained normal fluid and electrolyte balance, acid–base balance
3. Patient complied with treatment
4. Patient experienced no complications, or had early treatment of complications
5. Patient recovered from transplant surgery without complications

V. KIDNEY TUMORS

A. Assessment

1. Definition/pathophysiology: tumor in kidney that can be primary or secondary ascending from tumor lower in genitourinary system or as metastasis from another part of body; all malignant with no early signs and symptoms
2. Incidence: higher in males than females
3. Predisposing/precipitating factors
   a. unknown etiology
   b. tumor elsewhere in genitourinary system
   c. tumor metastasis elsewhere in body
4. Signs and symptoms
   a. in early stage usually none, often discovered secondary to radiograph for another reason
   b. in later stages
      (1) hematuria without pain
      (2) symptoms from metastatic process, depending on sites of invasion
      (3) weight loss
      (4) anemia
      (5) low-grade fever
5. Diagnostic tests
   a. history and physical examination
   b. intravenous pyelogram
   c. KUB radiograph
   d. CT scan
   e. renal biopsy: PN responsibilities
      (1) teach patient about procedure
      (2) vital signs preoperative and postoperative
      (3) intake and output
      (4) monitor for bleeding at incision site
      (5) position lying on biopsy site to apply pressure
      (6) blood-tinged urine is normal
      (7) no heavy lifting, exertion, hot baths for 2 weeks after biopsy
   f. CBC
   g. urinalysis

6. Complications
   a. kidney failure
   b. hemorrhage
   c. hypertension
   d. fluid and electrolyte imbalances
   e. acid–base imbalances
   f. metastasis
7. Usual treatment
   a. cancer chemotherapy (Tables 7-18 and 7-19)
   b. radiation therapy (Table 7-20)
   c. nephrectomy
   d. radical nephrectomy: kidney plus adjacent tissue and lymphatics
   e. peritoneal dialysis possible
   f. hemodialysis, as appropriate, particularly if both kidneys are affected
   g. intravenous therapy for hydration
   h. hyperalimentation feeding possible

B. Planning, Goals/ Expected Outcomes

1. Patient will identify need for and comply with treatment
2. Patient will maintain fluid, electrolyte, and acid–base balances
3. Patient will maintain energy levels
4. Patient will be free of pain
5. Patient will not develop complications of renal tumor

C. Implementation

1. Assist patient to understand purpose of surgery, chemotherapy, or radiation
2. Assist patient with activities of daily living while receiving treatments
3. Monitor intake and output, particularly drains after surgery, vital signs
4. Monitor for signs and symptoms of fluid and electrolyte balance, acid–base balance; report abnormalities to team leader
5. Provide medication for nausea, vomiting, and diarrhea as ordered (Table 7-32)
6. Assist patient to rest; provide diversional activities, space activities
7. Provide small, frequent meals; maintain intravenous therapy; assist RN with monitoring of hyperalimentation feeding
8. Provide emotional support to patient and significant others during diagnosis, treatment, and possible death
9. Administer pain medication as ordered (Table 7-8)

10. Monitor vital functions; monitor for hemorrhage; report abnormalities to team leader

D. Evaluation

1. Patient complied with treatment
2. Patient had tumor removed or diminished
3. Patient's fluid and electrolyte balance, acid–base balance maintained
4. Patient's energy levels maintained at optimum
5. Patient had no pain or pain controlled
6. Patient developed no complications
7. Patient and family coped with terminal prognosis

VI. BLADDER TUMORS

A. Assessment

1. Definition/pathophysiology: malignant tumors can range from no penetration beyond the bladder mucosa, to metastasis beyond the pelvis; benign tumors always premalignant
2. Incidence: more common in men than women, particularly in those over age 50 years
3. Predisposing/precipitating factors
   a. aging process
   b. cigarette smoking from toxins in smoke
   c. exposure to industrial dyes, particularly aniline dyes
4. Signs and symptoms
   a. painless hematuria that may come and go in early stages
   b. urinary frequency from diminished bladder capacity due to space-occupying tumor
   c. dysuria
   d. urgency
   e. in later stages gross hematuria may occur
   f. signs and symptoms of metastasis, such as weight loss and pain, depending on area of metastasis
   g. anemia
5. Diagnostic tests
   a. history and physical examination
   b. urinalysis
   c. urine culture and sensitivity
   d. CBC
   e. CT scan
   f. KUB radiograph
   g. IVP
   h. cystometrography: a sterile catheter is placed in the patient, then volumes and pressures are recorded systematically: PN responsibilities
      (1) teach patient about test
      (2) monitor for hematuria

      (3) monitor for signs of infection
      (4) catheter care if indwelling catheter in place
   i. cystoscopy with or without biopsy: PN responsibilities
      (1) teach patient about test
      (2) patient and significant support during diagnostic phase
      (3) cathartics and enemas night before per physician's order
      (4) NPO after midnight
      (5) monitor for hematuria, infection
      (6) symptomatic treatment of bladder spasms, such as warm baths if permitted
6. Complications
   a. obstruction of flow of urine
   b. hemorrhage
   c. anemia
   d. atonic bladder
   e. metastasis to other parts of urinary tract
   f. metastasis to other parts of body
7. Usual treatment
   a. in premalignant stage, electrocauterization of tumor via cystoscope
   b. segmental resection (partial resection) of bladder, particularly near trigone region of bladder or near sections where ureters enter bladder
   c. radical cystectomy: total removal of bladder and pelvic lymph nodes, resulting in impotence in males, combined with urinary diversion
   d. urinary diversion (Fig. 7-11): surgical rerouting of urinary output; types include:
      (1) ileal conduit: surgical resection of ileal segment of intestine, with blood supply and nerve endings left intact; proximal end sutured into pouch, and ureters sutured into ileal segment while distal end brought to outside of abdominal wall in right lower quadrant stoma; urine from kidneys drains down ureters into surgical pouch and spills out of stoma into collection pouch
      (2) ureterosigmoidoscopy: surgical implantation of ureters into sigmoid colon; urine drains right into sigmoid, liquefying stool and often producing incontinence; common danger is contamination, by *Escherichia coli*, of kidneys via ureters; rarely done now
      (3) cutaneous ureterostomy: surgical procedure in which one or both ureters brought to surface of abdominal wall in stoma; urine drains from kidney, down ureters and out stoma to drainage pouch; complications include infection and scar tissue that causes constriction of surgical opening; flow of urine onto skin can cause chemical burn; usually palliative procedure

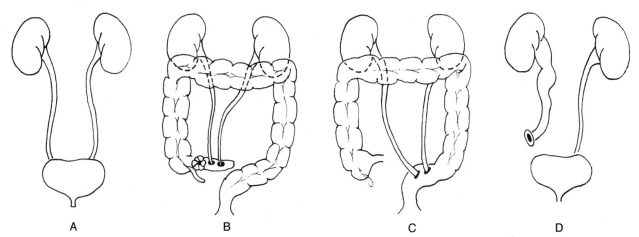

FIGURE 7–11. Urinary diversion. *A*, Normal urinary system. *B*, Ileal conduit. *C*, Ureterosigmoidostomy. *D*, Cutaneous ureterostomy.

B. Planning, Goals/ Expected Outcomes

1. Patient will identify and alleviate risk factors
2. Patient will understand the need for surgical procedure
3. Patient will have an uncomplicated surgical procedure and recovery
4. Patient will maintain skin integrity
5. Patient will maintain adequate intake and output
6. Patient will learn to care for own appliances
7. Patient will adjust to altered body image and impotence (males)

C. Implementation

1. Assist patient to stop smoking and avoid industrial dyes that can be toxic to bladder
2. Assist patient to understand need to treat irritating or obstructing conditions of bladder and other parts of urinary system
3. Assist patient to understand surgical procedure, including altered body image after surgery
4. Preoperative period
   a. teach patient to cough and deep breathe
   b. monitor intake and output
   c. monitor for hematuria, vital signs
   d. assist with diagnostic procedures
   e. provide emotional support for patient and significant others, especially sexual counseling for males
   f. administer cathartic, enemas night before surgery as ordered
   g. administer preoperative medications as ordered
5. Postoperative period
   a. monitor vital functions, especially intake and output

   b. monitor for bleeding, infection
   c. scrupulous skin care around stoma or rectal area, depending on procedure
   d. monitor intravenous hydration
   e. change disposable drainage pouches as needed; prevent fluid build-up
   f. ambulate early
   g. sterile technique for dressing change
   h. drainage pouches around stoma need to fit snugly to prevent urine drainage onto skin; change pouches immediately, preventing leakage onto skin
   i. monitor for bleeding, infection, scarring of the stoma
   j. change drainage pouch opening size appropriately as stoma shrinks
   k. monitor intake and output; do not give enemas or rectal suppositories with ureterosigmoidoscopy
   l. assist RN in teaching patient and significant others to care for appliances
   m. provide emotional support to patient and significant others
   n. if acceptable to physician and patient, have person with urostomy visit patient; make contact with ACS Ostomy Association

D. Evaluation

1. Patient eliminated risk factors
2. Patient complied with treatment
3. Patient recovered from surgery without complication
4. Patient's skin and mucous membrane intact
5. Patient able to care for self
6. Patient adjusted psychologically to altered body image

Questions

Mr. Andrews is admitted to your unit with a diagnosis of acute gastroenteritis. He has had nausea, vomiting, and diarrhea for the last 48 hours. You are the LPN caring for him.

1. One of the most important areas to assess Mr. Andrews for initially is:

   ① His knowledge of the hospital environment
   ② Fluid and electrolyte balance
   ③ Presence of a viral infection
   ④ His ability to withstand the stress of hospitalization

2. A priority of your ongoing assessment of Mr. Andrews would be:

   ① Vital signs
   ② Respiratory rate and breath sounds
   ③ Level of consciousness
   ④ Character and frequency of all stools

3. Besides the above assessment, another important area to assess would be:

   ① Total intake and output from all sources
   ② His ability to sleep through the night
   ③ The amount of IV fluid he receives each 24 hours
   ④ His former eating and elimination habits

4. Your goal for Mr. Andrews is to have him return to a normal elimination pattern. Which of the following would best reflect this goal in a measurable manner?

   ① The patient will have less frequent stools
   ② Diarrhea will be controlled and not recur
   ③ The patient will have no more than one stool per day
   ④ The patient will return to his normal bowel pattern

5. In order to achieve the above goal once the nausea has resolved, an appropriate intervention would be to:

   ① Allow food and fluids as desired
   ② Limit all fluids until diarrhea disappears
   ③ Administer liberal fluids and a bland diet
   ④ Give unlimited quantities of milk and fruit juice

6. You discover that Mr. Andrews has been admitted three times before for the same problem. An important assessment for the LPN to make would be:

   ① His usual bowel habits
   ② If anyone else in his family has the same symptoms
   ③ His usual eating pattern
   ④ Whether or not his wife does the cooking

7. The most common early sign of bladder cancer is:

   ① Painless hematuria
   ② Frequent urinary tract infections
   ③ Frequency and urgency without infection
   ④ Incontinence

Sara Miles is an obese 40-year-old mother of three who is admitted with a history of chronic cholecystitis.

8. She is ordered to receive vitamin K preoperatively. The reason for this drug is to improve:

   ① Digestion of fats
   ② Healing of tissues
   ③ Elimination of bile
   ④ Clotting of blood

9. Postoperatively, the best position for a cholecystectomy patient is:

   ① Side lying to prevent aspiration
   ② Semi-Fowler's to facilitate breathing
   ③ Supine to decrease strain on the incision line
   ④ On her abdomen to reduce nausea

10. Mrs. Miles has a T-tube in place after surgery. The purpose of the T-tube is to:

    ① Remove leaking bile from the incision
    ② Provide a means of irrigating the wound
    ③ Provide for drainage of bile from the common bile duct
    ④ Prevent rupture of the inflamed gallbladder

11. She was exhibiting some signs of a jaundice preoperatively. Common signs of jaundice include:

    ① Ascites
    ② Pruritus
    ③ Icteric sclera
    ④ Dark-colored stools

12. Prior to a paracentesis the patient must:

   ① Void to empty the bladder
   ② Receive cleansing enemas
   ③ Receive sedation
   ④ Be NPO for 8 hours

13. Diabetes mellitus is a deficiency condition with impaired ability to use:

   ① Fats
   ② Glucose
   ③ Protein
   ④ Minerals

14. Risk factors for cystitis include all of the following *except*:

   ① Being female
   ② Emptying the bladder every 8 hours
   ③ Drinking 2000 mL of fluid daily
   ④ Pregnancy

15. In teaching your female client to avoid recurrence of her chronic urinary tract infections, the most helpful instruction would be to:

   ① Decrease her sexual activity for a while
   ② Wipe carefully from front to back after voiding
   ③ Restrict her intake of fluids in the evening
   ④ Take all of the medication that is prescribed

Ellen Marks is a 42-year-old law student who has been complaining of fatigue, weight loss, thirst, and excessive urination. She is admitted by her doctor to be worked up for possible diabetes mellitus.

16. One of the first tests that the doctor orders is a glucose tolerance test. Preparation for this requires the patient to:

   ① Fast for 24 hours prior to the test
   ② Have no foods for 12 hours before the test
   ③ Take in approximately 100 G of glucose 2 hours before the test
   ④ No carbohydrates for 24 hours prior to the test

17. Miss Marks is diagnosed as having Type II diabetes mellitus. Diabetes is best defined as:

   ① An absence of insulin in the system
   ② Failure of the body to metabolize carbohydrates successfully
   ③ A complex condition related to the control of carbohydrate metabolism
   ④ A disease affecting the pancreas causing a lack of insulin

18. It is decided to control Ellen's condition with diet, exercise, and medication. The diabetic diet can be described as one that:

   ① Provides a well-balanced meal using an exchange list
   ② Severely limits carbohydrates but allows fats and protein
   ③ Limits the intake of carbohydrates slightly
   ④ Helps the patient lose the excess weight

19. Diabetics are much more prone to cardiovascular disease than the normal population. The most likely reason for this is:

   ① Diabetics have difficulty metabolizing fats and proteins, with the end-products of these accumulating in the vessels
   ② Diabetics are usually overweight, increasing the workload on the heart and blood vessels
   ③ Most diabetics are elderly persons who are more likely to have degenerative cardiovascular disease
   ④ Atherosclerotic changes occur in the blood vessels because of the high levels of glucose and fat with poor control

20. An exercise regimen would be helpful for Ellen because it would:

   ① Increase the rate of insulin secretion
   ② Lower the blood sugar by oxidizing carbohydrates
   ③ Prevent obesity
   ④ Help the insulin circulate in the body

21. It is important to teach Ellen proper foot care and methods of maintaining and improving circulation to the lower extremities because she:

   ① Is more prone to gangrene if she develops an infection of her foot
   ② Has no resistance to infection and can develop septicemia
   ③ Is a student and will therefore not take the time needed to do foot care
   ④ Has a lowered resistance to infection and increased bleeding tendencies

22. Prior to an upper intestinal tract radiograph, the nurse should:

   ① Administer a strong laxative
   ② Administer enemas until clear
   ③ Withhold food and fluids for 8 hours
   ④ Give a high fat dinner

23. A tubeless gastric analysis requires that the nurse:

① Obtain a urine specimen for testing
② Withhold food and fluids for 24 hours
③ Insert a nasogastric tube
④ Allow the patient to eat normally

Mary Weeks is a 34 year old who has been diagnosed with ulcerative colitis for about 5 years. She is admitted with severe diarrhea and fatigue.

24. Ulcerative colitis is best described as:

① Chronic constipation and spastic colon
② Chronic diarrhea due to improper diet
③ Inflammation and ulceration of the lining of the colon
④ Irritation of the small intestine

25. The cause of ulcerative colitis is unknown, but which of the following is thought to be a risk factor?

① Excessive bulk in the diet
② Stress and emotional tension
③ Overuse of laxatives
④ Excessive use of enemas

26. The chronic fatigue that Mary is experiencing is probably due to:

① Her lack of interest in activities outside her home
② Lack of appetite related to diarrhea
③ Failure to follow the prescribed diet
④ Anemia and malnutrition due to malabsorption and bleeding

27. The diet most usually recommended for people with ulcerative colitis is:

① High bulk and residue
② High protein, high vitamin
③ Bland, high carbohydrate
④ Low in fluids to decrease diarrhea

28. Mary is scheduled for an ileostomy. This is done to:

① Prevent possible perforation from the colitis
② Decrease the liquid feces
③ Control the odor from the diarrhea
④ Prevent intestinal obstruction

29. Which of the following would *not* be included in the preparation for surgery?

① Administration of antibiotics to cleanse the bowel
② Enemas until clear
③ Psychologic preparation concerning the stoma
④ Fluids and electrolytes to restore balance

30. Teaching that must be included in the discharge preparation of Mary would include:

① Information on stoma irrigation
② The need for sexual counseling
③ Care of the skin around the stoma
④ The need to restrict fluids

31. Mary must know the symptoms that would require her to notify the doctor. One of the most important signs of complication would be:

① Diarrhea or liquid stools for 3 days
② Daily stoma output more than 1500 mL/day for several days
③ Intolerance to high residue foods
④ A decrease in the size of her stoma

Elisa Mobile, age 32 years, has a history of ulcerative colitis for the past 5 years. She has been in her present job for 7 years and is described by her co-workers as a "go-getter."

32. Which of the following systems is involved for the client who is experiencing psychophysiologic distress?

① Autonomic nervous system
② Peripheral nervous system
③ Parasympathetic nervous system
④ Sympathetic nervous system

33. Which of the following is an appropriate opening greeting to a client experiencing psychophysiologic problems?

① "Good morning! You are looking terrific today!"
② "You mentioned pain yesterday. I'm wondering if it is there today?"
③ "You don't look like you feel good. Why don't you tell me about it?"
④ "Let me give you a hand with that. Then, we'll look at today's agenda."

34. Your patient is suffering from a deficiency of parathormone. The nurse knows to monitor the patient closely for:

① Muscular weakness
② An increase in the blood sugar
③ Muscle twitching and spasms of the voluntary muscles
④ Renal calculi

35. The above condition is caused because parathormone regulates:

① Acid–base balance
② Potassium secretion
③ Thyroid metabolism
④ Calcium metabolism

36. Cushing's syndrome is often associated with:

① Steroid therapy
② Adrenal atrophy
③ Hyperthyroidism
④ Decreased adrenocorticotropic hormone (ACTH) secretion

37. Nursing care for a patient with Cushing's syndrome would include:

① Giving a high carbohydrate, low protein diet
② Teaching the patient the signs of hypoglycemia
③ Helping the patient learn to avoid infections
④ Maintaining the patient on complete bedrest

Mrs. Baker is a 50-year-old mother of two admitted with a diagnosis of chronic glomerulonephritis and impending renal failure.

38. Upon admission, the doctor orders a blood urea nitrogen (BUN) to be done. This is done to measure the:

① Concentration of urine
② Amount of nitrogenous waste products accumulating in the urine
③ Waste products left in the blood as a result of renal failure
④ Amount of bacteria in the blood

39. Mrs. Baker begins to experience some muscle twitching. The nurse should be alert for:

① Other neurologic changes
② The need to increase her fluid intake
③ The presence of circulatory changes
④ An increase in her need for calcium

40. Treatment of chronic renal failure is aimed at:

① Increasing the urine output
② Preventing the loss of electrolytes
③ Increasing the concentration of electrolytes in the urine
④ Reducing the workload on the kidneys

41. Mrs. Baker is deteriorating and has begun to exhibit signs of renal failure and uremia. In order to help decrease the discomfort from the uremic frost on her skin, the nurse should:

① Provide cool alcohol baths and lotion
② Wash with diluted vinegar and apply lanolin lotion
③ Apply calamine or steroid cream
④ Wash with soap and apply mineral oil

Mr. Lane is admitted with a diagnosis of possible cancer of the colon.

42. The diagnostic test most helpful in diagnosing cancer of the colon would be a:

① Barium enema
② Stool for guaiac
③ Complete blood count
④ Colonoscopy and biopsy

43. A symptom that Mr. Lane may have noticed that led him to suspect colon cancer would be:

① Rectal bleeding and pain
② A change in the bowel habits
③ Persistent nausea and vomiting
④ Clay-colored stools

44. Mr. Lane is scheduled for a colon resection and a colostomy. Which of the following would be inappropriate in teaching Mr. Lane about his postsurgical care?

① Sexual counseling about inevitable impotence
② Care of the stoma
③ Irrigation and regulation of the bowel
④ Potential changes in his body image

45. In teaching Mr. Lane to irrigate his colostomy, the nurse should instruct him to:

① Use at least 1500 mL of warm tap water
② Stop irrigation and call the doctor if cramping occurs
③ Never irrigate if diarrhea is present
④ Irrigate at least twice a day, morning and night

46. After a hemorrhoidectomy, which of the following is most effective for the postoperative pain?

① Tylenol #3
✓② A sitz bath
③ Laxatives
④ Stool softeners

Mrs. Mayer is a 50-year-old Type I diabetic on insulin. She has been a diabetic for a number of years and is well controlled on insulin.

47. Recently Mrs. Mayer has been having marital difficulties that leave her emotionally upset. As a result of this stress, it is possible that she will exhibit:

① An insulin reaction more readily than usual
✓② An increase in her blood sugar
③ A need for less daily insulin
④ A need for more carbohydrates

48. The stress mentioned in the previous question leads to the increased production of glucocorticoids, which would tend to:

① Decrease the production of fatty acids and lower the blood sugar
② Increase the secretion of insulin and lower the blood sugar
✓③ Counteract the effects of insulin and raise the blood sugar
④ Increase the production of fatty acids and raise the blood sugar

49. Mrs. Mayer is receiving 40 U regular insulin at 7:30 AM daily. On the basis of this, you know that the most likely time for her to experience an insulin reaction is:

① By 8 AM
② At 4 PM
③ During the night
✓④ Around 11 AM

50. Mrs. Mayer received NPH insulin at 7:30 AM, the most likely time for the reaction to occur would be:

① By 8 AM
② At 4 PM
③ During the night
④ Around 11 AM

51. A characteristic symptom of insulin shock that should alert the nurse to an early insulin reaction would be:

① Diaphoresis
② Drowsiness
③ Severe thirst
④ Coma

Andy Jones, age 50 years, is admitted to the surgical floor with a history of gastric ulcers for several years. Recently he has begun having periods of severe nausea after eating and emesis of undigested food and bright red blood.

52. The doctor has scheduled him for a series of diagnostic tests, including radiographs. You know that these studies are:

① Usually not done preoperatively
② Ordered only if the doctor is not familiar with the patient and his history
③ Done preoperatively to confirm a diagnosis
④ Not useful in diagnosing gastric ulcers

53. Mr. Jones is scheduled for surgery 2 days later. In preparing him for a gastric resection, which of the following would *not* be appropriate to teach him?

① That a nasogastric tube will be in place several days after surgery
② To cough and deep breathe 10 times an hour after surgery
③ To exercise his leg hourly after surgery
✓④ That a Foley catheter will be in place for 1 week after surgery

54. On the night prior to surgery, Mr. Jones wants a "midnight snack," stating that he always has one when he is nervous. Your best response would be to tell him that:

① The kitchen has already closed for the night
② Food or fluids after midnight can lead to aspiration during surgery
③ Food or fluids will increase the risk of vomiting after surgery
④ Food or fluids will cause improper absorption of the anesthesia during surgery

55. Mr. Jones does not want to remove his wedding band prior to surgery. Your best action in this case would be to:

   ① Wrap tape around it once to secure it to his finger
   ② Tell him the surgery cannot be done if he does not remove it
   ③ Place a note on the chart stating that he refused to remove it
   ④ Remind the patient that the hospital will not be liable for any loss if he insists

56. The anesthesiologist has requested that Mr. Jones' dentures be left in when he is sent to surgery. The most likely reason for this request is that:

   ① Mr. Jones has requested it because he is vain
   ② Dentures do not have to be removed routinely for general anesthesia
   ✓③ Some forms of anesthesia are administered more easily if the dentures are left in place
   ④ There is less danger that the dentures will be misplaced if they are not removed during hospitalization

57. While the patient is under general anesthesia, there is loss of voluntary control of the sphincter muscles. For this reason, the nurse should:

   ① Insert a urinary catheter before the patient goes to surgery
   ② Withhold all fluids for 12 to 24 hours to decrease the amount of urine output
   ③ Awaken the patient frequently the night before surgery to empty his bladder
   ④ Have the patient void immediately before he leaves for surgery

58. Mr. Jones is complaining of nausea in the recovery room after his gastric resection. Your best priority action is to:

   ① Irrigate his nasogastric tube
   ✓② Notify the physician
   ③ Put him in semi-Fowler's so he will not aspirate
   ④ Medicate him with a narcotic analgesic

59. Mr. Jones, though awake and alert, complains that he is feeling cold when he returns to his room. The nurse should:

   ① Apply a heating pad to his back for warmth
   ② Recognize that this is a symptom of shock and notify the doctor
   ③ Realize that Mr. Jones is bleeding internally and call the doctor
   ④ Apply several blankets to maintain his body temperature at a normal level

60. On the first postoperative day, it is very important that Mr. Jones be out of bed and ambulate to a chair. The nurse knows that this is done to prevent the early postoperative complication of:

   ✓① Atelectasis
   ② Thrombophlebitis
   ③ Nausea and vomiting
   ④ Constipation

61. On the third postoperative day, Mr. Jones' nasogastric tube is draining bile-colored liquid containing coffee ground material. Your most appropriate action would be to:

   ✓① Continue simply to monitor the amount of drainage
   ② Irrigate the nasogastric tube with iced saline
   ③ Call the physician
   ④ Chart the information and ask the RN to irrigate the tube

62. When Mr. Jones is discharged, he will probably be placed on medication to prevent the recurrence of his ulcer. The most likely medication the doctor will order is:

   ① Tagamet
   ② Librium
   ③ Donnatal
   ④ Milk of magnesia

63. Because Mr. Jones had a gastric resection and a partial gastrectomy, several potential problems other than recurrence exist. If he developed symptoms of nausea, diaphoresis, and diarrhea about one-half hour after eating, the most likely cause would be:

   ① Pernicious anemia
   ② Pyloric obstruction
   ✓③ Dumping syndrome
   ④ Hyperemesis

64. The best treatment for the previous problem would be:

   ①   Weekly vitamin B_{12} injections

   ②   High carbohydrate, small meals

   ③   Dry meals with liquids between meals

   ④   Antiemetics before meals

Answers & Rationales

Guide to item identification (see pp. 3–5 for further details about each category)

I, II, III, or IV for the phase of the nursing process
1, 2, 3, or 4 for the category of client needs
A, B, C, D, E, F, or G for the category of human functioning
Specific content category by name; ie, cholecystectomy

1. ② Because of the prolonged nausea and vomiting, the most important area to assess is the fluid and electrolyte balance. This is the most potentially life-threatening area.
I, 2, F. GI.

2. ④ Because his presenting symptom is diarrhea, the number and consistency of stools are the most important factors to assess for this patient.
I, 2, F. GI.

3. ① With nausea, vomiting and diarrhea, fluid imbalance is one of the next most important assessments.
I, 2, F. GI.

4. ④ Goal setting is an important part of patient care planning. Goals should be specific and measurable and relate directly to the individual patient.
II, 2, F. GI.

5. ③ A bland diet will help prevent further nausea, and the fluids are needed to replace those lost.
III, 2, F. GI.

6. ② Because this is a recurrent problem, it would be helpful to know if anyone else in the family also had the problem. This could help to determine if something in the environment is contributing to the problem.
I, 2 & 4, F. GI.

7. ① The only early symptom of bladder cancer is painless blood in the urine.
I, 2, F. Bladder Cancer.

8. ④ Vitamin K increases blood clotting. Cholecystitis can decrease the absorption of vitamin K.
I, 2, F. Cholecystitis & Medications.

9. ② Semi-Fowler's increases lung expansion after a cholecystectomy.
III, 2, F & B. Cholecystectomy.

10. ③ A T-tube is used after a common bile duct exploration to maintain patency of the duct until healing can occur.
IV, 2, F. Cholecystectomy.

11. ③ Jaundice can occur if the common bile duct is obstructed with stones. Yellowish coloring around the eyes is a common symptom of jaundice.
I, 2, F. Cholecystitis.

12. ① The bladder can be punctured during a paracentesis if it is distended.
III, 2, F. Ascites.

13. ② Insulin is necessary for the utilization of glucose.
III, 2, F. Nutrition/Diabetes.

14. ③ Increased fluid intake helps to prevent, not cause, cystitis. All of the others are risk factors.
I, 2, C. Cystitis.

15. ② A common cause of urinary tract infections in women is contamination from the large intestine. Careful wiping can help to control this contamination.
III, 1, F. Cystitis.

16. ② The patient must be NPO for 12 hours, is then given a high carbohydrate source and tested for glucose in the blood and urine.
III, 1, F. Diabetes.

17. ③ Diabetes is a complex condition affecting carbohydrate metabolism.
I, 2, F. Diabetes.

18. ① The diabetic diet is a well-balanced diet with controlled amounts of food in the various exchange categories.
II, 2, F. Diabetes.

19. ④ With poor control of diabetes, levels of fat and glucose are high and cause atherosclerosis.
IV, 2, F. Diabetes.

20. ② Exercise acts to increase oxidation of carbohydrates without increases in insulin.
III, 2, F. Diabetes.

21. Diabetics have a decrease in the microcirculation, especially that of the lower extremities. If they suffer an injury, it is more likely to become gangrenous.
① III, 4, F. Diabetes.

22. For an upper GI study, food and fluid are withheld for 8 to 12 hours prior to the test so the stomach and small intestine are empty.
③ III, 1, F. Upper GI.

23. A tubeless test requires the urine to be tested for the presence of a dye, Diagnex blue, indicating the absence of hydrochloric acid in the stomach.
① III, 1, F. Peptic Ulcer.

24. Ulcerative colitis is characterized by inflammation and ulceration of the colon.
③ I, 2, F. Ulcerative Colitis.

25. Stress and emotional factors are thought to be a predisposing factor in ulcerative colitis.
② I, 2, F. Ulcerative Colitis.

26. Anemia and malabsorption leading to malnutrition are common problems in ulcerative colitis, both of which predispose to fatigue.
④ IV, 2, F. Ulcerative Colitis.

27. High protein levels are needed for healing and high vitamin levels for combatting the malabsorption. The diet is also usually high calorie, high potassium and low residue.
② III, 2, F. Ulcerative Colitis.

28. Colitis can eventually lead to perforation of the colon. In order to prevent it, if conservative medical therapy has failed, an ileostomy is done and the entire colon is removed.
① IV, 2, F. Ulcerative Colitis.

29. Enemas in a patient with ulcerative colitis can lead to megacolon or perforation. The bowel preparation for this patient usually is a single, gentle enema.
② III, 1, F. Ulcerative Colitis.

30. Care of the skin around the stoma is the most important aspect of care, because skin excoriation is a real risk and will lead to breakdown and further problems.
③ III, 1, F. Ulcerative Colitis.

31. The patient's stools always have a liquid consistency. The only way to determine diarrhea is the amount of drainage. The usual amount of drainage is 1200 mL per day.
② III, 1 & 2, F. Ulcerative Colitis.

32. "His (Franz Alexander) investigations revealed that (1) emotional states are accompanied by internal physiological processes of an adaptive nature; (2) these physiological processes are generally under the control of the autonomic nervous system. . . ." (Irving, 1983: 318)
① IV, 2, F and G. Ulcerative Colitis.

33. "The goal is to help the patient move in the direction of a state of interdependence rather than either extreme of dependence or independence." (Irving, 1983: 330)
④ III, 2, G. Ulcerative Colitis.

34. Parathormone controls calcium metabolism, and a decrease leads to hypocalcemia, which can cause muscle tetany.
③ III, 2, F. Endocrine Disorders.

35. Parathormone controls calcium metabolism.
④ I, 2, F. Endocrine Disorders.

36. Patients receiving steroids can develop Cushing's syndrome from the excessive amounts of cortisone.
① I & IV, 2, F. Cushing's Syndrome.

37. Steroids are immune suppressants, and the patient is more prone to infections.
③ III, 2, F. Cushing's Syndrome.

38. Normally the urea nitrogen is filtered out through the kidneys. With renal failure, it accumulates in the blood.
③ I, 2, F. Glomerulonephritis.

39. As the toxic waste products build up in the blood, central nervous system (CNS) changes can begin to occur. The nurse should monitor closely for neurologic changes.
① I, 2, C & F. Glomerulonephritis.

40. The goal in chronic renal failure is to prevent acute failure and maintain whatever function is left. This is best done by minimizing stress and workload on the kidneys.
④ IV, 2, F. Glomerulonephritis.

41. Diluted vinegar helps to neutralize the urea, and the lanolin softens the skin.
② III, 2, B, D, & F. Glomerulonephritis.

42. ④ The colonoscopy to visualize the lesion and a biopsy of that lesion are the only accurate diagnostic tests for colon cancer.
I, 2, F. Colon Cancer.

43. ② A change in bowel habits is one of the major early symptoms of colon cancer.
IV, 2, F. Colon Cancer.

44. ① Impotence does not occur after an abdominal–perineal resection and a sigmoid colostomy.
III, 2 & 4, F & G. Colon Cancer.

45. ③ The patient should never irrigate and cause further irritation when diarrhea is present.
III, 2 & 4, F. Colon Cancer.

46. ② A sitz bath is the most helpful for the pain of a hemorrhoidectomy.
III, 2, F. Hemorrhoidectomy.

47. ② Stress causes the adrenals to secrete more cortisol, leading to gluconeogenesis and insulin antagonism and raising the blood sugar.
IV, 2, F. Diabetes.

48. ③ Glucocorticoids are also insulin antagonists.
IV, 2, F. Diabetes.

49. ④ The peak of regular insulin is about 4 hours.
I, 2, F. Diabetes.

50. ② The peak for NPH is about 8 hours, and her blood sugar would also be low prior to dinner.
I, 2, F. Diabetes.

51. ① Diaphoresis and a shaky feeling are early signs of hypoglycemia.
I, 2, F. Diabetes.

52. ③ Radiographs are a common tool used by the doctor to confirm a diagnosis before the patient goes to surgery.
IV, 1, F. Gastric Ulcers.

53. ④ A Foley catheter is not a routine part of gastric surgery. Even if one is inserted in surgery to monitor output, it would not be left in for a week. The others are routine with this type of surgery.
III, 4, F. Gastric Surgery.

54. ② A patient receiving general anesthesia must be NPO for 8 to 12 hours to prevent vomiting and aspiration during surgery.
III, 1, F. Gastrectomy.

55. ① Dislodgement during surgery is the risk. If a patient absolutely refuses to remove a band, it must be safely and securely held in place.
III, 1, F. Gastrectomy.

56. ③ It is easier and safer to administer the anesthesia with certain types of dentures in place.
IV, 1, D & F. Gastrectomy.

57. ④ In order to decrease the risk of accidental voiding, have the patient void immediately before the preoperative medication is given.
III, 1, D & F. Gastrectomy.

58. ② The nasogastric tube should never be irrigated by the nurse following a gastric resection, only by the doctor. The only proper action is to notify the doctor that the tube probably needs irrigation.
III, 2, F & D. Gastrectomy.

59. ④ Chilling is normal after surgery because the temperature of the operating rooms is cool. Simply apply blankets to maintain the patient's body temperature.
III, 2, D. Gastrectomy.

60. ① Atelectasis is the most common early postoperative problem in patients with high abdominal incisions and general anesthesia. In order to facilitate lung expansion, the patient needs to be moved and gotten out of bed.
II, 2, D & F. Gastrectomy.

61. ① Coffee ground material is old blood. This is perfectly normal on the third postoperative day.
III, 2, F. Gastrectomy.

62. ① Tagamet blocks the release of gastric acid, thereby preventing the recurrence of ulcers.
II, 2, F. Gastrectomy.

63. ③ Dumping syndrome is a physiologic problem associated with too rapid movement of food through the remaining stomach. When this undigested hypertonic mass reaches the intestine, fluids are drawn to dilute it, resulting in hypotension.
I, 2, D & F. Postgastrectomy/Dumping Syndrome.

64. ③ Eating only dry, small meals, lying down after meals and low carbohydrate intake all helps decrease the symptoms of dumping syndrome.
III, 2, D & F. Postgastrectomy/Dumping Syndrome.

BIBLIOGRAPHY

GENERAL

Brill, E. & Kilts, D. (1986). *Foundations of Nursing, 2nd ed.* Appleton-Century-Crofts, East Norwalk, Connecticut.

Curren, A. (1983). *Clinical Nursing Skills.* Wallcur, San Diego.

Miller, B. & Keane, C. (1986). *Encyclopedia and Dictionary of Medicine, Nursing and Allied Health.* W.B. Saunders Co., Philadelphia.

Wolff-Lewis, L. (1984). *Fundamental Skills in Patient Care, 3rd ed.* J.B. Lippincott Co., Philadelphia.

REPRODUCTIVE DISORDERS IN WOMEN AND MEN

Keane, C.B. (1986). *Essentials of Medical-Surgical Nursing.* W.B. Saunders Co., Philadelphia.

The Nurses' Reference Library: Diseases. (1990). Nursing 90 Books. Intermed Communications, Springhouse, Pennsylvania.

The Nurses' Reference Library: Drugs. (1990). Nursing 90 Books. Intermed Communications, Springhouse, Pennsylvania.

CENTRAL NERVOUS SYSTEM DISORDERS

Keane, C.B. (1986). *Essentials of Medical-Surgical Nursing.* W.B. Saunders Co., Philadelphia.

The Nurses' Reference Library: Diseases. (1990). Nursing 90 Books, Intermed Communications, Springhouse, Pennsylvania.

The Nurses' Reference Library: Drugs. (1990). Nursing 90 Books. Intermed Communications, Springhouse, Pennsylvania.

AUDITORY/VISUAL DISORDERS

Hole, J. (1981). *Human Anatomy and Physiology, 2nd ed.* Wm. Brown Co., Dubuque, Iowa.

Milliken, M. & Campbell, G. (1985). *Essential Competencies for Patient Care.* C.V. Mosby Co., Princeton, New Jersey.

Scherer, J. (1986). *Introductory Medical-Surgical Nursing, 4th ed.* J.B. Lippincott Co., Philadelphia.

FLUID AND ELECTROLYTE IMBALANCES

Hole, J. (1981). *Human Anatomy and Physiology, 2nd ed.* Wm. Brown Co., Dubuque, Iowa.

Milliken, M. & Campbell, G. (1985). *Essential Competencies for Patient Care.* C.V. Mosby Co., Princeton, New Jersey.

Scherer, J. (1986). *Introductory Medical-Surgical Nursing, 4th ed.* J.B. Lippincott Co., Philadelphia.

CANCER

Keane, C.B. (1992). *Essentials of Medical-Surgical Nursing.* W.B. Saunders Co., Philadelphia.

The Nurses' Reference Library: Diseases. (1990). Nursing 90 Books. Intermed Communications, Springhouse, Pennsylvania.

The Nurses' Reference Library: Drugs. (1990). Nursing 90 Books. Intermed Communications, Springhouse, Pennsylvania

RENAL AND UROLOGIC DISORDERS

Nursing 84 Books. (1984). Springhouse Corporation, Springhouse, Pennsylvania.

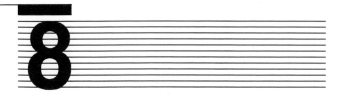

The Pediatric Patient

GROWTH AND DEVELOPMENT

■ Life Stages

I. THE INFANT (1 MONTH–1 YEAR)

A. Normal Physical Development

1. Appearance
   a. lifts head when prone by first month
   b. gains 2/3 oz/day for first 5 months, 1/2 oz/day for next 7; birth weight doubles by 5 to 6 months and triples by 1 year
   c. head size is 15.75 inches (38 cm) at 12 weeks, 16.5 inches (41 cm) at 20 weeks, 17 inches (42 cm) at 30 weeks, and 2/3 adult size by 1 year
   d. baby grows 1 foot first year
2. Nervous system
   a. under 4 months, objects are not followed out of line of vision
   b. by 7 to 8 weeks, eyes coordinated
   c. by 12 weeks, attends to and prefers novel stimuli
   d. full depth perception by 9 months
   e. touch important to help develop body image
3. Vital signs: by 1 year, pulse is 100–110; blood pressure, 96/66; respirations, 20–40; temperature, 99.7°F
4. Respiratory system
   a. increased susceptibility to infection, respiratory problems
   b. new alveoli developing up to 6 years of age
5. Gastrointestinal system
   a. matures to a degree after 2 to 3 months
   b. stomach emptying time slows
   c. teeth erupt at about 6 months
   d. peristalsis is more adult-like at about 8 months
6. Skin
   a. more prone to skin disorders
   b. sebaceous and sweat glands hypoactive
   c. ineffective for thermal regulation
7. Renal system
   a. reaches adult proportions in size by 5 months
   b. mature functional level at 1 year
   c. cannot handle excessive protein of cow's milk too early

8. Hemopoietic system
   a. inflammatory response immature
   b. ability to produce antibodies limited
   c. hemoglobin drops after 2 to 3 months, then gradually increases
   d. white blood cells (WBC) reach adult level by 1 year

B. Nutritional Needs

1. Breast milk all needed first 6 months
2. Solid foods added at varying times after 3 months
3. Iron stores may be low after 6 months
4. Self-feeding starts about 6 months
5. Food allergies common, so add foods one at a time

C. Sleep

1. By 6 weeks, infant has a nocturnal sleep pattern
2. By 7 to 8 months, infant sleeps through night without waking
3. By 1 year, infant sleeps 12 to 14 hours/night and 1 to 4 hours/day

D. Play

1. Solitary, with body parts
2. Touch, sight, and sound very important
3. Way of learning about self and environment and way of developing motor skills

E. Psychosocial Development

1. Erikson's stage of trust vs. mistrust
   a. feelings of comfort, safety, and security
   b. sense of trust in primary care giver
2. Piaget's stages of cognitive development
   a. neonate in reflex stage
   b. at 1 to 4 months, primary circular reactions
      (1) follows objects with eyes and follows sounds

(2) response to objects varies
(3) recognizes faces
  c. at 4 to 8 months, secondary circular reactions
    (1) beginning object permanence
    (2) imitates others
    (3) more oriented to environment
    (4) memory traces being developed
  d. at 8 to 12 months, coordination of secondary schemata
    (1) actions show intelligence and experimentation
    (2) increased sense of separateness
    (3) finds hidden objects
    (4) can attain small goals

F. Speech

1. Neonate cry undifferentiated
2. Cry differentiates at about 2 to 3 months
3. By 9 months, all universal sounds can be made
4. By 1 year, several words are spoken

G. Social Development

1. At 1 month, early recognition of faces
2. At 2 months, smiles in response to specific stimuli
3. At 4 months, recognizes primary care giver
4. At 7 to 8 months, shy with strangers
5. At 9 to 10 months, experiences separation anxiety

II. THE TODDLER (1–3 YEARS) (TABLES 8-1 AND 8-2)

A. Normal Physical Development

1. Appearance
   a. slower growth rate, but still cephalocaudal, proximal–distal, and general to specific
   b. all teeth in by 2 1/2 to 3 years
   c. chest circumference surpasses head
   d. birth weight quadrupled at 2 years
   e. approximately half of adult height by 2 years
   f. gross motor coordination improves, but still clumsy with fine motor coordination
   g. at 2 to 3 years, can pedal tricycle
2. Elimination
   a. toilet training at 2 to 3 years
   b. renal system functions normally
3. Other systems reach adult functions by 3 years

B. Nutritional Needs

1. 1000 cal daily by 1 year; 1300–1500 cal daily by 3 years

2. Is capable of and desires to self-feed
3. Likes and dislikes become obvious

C. Sleep

1. Needs 10 to 12 hours sleep at night plus nap
2. Nighttime rituals important

D. Play

1. How they learn about the world
2. Solitary, but parallel to others
3. Likes imitative activities
4. Loves to be read to

E. Psychosocial Development

1. Erikson's stage of autonomy vs. shame and doubt
   a. ability to gain self-control is main goal
   b. if unable to gain self-control, or if too controlled, develops shame and doubt
2. Piaget's stages of cognitive development
   a. by 12 to 18 months, fifth stage
      (1) begins to see space and time in new ways
      (2) finds hidden objects
      (3) manipulates new objects to learn
   b. by 18 to 24 months, sixth stage ends sensorimotor period and begins preoperational period
      (1) uses memory and imitation rather than trial and error
      (2) egocentric in thought and behavior
   c. by 2 to 7 years, preoperational stage
      (1) arrives at answers mentally instead of physically
      (2) uses symbolism
      (3) understands simple abstractions
      (4) increasing attention span
      (5) begins to understand cause and effect

F. Speech

1. Understands simple commands
2. Begins to put words together, and by age 3 years is speaking in sentences
3. Language development requires feeling of security

G. Social Development

1. Vacillates between need to be cuddled and need to show independence; tantrums are common
2. After 18 months, imitates parents' behavior (plays house)

TABLE 8–1. Summary of Toddler Growth and Development and Health Maintenance

Physical Competency GENERAL: FROM 1 TO 3 YEARS	Intellectual Competency	Emotional-Social Competency
Gains 5 kg (11 lb) Grows 20.3 cm (8 in) 12 teeth erupt Nutritional requirements Energy 100 Kcal/kg/day Fluid 115–125 mL/kg/day Protein 1.8 g/kg/day	Learns by exploring and experimenting Learns by imitating. Progresses from a vocabulary of three to four words at 12 months to about 900 words at 36 months.	Central crisis: to gain a sense of autonomy vs doubt and shame. Demonstrates independent behaviors. Exhibits attachment behavior strongly and regularly until third birthday. Fears persist of strange people, objects, and places and of aloneness and being abandoned. Egocentric in play (parallel play). Imitation of parents in household tasks and activities of daily living.
15 MONTHS Legs appear bowed. Walks alone, climbs, slides down stairs backwards. Stacks two blocks. Scribbles spontaneously. Grasps spoon but rotates it, holds cup with both hands. Takes off socks and shoes.	Trial and error method of learning. Experiments to see what will happen. Says at least three words. Uses expressive jargon.	Shows independence by trying to feed self and helps in undressing.
18 MONTHS Runs but still falls. Walks upstairs with help. Slides down stairs backwards. Stacks three to four blocks. Clumsily throws a ball. Unzips a large zipper. Takes off simple garments.	Begins to retain a mental image of an absent object. Concept of object permanence fully develops. Has vocabulary of ten or more words. Holophrastic speech (one word used to communicate whole ideas).	Fears the water. Temper tantrums may begin. Negativism and dawdling predominate. Bedtime rituals begin. Awareness of gender identity begins. Helps with undressing.
24 MONTHS Runs quickly and with fewer falls. Pulls toys and walks sideways. Walks downstairs hanging on a rail (does not alternate feet). Stacks six blocks. Turns pages of a book. Imitates vertical and circular strokes. Uses spoon with little spilling. Can feed self. Puts on simple garments. Can turn door knobs.	Enters into preconceptual phase of preoperational period: Symbolic thinking and symbolic play. Egocentric thinking, imagination, and pretending are common. Has vocabulary of about 300 words. Uses two-word sentences (telegraphic speech). Engages in monologue.	Fears the dark and animals. Temper tantrums may continue. Negativism and dawdling continue. Bedtime rituals continue. Sleep resisted overtly. Usually shows readiness to begin bowel and bladder control. Explores genitalia. Brushes teeth with help. Helps with dressing and undressing.
36 MONTHS Has set of deciduous teeth at about 30 months. Walks downstairs alternating feet. Rides tricycle. Walks with balance and runs well. Stacks eight to ten blocks. Can pour from a pitcher. Feeds self completely. Dresses self almost completely (does not know front from back). Cannot tie shoes.	Preconceptual phase of preoperational period as for 24 months. Uses around 900 words. Constructs complete sentences and uses all parts of speech.	Temper tantrums subside. Negativism and dawdling subside. Bedtime rituals subside. Self-care in feeding, elimination, and dressing enhances self-esteem.

Nutrition GENERAL: FROM 1 TO 3 YEARS	Play	Safety
Milk 16–24 oz. Appetite decreases. Wants to feed self. Has food jags. Never force food; give nutritious snacks. Give iron and vitamin supplementation only if poor intake.	Books at all ages. Needs physical and quiet activities, does not need expensive toys.	Never leave alone in tub. Keep poisons, including detergents and cleaning products, out of reach. Use car seat. Have ipecac in house.
15 MONTHS Vulnerable to iron deficiency anemia. Give table foods except for tough meat and hard vegetables. Wants to feed self.	Stuffed animals, dolls, music toys. Peek-a-boo, hide and seek. Water and sand play. Stacking toys. Roll ball on floor. Push toys on floor. Read to toddler.	Keep small items off floor (pins, buttons, clips). Child may choke on hard food. Cords and table cloths are a danger. Keep electrical outlets plugged and poisons locked away. Risk of kitchen accidents with toddler underfoot.
18 MONTHS Negativism may interfere with eating. Encourage self-feeding. Is easily distracted while eating. May play with food. High activity level interferes with eating.	Rocking horse. Nesting toys. Shape-sorting cube. Pencil or crayon. Pull toys. Four wheeled toy to ride. Throw ball. Running and chasing games. Rough-housing. Puzzles. Blocks. Hammer and peg board.	Falls: from riding toy in bathtub from running too fast Climbs up to get dangerous objects. Keep dangerous things out of wastebasket.
24 MONTHS Requests certain foods, therefore snacks should be controlled. Imitates eating habits of others. May still play with food and especially with utensils and dish (pouring, stacking).	Clay and Play-Doh. Finger paint. Brush paint. Record player with record and story book and song to sing along. Toys to take apart. Toy tea sets. Puppets. Puzzles.	May fall from outdoor large play equipment. Can reach farther than expected (knives, razors, and matches must be kept out of reach).

Table continued on following page

TABLE 8–1. Summary of Toddler Growth and Development and Health Maintenance *Continued*

Nutrition GENERAL: FROM 1 TO 3 YEARS	Play	Safety
36 MONTHS Sits in booster seat rather than high chair. Verbal about likes and dislikes.	Likes playing with other children, building toys, drawing and painting, doing puzzles. Imitation household objects for doll play. Nurse and doctor kits. Carpenter kits.	Protect from: turning on hot water falling from tricycle striking matches.

(From Foster, R.L., Hunsberger, M.M., & Anderson, J.J. Family-Centered Nursing Care of Children. Philadelphia, W.B. Saunders Company, 1989.)

TABLE 8–2. Developmental Needs and Nursing Strategies: Toddlers

PHYSICAL NEEDS

TO EXPLORE AND DEVELOP MUSCLE SKILL WITHIN A SAFE ENVIRONMENT

Assess prehospitalization exploratory activities.

Provide small manipulative toys (boxes with lids; stack toys; nesting toys; large beads; large puzzles; equipment to color, paint, and scribble).

Provide a crib with an enclosed see-through top when a child attempts to explore by reaching for dangerous objects or crawling out of the crib.

Permit supervised activities in a playroom to explore new toys and the unfamiliar environment.

Allow exploration in child's room under supervision.

TO HAVE OPPORTUNITY TO ENGAGE IN LARGE MUSCLE ACTIVITY WITHIN SAFE LIMITS

Assess degree of mobility attained.

Provide for supervised out-of-bed activities consistent with patterns at home as the child's condition permits.

Keep floors free of small objects.

Enforce rules about wearing of shoes or nonskid slippers when child is out of bed.

Provide toys for the large muscles (rocking horse, soft ball, indoor slide, push-and-pull toys).

TO MAINTAIN PHYSIOLOGIC FUNCTION THROUGH DEVELOPMENT OF SELF-CARE SKILLS

Assess level of self-care attained (eating, elimination, dressing, hygiene, bedtime care).

Provide opportunities for participation in self-care activities.

- Eating: Provide highchair or small table and chair, bib, and usual types of food; allow child to feed self in usual manner.
- Elimination: Provide a potty chair or diapers according to usual elimination patterns. Reinforce routine as established prehospitalization.
- Dressing: Permit child to assist with those activities he or she is capable of doing.
- Hygiene: Allow child to participate in handwashing, brushing teeth, manipulating own wash cloth in tub.

INTELLECTUAL NEEDS

TO HAVE OPPORTUNITY TO LEARN VIA SENSORIMOTOR EXPERIENCE AND EXPRESS SELF THROUGH IMITATION AND PRETENDING

TO ENGAGE IN CONVERSATION WITH ADULTS AND CHILDREN TO ENHANCE LANGUAGE DEVELOPMENT; TO HEAR PROPER LANGUAGE

AND BE ENCOURAGED TO EXPRESS SELF THROUGH LANGUAGE

Provide toys that encourage exploration and manipulation.

For older toddler, provide toys and equipment that can be used to reenact hospital experience.

Assess extent of child's vocabulary, especially key phrases and words pertaining to daily activities.

Allow child to complete sentences; avoid speaking for the child.

Reinforce words child has mastered and introduce new words.

Encourage group activities (play and eating) to encourage use of language among children.

TO RECEIVE EXPLANATIONS ABOUT PROCEDURES (TODDLERS CAN UNDERSTAND MORE THAN THEY CAN SAY)

Avoid speaking about children without explanations to them as well.

Explain procedures before doing them.

EMOTIONAL-SOCIAL NEEDS

TO DEVELOP SENSE OF AUTONOMY

Allow child to do things alone pertaining to own care.

Allow child to participate in the bedtime story, and preparation for bed according to home routines.

Give child control over some of own life: allow choices, restrain as little as possible, and praise for completed tasks.

TO LEARN TO SEPARATE FROM PARENT(S)

Encourage care by parents.

Assist family in coping with behaviors in response to hospitalization and separation.

Encourage parents to visit often even though child resists their leaving.

Provide primary nurse when parents cannot be present.

Keep image of parent in child's mind with a picture, personal belongings, or a tape recording

TO LEARN TO ADAPT SOCIALLY

Reinforce those socially acceptable behaviors mastered by the child before hospitalization (eating, elimination, play).

Provide play opportunities with other children.

TO MAINTAIN USUAL ROUTINES AND RITUALS FOR SENSE OF SECURITY

Assess important rituals and routines, especially regarding bedtime (provide security objects and maintain routine; reading story, hugging, use of night light, and other rituals).

Ask parents and child about preferences in foods, toys, routines regarding daily hygiene, elimination, and dressing.

Maintain as many home routines as possible.

(From Foster, R.L., Hunsberger, M.M., & Anderson, J.J. Family-Centered Nursing Care of Children. Philadelphia, W.B. Saunders Company, 1989.)

3. At 18 to 24 months, learns to undress self
4. By 2 to 3 years, learns to dress self with help
5. Territorial with belongings

III. THE PRESCHOOLER (3–5 YEARS) (TABLES 8-3 AND 8-4)

A. Normal Physical Development

1. Appearance
   a. becomes taller and thinner
   b. blood pressure, 90/60 pulse, 80–110; respirations, 30
   c. coordination and balance improve
   d. climbs and jumps rope by 5 years
2. Elimination
   a. toilet trained except for rare accidents by 3 years
   b. independent in toileting by 4 years
   c. in complete charge of needs by 5 years

B. Nutritional Needs

1. Growth slower; needs about 1700 calories per day
2. Needs four basic food groups
3. Eating habits simple
4. Definite food preferences

C. Sleep

1. Naps become less needed
2. 9 to 11 hours sleep/night
3. May have nightmares and fears of dark

D. Play

1. Cooperative
2. Imitative and dramatic in play
3. Likes creative toys that allow for imagination

E. Psychosocial Development

1. Erikson's stage of initiative vs. guilt
   a. increasing independence from parents
   b. assert themselves outside home
   c. involved in mastering new skills and tasks
2. Piaget's preconceptual and intuitive thought stages
   a. time, such as "tomorrow," has meaning
   b. decreased egocentricity
   c. cause and effect has magical quality

d. more social
e. thinks more without acting out

F. Speech

1. At 3 years, constantly asking how and why
2. By 5 years, uses adult-length sentences
3. Learning to read
4. Language has logic

G. Social Development

1. Socially capable of independence
2. Verbose even with strangers
3. Can share with others
4. May be more physical and aggressive

IV. THE SCHOOL-AGE CHILD (5–12 YEARS) (TABLES 8-5 AND 8-6)

A. Normal Physical Development

1. Appearance
   a. growth rate slow and steady, gaining 1 to 2 feet by 12 years
   b. a weight gain of about 10% per year
   c. by 12 years, about 84 lb and 59 inches tall
   d. growth spurt just before puberty for boys
   e. by 12 years, brain essentially adult size, with head circumference about 21 inches
   f. jaw expands so permanent teeth can erupt, usually all but third molar in by 12 years
2. Vital signs
   a. temperature, 98.6°F; pulse, 60–76; blood pressure, 94/56 to 112/60
   b. heart grows more slowly, more easily stressed because it is smaller in proportion to body size
3. General
   a. maturation of most body systems occurs by 12 years
   b. at 10 to 12 years, restless energy present
   c. secondary sexual characteristics develop at 10 to 12 years in girls and 12 to 14 years in boys

B. Nutritional Needs

1. Need 1600–2200 cal/day
2. Protein, vitamins, and minerals needed for growth
3. Become more influenced by others for food choices, more fads, and junk food
4. Obesity often becomes apparent

Text continued on page 275

TABLE 8–3. Growth, Development, and Health Promotion for Preschoolers

Physical Competency GENERAL: 3 TO 5 YEARS	Intellectual Competency	Emotional-Social Competency
Gains 4.5 kg (10 lb) Grows 15 cm (6 in) 20 teeth present Nutritional requirements: Energy: 1250–1600 cal/day (or 90–100 Kcal/kg/day) Fluid: 100–125 mL/kg/day Protein: 30 gm/day (or 3 gm/kg/day) Iron: 10 mg/day	Becomes increasingly aware of self and others Vocabulary increases from 900 to 2100 words Piaget's preoperational/intuitive period	Freud's phallic stage Oedipus complex—boy Electra complex—girl Erikson's stage of Initiative vs. Guilt
3 YEARS Runs, stops suddenly Walks backward Climbs steps Jumps Pedals tricycle Undresses self Unbuttons front buttons Feeds self well	Knows own sex Desires to please Sense of humor Language—900 words Follows simple direction Uses plurals Names figure in picture Uses adjectives/adverbs	Shifts between reality and imagination Bedtime rituals Negativism decreases Animism and realism: anything that moves is alive
4 YEARS Runs well, skips clumsily Hops on one foot Heel-toe walks Up and down steps without holding rail Jumps well Dresses and undresses Buttons well, needs help with zippers, bows Brushes teeth Bathes self Draws with some form and meaning	More aware of others Uses alibis to excuse behavior Bossy Language—1500 words Talks in sentences Knows nursery rhymes Counts to five Highly imaginative Name calling	Focuses on present Egocentrism/unable to see the viewpoint of others, unable to understand another's inability to see own viewpoint Does not comprehend anticipatory explanation Sexual curiosity Oedipus complex Electra complex
5 YEARS Runs skillfully Jumps 3–4 steps Jumps rope, hops, skips Begins dance Roller skates Dresses without assistance Tie shoelaces Hits nail on head with hammer Draws person—6 parts Prints first name	Aware of cultural differences Knows name and address More independent More sensible/less imaginative Copies triangle, draws rectangle Knows four or more colors Language—2100 words, meaningful sentences Understands kinship Counts to 10	Continues in egocentrism Fantasy and daydreams Resolution of Oedipus/Electra complex, girls identify with mother, boys with father Body image and body boundary especially important in illness Shows tension in nail-biting, nose-picking, whining, snuffling

Nutrition GENERAL: 3 TO 5 YEARS	Play	Safety
Carbohydrate intake approximately 40%–50% of calories Good food sources of essential vitamins and minerals Regular tooth brushing Parents are seen as examples, if parent won't eat it, child won't	Reading books is important at all ages Balance highly physical activities with quiet times Quiet rest period takes the place of nap time Provide sturdy play materials	Never leave alone in bath or swimming pool Keep poisons in locked cupboard; learn what household things are poisonous Use car seats and seatbelts Never leave child alone in car Remove doors from abandoned freezers and refrigerators
3 YEARS 1250 cal/day Due to increased sex identity and imitation, copies parents at table and will eat what they eat Different colors and shapes of foods can increase interest	Participates in simple games Cooperates, takes turns Plays with group Uses scissors, paper Likes crayons, coloring books Enjoys being read to and "reading" Plays "dress-up" and "house" Likes fire engines	Teach safety habits early Let water out of bathtub; don't stand in tub Caution against climbing in unsafe areas, onto or under cars, unsafe buildings, drainage pipes Insist on seatbelts worn at all times in cars
4 YEARS Good nutrition 1400 cal/day Nutritious between-meal snacks essential Emphasis on quality not quantity of food eaten Mealtime should be enjoyable, not for criticism As dexterity improves, neatness increases	Longer attention span with group activities "Dress-up" with more dramatic play Draws, pounds, paints Likes to make paper chains, sewing cards Scrapbooks Likes being read to, records, and rhythmic play "Helps" adults	Teach to stay out of streets, alleys Continually teach safety; child understands Teach how to handle scissors Teach what are poisons and why to avoid Never allow child to stand in moving car

Nutrition	Play	Safety
GENERAL: 3 TO 5 YEARS		
5 YEARS		
Good nutrition	Plays with trucks, cars, soldiers, dolls	Teach child how to cross streets safely
1600 cal/day	Likes simple games with letters or	Teach child not to speak to strangers or
Encourage regular tooth brushing	numbers	get into cars of strangers
Encourage quiet time before meals	Much gross motor activity: water, mud,	Insist on seatbelts
Can learn to cut own meat	snow, leaves, rocks	Teach child to swim
Frequent illnesses from increased exposure increases nutritional needs	Matching picture games	

(From Foster, R.L., Hunsberger, M.M., & Anderson, J.J. Family-Centered Nursing Care of Children. Philadelphia, W.B. Saunders Company, 1989.)

TABLE 8–4. Developmental Needs and Nursing Strategies: Preschoolers

PHYSICAL NEEDS

TO MAINTAIN CONTROL OF BODY FUNCTIONS

Assess prehospitalization level of control and patterns for eating, elimination, and sleep. Assess words used to describe functions.

Allow normal patterns as much as possible.

Reassure when accidents in elimination occur; do not reprimand or punish.

Praise successes in self-control.

Provide age-appropriate motor stimulation.

TO MAINTAIN PHYSIOLOGIC FUNCTION THROUGH INCREASED DEVELOPMENT OF SELF-CARE SKILLS

Assess prehospitalization self-care tasks.

Allow continued self-care when possible; provide some opportunities for decisions on care, especially in aspects of care in which condition or treatment prohibits self-care.

Allow usual eating practices: provide foods child is used to, finger foods, favorite foods, and eating utensils from home; allow family members to eat with child if isolated or to feed if child must be fed; if not isolated, allow eating at child-sized table with hospitalized peers; follow child's usual rituals, such as prayer before eating.

Allow usual elimination practices: provide potty chair (from home if preferred) or regular toilet as child is accustomed to; if mobility is restricted, offer to assist child to toilet or bedpan at usual eliminating times. Keep call bell near so child may get prompt assistance at other times. (Preschoolers still have difficulty "holding off" elimination processes.) Stay with child or provide privacy as child is accustomed.

Allow usual rest and sleep practices. Allow night light if child is used to one or requests one; provide quiet, uninterrupted period during child's usual nap or rest time if nap still taken; allow usual sleep time attire to be worn; if not contraindicated, allow usual sleep position and amount of cover and pillows used at home; bring any special sleep items (blanket, pacifier, toy) from home.

Permit child to dress at least partially in own clothing during daytime.

INTELLECTUAL NEEDS

TO BE PROTECTED FROM SENSE OF GUILT, WHICH CAN OCCUR AS A RESULT OF EGOCENTRIC THINKING

Reassure repeatedly that no one is to blame for the condition or hospitalization.

Reassure that only necessary treatments will be done, and they will not be done without telling the child first.

Provide activities (play, arts and crafts, stories) that stimulate intellectual development.

TO BE PROTECTED FROM FEARS CREATED BY PREOPERATIONAL THINKING (INTUITIVE, MAGICAL THOUGHTS)

Explain all procedures, especially describing what child can expect to experience through the senses, before doing them.

Provide for dramatic and therapeutic play; make available safe procedural equipment and dolls during education sessions, in playroom, at bedside.

Do not talk about the child unless child is included in the conversation.

TO HAVE OPPORTUNITY TO USE EXPRESSIVE LANGUAGE

Encourage questions and ask questions to learn fears, fantasies, and misperceptions (correct these when possible). Give opportunity for verbal expressions during stress.

Encourage child to tell stories about drawings or to tell you a "story" about hospital procedures or experiences.

Teach new words related to simple anatomy and physiology, the disease or treatment, and hospital equipment and personnel.

EMOTIONAL-SOCIAL NEEDS

TO MASTER CONTROL OF THE ENVIRONMENT AND DEVELOP INDEPENDENCE

Encourage self-care in hygiene and participation in medical care and treatments. (The preschooler can cooperate if given adequate instruction and permission to participate.)

Observe safety precautions.

Promptly remove offensive smells and preserve orderliness. As a result of having mastered toilet functions, the preschooler is keenly aware of smells and disorder and is upset by them.

Permit and encourage child's own decision making regarding care and treatments when choices exist.

Praise evidence of competence in all areas of development (self-care, learning new words, helping with a treatment, cooperation during stressful procedures).

Solicit and respect child's suggestions regarding care, room environment changes, toys in room, etc.

TO EXPERIENCE LIMITS WITHIN ENVIRONMENT TO FEEL SECURITY

Enforce safety rules; give simple explanations for rules (child must be in crib or bed with rails up even if used to big bed without rails at home).

Define limits on activity due to illness (isolation from other children while disease is communicable). Since time concept is undeveloped, give idea of how long the limitation will be by associating it with concrete things ("You can go to the playroom Saturday. That is the day that cartoons are on TV all morning" or "You can drink water and other drinks again when Nurse Smith comes to care for you this afternoon").

Learn during admission interview if parents want any home rules continued during hospitalization (only certain TV shows may be watched or TV is allowed only so many hours a day, teeth are to be brushed after each meal, limited beverages are allowed after suppertime) and enforce those not in conflict with treatment regimen.

Explain to parents reasons any cannot be enforced.

TO ENGAGE IN RITUALS TO FEEL SECURE

Assess usual routines and rituals during interview. Integrate rituals into care plan as possible.

Encourage parents or other family members acquainted with the rituals to be present and help child carry out mealtime, bedtime, other significant rituals.

Ask parents to bring from home those objects related to child's rituals and other security items.

TO LEARN TO SEPARATE WITHOUT CONFLICT

Provide for a primary nurse for each shift.

Permit and encourage unlimited parental visits and participation in planning and giving care.

Table continued on following page

TABLE 8–4. Developmental Needs and Nursing Strategies: Preschoolers *Continued*

Allow parents to remain and comfort child, if desired during treatments or procedures parents cannot or do not wish to do. Primary nurse is present as parent surrogate to stay with and comfort child.

Let parents do as many of the "caretaking" tasks as possible.

Ask parents to bring in familiar toys, family photos, personal belongings that can be left with child as reminders of them during their absence.

During care, make up pleasant stories about home activities, including names of family members in the stories, or encourage child to tell stories about home and family activities.

Provide opportunities for child to become acquainted with other children and parents who may "fill in" as sources of comfort during parental and sibling separations.

Help parents identify ways to keep child in contact with siblings or peers who cannot visit (phone call, tape recordings, notes, pictures).

TO ACHIEVE SEXUAL IDENTITY AND COMFORT WITH SEXUAL SENSATIONS AND FEELINGS

Give thorough explanations and continued reassurance about what will happen to the child's body as a result of a treatment or procedure; it is especially important to reassure of continued presence and intactness of genitals when these body parts are involved.

Handle genitalia as little as possible and use gentleness when handling is necessary. Some children respond better if their hand is used with the nurse's in handling the genitalia.

Avoid use of intrusive procedures or treatments whenever possible (preschoolers cope with axillary or oral thermometers better than rectal).

(From Foster, R.L., Hunsberger, M.M., & Anderson, J.J. Family-Centered Nursing Care of Children. Philadelphia, W.B. Saunders Company, 1989.)

TABLE 8–5. Competency Development of the School-Age Child

Physical Competency	Intellectual Competency	Emotional-Social Competency
GENERAL: 6 TO 12 YEARS		
Gains an average of 2.5–3.2 kg/year (5½–7 lb/year). Overall height gains of 5.5 cm (2 inches) per year; growth occurs in spurts and is mainly in trunk and extremities. Loses deciduous teeth; most of permanent teeth erupt. Progressively more coordinated in both gross and fine motor skills. Caloric needs increase with growth spurts.	Masters concrete operations. Moves from egocentrism; learns he or she is not always right. Learns grammar and expression of emotions and thoughts. Vocabulary increases to 3000 words or more; handles complex sentences.	Central crisis; industry vs. inferiority; wants to do and make things. Progressive sex education needed. Wants to be like friends; competition important. Fears body mutilation, alterations in body image; earlier phobias may recur, nightmares; fears death. Nervous habits common.
6 TO 7 YEARS		
Gross motor skill exceeds fine motor coordination. Balance and rhythm are good—runs, skips, jumps, climbs, gallops. Throws and catches ball. Dresses self with little or no help.	Vocabulary of 2500 words. Learning to read and print; beginning concrete concepts of numbers, general classification of items. Knows concepts of right and left; morning, afternoon, and evening; coinage. Intuitive thought process. Verbally aggressive, bossy, opinionated; argumentative. Likes simple games with basic rules.	Boisterous, outgoing, and a know-it-all, whiney; parents should sidestep power struggles, offer choices. Becomes quiet and reflective during seventh year; very sensitive. Can use telephone. Likes to make things: starts many, finishes few. Give some responsibility for household duties.
8 TO 10 YEARS		
Myopia may appear. Secondary sex characteristics begin in girls. Hand–eye coordination and fine motor skills well established. Movements are graceful, coordinated. Cares for own physical needs completely. Constantly on move; plays and works hard; enforce balance in rest and activity.	Learning correct grammar and to express feelings in words. Likes books he or she can read alone; will read funny papers, scan newspaper. Enjoys making detailed drawings. Mastering classification, seriation, spatial and temporal, numerical concepts. Uses language as a tool; likes riddles, jokes, chants, word games. Rules guiding force in life now. Very interested in how things work, what and how weather, seasons, etc., are made.	Strong preference for same-sex peers; antagonizes opposite-sex peers. Self-assured and pragmatic at home; questions parental values and ideas. Has a strong sense of humor. Enjoys clubs, group projects, outings, large groups, camp. Modesty about own body increases over time; sex conscious. Works diligently to perfect skills he or she does best. Happy, cooperative, relaxed and casual in relationships. Increasingly courteous and well-mannered with adults. Gang stage at a peak; secret codes and rituals prevail. Responds better to suggestion than dictatorial approach.
11 TO 12 YEARS		
Vital signs approximate adult norms. Growth spurt for girls; inequalities between sexes are increasingly noticeable; boys greater physical strength. Eruption of permanent teeth complete except for third molars. Secondary sex characteristics begin in boys. Menstruation may begin.	Able to think about social problems and prejudices; sees others' points of view. Enjoys reading mysteries, love stories. Begins playing with abstract ideas. Interested in whys of health measures and understands human reproduction. Very moralistic; religious commitment often made during this time.	Intense team loyalty; boys begin teasing girls and girls flirt with boys for attention; best friend period. Wants unreasonable independence. Rebellious about routines; wide mood swings; needs some times daily for privacy. Very critical of own work. Hero worship prevails. "Facts of life" chats with friends prevail; masturbation increases. Appears under constant tension.

TABLE 8–5. Competency Development of the School-Age Child *Continued*

Nutrition GENERAL: 6 to 12 YEARS	Play	Safety
Fluctuations in appetite due to uneven growth pattern and tendency to get involved in activities. Tendency to neglect breakfast due to rush of getting to school. Though school lunch is provided in most schools, child does not always eat it.	Plays in groups, mostly of same sex; "gang" activities predominate. Books for all ages. Bicycles important. Sports equipment. Cards, board and table games. Most of play is active games requiring little or no equipment.	Enforce continued use of safety belts during car travel. Bicycle safety must be taught and enforced. Teach safety related to hobbies, handicrafts, mechanical equipment.
6 TO 7 YEARS Preschool food dislikes persist. Tendency for deficiencies in iron, vitamin A, and riboflavin. 100 mL/kg of water per day. 3 g/kg protein daily.	Still enjoys dolls, cars and trucks. Plays well alone but enjoys small groups of both sexes; begins to prefer same sex peer during 7th year. Ready to learn how to ride a bicycle. Prefers imaginary, dramatic play with real costumes. Begins collecting for quantity, not quality. Enjoys active games such as hide-and-seek, tag, jump-rope, roller skating, kickball. Ready for lessons in dancing, gymnastics, music. Restrict TV time to 1–2 hours/day.	Teach and reinforce traffic safety. Still needs adult supervision of play. Teach to avoid strangers, never take anything from strangers. Teach illness prevention and reinforce continued practice of other health habits. Restrict bicycle use to home ground; no traffic areas; teach bicycle safety. Teach and set examples re harmful use of drugs, alcohol, smoking.
8 TO 10 YEARS Needs about 2100 cal/day; nutritious snacks. Tends to be too busy to bother to eat. Tendency for deficiencies in calcium, iron, and thiamine. Problem of obesity may begin now. Good table manners. Able to help with food preparation.	Likes hiking, sports. Enjoys cooking, woodworking, crafts. Enjoys cards and table games. Likes radio and records. Begins qualitative collecting now. Continue restriction on TV time.	Stress safety with firearms. Keep them out of reach and allow use only with adult supervision. Know who the child's friends are; parents should still have some control over friend selection. Teach water safety; swimming should be supervised by an adult.
11 TO 12 YEARS Male needs 2500 cal per day; female needs 2250 (70 cal/kg/day). 75 mL/kg of water per day. 2 g/kg protein daily.	Enjoys projects and working with hands. Likes to do errands and jobs to earn money. Very involved in sports, dancing, talking on phone. Enjoys all aspects of acting and drama.	Continue monitoring friends. Stress bicycle safety on streets and in traffic.

(From Foster, R.L., Hunsberger, M.M., & Anderson, J.J. Family-Centered Nursing Care of Children. Philadelphia, W.B. Saunders Company, 1989.)

C. Rest/Activity Needs

1. At 6 years, about 11 hours sleep; at 11 years, about 9 hours
2. Exercise essential for growth and muscle development

D. Safety Needs

1. Major concern for this group with its increased independence and abilities
2. Boys more accident-prone than girls
3. Must be taught safety precautions because accidents are leading cause of death in this age group

E. Psychosocial Development

1. Erikson's stage of industry vs. inferiority
   a. sense of accomplishment at school and play
   b. fear of failure may develop
   c. much more competitive
2. Piaget's stage of concrete operations
   a. systematic reasoning about tangible or familiar situations

   b. decenters: considers more than one characteristic at a time
   c. reverses: images process in reverse
   d. conservation: see consistency in patterns
   e. reasons logically: thinks through situations and anticipates outcomes

F. Communication

1. At 6 years, uses language more as tool; swears and uses slang to test others' reactions
2. At 7 years, can print
3. At 8 years, writes cursive
4. By 9 years, participates in discussions
5. Preadolescent seems less communicative, often finding one close friend to share feelings with

G. Social Development

1. Friends more important than family; usually one special friend
2. Begins to develop relationships with adults other than parents

TABLE 8–6. Developmental Needs and Nursing Strategies: School-Age Children

PHYSICAL NEEDS

To COMPLETE CONTROL OF BODY FUNCTIONS AND SELF-CARE

Assess and maintain usual routines related to body function and self-care.

Allow independent self-care to extent feasible by treatment restrictions and child's tolerance.

Praise whatever self-care child does perform.

To DEVELOP FINE MOTOR SKILLS

Provide materials for fine motor activities (pencils and crayons, scissors, Lego, computer games, hospital equipment safe for play that requires finger manipulation).

Encourage drawing pictures of body and body parts during discussions of disease and treatment. This gives nurse feedback on the accuracy of the child's interpretation of information.

Encourage child to "take notes" during patient education sessions—gives practice in fine motor dexterity for printing or writing.

Teach child to participate in treatments that give practice in fine motor skills.

INTELLECTUAL NEEDS

To DEVELOP RATIONAL THINKING, REALITY ORIENTATION

Provide scientific descriptions of the child's disease and body responses during educational sessions or in reply to questions.

Offer a rationale for each procedure before doing it to help the child to maintain self-control during procedures and to participate when feasible.

Provide children with rules about what they may and may not do during hospitalization, because of the disease or during a treatment. Suggest writing out a list of rules to post at bedside.

Assess whether child perceives hospitalization as a punishment; intervene as for preschooler if so.

Provide opportunities for child to make decisions about routine, treatments, and daily care whenever choices actually exist. Encourage middle school-age child to help devise a care plan.

To MASTER CONCEPTS OF CONSERVATION, CONSTANCY, AND REVERSIBILITY AND TO DEVELOP SKILLS IN CLASSIFICATION AND CATEGORIZATION

Allow child to participate in care by helping keep track on intake and output, writing down vital signs, counting the seconds or adding up the minutes it takes to complete a procedure.

Encourage the child who can tell time to inform the nurse when it is time for a procedure or when it is time to stop the procedure (when to take out thermometer, when to take off soaks, etc.).

Encourage scrapbook making, collection, diary keeping (according to child's interests) during hospital stay.

Utilize these concepts in teaching sessions.

Provide games that require use of these concepts (card games, board games).

Provide hospital school or tutor schoolwork.

To VOCALIZE FEELINGS DURING STRESS

Encourage verbalization of feelings associated with hospitalization, disease, procedures by asking questions ("How does it make you feel to have to miss school and be away from your friends?" or "Tell me what it is like to have to lie still for 30 minutes while those compresses are on").

Schedule time to talk with child, time not associated with any specific care or procedure. Let child know this is a time she or he can talk about anything or ask any questions. Encourage parents to do the same.

EMOTIONAL-SOCIAL NEEDS

To HAVE THE OPPORTUNITY TO CHANNEL DRIVES INTO SOCIALLY ACCEPTABLE BEHAVIORS

Do not place girls and boys in the same room.

Provide opportunities to interact with other hospitalized school-age children.

Assess for preschool residual concerns re genitalia; manage as for preschooler.

Help maintain peer group contact via phone calls, letter writing, tape recordings, peer visitation, photo exchanges. (Teachers and parents are usually willing to help arrange these things.)

Arrange group education sessions for children with similar problems. Include discussions of how problems are similar and how they differ. Involve children in teaching each other about anatomy and physiology, disease process, treatment, under nurse supervision.

Treat any separation anxiety as for preschooler.

Encourage parents to express affection toward their hospitalized school-age children and to continue setting limits as before hospitalization.

To ACHIEVE INDUSTRY AND ASSOCIATED DEVELOPING SELF-CONCEPT

Praise cooperation efforts, self-care accomplishments, participation in treatments, and any other achievements. Praise honestly and often.

Provide opportunities for built-in successes several times daily. (Assign tasks the child is known to be able to accomplish.)

Provide opportunities for peer cooperation (solicit roommate's help in entertaining an immobilized child).

Actively involve child in care and treatments.

Balance quiet and solitary activity with action and peer interaction as tolerated.

(From Foster, R.L., Hunsberger, M.M., & Anderson, J.J. Family-Centered Nursing Care of Children. Philadelphia, W.B. Saunders Company, 1989.)

3. Increased social skills
4. More cooperative, but still may be highly competitive

V. THE ADOLESCENT (12–19 YEARS) (TABLE 8-7)

A. Normal Physical Development

1. Appearance
   a. second major period of rapid growth
   b. girls average 2.5 to 5 inches, and boys 3 to 6 inches
   c. developmental spurt also with puberty and development of adult reproductive status
   d. more clumsy because bones outgrow muscles
2. Other systems
   a. heart grows more slowly than rest of body, causing fatigue
   b. blood pressure, 100–120/50–70; pulse, 60–68; respirations, 16–20; girls have slightly higher basal temperature
   c. all teeth by 20 to 21 years
   d. auditory acuity peaks at 13 years and decreases thereafter

B. Nutritional Needs

1. Increased appetite
2. Females need 2100–2400 calories/day; males, 2800–3000 calories
3. Iron, calcium, and protein needs increase
4. Eating greatly influenced by peer group, fad diets, eating disorders

TABLE 8–7. Developmental Needs and Nursing Strategies: Adolescents

PHYSICAL NEEDS
SUPPORT OF RAPID SKELETAL GROWTH
Provide nutritional information on diet, snacks, and weight control.
Refer to dietitian for special dietary needs.
Encourage consumption of nutritional snacks, rather than "empty calories."
TO PERFORM SELF-CARE SKILLS ASSOCIATED WITH ONSET OF PUBERTY
Provide information on hygiene measures; means of independent bathing.
Answer questions and provide counseling on reproductive system and function.
Provide anticipatory guidance on preventive health maintenance, breast examinations, birth control.
PHYSICAL EXERCISE AND MOBILITY
Assist to move out of bed and around the unit.
Recreation activities suitable to age and size.
Acknowledge need for physical expression of frustration and provide innovative means.
Encourage physical and occupational therapy to increase independence, muscle strength, and mobility.

INTELLECTUAL NEEDS
TO RECEIVE SCIENTIFIC EXPLANATIONS
Thorough explanation and preparation for procedures and instructions.
Use scientific terminology to explain illness.
TO PARTICIPATE IN HEALTH CARE MANAGEMENT DECISIONS
Include client in planning guide.
Give all instructions to client as well as parent. Orient to environment, routines, and expectations.
TO ACHIEVE IN ACADEMICS AND STRIVE TOWARD CAREER GOALS
Provide opportunity to complete schoolwork while hospitalized.

Involve school teachers in health care planning.
Reinforce realistic career goals.

EMOTIONAL-SOCIAL NEEDS
TO DEVELOP HEALTHY ATTITUDES ABOUT BODY IMAGE AND SEXUALITY
Encourage verbalization of fears and concerns.
Provide privacy.
Let youth have own belongings and wear own clothes.
Assist with grooming needs (eg, hair washing, nails).
TO ACHIEVE INDEPENDENCE
Compliment the adolescent's strengths.
Encourage self-care.
Provide flexible limits.
Provide opportunities to participate in setting goals, planning care, and choosing options.
Provide opportunities for appropriate decisions and control.
TO HAVE PEER CONTACT AND APPROVAL
Provide opportunities for friends to visit and call.
Suggest recreation activities that stimulate adolescents to gather.
Arrange for unit meeting for adolescents.
Suggest passes to go home or to school or social functions.
Opportunities for appropriate calls to friends.
TO RECEIVE FAMILY SUPPORT
Encourage parents to visit and stay when adolescent needs or wants them.
Provide opportunities for meetings where parents can discuss issues and get support.
Encourage sibling visits.
Give support to maintain the family unit.
Encourage chaplain visits.
Encourage use of appropriate community resources.
Provide community agency referrals.

(From Foster, R.L., Hunsberger, M.M., & Anderson, J.J. Family-Centered Nursing Care of Children. Philadelphia, W.B. Saunders Company, 1989.)

C. Rest/Activity Needs

1. Activities consistent with peer group
2. Many competitive activities
3. Need more rest and sleep

D. Psychosocial Development

1. Erikson's stage of identity formation vs. identity diffusion
   a. asks "Who am I? What am I going to do with my life?"
   b. work to become independent of parents and find their own place in world
   c. also develop sexual identity

   d. without success, youth becomes alienated and disillusioned
2. Piaget's stage of formal operations
   a. abstract and analytical thinking
   b. becomes philosophical

E. Social Development

1. May have difficulty with adults, authority figures
2. Still need parental figures
3. Becomes sexually attracted and may be sexually active
4. Needs peer group to identify with
5. Has close friends of same sex

Questions

Your friend, Beverly, has expressed concern about her daughter, Maria, who has recently celebrated her second birthday. She states that Maria will not play with other children and has suddenly become extremely possessive of her belongings.

1. An appropriate response to Beverly would be:

① "It is never too early to begin counseling."
✓② "Maria is demonstrating normal behavior for a child of her age."
③ "Maria has probably inherited her daddy's personality."
④ "You should strongly encourage Maria to interact with others and share her toys so that future problems can be prevented."

2. Maria is also beginning to use the word "no" in response to almost all requests and insists upon doing things by herself. According to Erikson, the developmental stage that must be achieved by Maria at this age is

✓① Autonomy
② Initiative
③ Industry
④ Identity

3. Freud referred to late childhood as the period of:

① The oral stage
② The anal stage
③ The Oedipal stage
✓④ The latent stage

4. The resting time between early childhood and adolescence when the sex drives are repressed is termed:

① The anal stage
② The Oedipal stage
✓③ Latency
④ Puberty

5. Generally the sexual development of girls compared with boys is:

✓① Earlier
② Later
③ The same
④ Individualized

6. Erik Erikson designates the late childhood as a time of:

① Trust
② Autonomy
③ Initiative
✓④ Industry

7. The school-age child's loyalty is placed on the following:

① The individual
✓② The family
③ The peers
④ The church

8. Intellectual development of a school-age child becomes more flexible and systematic. Piaget termed this operation as:

① Sensory-motor
② Preoperational
✓③ Concrete
④ Formal

9. Knowing that there is as much water in a low quart container as in a tall quart container is an example of which of Piaget's stages:

① Preoperational
✓② Concrete
③ Formal
④ Generativity

10. Physical growth is slowest during the period of:

① Infancy
② Preschool
✓③ School age
④ Adolescence

11. The ability of a child to know that a ball of clay flattened out into a pancake or a long string is not really bigger is called:

① Reversibility
✓② Conservation
③ Configuration
④ Seriation

12. The ability to arrange articles according to size is called:

① Preconstruction
✓② Seriation
③ Configuration
④ Reversibility

13. The ability to understand that shapes can be reversed or that sequences have a beginning and an end and can be rerun is termed:

① Reversibility
② Conservation
③ Transposition
④ Seriation

14. Shyness in a school-age child may be produced by:

① Shaming
② Encouraging
③ Lying
④ Ignoring

15. One remedy for decreasing shyness in children is:

① Finding ways to increase self-esteem
② Giving them adult responsibilities
③ Forcing them to meet strangers
④ Doing all their tasks for them

16. A parent who says to a child, "Do as you are told because I said so," is an example of a person who is:

① Authoritative
② Permissive
③ Authoritarian
④ Submissive

17. A parent who offers no guidelines, thus allowing the child to make his or her own decisions, is an example of:

① Authoritarian
② Authoritative
③ Submissive
④ Permissive

18. Which age group has the most difficulty coping with divorce in the family?

① Infant
② Early childhood
③ School-age child
④ Adolescent

19. Motor coordination in the school-age child:

① Increases
② Decreases
③ Stagnates
④ Fluctuates

20. Gross motor coordination is demonstrated by:

① Running
② Tying
③ Writing
④ Sewing

21. Emotionally, the 7–12 year span is one of relationships of:

① Gangs with the same sex
② Opposite sex and intimacy
③ Oedipus complex
④ Electra complex

22. The girl's first menstrual period is termed:

① Prepubescence
② Socialization
③ Menarche
④ Maturation

23. You are caring for a 26-month-old boy who was admitted for severe diarrhea. The child is doing well and will be discharged tomorrow. His mother states that he does not usually nap at home. The most appropriate action during nap time would be to:

① Insist that he take a nap with all the children
② Put him down for a nap and turn out the lights
③ Hold him and rock him until he sleeps
④ Allow him simply to play quietly in his crib

24. Your patient is a preschool child who is admitted for surgery. The nurse should tell the patient that:

① Surgery will be painless
② The child should not be afraid
③ Everyone is afraid at times
④ Crying is a sign of "babyishness"

Answers & Rationales

Guide to item identification (see pp. 3–5 for further details about each category)

I, II, III, or IV for the phase of the nursing process
1, 2, 3, or 4 for the category of client needs
A, B, C, D, E, F, or G for the category of human functioning
Specific content category by name; ie, cholecystectomy

1. The toddler requires instant gratification of desires and at this age has no comprehension of sharing or desire to share. She also prefers to play next to, rather than with, other children —"parallel play."
② III & IV, 4, A. Peds Growth and Development.

2. The toddler begins to realize she has some measure of control over her surroundings and begins to test the extent of her power by use of the word "no."
① I, 4, A. Peds Growth and Development.

3. Latency means quiet time or time without obvious changes.
④ I, 4, A. Peds Growth and Development.

4. The hormone balance is similar in both sexes.
③ I, 4, A. Peds Growth and Development.

5. The pituitary gland activates the female hormones in preparation for menarche.
① I & IV, 4, A. Peds Growth and Development.

6. Energy is channeled into learning.
④ I & IV, 4, A. Peds Growth and Development.

7. Family continues to serve as a guide and security factor.
② I & IV, 4, A. Peds Growth and Development.

8. The ability to see an organized "whole" and its parts for application is developing.
③ I, 4, A. Peds Growth and Development.

9. The ability to transfer and conserve a volume is developed.
② I, 4, A. Peds Growth and Development.

10. This time is used to prepare the body for sexual development.
③ I, 4, A. Peds Growth and Development.

11. Transfer of volume and its application to change are developed.
② I, 4, A. Peds Growth and Development.

12. The ability to relate small to large is developing.
② I, 4, A. Peds Growth and Development.

13. Control of a physical world is present.
① I, 4, D. Peds Growth and Development.

14. The school-age child listens to the significant "other's" negative remarks and internalizes them to be true, preventing a positive self-image.
① I, 4, A. Peds Growth and Development.

15. Shyness results from derogatory remarks being internalized. In order to decrease shyness, a child needs to develop a positive sense of self.
① I, 4, A. Peds Growth and Development.

16. An authoritarian figure does not consider the child or the situation and needs control over both rather than teaching self-control.
③ I, 4, A. Peds Growth and Development.

17. The parent has a low self-esteem, and giving the responsibility and control to the child assures the parent of being accepted by the child.
④ IV, 4, A. Peds Growth and Development.

18. The school-age child questions the reason for the divorce and sees self as a possible cause.
③ IV, 4, A. Peds Growth and Development.

19. The development of muscles and bones coincides with neurological development; therefore, physical control is observed.
① I, 4, A & F. Peds Growth and Development.

20. Large muscle groups of the legs are demonstrated in running. Small muscle groups are used for the other activities.
① I, 4, F. Peds Growth and Development.

21. Resolution of the Electra and Oedipus complex permits an acceptance of one's own sexual orientation.
① IV, 4, A. Peds Growth and Development.

22. *Mena* means monthly and *arche* means first—subsequently "first monthly."
③ I, 4, D. Peds Growth and Development.

23. Trying to force a toddler to take a nap is futile.
④ Allowing quiet play in the crib allows for rest without unduly upsetting the child's routine.
III, 3, A. Peds Growth and Development.

24. The child needs reassurance that what he or she
③ is feeling is perfectly normal and that it is all right to be afraid.
III, 4, A. Peds Growth and Development.

OXYGENATION

■ Cardiovascular Disorders

I. CONGENITAL: ACYANOTIC HEART DEFECTS

A. Septal Defects (Fig. 8-1)

1. Assessment
   a. definitions
      (1) ventricular septal defect: abnormal opening between right and left ventricles; causes left to right shunting of blood; can vary in size from tiny to complete absence of septum
      (2) atrial septal defect: abnormal opening between two atria; may also be patent foramen ovale; causes left to right shunting of blood
   b. cyanosis on exertion
   c. history of frequent upper respiratory infections
   d. loud murmur hear on auscultation
   e. congestive heart failure (CHF) frequent complaint with severe defects
2. Planning, goals/expected outcomes
   a. family/infant will be prepared for surgery
   b. family/infant will be supported emotionally
   c. family will cope with infant's problem
3. Implementation
   a. prepare infant/parents for surgery to close defect
   b. provide emotional support to infant and family
   c. teach family to cope with reality of defect; surgical closure may be delayed to maximize child's growth before intervention
   d. prevent infection
4. Evaluation
   a. family/infant prepared for surgery
   b. family/infant supported emotionally
   c. family coped with infant's problem
   d. no CHF developed

B. Patent Ductus Arteriosus

Failure of fetal ductus arteriosus to close after birth; causes murmur, and overload of left ventricle (Fig. 8-1)

1. Assessment: signs and symptoms
   a. widened pulse pressure
   b. loud murmur on auscultation
   c. cyanosis on exertion
   d. growth below expected norm
2. Planning, goals/expected outcomes
   a. child/parents will be adequately prepared for surgery

   b. symptoms will be controlled until surgery
   c. family will cope with child's problem
3. Implementation
   a. surgery to close defect performed when symptoms indicate, usually after 1 year of age
   b. provide emotional support to child and family
   c. teach family to cope with symptoms
   d. preoperative preparation and postoperative care as appropriate
   e. mortality rate for elective closure very low
   f. prevent infection
4. Evaluation
   a. child/parents adequately prepared for surgery
   b. symptoms controlled until surgery
   c. family coped with child's problem
   d. child recovered from surgery without complications

C. Coarctation of Aorta

Narrowing of aorta; usually causes hypertension in upper body and hypotension in lower body (Fig. 8-1)

1. Assessment
   a. hypertension in arms and hypotension in legs
   b. history of cephalgia and epistaxis
   c. auscultation may not reveal any murmurs
2. Planning, goals/expected outcomes
   a. surgery will be delayed to allow child to grow
   b. child/parents will be adequately prepared for surgery
   c. child will recover from surgery without complications
3. Implementation
   a. surgery to resect aorta or to insert graft, treatment of choice
   b. teach parents care of child
   c. preoperative and postoperative care as appropriate
   d. prevent infection
4. Evaluation
   a. surgery delayed to allow child to grow
   b. child/parents adequately prepared for surgery
   c. child recovered from surgery without complications

II. CONGENITAL: CYANOTIC HEART DEFECTS

A. Tetralogy of Fallot

Consists of four defects: (1) ventricular septal defect; (2) right ventricular hypertrophy; (3) pulmonary stenosis; and (4) overriding of aorta (Fig. 8-1)

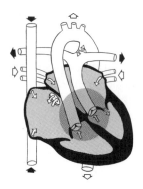

Complete transposition of the great vessels.
The aorta originates from the right ventricle and the pulmonary artery from the left ventricle; the aorta arises anterior to the pulmonary artery. This malformation results in two separate circulations. The systemic venous blood returns to the right-sided cardiac chambers, is then ejected into the aorta, and supplies the systemic circulation. The pulmonary venous blood returns to the left-sided cardiac chambers and is ejected into the pulmonary artery, supplying the pulmonary circulation.

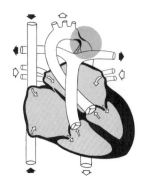

Coarctation of the aorta.
It consists of a narrowed aortic lumen, usually at the entrance of the ductus arteriosus. A long, narrowed area (hypoplastic segment) may be located proximally to the coarctation and coexists with additional intracardiac defects. A bicuspid aortic valve coexists in at least half of patients. The constricted segment of the aorta obstructs blood flow, causing a difference in pressure across the segment. The elevation of pressure that occurs proximally increases left ventricular systolic pressure, which is accompanied by hypertrophy and, in symptomatic infants, dilation.

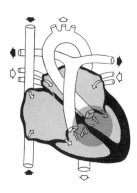

Ventricular septal defect.
An abnormal opening exists between the right and left ventricles. Ventricular septal defects can occur anywhere in the ventricular septum, but most commonly involve its membranous portion. Occasionally, more than one defect is present. Because the pressure is higher in the left ventricle than in the right and the systemic vascular resistance is greater than the pulmonary vascular resistance, blood shunts from left to right through the defect. Size of the defect is more important than its location. The clinical and laboratory features, treatment, and natural history vary with the size of the defect. The defects are classified as small and large.

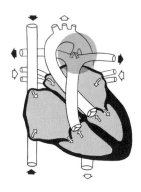

Patent ductus arteriosus.
Vascular communication persists that short-circuits the pulmonary vascular bed and directs blood from the pulmonary artery to the aorta during fetal life. Functional closure of the ductus normally occurs soon after birth. If the ductus remains patent after birth, the direction of flow through the ductus is the opposite of that in the fetus, passing instead from the aorta into the pulmonary artery.

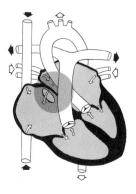

Atrial septal defect.
A hole in the atrial septum permits blood to flow between the atria. Before birth, blood flows from the right to the left atrium through the foramen ovale. This trapdoor-like opening in the septum normally closes after birth when left atrial pressure exceeds right atrial pressure. The foramen ovale then gradually undergoes anatomic fusion in infancy. However, if the foramen ovale retains its patency instead of becoming anatomically fused and is subsequently subjected to tension, it may gap open, permitting a right-to-left shunt. Likewise, if the left atrium dilates because of a large blood flow, the foramen ovale may be stretched, permitting a left-to-right shunt.

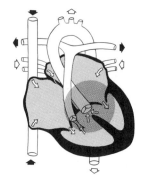

Tetralogy of Fallot.
Four conditions are present: pulmonary stenosis, ventricular septal defect, overriding aorta, and hypertrophy of the right ventricle. The obstruction can be located in the outflow area (infundibulum) of the right ventricle or at the pulmonary valve or valve ring. Or the pulmonary arteries may be reduced in caliber. A combination of these obstructions is usually present. The ventricular defect is usually large, causing equalization of pressure between the two ventricles. Because of the obstruction to blood flow from the right ventricle into the pulmonary artery, unsaturated blood flows through the ventricular septal defect into the aorta.

FIGURE 8–1. Congenital heart abnormalities. (From Congenital Heart Abnormalities. Clinical Education Aid No. 7. Ross Laboratories, Columbus, Ohio.)

1. Assessment: signs and symptoms
   a. cyanosis, periodic loss of consciousness, convulsions
   b. child assumes characteristic squatting position to facilitate breathing; preference for squatting position as child's activity increases
   c. clubbing of fingers
   d. growth and development below expected norm

2. Planning, goals/expected outcomes
   a. preoperative cyanosis will be minimized
   b. child/parents will be adequately prepared for surgery
   c. child will recover from surgery without complications

3. Implementation
   a. assist with best position for breathing

b. provide emotional support to child and family
c. teach child/parent to cope with symptoms
d. preoperative preparation and postoperative care as appropriate
e. prevent infection
f. surgery delayed to permit child to grow
4. Evaluation
   a. preoperative cyanosis minimized
   b. child/parents adequately prepared for surgery
   c. child recovered from surgery without complications

B. Transposition of Great Vessels

Pulmonary artery leaves left ventricle, and aorta leaves right ventricle (Fig. 8-1)

1. Assessment: signs and symptoms
   a. dyspnea and cyanosis
   b. tachycardia and tachypnea
2. Planning, goals/expected outcomes
   a. preoperative cyanosis will be minimized
   b. child/parents will be adequately prepared for surgery
   c. child will recover from surgery without complications
3. Implementation
   a. prevent infection
   b. monitor vital signs
   c. provide preoperative and postoperative care, as appropriate
   d. provide emotional support for child and family
   e. temporary shunt for oxygenated blood into general circulation may be done in infancy with surgical repair scheduled later
4. Evaluation
   a. preoperative cyanosis minimized
   b. child/parents adequately prepared for surgery
   c. child recovered from surgery without complications

III. CARDIAC SURGERY

A. Assessment

1. Preoperative observations
   a. vital signs to detect infection or CHF
   b. sleep/activity schedule to lessen stress in postoperative period
   c. bowel and bladder elimination
   d. fluid and food intake patterns to identify preferences and pattern of consumption
2. Most commonly done for infants and toddlers with congenital heart abnormality

B. Planning, Goals/Expected Outcomes

1. Child will be adequately prepared for surgery
2. Child will recover from surgery without complications

C. Implementation

1. Preoperatively
   a. familiarize child with environment, equipment, nursing personnel, and procedures
   b. use therapeutic play to practice postoperative procedures
   c. maintain preoperative schedule for least disruption
2. Postoperatively
   a. monitor vital signs continuously to detect pneumothorax, dehydration, and infection
   b. maintain patent airway
   c. monitor dressings for bleeding
   d. care for special apparatus, such as waterseal drainage (see Fig. 7-1)
   e. monitor hydration, intravenous and oral fluids
   f. increase activity as tolerated and appropriate for age
   g. provide emotional support for child and family
   h. discharge planning: foster independence, provide discharge teaching
   i. refer to follow-up agency

D. Evaluation

1. Child adequately prepared for surgery
2. Child recovered from surgery without complications

IV. CHRONIC CONDITIONS

A. Congestive Heart Failure

Failure of myocardium resulting in engorgement of heart and blood vessels; eventually increased pressure in pulmonary or venous systems

1. Assessment
   a. assess vital signs as indicated by condition; changes in pulse and respiration can mean decompensation
   b. assess edema by checking weight gain, visible edema in dependent tissues and periorbital area of infants
   c. most common in infant with congenital abnormalities

2. Planning, goals/expected outcomes
   a. child's heart will be maintained in compensated state
   b. child's condition will not deteriorate
   c. child/parents will understand and comply with therapeutic regimen
3. Implementation
   a. decrease cardiac demands by controlling activity, providing rest, and conserving energy; anticipate child's needs to avoid crying; decrease anxiety by teaching; maintain quiet environment
   b. reduce respiratory distress by using semi-Fowler's or Fowler's position; oxygen and humidity as ordered
   c. maintain nutritional status with small, frequent feedings and selection of nutritious, easily consumed, and easily digested foods
   d. administer digitalis (Table 7-5): count apical pulse for 1 full minute prior to administration; assess for toxicity and report vomiting, bradycardia, arrhythmias, pulse deficit; monitor potassium levels
   e. administer diuretics (Table 7-3): accurate intake and output; daily weights; encourage intake of potassium-rich foods, such as orange juice and bananas (Table 5-4)
   f. restrict fluids; record child's usual pattern of intake and schedule restricted fluids in accordance with usual drinking habits; administer fluids in small container; educate child/parents
   g. restrict salt; monitor diet selection; educate parents/child (Table 5-3)
   h. provide emotional support: keep parents informed of child's condition and scheduled therapies; encourage parental participation in child's care
   i. may be terminal condition: support parents' grief and remain with them; make child as comfortable as possible
4. Evaluation
   a. child's heart returned to compensated state
   b. child's condition did not deteriorate
   c. child/parents understood and complied with therapeutic regimen

B. Rheumatic Fever

General systemic and chronic disease affecting connective tissues of heart, lungs, brain, and joints caused by antigen–antibody reaction to beta-hemolytic streptococcus; usually follows streptococcal infection that occurred elsewhere in body

1. Assessment
   a. between 1 and 5 weeks following initial infection, symptoms begin: lethargy, low-grade fever, anorexia, muscle and joint pain, carditis, chorea, polyarthritis
   b. laboratory studies confirm diagnosis: C-reactive blood protein, positive throat culture for group A streptococcus, increased titer of antistreptococcal antibodies, increased erythrocyte sedimentation rate (ESR)
   c. most common in school-age child
2. Planning, goals/expected outcomes
   a. infection will be detected early
   b. child will recover from infection without complications
   c. child/parents will understand and follow therapeutic regimen
3. Implementation
   a. maintain bed rest with continuous cardiac monitoring
   b. position comfortably with good body alignment and support
   c. provide age-appropriate and nonstressful diversional activities
   d. continue observation on vital signs
   e. select nutritious, appetizing meals
   f. support child during frequent laboratory tests
   g. provide emotional support and preparation for discharge that emphasizes balance of rest and activity periods
   h. administer medications, especially salicylates for joint pain, steroids for inflammation, and antibiotics for infection; educate parents and child concerning medications
4. Evaluation
   a. infection detected early
   b. child recovered from infection without complications
   c. child/parents understood and followed therapeutic regimen

V. CARDIOPULMONARY RESUSCITATION (CPR)

A. Assessment/Implementation

1. *Airway*
   a. assess patency
   b. if occluded, clean out mouth and open airway using head-tilt/chin-thrust maneuver
2. *Breathing*
   a. determine if child is breathing
   b. if not, ventilate twice using mouth-to-mouth respiration
3. *Circulation*
   a. after two breaths, check for carotid pulse (brachial pulse in infant)

b. if no pulse, using 5:1 ratio, compress chest five times, then ventilate
c. for infants, compress at 100 times/minute; for children age 1 to 8 years, rate 80 to 100 times/minute

■ Diseases of the Blood

I. SICKLE CELL ANEMIA

Hereditary trait causing breakdown of red blood cells carrying abnormal hemoglobin S

A. Assessment (Fig. 8-2)

1. Defect leads to severe hemolytic anemia
2. Cells tend to be crescent shaped when under low oxygen tension
3. Transmitted as autosomal recessive trait, particularly among blacks

4. Noncrisis state: symptoms of severe chronic anemia, enlarged spleen, jaundice from excessive red blood cell destruction
5. Crisis state: symptoms of thrombocytic crisis with occlusion of small blood vessels producing swelling of hands and feet, swelling of large joints and surrounding tissues with severe pain, severely distended abdomen, fever

B. Planning, Goals/Expected Outcomes

1. Early detection of children with sickle cell disease
2. Long-term complications will be minimized

C. Implementation

1. Prepare for laboratory studies, including sickle cell slide test, sickle cell turbidity test, and hemoglobin electrophoresis

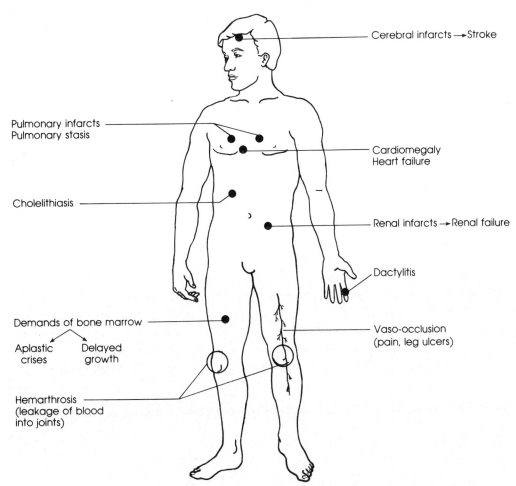

Cerebral infarcts →Stroke

Pulmonary infarcts
Pulmonary stasis

Cardiomegaly
Heart failure

Cholelithiasis

Renal infarcts →Renal failure

Dactylitis

Demands of bone marrow

Aplastic   Delayed
crises   growth

Vaso-occlusion
(pain, leg ulcers)

Hemarthrosis
(leakage of blood
into joints)

FIGURE 8–2. Potential effects of episodes of sickling. The fragility of the abnormal red blood cells results in their destruction and the formation of emboli and infarcts, and the leakage of blood into the joints. Virtually every system of the body can be adversely affected. (From Keane, C.B.: Essentials of Medical-Surgical Nursing. 2nd ed. Philadelphia, W.B. Saunders Company, 1986.)

2. Provide supportive care with IV and oral fluids
3. Monitor blood transfusions as ordered
4. Administer analgesics as ordered
5. Teach child and parents concerning disease and therapy
6. Teach parents about availability of genetic counseling

D. Evaluation

1. Sickle cell disease detected early
2. Long-term complications minimized

II. LEUKEMIA

Malignant blood disorder in which immature white blood cells increase in number, causing decrease in red blood cells and platelets in bone marrow

A. Assessment

1. Most common cancer in children, with acute lymphocytic leukemia the most common type
2. Signs and symptoms: anorexia, nausea and vomiting, weight loss, fatigue, pallor, fever, bone and joint pain, abdominal pain, petechiae and bruises, and enlarged spleen and liver
3. Diagnosed by presence of immature white blood cells, called blast cells, in blood and bone marrow
4. Most common in preschool children

B. Planning, Goals/Expected Outcomes

1. Leukemia will be diagnosed early
2. Child/parents will be adequately prepared for treatment regimen
3. Child/parents will be adequately prepared and will cope with prognosis

C. Implementation

1. Prepare for diagnostic tests
2. Provide support during bone marrow biopsy
3. Provide supportive and symptomatic care
4. Provide emotional support to child/parents to handle chronic, sometimes fatal, disease
5. Support during administration of antineoplastic drugs (Tables 7-22 and 7-23)
6. Observe meticulous medical asepsis to prevent infection

7. Maintain good nutrition
8. Provide careful skin and mouth care

D. Evaluation

1. Leukemia diagnosed early
2. Child/parents adequately prepared for treatment regimen
3. Child/parents adequately prepared and coped with terminal prognosis

III. HODGKIN'S DISEASE

Malignancy of lymph system characterized by presence of large, primitive, malignant cell

A. Assessment

1. History of frequent infections
2. Physical examination reveals enlarged, painless lymph nodes, especially cervical or groin
3. Most common in adolescents and young adults, rare before age 5 years
4. Very curable cancer with early diagnosis and treatment

B. Planning, Goals/Expected Outcomes

1. Patient will be diagnosed early
2. Patient will be prepared for treatment regimen including surgery, radiation therapy, and chemotherapy

C. Implementation

1. Prepare child for diagnostic tests, such as radiographs, lymph node biopsy, and lymphangiogram
2. Prevent infection
3. Provide emotional support to child and family to cope with debilitating and sometimes fatal disease

D. Evaluation

1. Patient diagnosed early
2. Child/parents complied with therapeutic regimen

IV. HEMOPHILIA

Sex-linked autosomal recessive hereditary disorder of delayed blood coagulation due to absence of clotting factor

A. Assessment

1. Easy bruising and bleeding into tissues
2. Diagnostic tests: bleeding time and clotting time show prolonged intervals
3. Injured areas show marked swelling and bruising
4. More common in boys

B. Planning, Goals/Expected Outcomes

1. Child will be diagnosed early
2. Child will develop minimal complications
3. Child/parents will understand and follow therapeutic regimen
4. Child/parents will cope with chronic, usually fatal illness

C. Implementation

1. Provide support during frequent laboratory tests
2. Prevent injury
3. Teach child/parents to understand nature of disease and factors to control
4. Provide support during blood transfusions
5. Refer to community agencies or support groups

D. Evaluation

1. Child diagnosed early
2. Child developed minimal complications
3. Child/parents understood and complied with therapeutic regimen
4. Child/parents coped with chronic, usually fatal illness

V. INFECTIOUS MONONUCLEOSIS

Infectious disease, believed to be caused by virus, results in increase in mononuclear white blood cells and signs of a general infection; thought to be only mildly contagious and spread by oral contact (sometimes called "kissing disease")

A. Assessment

1. History of exposure; incubation period around 10 to 14 days
2. Signs and symptoms: malaise; sore throat with pharyngitis; fever; enlarged liver, spleen, and lymph glands; lack of energy
3. Macular type of skin rash on trunk
4. Positive Monospot test
5. Most common in adolescents

B. Planning, Goals/Expected Outcomes

1. Transmission of virus will be minimized
2. Child will recover from disease without complications

C. Implementation

1. Maintain bed rest as necessary and gradually increase activity as symptoms decrease
2. Administer antibiotics as ordered
3. Administer nonsalicylate antipyretics as ordered
4. Maintain hydration with oral or IV fluids
5. Maintain good nutrition and provide diet as tolerated
6. Teach child and parents regarding need for rest and sleep
7. Maintain medical asepsis, isolation usually not necessary

D. Evaluation

1. Transmission of virus minimized
2. Child recovered from disease without complications

■ Pulmonary Disorders

I. ACUTE DISORDERS

A. Upper Respiratory Infection (URI)

Viral or bacterial infection affecting upper respiratory tract; also called nasopharyngitis or "common cold"

1. Assessment
   a. common in children of all ages
   b. signs and symptoms: fever, nasal congestion, sore throat, sneezing, cough, anorexia, irritability

c. laboratory tests, such as throat culture, rarely done (mainly to rule out streptococcal infections)
2. Planning, goals/expected outcomes: child will recover without complications
3. Implementation
   a. maintain bed rest or quiet environment until fever subsides
   b. maintain hydration with oral fluids
   c. administer antipyretics and decongestants as ordered (not aspirin because of risk of Reye's syndrome)
   d. humidify air to assist in decreasing congestion
   e. maintain adequate nutrition
4. Evaluation: child recovered without complications

B. Acute Otitis Media

Inflammation and infection of middle ear, frequently caused by infection-producing organism traveling through infant's shortened, widened eustachian tubes

1. Assessment
   a. signs and symptoms: fever, pain in ears, irritability, restlessness, pulling or rubbing ears, convulsions with high fever
   b. history of URI
   c. most common in infants
2. Planning, goals/expected outcomes
   a. condition will be diagnosed and treatment begun early
   b. child/parents will understand and follow therapeutic regimen
3. Implementation
   a. administer antibiotics and ear drops as ordered
   b. monitor vital signs
   c. encourage oral fluids to maintain hydration
   d. observe for ear drainage
   e. provide good skin care and cleanliness
   f. prepare for myringotomy as indicated: incision that opens tympanic membrane for drainage; may also include insertion of tubes to maintain patent incision for drainage
   g. teach child and family about cause and treatment of otitis media
4. Evaluation
   a. condition diagnosed and treatment begun early
   b. child/parents understood and complied with therapeutic regimen
   c. no hearing loss occurred

C. Bronchiolitis

Inflammation of bronchioles usually caused by virus; results in thick mucus plugging bronchioles and

trapping air in alveoli, leading to poor air exchange and difficulty in expelling air from lungs

1. Assessment
   a. signs and symptoms: dry, nonproductive cough, shallow respirations, air hunger and cyanosis, dyspnea, irritability, retractions, rapid respirations
   b. slight fever
   c. most common in infants
2. Planning, goals/expected outcomes
   a. child will recover without complications
   b. child will not have recurrence of disease
3. Implementations
   a. maintain patent airway
   b. position for comfort and to ease respirations (Fowler's position or raise head of crib)
   c. humidify air and give oxygen as ordered
   d. monitor vital signs frequently
   e. maintain hydration with IV or oral fluids and feedings as indicated by dyspnea
   f. conserve energy: provide rest and activity as tolerated
4. Evaluation
   a. child recovered without complications
   b. child did not have recurrence of disease

D. Bronchitis

Inflammation of mucous membrane of bronchial tubes **without** obstruction

1. Assessment
   a. history of URI
   b. signs and symptoms: dry, nonproductive cough, irritability, fever
   c. most common in infants
2. Planning, goals/expected outcomes
   a. child will recover without complications
   b. child will not have recurrence of disease
3. Implementation
   a. humidify air
   b. maintain hydration by encouraging oral fluids
   c. monitor vital signs
   d. perform postural drainage as ordered
4. Evaluation
   a. child recovered without complications
   b. child did not have recurrence of disease

E. Pneumonia

Localized inflammation of lung tissues caused by primarily bacteria or viruses; may also be from aspiration

1. Assessment
   a. signs and symptoms: nonproductive cough, fe-

ver, vomiting, diarrhea, convulsions with high fever, increased pulse and respirations
    b. laboratory tests showing increased white blood cell count
    c. chest radiograph positive for infiltrates
    d. most common in infants and toddlers
2. Planning, goals/expected outcomes
    a. child will recover without complications
    b. child/parents will understand and follow therapeutic regimen
3. Implementation
    a. bed rest until fever diminishes
    b. maintain Fowler's position or elevate head of crib for comfort
    c. monitor vital signs frequently
    d. maintain hydration by encouraging oral fluids
    e. administer antipyretics and antibiotics (Table 7-10) as ordered (not aspirin, which might lead to Reye's syndrome)
    f. control fever with sponge baths
    g. humidify air
    h. activity as tolerated, but prevent dyspnea
4. Evaluation
    a. child recovered without complications
    b. child/parents understood and complied with therapeutic regimen

F. Croup

Sudden attack of group of symptoms resulting from laryngospasm or obstruction of larynx; also called spastic laryngitis

1. Assessment
    a. history of runny nose or hoarseness
    b. signs and symptoms: barking cough, inspiratory stridor, retractions, restlessness, rapid respirations
    c. sudden onset of symptoms
    d. assess for symptoms of asphyxia
    e. fever may or may not be present
    f. usually occurs in children under age 5 years
2. Planning, goals/expected outcomes
    a. child will recover without complications
    b. child/parents will understand and follow therapeutic regimen
3. Implementation
    a. monitor vital signs frequently
    b. provide croup tent or mist tent for humidified oxygen
    c. maintain calm manner and environment to avoid upsetting child
    d. have tracheostomy tray at bedside for emergencies
    e. provide emotional support to child and family
    f. teach parents about emergency care at home;

inhaling humidified air from steamy bathroom shower may relieve acute symptoms
4. Evaluation
    a. child recovered without complications
    b. child/parents understood and complied with therapeutic regimen

G. Tonsillitis and Adenoiditis

Inflammation of tonsils and adenoids, caused by either bacteria or viruses and often accompanied by frequent URI

1. Assessment
    a. signs and symptoms: sore throat, difficulty in swallowing, hoarseness, nonproductive cough
    b. noisy breathing or difficulty in breathing, "mouth breathers"
    c. direct visualization of throat will show presence of redness and swelling of tonsils and adenoids
    d. most common in preschoolers
2. Planning, goals/expected outcomes
    a. child will be adequately prepared for surgery
    b. child/parents will understand and follow therapeutic regimen
    c. child will recover without complications
3. Implementation
    a. administer antibiotics as ordered
    b. provide supportive care of warm, salt-water gargles as age of child permits
    c. maintain hydration by encouraging oral fluids as tolerated
    d. prepare child/parents for surgery if chronic infections present
    e. postoperative care: monitor vital signs, check throat and nares for bleeding, observe for frequent swallowing that may indicate bleeding, prone or flat with head to side initially
    f. discharge instructions following surgery to include teaching child and parents concerning diet, fluids, activity, prevention of infections, delayed hemorrhage due to tissue sloughing
4. Evaluation
    a. child adequately prepared for surgery
    b. child/parents understood and complied with therapeutic regimen
    c. child recovered without complications

H. Sudden Infant Death Syndrome (SIDS)

Sudden, unexplained death of infant who was apparently healthy immediately before death; also known as "crib death"

1. Assessment
   a. often parent puts infant to bed and infant later discovered dead or infantile apnea noted (near-miss baby)
   b. assess for any physical cause; autopsy usually rules out any preventable cause
   c. research has not yet discovered cause for this syndrome
   d. evaluate apnea in near-miss baby
2. Planning, goal/expected outcome
   a. parents will cope with loss
   b. parents will learn care for near-miss SIDS baby
3. Implementation
   a. emotional support crucial to family; parents often feel tremendous guilt
   b. encourage psychologic counseling for parents, siblings, other family members, and care givers
   c. monitor for apnea/bradycardia continuously
   d. teach parents continuous monitoring of near-miss SIDS baby
   e. teach parents CPR
   f. emotional support to parents of near-miss SIDS baby
4. Evaluation
   a. parents coped with loss
   b. parents verbalized and demonstrated care of near-miss SIDS baby

II. CHRONIC DISORDERS

A. Cystic Fibrosis

Autosomal recessive hereditary disease caused by error in metabolism; generalized dysfunction of exocrine glands of lungs, pancreas, and liver; excessive amounts of mucus and sweat are produced, and these organs become obstructed

1. Assessment
   a. pancreatic involvement results in copious, bulky, greasy, foul-smelling stools containing large amounts of fat but no trypsin; infants eat well but do not gain weight
   b. lung involvement consists of chronic cough and frequent URI
   c. sweat gland involvement results in increased sweat chloride test over 60 mEq/L; salty "taste" to skin
   d. poor absorption of fat-soluble vitamin D can lead to osteoporosis
   e. pancreatic damage can lead to diabetes mellitus
   f. prognosis: chronic disease that may shorten lifespan, but many children now survive to adulthood
   g. family history of disease
2. Planning, goals/expected outcomes
   a. child will be diagnosed early
   b. child/parents will understand and follow therapeutic regimen
   c. child/family will be prepared for possible shortened lifespan
3. Implementation
   a. provide special nutrients and foods (especially pancreatic enzymes with food intake, vitamins, low fat and high protein diet, and additional salt during hot weather)
   b. prevent respiratory infection
   c. provide inhalation therapy, humidified air, percussion and postural drainage, breathing exercises, and mucolytic drugs as ordered to help break up mucus and keep lungs clear
   d. provide meticulous skin care to prevent irritation
   e. teach family concerning special care procedures, diet, and medications
   f. provide emotional support to family and child to accept and cope with this condition
   g. refer to Cystic Fibrosis Foundation and other community agencies
4. Evaluation
   a. child diagnosed early
   b. child/parents understood and complied with therapeutic regimen
   c. child/family prepared for possible shortened lifespan

B. Asthma

Obstructive airway disease caused by spasms of bronchioles due to hypersensitivity of airways

1. Assessment
   a. often caused by allergic response to pollen, food, animal fur; can also be triggered by emotional upset
   b. history of respiratory problems in family
   c. chest radiograph rules out other causes
   d. most common in school-age children
2. Planning, goals/expected outcomes
   a. child's asthma will be controlled
   b. child/parents will understand and follow therapeutic regimen
3. Implementation
   a. do environmental study to remove allergens as much as possible
   b. administer bronchodilators as ordered (Table 7-13)
   c. steroids may be given briefly to reduce inflammation, with care
   d. maintain hydration by encouraging fluids
   e. administer inhalation therapy and breathing exercises to maintain patency of bronchial tubes

f. monitor theophylline levels
g. teach child and parents to cope with condition
4. Evaluation
   a. child's asthma controlled
   b. child/parents understood and complied with therapeutic regimen

C. Allergic Rhinitis (Hay Fever)

Allergic response to allergen, such as pollen, dust, fur, or food

1. Assessment
   a. signs and symptoms: sneezing, watery and itchy eyes, runny nose, postnasal drip
   b. history of previous response to allergen
   c. allergy testing may be done
   d. most common in school-age children and adolescents
2. Planning, goals/expected outcomes
   a. child's symptoms will be controlled
   b. child/parents will understand and follow therapeutic regimen
3. Implementation
   a. do environmental study to remove allergens, if possible
   b. provide supportive therapy of decongestants and antihistamines as ordered
4. Evaluation
   a. child's symptoms controlled
   b. child/parents understood and complied with therapeutic regimen

■ Fluid and Electrolyte Balance

I. NORMAL FLUID AND ELECTROLYTE BALANCE

A. Assessment

1. Observe hydration of child; 73% of infant's weight is water
2. Laboratory tests for fluid and electrolyte levels

B. Planning, Goal/Expected Outcome

Child's fluid and electrolyte balance will be maintained in homeostatic state

C. Implementation

1. Provide proper balance of electrolytes for homeostasis

2. Provide adequate hydration for proper body functioning

D. Evaluation

Child remained in healthy homeostasis with correct fluid and electrolyte balance

II. FAILURE TO THRIVE

Failure to grow and develop within normal range; no apparent cause

A. Assessment

1. Below 5th percentile for height and weight
2. Malaise, listlessness
3. Poor appetite, poor eating habits
4. Unresponsive to being held and cuddled
5. Laboratory tests will rule out any specific disease entity
6. Evident in first few months of life

B. Planning, Goals/Expected Outcomes

1. Parents will learn effective parenting skills
2. Infant will have condition diagnosed early
3. Infant will begin to grow at normal rate

C. Implementation

1. Provide tender, loving care
2. Provide sensory stimulation: visual, auditory, and tactile stimulation needed
3. Give small, frequent feedings for weight gain; IV or nasogastric feedings may also have to be given
4. Provide emotional support to family
5. Encourage parents to assist in care; teach parents effective care of infant

D. Evaluation

1. Parents learned effective parenting skills
2. Infant had condition diagnosed early
3. Infant began to grow at normal rate

Questions

Sam is a 6-year-old admitted to the hospital for a diagnostic work-up. He has been experiencing a low-grade fever, weight loss, and pain in his arms and legs. His admitting diagnosis is rheumatic fever.

1. The pain most often associated with rheumatic fever:

  ① Results from involuntary muscle spasms
  ② Is located in the joints and migrates from one to the other
  ③ Is never associated with swelling or any other obvious symptom of the disease
  ④ May cause paralysis of the lower extremities

2. Rheumatic fever usually follows:

  ① Infections caused by beta-hemolytic streptococci
  ② Violent trauma to the body
  ③ Viral upper respiratory infections
  ④ Osteomyelitis

3. Sam is placed on complete bed rest after the diagnosis has been confirmed. The nurse can best explain this to Sam by telling him that:

  ① He must stay in bed or he will damage his heart and might die
  ② The doctor wants him in bed even if we have to restrain him
  ③ He must rest in bed while we will bring him everything he needs so he can get well
  ④ He can play quietly in his room as long as he rests whenever he is even slightly tired

4. The doctor orders aspirin every 4 hours for Sam. Salicylates are given to treat rheumatic fever because they:

  ① Help destroy the bacteria causing it
  ② Keep the body temperature subnormal
  ③ Prevent cardiac involvement
  ④ Relieve the joint pain

5. The most potentially serious complication from rheumatic fever is:

  ① Cardiac involvement
  ② Disintegration of the joints
  ③ Rheumatoid arthritis
  ④ Cerebral involvement

6. Maternal factors that may possibly predispose to the birth of a child with a heart defect include:

  ① Early maternal age
  ② Tuberculosis in remission
  ③ Excessive weight gain
  ④ Rubella during the first trimester of pregnancy

7. A symptom *not* associated with prolonged vomiting in infants is:

  ① Decreased skin turgor
  ② Increased urine output
  ③ Metabolic alkalosis
  ④ Decreased blood volume

8. Mary has returned to her room following a tonsillectomy. A symptom that does *not* indicate hemorrhage is:

  ① Increased pulse and respiration
  ② Frequent swallowing
  ③ Complaint of sore throat
  ④ Vomiting bright red blood

9. Tony, age 5 months, is diagnosed with asthma and placed on bronchodilators and steroids. Because Tony is receiving steroids, the nurse should assess for:

  ① Increased respirations
  ② Decreased respirations
  ③ Fluid retention
  ④ Increased fluid output

10. Infants under evaluation for prolonged periods of coughing and episodes of large bulky stools may undergo which of the following diagnostic studies?

  ① Sweat electrolytes for cystic fibrosis
  ② Gastric pH for gastroesophageal reflux
  ③ Barium enema for intussusception
  ④ Arterial blood gases to determine oxygenation

11. Alecia, age 2 years, is brought to the emergency room after waking up with a barky cough and stridor. On arrival to the emergency room, she is in no respiratory distress and afebrile. The diagnosis is spasmodic croup. The nurse instructs the parents to:

  ① Perform percussion and postural drainage before putting Alecia to bed
  ② Encourage frequent coughing and deep breathing
  ③ Run a cool mist vaporizer in her room at night
  ④ Follow the schedule of antibiotic therapy

12. Tara, age 3 years, is admitted to the pediatric unit with a left lower lobe pneumonia. She has a temperature of 39.5°C and is complaining of chest pain. Respirations are shallow with a rate of 60. Nursing interventions for Tara would include:

   ① Forcing oral fluids
   ② Positioning Tara on her left side with head elevated
   ③ Administering IV morphine for pain
   ④ Provision of a high caloric diet

13. What is the primary factor that causes the observable clinical signs in cystic fibrosis?

   ① Abnormal secretion of most of the exocrine glands
   ② Hyperactivity of the parasympathetic nervous system
   ③ Mechanical obstruction of gland secretion
   ④ Hypoactivity of the sweat glands

14. Which of the following best describes why cystic fibrosis can predispose a child to bronchitis?

   ① Elevated sodium in saliva can irritate the mucous membranes in the nasopharynx
   ② Related cardiac defects and congestive heart failure can cause increased respiratory distress
   ③ Neuromuscular irritability can cause constriction of the bronchioles
   ④ Thick secretions block the respiratory tract, causing impaired drainage from the bronchi

15. The preschooler with allergic rhinitis would most likely *not* experience symptoms when:

   ① Eating eggs
   ② Playing with the dog
   ③ Rolling in the grass
   ④ Lying on the rug watching TV

16. During an asthmatic attack, proper positioning can facilitate respirations. Respiratory effort is assisted if the child:

   ① Lies flat and is turned side to side frequently
   ② Sits upright and leans over a table
   ③ Lies on his or her side with head up 30 degrees
   ④ Lies flat with legs raised to promote venous return

Answers & Rationales

Guide to item identification (see pp. 3–5 for further details about each category)

I, II, III, or IV for the phase of the nursing process
1, 2, 3, or 4 for the category of client needs
A, B, C, D, E, F, or G for the category of human functioning
Specific content category by name; ie, cholecystectomy

1. ② Migratory polyarthritis is a common symptom that does not cause permanent joint destruction.
IV, 2, B & E. Rheumatic Fever.

2. ① The causative agent for rheumatic fever is the beta-hemolytic streptococcus.
IV, 2, B & E. Rheumatic Fever.

3. ③ A child will cooperate better if he knows the reason for the restrictions and also knows that all of his needs will be met.
III, 2, B & E. Rheumatic Fever.

4. ④ Aspirin is a nonsteroidal antiinflammatory that helps relieve the joint pain.
IV, 2, B & E. Rheumatic Fever.

5. ① Valvular heart damage is common following rheumatic fever, especially mitral valve disease.
IV, 2, B & E. Rheumatic Fever.

6. ④ Rubella or measles during the first trimester in the mother can lead to serious heart defects in the fetus.
IV, 4, B. Rubella.

7. ② The fluid and electrolyte imbalance from prolonged vomiting in an infant would lead to a decrease in the urine output.
I, 4, B. Fluid & Electrolytes.

8. ③ A complaint of a sore throat, while a normal postoperative complaint, does not signify hemorrhage.
I, 2, B. Tonsillitis.

9. ③ Steroids often cause the child to retain sodium and fluid.
IV, 2, B. Asthma.

10. ① Sweat electrolytes are elevated in children with cystic fibrosis. These children demonstrate coughing as well as unusual stooling as first signs and symptoms of the disease.
I, 1, B. Cystic Fibrosis.

11. ③ Laryngeal spasm is relieved by provision of a high-humidity atmosphere, especially at night.
III, 2, B. Croup.

12. ② Children are generally more comfortable semi-erect, lying on the affected side to splint the chest wall and to reduce painful pleural rubbing. Children who are dyspneic are given nothing by mouth because of the danger of aspiration.
III, 2, B. Pneumonia.

13. ① The primary abnormality in cystic fibrosis is an abnormality in the secretions of the exocrine glands, resulting in a thick mucus production.
I, 2, B. Cystic Fibrosis.

14. ④ Thick secretions cause impaired drainage from the bronchi, leading to chronic cough, bronchitis, and bronchopneumonia.
I, 2, B. Cystic Fibrosis.

15. ① Allergic rhinitis results from inhalation of certain airborne particles.
I, 1, B. Allergic Rhinitis.

16. ② The child in respiratory distress is better able to breathe in a sitting position.
III, 2, B. Asthma.

SENSORY/PERCEPTUAL ALTERATIONS

■ Disorders of the Cerebral/Central Nervous System

I. SEIZURE DISORDERS

A. Epilepsy

Recurrent, transient attacks of disturbed brain function resulting in convulsive symptoms of general or localized nature

1. Assessment
   a. idiopathic epilepsy: no identifiable cause; genetic defect in metabolism in brain thought to be related
   b. organic epilepsy: history of phenylketonuria, hypoglycemia; prenatal birth or postnatal injury, CNS infection; trauma; genetic influences; toxic effects; brain tumors
   c. careful observation and recording of convulsions will help specify type of disorder and appropriate treatment
   d. classification of seizures
      (1) generalized seizures
         (a) absence seizure (petit mal): brief loss of consciousness; "staring" expression with immediate return to alert state
         (b) tonic-clonic seizure (grand mal): tonic (stiffening) and clonic (twitching) phases; may be accompanied by aura; loss of consciousness; incontinence; may be apneic with cyanosis; can progress to status epilepticus, a prolonged seizure and medical emergency
         (c) myoclonic seizure: single or repetitive muscle flexion spasms
         (d) atonic seizure: brief loss of posture or muscle tone
         (e) infantile spasms: massive myoclonus; occurs in infants 3 to 8 months of age
      (2) partial seizures: involved a localized area of cerebral cortex
         (a) simple partial: localized motor or sensory disturbance, usually without loss of consciousness
         (b) complex partial: psychomotor, temporal lobe seizures; often accompanied by tongue, hand, feet and/or trunk; may or may not involve loss of consciousness
   e. preparation and support during electroencephalogram
   f. observation of neurologic signs
2. Planning, goals/expected outcomes
   a. child will be diagnosed early
   b. child/parents will understand and follow therapeutic regimen
   c. child will not suffer injuries from seizures
   d. child/family will cope with chronic illness
3. Implementation
   a. provide safe environment for child: safe toys; quiet surroundings; protect during seizure
   b. teach parent and child concerning nature of disorder, self-help activities, safety, medication administration, emergency procedures
   c. provide emotional support to understand disorder and cope with long-term care
   d. administer anticonvulsant medications (Table 8-8)
   e. have emergency equipment available for resuscitation, suction, CPR
   f. refer to national foundations and community support groups
4. Evaluation
   a. child diagnosed early
   b. child/parents complied with therapeutic regimen

TABLE 8–8. Properties of Some Commonly Used Anticonvulsant Drugs

Drug	Side Effects	Comments
Luminal (phenobarbital)	Drowsiness, irritability, hyperactivity	Safest overall medication; bitter, often combined with other drugs
Dilantin (phenytoin)	Ataxia, insomnia, motor twitching, gum overgrowth, hirsutism (hairiness), rash, nausea, vitamin D and folic acid deficiencies	Generally effective and safe; regular massaging of gums decreases hyperplasia; used in combination with phenobarbital or primidone
Depakene (valproic acid)	Gastrointestinal disturbance, altered bleeding time, liver toxicity	Monitor blood counts; take with food or use enteric-coated preparations; potentiates action of phenobarbital and other drugs
Mysoline (primidone)	Ataxia, vertigo, anorexia, fatigue, hyperirritability, dermatitis	May be used alone or in combination; side effects minimized by starting with small amounts
Valium (diazepam)	Headache, tremor, fatigue, depression	Used in combination or alone
Clonopin (clonazepam)	Behavior changes, ataxia, anorexia, nystagmus	Effective for most minor motor seizures

Note: The physician determines the child's medication by the type of seizure and other factors. The goal is to achieve the best control with the minimum dosage and the least number of side effects. An important aspect of nursing intervention includes reinforcing the need for drug supervision and compliance.
(From Thompson, E. D.: Introduction to Maternity and Pediatric Nursing. Philadelphia, W.B. Saunders Company, 1990, p. 578.)

c. child did not suffer injuries from seizures

d. child developed normally and coped with chronic disease

B. Febrile Seizures

Seizures caused by high temperature (above 102°F or 38.8°C)

1. Assessment
   a. generalized seizure characterized by tonic and clonic movements and loss of consciousness
   b. significantly elevated temperature
   c. history of recent infection or illness or fever
2. Planning, goals/expected outcomes
   a. child/parents will understand and follow therapeutic regimen
   b. child will recover from disease without complications
3. Implementation
   a. prevent injury and ensure safety during seizure
   b. monitor vital signs continuously
   c. medicate as ordered, antipyretics (Tylenol)
   d. use nursing measures to lower temperature; eg, tepid sponge baths
   e. have emergency equipment for suctioning and resuscitation at bedside
   f. provide emotional support to child and family
   g. teach parent care during seizure and prevention of injury
4. Evaluation
   a. child/parents complied with therapeutic regimen
   b. child recovers without complications

II. CONGENITAL DISORDERS

A. Cerebral Palsy

Group of disorders caused by disruption of motor centers in brain; cause usually interruption of oxygen supply to brain occurring prenatally, during birth, or from accident or disease

1. Assessment
   a. motor development, difficulty with voluntary motor movements, developmental delays
   b. involuntary, random movements may be present
   c. history of mother, prenatally and during labor and delivery
   d. history of childhood accident or serious illness
   e. observation of weakness and spasticity of the extremities
   f. vision and hearing disabilities may also be present

   g. cerebral palsy from disease or accident can be manifested at any age
2. Planning, goals/expected outcomes
   a. diagnosis of disease will be made early
   b. child/parents will understand and follow therapeutic regimen
   c. child/family will cope with chronic disease
3. Implementation
   a. individualize care to specific needs of child
   b. maintain good body alignment, prevention of contractures, reinforcement of physical therapy or other ordered exercises
   c. maintain good nutrition
   d. prevent infection
   e. provide emotional support to child and family to accept long-term care; no cure
   f. teach parents and child concerning supportive appliances (eg, braces), activities of daily living, expected growth and development
   g. refer to national organizations and local support groups for assistance
4. Evaluation
   a. prenatal or birth injury diagnosed in infancy
   b. child/parents complied with therapeutic regimen
   c. child coped with disorder and altered life style

B. Hydrocephalus

Increased intracranial pressure due to overabundance of cerebrospinal fluid (CSF) within brain; this accumulation may be due to blockage of flow of CSF or to inadequate absorption, producing enlarged head and possible brain damage and retardation

1. Assessment
   a. increased head circumference and change in shape
   b. separating suture lines and bulging fontanels in infant
   c. eye abnormalities may be present: strabismus, nystagmus, and "sunset sign" (sclera visible around iris)
   d. malaise, lethargy may be present
   e. poor neck control; inability to support head in upright position
   f. feeding problems, anorexia, projectile vomiting
   g. diagnostic tests, may include computed tomography (CT) scan
2. Planning, goals/expected outcomes
   a. child/parents adequately prepared for surgery
   b. child will suffer minimal complications from disease
3. Implementation
   a. if surgery to implant ventriculoperitoneal shunt planned, preoperative care intended to prevent

infection, maintain good nutrition, provide for emotional support of child and family, and make the child as comfortable as possible

b. postoperative care will include maintenance of patent airway, observing neurologic and vital signs closely, supporting head and neck during any movement, prevention of infection, and emotional support to child and family

c. prevention of complications important during all phases of care

4. Evaluation
   a. child recovers from surgery without complications
   b. child suffered from minimal complications from disorder

C. Down's Syndrome

Chromosomal defect (trisomy 21, or extra chromosome), resulting in characteristic physical changes and mental retardation

1. Assessment
   a. history of mother: Down's syndrome often associated with advanced maternal age
   b. presence of particular physical characteristics, such as round face; thick, protruding tongue; almond-shaped eyes (origin of "mongoloid" description); small, flat nose
   c. developmental tests will show slow motor development and varying degrees of mental retardation
   d. hands show transverse palmar crease (simian crease)
   e. integumentary system usually shows dry, cracked skin
   f. child usually very happy and smiling
   g. usually diagnosed at birth or shortly after

2. Planning, goals/expected outcomes
   a. child/family will cope with diagnosis
   b. child will develop to maximal potential

3. Implementation
   a. individualize all care according to the needs of the child
   b. emotionally support parents, who expected "perfect baby"
   c. teach parents and family about syndrome and reasonable expectations and goals for child
   d. teach about normal growth and development and expectations for their child
   e. prevent infection; parent teaching to prevent infection
   f. provide stimulation for child
   g. teach parents care of child at home
   h. genetic counseling for future pregnancies
   i. refer to local agencies and support groups

4. Evaluation
   a. child/family coped with diagnosis
   b. child developed to maximal potential

D. Mentally Retarded Child

Impairment of intelligence from unknown cause or injury or disease

1. Assessment
   a. developmental testing will result in classification according to intelligence quotient (IQ):
      (1) educable mentally retarded: IQ between 50 and 75; capable of simple basic learning, social and sensorimotor skills can be developed; can learn activities of daily living
      (2) trainable mentally retarded: IQ between 35 and 50, can usually learn to communicate and interact on basic level; can learn independence with supervision
      (3) severely retarded: IQ between 20 and 35, constant supervision necessary; learning ability very poor
      (4) profoundly retarded: IQ below 20, minimal capacity to function at most basic level; requires custodial care
   b. history of child and family for disease or injury
   c. usually evident in infancy; may be diagnosed anytime during childhood depending on cause

2. Planning, goals/expected outcomes
   a. parents/child will cope with diagnosis
   b. child will develop to maximal potential

3. Implementation
   a. nursing care must be provided for child's developmental age, not chronologic age
   b. provide stimulation
   c. prevent infection
   d. techniques of behavior modification often useful
   e. provide emotional support to child and family
   f. teach family to cope with child's permanent condition and maximize his or her potential
   g. refer to local support agencies

4. Evaluation
   a. parents/child coped with diagnosis
   b. child developed to maximal potential

E. Spina Bifida

Spinal defect caused by failure of laminae to fuse or by absence of laminae; usually occurs in lumbosacral area; complications from involvement of spinal cord may occur

1. Assessment
   a. visual observation of defect and resulting spinal cord involvement

(1) spina bifida occulta: bony defect of laminae with visible dimple or indentation
(2) meningocele: bony defect of laminae with protrusion of meninges and cerebrospinal fluid into membranous sac
(3) myelomeningocele: bony defect with protrusion of meninges, cerebrospinal fluid, spinal cord, and spinal nerves into membranous sac; paralysis below level of defect usually occurs

b. observation of involvement of lower extremities, bowel and bladder function

2. Planning, goals/expected outcomes
   a. child/parents will be prepared for surgery
   b. child/family will cope with permanent deficits
3. Implementation
   a. if surgical closure of defect planned, preoperative care will include optimum skin care, nutrition, hydration, prevention of infection, and position of comfort to prevent pressure on sac
   b. postoperative care will include prevention of infection, optimum skin care, nutrition, hydration, and position of comfort with good body alignment
   c. do range of motion exercises to lower extremities
   d. provide bladder care, including Credé's method of expelling urine as appropriate
   e. provide emotional support to child and family to accept condition and resultant lengthy treatment
4. Evaluation
   a. child recovered from surgery without complications
   b. child and family coped with permanent deficits

III. INFECTIOUS DISORDERS

A. Meningitis

Viral or bacterial infection of meninges and cerebrospinal fluid

1. Assessment
   a. fever
   b. high-pitched cry, irritability
   c. physical examination will reveal nuchal rigidity
   d. seizures likely
   e. most common in infancy
2. Planning, goals/expected outcomes
   a. child/family will understand and follow therapeutic regimen
   b. child will recover from disease without complications
3. Implementation
   a. prepare for and assist with lumbar puncture; white blood cells and bacteria may be present

b. administer antibiotics as ordered; initially IV route may be used to assure optimum immediate dosage; IM and oral doses will follow as child's condition improves
   c. monitor vital signs
   d. monitor neurologic signs and level of consciousness
   e. IV may be used to give fluids and as vehicle for drug administration
   f. fluids restricted to prevent increased intracranial pressure
   g. sponge baths to reduce high fever
   h. maintain quiet environment when irritable
   i. provide emotional support for child and family
4. Evaluation
   a. child/parents complied with therapeutic regimen
   b. child recovered without complications

B. Reye's Syndrome

Acute encephalopathy following apparent improvement of viral infection

1. Assessment
   a. history of characteristic symptom of severe and persistent vomiting 1–7 days after onset of viral illness, such as influenza or chickenpox
   b. progression of symptoms to alteration in mental functioning, such as extreme sleepiness, disorientation, hostility or combativeness, loss of consciousness
   c. history of aspirin use has been connected with increase in severity of Reye's syndrome
   d. can occur repeatedly in one individual or in several children in one family
   e. most survivors recover completely, but some suffer from minor to severe brain damage and resultant disability
2. Planning, goals/expected outcomes
   a. parents will understand nature of illness and institute preventive measures
   b. diagnosis will be made early
   c. child/parents will understand and follow therapeutic regimen
   d. child/family will cope with residual deficits
3. Implementation
   a. quickly recognize symptoms, make accurate diagnosis, and begin immediate supportive care (extremely important); once mental changes have begun, progression may be very rapid and may lead to death
   b. maintain hydration with IV fluids as ordered
   c. emergency equipment needed to assist respiration should be at the bedside
   d. maintain convulsion precautions
   e. make accurate recording of signs, symptoms,

and history; Reye's syndrome can be mistaken for encephalitis, meningitis, diabetic acidosis, poisoning, or drug overdose

    f. provide emotional support to the child and family; Reye's syndrome can lead to death in 3 to 5 days from the onset of vomiting

    g. teach parents regarding signs and symptoms to be alert for and what to report to doctor

    h. provide preventive teaching complications of viral illness for all parents; Reye's syndrome **not** communicable but occurs following viral infection

4. Evaluation
   a. syndrome did not occur
   b. diagnosis made early
   c. child/parents complied with therapeutic regimen
   d. child/family coped with residual deficits

IV. BRAIN TUMORS

Abnormal growth within cranium; may be benign or malignant, but always treated surgically

A. Assessment

1. Signs of increased intracranial pressure, including vomiting, headache, irritability, malaise, widening pulse pressure
2. Neuromuscular changes, including unsteady ambulation and incoordination
3. Sensory loss in sight, hearing, perception
4. Specific symptoms can assist in locating tumor site within brain
5. Most common in school-age years

B. Planning, Goals/ Expected Outcomes

1. Child will have increased intracranial pressure diagnosed and treated early
2. Child/parent will be adequately prepared for surgery and follow-up therapy
3. Child will cope with any residual deficits

C. Implementation

1. With surgical removal, preoperative care involves maintenance of hydration, fluid restriction if indicated, good nutrition, safety and specific care for individual symptoms
2. Postoperative care will include prevention of infection and continuation of preoperative care

3. Monitor vital signs and signs of increased intracranial pressure continually
4. Control of fever with sponging
5. Observe seizures
6. Prepare chemotherapy and support during course of medication administration
7. Prepare for radiation therapy and support during therapy
8. Provide emotional support for child and family; acceptance of condition and realistic future goals for child

D. Evaluation

1. Child's increased intracranial pressure diagnosed and treated early
2. Child recovered without complications
3. Child coped with any residual deficits

V. DEGENERATIVE DISORDERS

A. Lead Poisoning

Poisoning from ingestion of lead from lead-based paints, plaster, and exhaust accumulation

1. Assessment
   a. central nervous system symptoms appear gradually: irritability, drowsiness, convulsions, weakness, vomiting, abdominal pain, constipation
   b. symptoms of encephalitis
   c. history reveals pica or eating of nonfood substances
   d. death may occur; residual mental retardation possible
2. Planning, goals/expected outcomes
   a. child will not continue to ingest lead
   b. child will recover without permanent damage
3. Implementation
   a. collect urine and blood specimens for tests to determine amount of lead in child's body
   b. tell parents to study environment and remove sources of ingested lead
   c. administer anti–lead-absorbing medications (chelation therapy); quantities of milk also sometimes used to form insoluble lead compound that is then excreted
   d. teach child and family concerning sources of lead and substitute safe chew toys and objects
   e. refer to community agencies for ongoing follow-up
4. Evaluation
   a. child's environment modified so lead ingestion does not continue
   b. child recovered without permanent damage

■ Vision/Hearing/Speech

I. AMBLYOPIA

"Lazy eye," reduced visual acuity in one eye caused by inability of eyes to focus and work together for binocular vision; without treatment blindness may occur in affected eye

A. Assessment

1. History of blurred vision, double vision, problems with "blind spot"
2. Examination with Snellen eye chart will pinpoint problem eye if child old enough to cooperate

B. Planning, Goals/ Expected Outcomes

1. Child/parents will understand and follow therapeutic regimen
2. Child will recover without complications

C. Implementation

1. Treatment usually application of patch to good eye so that child must use weak eye; this use will focus and strengthen weaker eye; length of treatment depends on severity and response to treatment
2. Provide emotional support to child and family; assistance with coping mechanisms
3. Teach child and family importance of following treatment regimen faithfully
4. Response to treatment best during preschool years

D. Evaluation

1. Child/parents complied with therapeutic regimen
2. Vision returned to normal

II. STRABISMUS

"Cross-eyed," failure of eyes to work together and focus on same object at same time for binocular vision

A. Assessment

1. Assess for eye deviations
2. History of problems with vision
3. Defect responds best to treatment during the preschool years

B. Planning, Goals/ Expected Outcomes

1. Child/parents will understand and follow therapeutic regimen
2. Child's vision will be normal

C. Implementation

1. Apply patch to stronger eye to force weaker eye to focus
2. Corrective lenses and exercises may be prescribed
3. If conservative therapy does not correct problem, surgical intervention to correct muscle defects may be indicated
4. Provide emotional support to child and family to follow treatment regimen exactly
5. Teach patient and family to understand the defect and methods to correct it for normal binocular vision

D. Evaluation

1. Child/parents complied with therapeutic regimen
2. Vision returned to normal level

Questions

1. When a congenital defect results in an increase in the intracranial pressure and size of the child's head, the child is said to have:

  ① Hydrocephalus
  ② Microcephalus
  ③ Anencephaly
  ④ A hydrocele

2. A symptom exhibited by infants with a cold that is rare in adults is:

  ① Nasal congestion
  ② Nasal discharge
  ③ A sore throat
  ④ A high fever

Sally Ponds, 4 days old, is admitted to the pediatric unit from the nursery with a diagnosis of Down's syndrome.

3. Which of the following are problems expected to develop in Sally?

  ① Slowed development once she reaches 1 or 2 years of age
  ② Profound mental retardation
  ③ More respiratory tract infections
  ④ Hearing problems

4. The symptom of Down's syndrome most evident during the initial newborn assessment would be:

  ① Asymmetry of the gluteal folds
  ② Hypertonicity of the skeletal muscles
  ③ A rounded occiput
  ④ Simian creases on the palms and soles

5. Which of the following would Sally need more than most babies?

  ① Frequent handling and rocking to keep her from crying
  ② Helping her parents learn to care for and about her
  ③ Teaching her parents to nipple-feed her
  ④ Preventing aspiration of formula by frequent burping

6. A common defect associated with Down's syndrome is:

  ① Deafness
  ② Congenital heart defects
  ③ Hydrocephaly
  ④ Muscular hypertonicity

7. As Sally grows, her development lags and it is found that she is moderately retarded. Which of the following activities is best for her?

  ① Challenging, competitive situations
  ② Simple, repetitive tasks
  ③ Detailed tasks
  ④ Tasks that can be accomplished in less than 1 hour

Mary Spring, 7 years old, has spastic cerebral palsy involving all extremities, and a history of grand mal seizures. She is admitted to the pediatric unit accompanied by her parents, with a diagnosis of bronchopneumonia.

8. Which of the following information is most essential to plan her nursing care?

  ① Abilities to perform activities of daily living
  ② Immunizations received
  ③ Family history of illnesses
  ④ Reactions to previous hospitalizations

9. Mary's rectal temperature is 103.6°F. In order to decrease her temperature, the PN should:

  ① Put her in a cool mist croupette with compressed air
  ② Sponge her trunk and extremities with tepid water
  ③ Encourage her to take clear liquids such as apple juice
  ④ Sponge her with a half water and half alcohol solution

10. Mary had a tonic-clonic seizure (grand mal seizure). Which of the following interventions would be done first:

  ① Loosen her clothing and protect her from injury by padding the crib
  ② Maintain a patent airway by turning her head to the side and suction her if necessary
  ③ Remain with her and administer anticonvulsant medications as ordered by the physician
  ④ Describe and record events before the onset of the seizure, during the seizure, and after the seizure

11. Mary is on a puréed diet. While feeding her, the PN sees that she has trouble eating because of?

　① Weakness of the muscles used in sucking and swallowing
　② Delayed eruption of the lateral and central incisors
　③ Inability to relax completely during meal time
　④ Loss of appetite due to bronchopneumonia

12. Which of the following interventions should the PN plan to implement each day prior to Mary's physical therapy?

　① Decrease the tension in her muscles by placing her in a warm bath
　② Administer a muscle relaxant as prescribed by the pediatrician
　③ Provide a rest period in a quiet room with decreased stimulation
　④ Decrease the tension in her muscles by massaging her extremities

13. Mary's mother states, "Mary is not progressing. I'm going to take her to another doctor who will take better care of her and help her get well." This comment probably reflects her mother's:

　① Anger at the health care team
　② Denial of Mary's condition
　③ Guilt feelings about Mary
　④ A lack of understanding of cerebral palsy

14. Rapid diagnosis of Reye's syndrome is essential. What health teaching can possibly prevent this life-threatening disorder?

　① It is associated with all viral infections and occurs primarily during the warmer months.
　② Children recovering from a viral infection will suddenly begin to vomit.
　③ It is a self-limiting disorder that may precipitate liver failure
　④ Aspirin administration during the febrile period seems to decrease long-term complications

15. Children receiving Dilantin to control seizures are instructed to:

　① Take it with Maalox to reduce gastric upset
　② Brush teeth frequently and see dentist regularly
　③ Eat a high fiber diet to reduce constipation
　④ Stay away from known sources of infection

Answers & Rationales

Guide to item identification (see pp. 3–5 for further details about each category)

I, II, III, or IV for the phase of the nursing process
1, 2, 3, or 4 for the category of client needs
A, B, C, D, E, F, or G for the category of human
  functioning
Specific content category by name; ie, cholecystectomy

1. ① The condition resulting when fluid causes an increase in the size of the skull and increased intracranial pressure is called hydrocephalus.
I, 4, C. Hydrocephalus.

2. ④ Infants are much more likely to develop high fevers from a trivial cold than an adult.
I, 4, C. Febrile Seizures.

3. ③ Babies with Down's syndrome have decreased muscle tone, which compromises breathing and coughing, leading to a likelihood of upper respiratory tract infections.
I, 2, B & C. Down's Syndrome.

4. ④ Simian creases are the only symptom always observable. Other physical characteristics may suggest Down's syndrome.
I, 4, B & E. Down's Syndrome.

5. ② Parents' response to the child may greatly influence their ability to care for child. Learning about the child and Down's syndrome may help them give better care.
III, 3, C. Down's Syndrome.

6. ② Babies with Down's syndrome have a high incidence of congenital heart disease, especially atrial defects.
I, 2, B & C. Down's Syndrome.

7. ② A child who is moderately retarded is unable to follow complicated procedures or remember detailed directions. Simple repetitive tasks provide all the challenge needed.
III, 4, A & C. Down's Syndrome.

8. ① When a child with cerebral palsy is hospitalized, routines used at home should be followed, so it is very important to know her abilities.
II, 1, C. Cerebral Palsy.

9. ② Tepid sponge baths reduce temperature by promoting evaporation. Alcohol baths may reduce temperature too rapidly, leading to vascular collapse/vasoconstriction, which defeats the purpose of the cool applications.
II, 1, D & C. Cerebral Palsy.

10. ② The most important action during a grand mal seizure is to maintain a patent airway. Accumulated secretions must be removed from the nasopharynx.
II, 1, B & C. Seizures.

11. ① Children with cerebral palsy often have feeding difficulties due to poor sucking ability and persistent tongue thrust. She needs to sit up to promote swallowing.
I, 1, C & F. Cerebral Palsy.

12. ③ Children with cerebral palsy tire easily but find it difficult to relax. A period of rest should be provided before physical therapy.
III, 1, C. Cerebral Palsy.

13. ② Parents of handicapped children experience a period of mourning for the normal child they were expecting. Denial of the child's condition is expressed by consulting a variety of physicians, one of whom, it is hoped, will change the child's diagnosis.
IV, 3, G. Cerebral Palsy.

14. ② Reye's syndrome appears to follow a mild viral infection from which the child is recovering. He then begins to vomit suddenly.
III, 1, C. Reye's Syndrome.

15. ② A common side effect of prolonged Dilantin administration is gum hyperplasia.
III, 2, C. Seizures/Medications.

PROTECTIVE FUNCTIONS

■ Immunization (Table 8-9)
■ Trauma/Accidents (Table 8-10)

I. ACCIDENTS

A. Assessment

1. Major cause of death of children; as independence increases during toddler and preschool years, risk of accidents increases; as environment broadens during school-age years and adolescence, accidents continue to be major threat
2. Determination of risk of environment
3. Determination of risk due to age and growth and developmental level of child

B. Planning, Goals/Expected Outcomes

1. Parents will understand risk of accidents and help prevent them
2. Child will not suffer injury

C. Implementation

1. Teach parents concerning accident prevention and supervision
2. Provide specific teaching concerning vehicle safety, home safety, water safety
3. Teach emergency first aid, poison control information, rescue squad information
4. Guide parents to teach children safety

D. Evaluation

1. Parents decreased risk of accidents
2. Child was not injured

■ Communicable Diseases (Table 8-11)

I. VIRAL DISEASES

A. Measles (Rubeola)

1. Assessment
   a. assess for clinical manifestations
   b. spread by direct contact with droplets; incubation period of 10 to 14 days
   c. prodromal symptoms of fever, malaise, cough, coryza, Koplik's spots
   d. preventable by immunization
   e. rash maculopapular
2. Planning, goals/expected outcomes
   a. child will be immunized
   b. child will recover without complications
3. Implementation
   a. provide supportive care during fever; administer antipyretics, sponge to lower temperature
   b. provide quiet environment; dim room if photophobia present
   c. humidify air to ease coryza and cough
   d. provide gentle skin care; keep skin clean
   e. maintain respiratory isolation to prevent spread of virus
   f. observe for complications of otitis media, pneumonia, croup, encephalitis
4. Evaluation
   a. child immunized
   b. child recovered without complications

B. Rubella (German Measles)

1. Assessment
   a. low-grade fever, malaise, conjunctivitis, coryza, sore throat, cough, swollen lymph glands; rash pinkish red and maculopapular

TABLE 8–9. Immunization Guide

Age	Immunization
2 months	Diphtheria ⎫ Pertussis ⎬ DPT Tetanus ⎭ Oral poliovirus vaccine (trivalent)
4 months	Diphtheria ⎫ Pertussis ⎬ DPT Tetanus ⎭ Oral poliovirus vaccine (trivalent)
6 months	Diphtheria ⎫ Pertussis ⎬ DPT Tetanus ⎭ Oral poliovirus vaccine (trivalent) (given in high risk areas)
15 months	Tuberculin test (at or preceding measles vaccine) Measles ⎫ MMR Mumps ⎬ Singly or combined Rubella ⎭
18 months	Diphteria ⎫ Pertussis ⎬ DPT Tetanus ⎭ Oral poliovirus vaccine (trivalent)
24 months	Hemophilus b polysaccharide vaccine (HBPV)
4–6 years	Diphtheria ⎫ Pertussis ⎬ DPT Tetanus ⎭ Oral poliovirus vaccine (trivalent)
14–16 years	Tetanus ⎫ Diphtheria ⎬ TD (every 10 years) (adult form) ⎭

TABLE 8–10. Typical Accidents According to Developmental Age and Prevention Strategies

Prevention Strategies Requiring Repeated Monitoring Across Various Ages

Automobile:	Use of child-restraint device in automobile (check at *each* visit)
	Never leave child alone in car
Burns:	Reduce hot water temperature
	Purchase and install smoke alarm
	Use nonflammable clothing and toys
Poisonings:	Safe storage of drugs, corrosives, and chemicals
	Use child-resistant caps on drugs
	Syrup of ipecac in the home
	Poison Control Number placed at telephone
Play:	Monitor safety of toys, activities, and sports appropriate to age
Drowning:	Supervise children around water
	Encourage swimming lessons

Developmental Landmarks	Event and Preventive Strategies

INFANT (0 TO 4 MONTHS)
Can roll, reach, grasp, and mouth objects
	Motor Vehicle Accidents
	    Child-restraint device
	Falls
	    Protect from falls during dressing, etc.
	    Keep one hand on baby
	Suffocation/Aspiration
	    Avoid use of plastic bags in and near crib and playing area
	    Avoid bottle propping
	    Check crib safety
	    Do not tie pacifier around neck
	    Keep small objects and toys with removable parts out of crib
	    Do not use pillows or excess blankets
	Burns
	    Water temperature of bath should be checked with wrist or
	        back of hand
	    Avoid handling hot foods or liquids near baby
	Drowning
	    Nonskid bottom in tub
	    Keep hand on baby in tub at all times

INFANT (4 TO 6 MONTHS)
Is mobile and is developing some fine motor skills
Can roll over
Touches, reaches, and grasps to learn about environment
Begins to understand off-limit areas (e.g., stove)
	Motor Vehicle Accidents
	    Continue use of child-restraint device
	Falls
	    Discourage use of walkers
	    Use gates at stairs
	    Highchair safety
	Suffocation, Aspiration, Strangulation
	    Keep drapery cords and mobiles out of reach
	    Avoid hard foods, such as raw vegetables, peanuts, popcorn
	    Avoid use of toys with small parts
	Ingestions, Poisonings
	    Place all harmful products out of reach
	    Remove poisonous plants from child's reach
	Burns
	    Begin to teach meaning of "hot" and off-limit areas
	Drowning
	    Never leave child alone in tub

INFANT (6 TO 12 MONTHS)
Creeps, crawls, is inquisitive
Pincer grasp has developed by 8 months
Pulls self up and other things down
May begin table foods around 8–9 months
Holds own bottle and begins to drink from cup
Teeth are developing
Has the capability to chew a teething biscuit and soft cooked
    foods
	Motor Vehicle Accidents
	    Continue use of child-restraint device
	Falls (from windows, down stairs, and from outdoor play
	    equipment)
	    Keep crib away from window
	    Constant supervision is required to prevent falls
	Suffocation, Aspiration, Strangulation
	    Child should sit when eating to prevent aspiration
	    Continue to avoid hard foods
	    Cut foods into small pieces
	Burns
	    Keep vaporizer beyond child's reach
	    Supervise constantly, especially in kitchen and bathroom
	Drowning
	    Same as for 0–6 months

Table continued on following page

TABLE 8–10. Typical Accidents According to Developmental Age and Prevention Strategies *Continued*

Developmental Landmarks	Event and Preventive Strategies

TODDLER (1 TO 3 YEARS)
Walks, runs quickly, and often darts onto the street
Is more independent and developing autonomy (will stray farther from a parent)
Not aware of dangers but is intent on exploration
Has unsteady gait
By 3 years has full set of deciduous teeth
Can reach higher and open lids, can turn doorknobs
May be learning to swim but continues to need supervision
	Teaching of child should begin at this age
	Motor Vehicle Accidents (as a passenger, cyclist, and pedestrian)
	    Reaffirm importance of car seat even if toddler resists
	    Ride in center of back seat (restrained)
	    Teach to stay off streets with riding toys and tricycle
	    Cannot be trusted, therefore requires supervision
	    Provide a fenced-in play area if possible
	Falls
	    Open windows from the top
	    Remove objects from crib that child could stand on to climb out window
	Suffocation, Aspiration
	    Table foods can be given but avoid nuts and other small, hard foods
	    Teach the danger of plastic bags and similar items
	    Teach the child not to run with popsicle sticks or lollipops in mouth
	Burns
	    Expand on teaching about hot things. Especially teach about hot water, the stove, and hot food on the stove
	Ingestions, Poisonings, Trauma
	    Reevaluate placement of poisons and medicines
	    Keep sharp objects out of reach
	    Use only child-resistant containers for poisons and medicines
	    Teach child about poisons
	Drowning
	    Close supervision around water
	    Teach not to run around pools or other bodies of water
	    Supervise in tub

PRESCHOOL (3 TO 5 YEARS)
Eager to learn and capable of understanding simple explanations
Has the motor and coordination skills to ride a tricycle and is learning to ride a bicycle
Curious and explorative, particularly outdoors
Active in playground and outdoor play
Motor abilities exceed cognitive skills, therefore, child engages in physical activities without foreseeing danger
Is more independent and may walk or ride bike in the neighborhood with less supervision than when a toddler
Engages in sex play
Engages in dramatic play
	All aspects of safety should be taught to child
	Motor Vehicle, Pedestrian, Cycle Accidents
	    Begin to teach how to cross street safely
	    Teach rules of the road
	    Teach purpose of car seats and seat belts
	Falls, Trauma
	    Caution against climbing into unsafe areas, marshy lands, drainage pipes, unsafe buildings
	    Teach child how to handle scissors
	Suffocation, Aspiration
	    Teach child not to run while eating
	    Teach child not to crawl into areas where he or she could be entrapped (refrigerators, drainage pipes, excavation areas)
	Burns
	    Teach fire escape rules
	    Caution child against playing with matches
	    Keep matches out of reach
	Drowning
	    Begin organized swimming lessons
	    Never leave alone in bath or while swimming
	Street Safety
	    Teach child not to accept rides or foods without permission of parents
	Bodily Injury
	    Teach child not to insert objects into body orifices
	Ingestion, Inhalation
	    Expand on teaching about poisons and medicines
	    Include teaching about cosmetics and sprays, which child may use in playing house

SCHOOL-AGE (6 TO 12 YEARS)
More coordination in motor skills
Runs, skips, jumps, climbs, constantly on the move
Active in sports
Increasing independence and need for peer acceptance
Curiosity about sexuality
	All aspects of safety should be taught to child
	Motor Vehicle Accidents
	    Pedestrian safety needs to be repeated
	    Bicycle safety must be emphasized
	Bodily Injury, Fractures
	    Teach how to prevent injury from cold
	    Teach safety related to hobbies, handicrafts, sports, mechanical equipment

TABLE 8–10. Typical Accidents According to Developmental Age and Prevention Strategies *Continued*

Developmental Landmarks	Event and Preventive Strategies
	Drowning
	Water safety
	Supervise water sports
	Burns
	Teach child appropriate use of matches and campfires
	Firearms
	Teach respect of firearms
	Avoid keeping a loaded weapon in house
	Bodily Harm and Trauma
	Reinforce to avoid taking things or getting into a car of anyone without parents' knowledge
	Teach child about harmful use of drugs, alcohol, and cigarettes
	Sex education to make child aware of "good touching" and "bad touching" to prevent sexual abuse
ADOLESCENT (13 TO 18 YEARS)	
Drive motor vehicles (cars, motorcycles)	All aspects of safety should be taught to adolescent
Peer pressure and their acceptance predominates	Motor Vehicle Accidents
Risk-taking to establish self with peers is common	Reemphasize use of seat belts
Activities in work and sports involve dangerous equipment	Emphasize the danger of alcohol and drug use (especially related to motor vehicle accidents)
Independence in all activities	Bodily Injury and Trauma
	Teach proper use of equipment and maintenance of equipment
	Drowning
	Teach water safety
	Instruct in the use of emergency care equipment
	Teach CPR
	Firearms
	Close supervision regarding firearms is required
	No loaded weapon in house

(From Foster, R.L., Hunsberger, M.M., & Anderson, J.J. Family-Centered Nursing Care of Children. Philadelphia, W.B. Saunders Company, 1989.)

   b. preventable by immunization
2. Planning, goals/expected outcomes
   a. child will be immunized
   b. child will recover without complications
3. Implementation
   a. administer antipyretics for fever
   b. provide supportive care for comfort
   c. teach child and family to avoid contact with pregnant women
4. Evaluation
   a. child immunized
   b. child recovered without complications

C. Roseola (Exanthema Subitum)

1. Assessment
   a. observation for persistent high fever; maculopapular rash appears as fever subsides
   b. most common in infant under 1 year; no immunization available
2. Planning, goals/expected outcome: child will recover without complications
3. Implementation
   a. observe for febrile seizures; take seizure precautions
   b. administer antipyretics; anticonvulsants may also be given (avoid aspirin)

   c. teach family to lower fever with tepid sponge bath
4. Evaluation: child recovered without complications

D. Varicella Zoster (Chickenpox)

1. Assessment
   a. prodromal symptoms of malaise, anorexia
   b. rash appears first as macule, then papule, then vesicle; itching intense
   c. no immunization available
2. Planning, goal/expected outcome: child will recover without complications
3. Implementation
   a. skin care important to prevent secondary bacterial infection
   b. administer Benadryl or antihistamines to ease itching
   c. teach child and family concerning scratching; pressure, calamine lotion, baths, and fresh linen will help
   d. observe for complications of encephalitis, pneumonia, sepsis
   e. isolate to prevent spread until vesicles dried
4. Evaluation: child recovered without complications

TABLE 8–11. Clinical Presentation of Infection

System Involved	Signs and Symptoms
Central nervous system	Lethargy or irritability
	Jitteriness or hyporeflexia
	Tremors or seizures
	Coma
	Full fontanel
	Abnormal eye movements
	Hypotonia or increased tone
Respiratory system	Cyanosis
	Grunting
	Irregular respirations
	Tachypnea or apnea
	Retractions
Gastrointestinal tract	Poor feeding
	Vomiting (may be bile stained)
	Diarrhea or decreased stools
	Abdominal distention
	Edema or erythema of abdominal wall
	Hepatomegaly
Skin	Rashes or erythema
	Purpura
	Pustules or paronychia
	Omphalitis
	Sclerema
Hematopoietic system	Jaundice
	Bleeding
	Purpura or ecchymosis
	Splenomegaly
Circulatory system	Pallor, cyanosis, or mottling
	Cold, clammy skin
	Tachycardia or arrhythmia
	Hypotension
	Edema
Whole-body system	"Not doing well"
	Poor temperature control (fever or hypothermia)

(From Klaus, M., & Fanaroff, A. Care of the High Risk Neonate, 2nd ed. Philadelphia, W.B. Saunders Company, 1979. Adapted from Gotoff, S., & Behrman, R. Neonatal septicemia. J. Pediatr. 16:142, 1972.)

E. Mumps

1. Assessment
   a. prodromal symptoms: fever, headache, earache aggravated by chewing and talking
   b. enlarged parotid gland(s); tender and painful
   c. preventable by immunization
2. Planning goals/expected outcome
   a. child will be immunized
   b. child will recover without complications
3. Implementation
   a. diet and fluids for bland, nonirritating, palatable foods
   b. administer analgesics and antipyretics as necessary; elixirs may be more easily tolerated than tablets (do not use aspirin)
   c. if orchitis develops, scrotal support may ease discomfort
   d. observe for complications of encephalitis, hepatitis, deafness, sterility (adult male)

4. Evaluation
   a. child immunized
   b. child recovered without complications

F. Poliomyelitis

1. Assessment
   a. observe for symptoms of fever, sore throat, vomiting, anorexia, abdominal pain
   b. symptoms may disappear with apparent recovery, but then central nervous system paralysis appears
   c. preventable by immunization
   d. postpolio syndrome may occur 30 to 40 years later
2. Planning, goals/expected outcomes
   a. child will be immunized
   b. child/parents will understand and follow therapeutic regimen
   c. child will recover without complications
   d. child/family will cope with resultant deficits
3. Implementation
   a. provide supportive care; bed rest as appropriate
   b. assist with ventilation as necessary
   c. assist with physical therapy as necessary
   d. position for good body alignment and support
   e. monitor for complications: respiratory arrest, permanent paralysis
4. Evaluation
   a. child immunized
   b. child/parents complied with therapeutic regimen
   c. child recovered without complications
   d. child/family coped with resultant deficits

II. BACTERIAL DISEASES

A. Diphtheria

Causative organism *Corynebacterium diphtheriae*

1. Assessment
   a. signs and symptoms: coryza without generalized symptoms of common cold; epistaxis, sore throat, fever
   b. physical examination for whitish gray membrane on tonsils or larynx
   c. preventable by immunization
2. Planning, goals/expected outcomes
   a. child will be immunized
   b. child will recover from illness without complications
3. Implementation
   a. maintain strict isolation
   b. maintain bed rest

c. humidify air

d. administer antibiotics: usually penicillin or erythromycin (Table 7-10)

e. monitor for respiratory obstruction: tracheostomy tray at bedside

4. Evaluation

a. child immunized

b. child recovered without complications

B. Pertussis (Whooping Cough)

Causative organism *Bordetella pertussis*

1. Assessment

a. symptoms similar to those of URI

b. cough that becomes more severe and paroxysmal

c. preventable by immunization

2. Planning, goals/expected outcomes

a. child will be immunized

b. child will recover without complications

3. Implementation

a. maintain bed rest and quiet environment when fever present

b. humidify air

c. maintain adequate hydration and nutrition

d. observe for signs of airway obstruction

e. provide emotional support for child and family

4. Evaluation

a. child immunized

b. child recovered without complications

C. Scarlet Fever

Causative organism group A beta-hemolytic streptococcus

1. Assessment

a. prodromal symptoms of high fever, tachycardia, headache, chills, vomiting, malaise

b. physical examination for red, enlarged tonsils and strawberry red tongue

c. no immunization available

2. Planning, goals/expected outcomes

a. child will be diagnosed early

b. child/parents will understand and follow therapeutic regimen

c. child will recover from infection without complications

3. Implementation

a. maintain bed rest during fever

b. administer antibiotics; usually IM penicillin, progressing to oral penicillin

c. teach child and family emphasizing importance of antibiotic therapy

d. administer analgesics as indicated; gargles and lozenges may also be used to ease sore throat

e. maintain adequate hydration by encouraging nonirritating fluids and bland foods

f. observe for complications, such as otitis media, rheumatic fever, glomerulonephritis, peritonsillar abscess

g. prophylactic antibiotic therapy may be indicated for contacts

4. Evaluation

a. child diagnosed early

b. child/parents complied with therapeutic regimen

■ Abuse

I. ABUSE OF CHILDREN

Physical, sexual, nutritional or emotional maltreatment or negligence of children by parents or others in position of care giver (see Chapter 10)

A. Assessment

1. Risk factors: unplanned pregnancy, premature birth, stepchildren, high expectations of children, parents themselves were often abused as children

2. Physical examination of child: unexplained scars, bruises, burns, and other injuries

3. Discrepancies in accounts from parents, child and others as to how injury occurred

4. Emotional interaction with child difficult; child withdraws from contact; passive, noncommunicative

5. Incidence of child abuse epidemic proportions

B. Planning, Goals/ Expected Outcomes

1. Abuse will be prevented

2. Abuse will be detected early

C. Implementation

1. Nurses have legal responsibility to report incidents of suspected abuse to proper authorities

2. Optimize bonding of infant and parents at every opportunity

3. Teach growth and development and reasonable expectations to parents

4. Be nonjudgmental but also fulfill legal obligations

5. Provide physical and emotional care for the child, including a safe environment and nonthreatening interaction

D. Evaluation

1. Abuse prevented
2. Abuse detected

■ Poisoning

I. Poisoning in Children

A. Assessment

Unusual behavior or evidence of empty container near children

B. Planning, Goal/ Expected Outcome

Poisoning will be prevented

C. Implementation

1. Teach family to prevent poisonings by locking medicines and dangerous chemicals out of child's reach
2. Contact nearest poison control center for important information when poisoning suspected; current first aid standard to contact poison center for any directions
3. Teach child beginning in infancy to avoid dangers

D. Evaluation

Accidental poisoning prevented

■ Skin Disorders

I. BURNS

Destruction of body tissue caused by coagulation of cells; most frequent accidental injury to infants and young children

A. Assessment

1. First degree: superficial, involving only epidermis; symptoms of redness, swelling, and pain
2. Second degree: involves epidermis and dermis; symptoms of redness, swelling, blisters, and pain; may result in scarring
3. Third degree: involves epidermis, dermis, and sometimes underlying subcutaneous tissues; can also involve deeper muscle and bone; symptoms of charring and destruction of nerve endings, sudoriferous glands, hair follicles; skin grafts necessary

B. Planning, Goals/ Expected Outcomes

1. Burns will be prevented
2. Child will recover from burns without complications
3. Child will regain maximal function

C. Implementation

1. Prevent infection
2. Maintain alignment and support to all extremities
3. Maintain adequate nutrition and hydration; IV fluids may be used initially
4. Choice of treatment will depend on type, extent, and depth of burn; open method with reverse isolation, sterile wet dressings (silver nitrate or similar drug), cream, skin grafts may be used

D. Evaluation

1. Burns prevented
2. Child recovered from burns without complications
3. Child regained maximal functioning

II. INFANTILE ECZEMA

Inflammation of skin (atopic dermatitis) due to allergic reaction to some allergen

A. Assessment

1. Observe skin for redness, swelling, papules, vesicles
2. Rash accompanied by itching, oozing, crusting; can occur on any part of body
3. Usually before age 2 years

B. Planning, Goals/ Expected Outcomes

1. Allergens will be identified and attacks prevented
2. Child will understand and follow therapeutic regimen
3. Child will recover without complications

C. Implementation

1. Provide meticulous skin care to keep affected area clean and dry
2. Apply local ointments, creams, corn starch for itching
3. Prevent scratching with adequate stimulation and cuddling; "mittens" to cover hands and elbow restraints only as necessary
4. Coordinate environmental study to find allergen and control or eliminate it as possible
5. Provide emotional support to child and family

D. Evaluation

1. Further attacks prevented
2. Child complied with therapeutic regimen
3. Child recovered without complications

III. IMPETIGO

Skin infection caused by *Streptococcus* or *Staphylococcus* bacteria

A. Assessment

1. Observe skin for red vesicles and pustules
2. Assist with collection of culture for positive diagnosis
3. Can occur as break in hand-washing technique in hospital nursery or pediatric unit

B. Planning, Goals/ Expected Outcomes

1. Infection will be prevented
2. Child will recover without complications

C. Implementation

1. Follow strict hand-washing technique
2. Isolate child
3. Administer parenteral, oral, or local antibiotics as ordered
4. Provide meticulous skin care
5. Provide emotional support to child and family

D. Evaluation

1. Infection prevented
2. Child recovered without complications

IV. RINGWORM

(*scalp—tinea capitis; body—tinea corporis; feet—tinea pedis*): fungal infection spread by direct contact

A. Assessment

1. Observe for papules, dry scales; itching
2. Commonly spread in close proximity of daycare or classroom situations

B. Planning, Goals/ Expected Outcomes

Child will recover without complications

C. Implementation

1. Provide meticulous skin care; remove crusts after washing
2. Apply antifungal ointments as ordered; antifungal medication may also be given orally

D. Evaluation

Child recovered without complications

V. PEDICULOSIS

Presence of lice on scalp and other hairy areas of body

A. Assessment

1. Observe for nits or mature lice on examination of scalp and hairlines
2. History of intense itching, known contact
3. Will recur without treatment of all infected family members and environment

B. Planning, Goals/ Expected Outcomes

1. Lice will be prevented
2. Child will recover from infestation without complications

C. Implementation

1. Shampoo and wash with special solution, such as Kwell or Rid
2. Wash all clothing, hats, bed linens in hot wash to destroy nits and eggs
3. Teach child and family to prevent recurrence
4. Provide emotional support to child and family

D. Evaluation

1. Lice prevented
2. Child recovered without complications

VI. HIVES (URTICARIA)

Allergic reaction to food, drugs, or other allergen

A. Assessment

1. Observe bright red, raised rash in patches; intense itching of affected areas
2. History of exposure to known allergen
3. Assist with allergy testing to identify specific allergen
4. Assess for progression of hives to anaphylactic shock (emergency situation)

B. Planning, Goals/ Expected Outcomes

1. Allergens will be identified
2. Child/family will understand and follow therapeutic regimen
3. Child will recover without complications

C. Implementation

1. Assist with environmental study to isolate and remove allergen if possible
2. Administer antihistamines or Benadryl to decrease inflammation and itching
3. Provide meticulous skin care to prevent infection
4. Teach child and family
5. Provide emotional support to child and family
6. Desensitization may be useful to prevent recurrence

D. Evaluation

1. Allergens identified
2. Child/family complied with therapeutic regimen

VII. ACNE VULGARIS

Inflammation of sebaceous glands; overactive sebaceous glands become blocked with sebum

A. Assessment

1. Observe face, chest, and back for comedones (noninflamed impacted sebaceous glands) or papules and pustules (inflamed glands)
2. History of patient's age and diet
3. Usually occurs during adolesence

B. Planning, Goals/ Expected Outcomes

Child will recover without complications

C. Implementation

1. Provide meticulous skin care to keep affected areas clean and dry
2. Teach patient concerning hygiene, and avoidance of stress
3. Administer oral medications or local creams and ointments as ordered
4. Provide emotional support to adolescent and family

D. Evaluation

Child recovers without complications

■ PERIOPERATIVE PERIOD

I. PREOPERATIVE PREPARATION (TABLE 8-12)

A. Assessment

1. Assess child's developmental level and choose activities and words appropriate to that level
2. Assess the child's knowledge of what to expect
3. Postoperative period can be less stressful and uncomfortable if the child has been prepared preoperatively

B. Planning, Goals/ Expected Outcomes

1. Child/parents will be adequately prepared for surgery

TABLE 8–12. Summary of Preparation of the Child for Surgery

Procedure	Modification
Consent	Parent or legal guardian
Blood work	Age appropriate restraint
Urinalysis	Age appropriate collection (U-bag)
	Assist school-age child
	Age appropriate instructions
Evaluate for respiratory infection, nutritional status	Utilize more objective observations in infants and toddlers because of child's limited verbal skills
Allergies	Indicate clearly on chart
NPO	Increase fluids prior to NPO
	Length of time may vary with age and surgery (6–12 hours)
	If surgery is late, place appropriate notice on child—"Do not feed me"
	Remove goodies from bedside stand—no gum
	Supervise hungry, ambulatory patients carefully
Vital signs	Approach child carefully, explain, demonstrate, allow more time
Void before surgery	Not always possible in infants and toddlers
Bath	Hospital gown—also may wear underwear or pajama bottoms depending on age, type of surgery
Identification	Ident-a band
Teeth	Check for loose teeth, orthodontic appliances
Skin prep	May be done in operating room (OR)
Nails	Trim, remove nail polish
Enemas	Not routine
Transportation	Crib or stretcher—parents may accompany to OR door
Emotional preparation	Preoperative tour
	Group and individual puppet play
	Body drawings of parts involved
	Play selected by child as mode of expression
	Support parents during surgery
Sedation	Usually 20 minutes prior to surgery
Record all pertinent data	Essentially the same, with pediatric modifications as indicated by the above

2. Child will recover from surgery without complications

C. Implementation

1. Since fear increases tension and pain, basic principle for preparation for hospitalization is to decrease fear of unknown
2. All hospital procedures should be explained in way geared to child's level of comprehension
3. Involve family members in child's care to lessen anxiety of both parents and child
4. As child's development permits, let child participate in decision making; give child choices to make; avoid yes-no answers
5. Be truthful in explanations; explain at level of child's understanding, but do not lie to child
6. Therapeutic plan can assist child to handle anxiety and fear
7. Maintain familiar routine with familiar objects and toys
8. Safety important at all times; appropriate restraints should be used as necessary for child's safety

9. Medication administration should be matter of fact and cheerful; allowing child to choose if injection to be given "in this leg or your other leg" makes child feel able to exercise some control over stressful situation
10. Preoperative teaching for specific surgeries should be geared to developmental level of child; describing anesthesia as "sleepy air," and assuring children they will not feel any pain can lessen anxiety
11. Telling child all details specific to surgery, such as IV infusions, dressings, tubes, medications, casts, traction, limitations of movement after surgery, where pain will be felt, limitations in diet, and frequent vital sign checks, will avoid surprise when the child awakens in recovery room
12. Answer all child's questions honestly at child's comprehension level
13. Provide emotional support to both child and family to lessen anxiety

D. Evaluation

1. Child adequately prepared for surgery
2. Fewer postoperative complications occurred

II. POSTOPERATIVE PERIOD (TABLES 8-13 AND 8-14)

A. Assessment

1. Determine how well the child has been prepared preoperatively and fill in the gaps in child's knowledge
2. Assess vital signs, wounds, IVs, pain, and any postoperative complications

B. Planning, Goals/ Expected Outcomes

1. Child will be adequately prepared for surgery and recovery based on developmental level
2. Child will recover from surgery without complications

C. Implementation

1. Continuity of nursing personnel will lessen anxiety of children
2. All procedures should be explained; use words appropriate to child's vocabulary and provide demonstrations with puppets or dolls to increase understanding
3. Teach family how to participate in child's care
4. Honestly tell child when to expect pain; administer pain medication as needed
5. Provide basic postoperative care, such as vital sign checks, observation of dressings, intake and output, IV infusion, Foley catheters, nasogastric (NG) tubes, diet limitation, and assessment of level of consciousness will be pertinent to the child's surgical procedure
6. Maintain safety at all times
7. Provide emotional support to child and family

TABLE 8–13. Hospital Play Nursing Intervention for Various Age Levels

Age	Play	Nursing Intervention
1 to 3 months	Rattle, music boxes, mobiles. Do not discourage finger-mouth activity. Allow free movements when possible.	Cuddle, rock, talk softly. Encourage liberal parent contact. Anticipate needs.
3 to 6 months	Play peek-a-boo, provide soft toys, squeaky toys, music boxes.	Smile, talk softly. Provide same caregiver. Use pacifier if oral feedings are restricted.
6 to 18 months	If child has own toy or blanket, encourage keeping it with child. Use mirror reflectors for immobilized child. Play identifying parts of body. Provide toys that child can mouth safely. Supervised crawling and walking when possible. Use sterilizable toys. Play give and take games. Toy telephone, cloth books, pots and pans.	Nurture growth and development by encouraging participation in care; eg, holding own bottle, but do not insist. Provide finger foods. Allow as much movement and exploring as environment and therapy allow.
18 to 24 months	Books, building toys, pictures, magic slates, action toys, foam blocks, toy telephones. Play games that show understanding of positive and negative demands.	Nurse or volunteer can read to child at child's level. Have child mimic word meanings. Use potty chair when possible. Allow child to help with daily care.
2 to 3 years	Read books and stories concerning separation and returning of visiting family. Coloring books, active and passive exercises, dolls, cars, clay, cuddly toys.	Provide alternatives instead of criticism. Understand and accept ritualistic behavior needs. Provide choices when possible. Allow child to assist with care. Use familiar terms for urination, defecation, pacifier, etc. Use potty chair when possible.
3 to 6 years	Tape recorders can be used to listen to familiar voices or songs. Dolls, cars, television, radio, cuddly toys, picture books, easily won games, simple puzzles, pop-up books. Encourage peer contact when possible. Use doctor-nurse dress-up clothes.	Encourage independence when possible. Allow child to participate in planning and carrying out routine care.
6 to 12 years	Provide school activities when possible to keep up with peers. Write cards to friends and classmates. Play show-and-tell to explain equipment and procedures. Provide visual and verbal contact with peers. Electronic games, books, checkers, card games, paint, drawing pad, baseball cards, television, radio, crafts, toys involving large muscle coordination, weaving.	Separate male and female when appropriate and possible. Provide for privacy needs. Have child participate in decision making when possible and in self care. Use reason and logic with child. Encourage self-expression. Hang up pictures child drew or painted. Provide private nook for personal items.
12 to 18 years	Provide school activities to avoid school problems on discharge. Write cards to friends and teachers. Provide hairstyling, deodorant, and pretty bedjacket when possible to enhance body image. Electronic games, checkers, chess, card games, puzzles, television, radio, crafts, weaving.	Separate sexes when possible. Have child help with ward activities when possible to feel useful. Set realistic standards and rules that may be required by diagnoses and therapy prescribed. Treat as an adult, do not talk down or order child. Provide private nook for personal items. Allow snack foods to be brought in.

(From Leifer, G. Principles and Techniques in Pediatric Nursing, 4th ed. Philadelphia, W.B. Saunders Company, 1982.)

TABLE 8–14. Summary of Postoperative Care of the Child

Procedure	Modification
Return from recovery room	Notify parents
	Smaller patients generally in crib
	Age appropriate safety precautions
Note general condition, alertness	Infant and toddler cannot verbalize fear or pain
Vital signs	Every 15–30 minutes until stable
	Blood pressure is sometimes omitted in infant
Evaluate for shock	Essentially same
Assess operative site for bleeding, dressing intactness	Essentially same
	Elevate casted extremities
	Circle drainage
Restraints	May be necessary to protect IV
	Remove periodically for ROM
Connect dependent drainage (urinary catheter, Levin tubes, oxygen)	Prepare child for sight and noises of equipment, draw pictures to clarify purpose
Position patient	Abdomen or side unless contraindicated; no pillow
IV	Should have pediatric adapting device
	Monitor rate meticulously as infants and small children respond quickly to fluid shifts
	Measure and record intake and output
Assess elminination	Bowel and bladder
Relief of pain	Hold, comfort small children unless contraindicated
	Be sensitive to behavioral changes, such as increase in irritability, crying, regression, nail biting passivity, withdrawal
	Administer pain relievers
	Involve parents in care
	Provide transitional object such as blanket, favorite toy, pacifier
	Be aware of transcultural considerations that provide familiarity and comfort
NPO	Until fully awake, babies are started on clear fluids by bottle unless contraindicated
	Avoid brown- or red-colored liquids, which may be confused with old or fresh blood
	Monitor bowel sounds
Consider diet	Advance clear, full liquids, soft regular
Observe for complications	Turn, cough, deep breathe, dangle feet, early ambulation—less of a problem in children
	Splint operative site with hands when child coughs

8. Referrals to community agencies and support groups should be made as appropriate to the child's surgical procedure
9. Provide care per developmental level
   a. infant: separation anxiety threatening; provide sensory stimulation; provide tender, loving care and cuddling and encourage parents to participate in care
   b. toddler: developmental stages may be disrupted during hospitalization; maintain rituals and routines to give child sense of control over frightening situations; explain to family that regression is normal behavior
   c. preschool child: sense of independence may be disrupted during hospitalization; therapeutic play and puppets can help work through anxiety, frustration, and painful experiences; answer questions honestly and encourage parents to do same; child-size wheelchairs, stretchers, and carts help to avoid feeling of being overwhelmed; regression is normal behavior
   d. school-age child: honest explanations important; children of this age value privacy; absence from peer group increases anxiety; opportunities for choices help foster sense of control; as child's condition permits, tutor or schoolwork assignments will help child keep pace with class; provide outlets for frustration through physical activity as appropriate
   e. adolescent: absence from peer group and social activities very threatening; body image fragile; privacy very important; maintain independence as much as possible; access to telephone and privacy for conversations may lessen resentment at separation from peer group; answer all questions honestly; heterosexual relationships important at this age; depending on seriousness of adolescent's condition, concern for future may produce anxiety

D. Evaluation

Child recovered from surgery without complications

■ Immune Disorders

I. HUMAN IMMUNODEFICIENCY VIRUS (HIV) AND ACQUIRED IMMUNODEFICIENCY SYNDROME (AIDS)

A. Assessment

1. Symptoms vague and nonspecific
2. Blood serotest reveals presence of HIV
3. Often transmitted in utero from mother
4. May be from transfusions

B. Planning, Goals/ Expected Outcomes

1. Child will be supported throughout disease
2. Child will not develop opportunistic infections
3. Child/family will understand and cope with terminal nature of illness

C. Implementation

1. Provide emotional support for child and family
2. Educate concerning ways HIV transmitted and how to prevent transmission
3. Provide supportive care for symptoms
4. Prevent secondary infections

D. Evaluation

1. Child supported throughout disease
2. Child did not develop opportunistic infections
3. Child/family understood and coped with terminal nature of illness

Questions

Bradley Mustin, age 2 years, has been brought to the nurse's home by his mother for an unexplained swollen arm. While assessing Bradley, the nurse notes several bruises over Bradley's shoulders, arms, legs, and buttocks in various stages of healing. Bradley is very quiet and refuses to look at the nurse. He also turns away from his mother.

1. The nurse suspects Bradley is a victim of child abuse. The nurse should report her findings to:

   ① The doctor
   ② The visiting nursing service
   ③ The county prosecutor
   ④ The county children's services agency

2. The first step of treatment of the family suffering from child abuse is:

   ① Assessment of the situation
   ② Immediate removal of the child from the home
   ③ Beginning criminal prosecution
   ④ Encouraging parent to attend support groups

3. The nurse assesses the mother and child for a negative parent–child fit. Which of the following statements by the mother may indicate a negative fit?

   ① "He's such a quiet child. He never gives me any trouble."
   ② "He really knows his own mind."
   ③ "He never tells me when his diaper is wet until it's too late. You'd think he'd learn."
   ④ "He didn't inherit my blue eyes. His are a light brown."

4. In her assessment, the nurse takes note of Bradley's age. She knows toddlers are the most common age group in which child abuse occurs. Erikson's developmental theory places the toddler in a conflict between:

   ① Trust vs. mistrust
   ② Autonomy vs. shame and doubt
   ③ Dependence vs. independence
   ④ Initiative vs. guilt

Jimmy Rogers, 5 years old, has had numerous upper respiratory infections (URI), complicated with middle ear infections. The pediatrician has recommended that he have his tonsils and adenoids removed.

5. Which of the following should the PN tell the surgeon about preoperatively?

   ① Jimmy's pulse is 92, respiratory rate is 24.
   ② Jimmy sometimes has difficulty swallowing.
   ③ Jimmy's upper right lateral incisor is loose.
   ④ Jimmy had an upper respiratory infection 2 weeks ago.

6. The PN plans to explain the experience to Jimmy. What should the PN do first?

   ① Explain to Jimmy the need for preoperative medications
   ② Tell Jimmy that his parents will be waiting in his room after surgery
   ③ Describe the appearance of the recovery room and the operating room
   ④ Ask Jimmy to tell you what he knows about the procedure

7. The PN is going to give Jimmy his preoperative medication. Jimmy asks, "Is it going to hurt?" The PN should reply:

   ① "If you lie very still, it won't hurt."
   ② "Shots don't hurt brave little boys."
   ③ "Yes, it will, but I'll stay with you until it stops."
   ④ "Yes, but it will only hurt for a little while."

8. Jimmy arrives in the recovery room after surgery. The best position for him is:

   ① Semi-Fowler's with his head turned to the side
   ② Prone with the head of the bed slightly elevated
   ③ On his back with his head turned to the right side
   ④ On his abdomen with his head turned to the side

9. When Jimmy starts to take fluids, which is best given first?

   ① Cool water
   ② Cranberry juice
   ③ Milk
   ④ Orange juice

10. Which of the following should the parents be told to report to the doctor after Jimmy's discharge?

   ① If he develops a heavy, dirty gray membrane over the tonsilar area
   ② If he complains of a sore throat on the sixth postoperative day
   ③ If he complains of an earache without fever
   ④ If he develops bleeding in the throat on the sixth postoperative day

11. A priority intervention for the child who has ingested Lysol is:

   ① Maintenance of hydration
   ② Removal of gastric contents by lavage
   ③ Observation for seizure activity
   ④ Prevention of vomiting

12. The long-term effects of lead poisoning are primarily related to:

   ① Neurologic damage due to cortical atrophy
   ② Prolonged anemia producing congestive heart failure
   ③ Decalcification of bones causing fractures
   ④ Kidney failure related to nephron damage

13. The nurse instructs the mother of a child with varicella to do all of the following **except**:

   ① Administer aspirin for temperature above 101°F
   ② Keep fingernails short
   ③ Apply Calamine lotion for itching
   ④ Encourage child's favorite liquids

14. When caring for Mark, who has varicella, the nurse prevents spread of the disease to other children by:

   ① Keeping Mark confined to his bed
   ② Placing Mark in a single room with the door closed
   ③ Wearing a mask whenever caring for Mark
   ④ Instructing all child who play with Mark to wash their hands

15. The most common cause of adolescent accidental injury involves:

   ① Motor vehicles
   ② Handguns
   ③ Skateboards
   ④ Alcohol

16. Gary has recently developed acne on his face. He asks you what happens to cause it to appear.

   ① Acne results from overactive estrogen that is eliminated through the pores in the skin.
   ② Acne is an inherited disorder that is transmitted via an autosomal recessive trait.
   ③ Acne is related to the overproduction of sebum, which blocks the sebaceous glands.
   ④ Acne is related directly to the excessive amount of masturbation engaged in by the adolescent.

Answers & Rationales

Guide to item identification (see pp. 3–5 for further details about each category)

I, II, III, or IV for the phase of the nursing process
1, 2, 3, or 4 for the category of client needs
A, B, C, D, E, F, or G for the category of human functioning
Specific content category by name; ie, cholecystectomy

1. The law requires all medical professionals to
④ report any suspected child abuse to the children's services department. If it is after hours, they often may be contacted through the sheriff's department.
III, 3, D. Child Abuse.

2. Without knowing the details of the situation,
① the nurse will not be able to decide the next action adequately. Removal from the parents is traumatic to the child and is therefore reserved as a last resort. Criminal procedures have proven fairly ineffective in changing the parents' behavior. Instead, they often blame the child for their trouble with the law. Without knowing the cause, the nurse cannot direct the parent to the correct support group.
I, 3, D. Child Abuse.

3. This indicates a normal behavior on the part of
③ the child that the parent sees in a negative and even unrealistic way.
I, 3, D & G. Child Abuse.

4. Because the toddler is striving for autonomy, he
② often ignores adult directives. If the parents are unaware of this normal reaction, they may find it frustrating and intolerable.
I, 3, A & D. Child Abuse.

5. Loose teeth are potential hazards during the
③ anesthetic procedure. They may become dislodged and aspirated by the child.
III, 1, D. Perioperative Care.

6. The first step in the teaching/learning process is
④ to determine the child's present knowledge. Further explanations are then planned accordingly.
I, IV, D. Perioperative Care.

7. Simple, truthful explanations of procedures

③ provide a basis for establishing trust with the school-age child. The nurse should remain with Jimmy after the shot in order to encourage him to verbalize his feelings.
III, 1, A, G, & E. Perioperative Care.

8. Before the child is fully awake, he should be
④ placed on his abdomen with his head turned to the side to promote the drainage of secretions and to prevent aspiration. When alert, he may sit up, but should remain in bed for the rest of the day.
III, 1, D. Perioperative Care.

9. Cool water or synthetic fruit juices are offered
① first. Red juices are avoided so that fresh blood in the emesis can be distinguished from ingested fluid. Citrus juices are avoided because they are irritating. Milk coats the throat, causing the child to clear his throat often, which may lead to bleeding.
III, 2, D. Perioperative Care.

10. Bleeding from 5 to 10 days postoperatively is a
④ possible complication of a tonsillectomy and adenoidectomy. This is the time when there is tissue sloughing as healing occurs. The sign noted is frequent swallowing and it requires immediate medical attention.
III, 2, B & D. Perioperative Care.

11. To prevent re-exposing the mucous mem-
④ branes, corrosive chemicals should not be removed from the stomach by emesis or lavage.
II, 1, D. Poisoning.

12. Late effects include learning problems, sei-
① zures, mental retardation, and cerebral palsy.
I, 1, D. Lead Poisoning.

13. Aspirin should not be given owing to high risk
① of Reye's syndrome.
III, 2, D. Varicella/Reye's Syndrome.

14. Varicella is spread via droplets by direct or indi-
② rect contact.
III, 1, D. Varicella.

15. Motor vehicles continue to be the leading cause
① of death in the adolescent period.
I, 1, D. Trauma/Accidents.

16. Acne is an inflammatory condition that in-
③ volves overactive sebaceous glands that become blocked with sebum.
III, 2, D. Acne Vulgaris.

MOBILITY

I. CONGENITAL MUSCULOSKELETAL DISORDERS

A. Congenital Clubfoot (Talipes Equinovarus)

Congenital malformation in which foot twisted inward; may affect one or both feet (Fig. 8-3)

1. Assessment
   a. physical examination shows obvious defect; foot turns inward and adducted
   b. usually diagnosed at birth or in early infancy
2. Planning, goals/expected outcomes
   a. child will be diagnosed early
   b. child will recover without complications
3. Implementation
   a. teach family to explain the condition to others
   b. treatment should begin as soon as possible; if not treated, bones, muscles, and tendons continue to develop abnormally
   c. less severe defects treated with application of Denis Browne splint for rotation, eversion, and dorsiflexion
   d. casts and surgery also used
   e. preoperative and postoperative care as appropriate
   f. teach family to continue prescribed routine after discharge
4. Evaluation
   a. child diagnosed early
   b. child recovered without complications

B. Congenital Dislocation of Hip

Congenital defect caused by shallow acetabulum, resulting in partial or complete displacement of head of femur; usually bilateral

1. Assessment
   a. observe asymmetry of gluteal and thigh folds on affected side
   b. observe limitation of movement and abduction on affected side
   c. usually diagnosed when child is a newborn or is 1–2 months of age
2. Planning, goals/expected outcomes: child will recover without complications
3. Implementation
   a. double diapering can be sufficient to maintain abduction in the newborn
   b. apply hip spica cast to maintain abduction in older infant; brace or splint may also be used
   c. teach family care of infant, important for successful treatment
   d. provide emotional support to infant and family
4. Evaluation: child recovered without complications

II. TRAUMA

A. Fractures

1. Assessment
   a. signs and symptoms of fracture: limitation of movement, displacement, pain, swelling, dis-

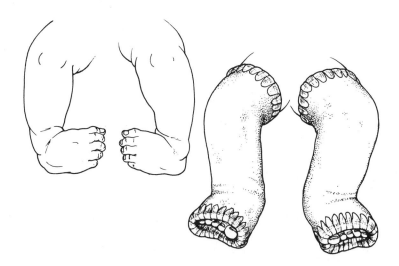

FIGURE 8–3. Bilateral talipes equinovarus (clubfoot) before and after application of plaster casts. Adhesive "petals" have been placed around the ends of the casts in order to prevent plaster from irritating the skin. (From Thompson, E.D.: Introduction to Maternity and Pediatric Nursing. Philadelphia, W.B. Saunders Company, 1990.)

coloration, bone fragment protruding through the skin (compound)
    b. history of fall or traumatic injury
    c. accidents leading cause of death in children of all ages
2. Planning, goals/expected outcomes
    a. fractures will be prevented
    b. fractures will be treated and heal without complications
3. Implementation
    a. provide emotional support to child and family
    b. maintain safety
    c. prepare for closed or open reduction as ordered
4. Evaluation
    a. fractures prevented
    b. fractures treated and heal without complications

B. Casts

1. Assessment
    a. observe extremity distal to cast for color, motion, sensation, edema, and irritation
    b. observe for unusual odor, bleeding
2. Planning, goals/expected outcomes
    a. circulation will remain adequate
    b. fracture will heal without complications
3. Implementation
    a. handle damp cast with palms to avoid fingertip indentations
    b. check pulse distal to cast; check capillary refill; check motion of phalanges; check sensation distal to cast
    c. protect cast from water, urine, feces
    d. teach child and family concerning safety while fracture heals; how to cope with itching and irritation; importance of not putting or poking anything into cast
4. Evaluation
    a. circulation remained adequate
    b. fracture healed without complications

C. Traction

1. Types of traction (Fig. 8-4)
    a. skeletal: pins, wires, or tongs for attachment
    b. skin: tape, moleskin, or bandages for attachment
    c. Bryant's: particular type of skin traction commonly used for infants and young children to treat fractured femur
2. Care of child in traction

a. maintain traction alignment and constant pull
    b. maintain good body alignment and support
    c. teach child and family to allay anxiety
    d. provide meticulous skin care to avoid breakdown
    e. maintain hydration and good nutrition for healing and growth
    f. encourage exercises as ordered to prevent decalcification, contractures, and atrophy during immobilization
    g. observe affected extremity for color, motion, sensation, edema, and movement
    h. administer pain medications as necessary

III. OTHER DISORDERS

A. Juvenile Rheumatoid Arthritis (JRA)

Systemic disease with chronic inflammation of one or more joints

1. Assessment
    a. both infectious and autoimmune theories presented for etiology
    b. symptoms of edema, congestion, and visible swelling of joints and synovial tissues
    c. assess joint movement, limitation, and pain as disease progresses
    d. redness and warmth at involved joints
    e. intermittent rheumatoid rash (macules)
2. Planning, goals/expected outcomes
    a. child/parents will understand and follow therapeutic regimen
    b. child will maintain functional ability
    c. child will adjust to chronic disease and disability
3. Implementation
    a. observe involvement of individual joints, systemic symptoms, and progression of symptoms
    b. monitor fever
    c. monitor affected joint warmth, redness, stiffness, and painful movement
    d. observe for involvement of eyes: photophobia, redness, discomfort, and vision problems; report them to physician
    e. provide exercise as ordered in nonacute states, with support to all joints
    f. provide emotional support to child and family
4. Evaluation
    a. child/parents understood and complied with therapeutic regimen
    b. child maintained functional ability
    c. child adjusted to chronic disease and disability

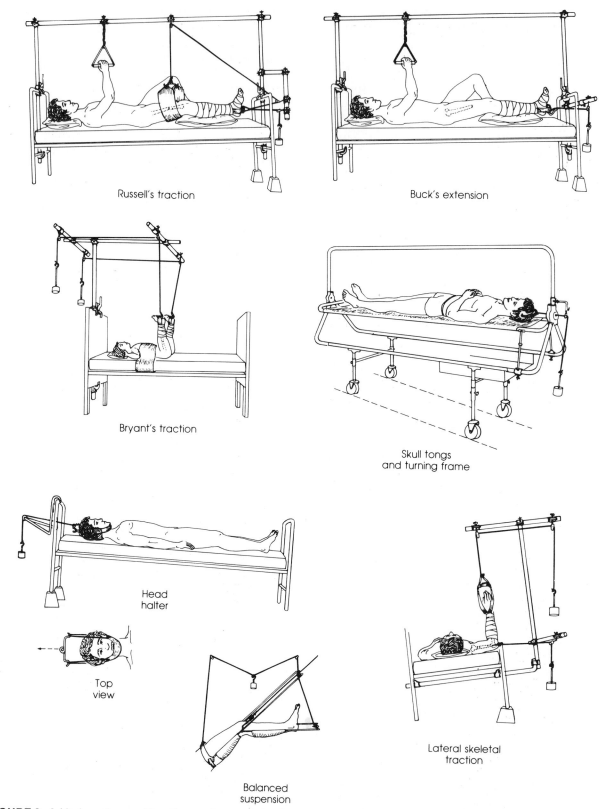

Russell's traction

Buck's extension

Bryant's traction

Skull tongs
and turning frame

Head
halter

Top
view

Balanced
suspension

Lateral skeletal
traction

FIGURE 8–4. Various types of traction and suspension. (From Keane, C.B.: Essentials of Medical-Surgical Nursing, 2nd ed. Philadelphia, W.B. Saunders Company, 1986.)

B. Scoliosis

Lateral "S" shaped spinal curvature that occurs during growth spurt at puberty

1. Assessment
   a. one shoulder or one hip higher than other, especially when child bends at waist
   b. one leg shorter than other
   c. complaints by child that clothes do not fit well or "look right"
   d. poor posture
   e. noticeable spinal curvature on examination of back
   f. more common in girls
2. Planning, goals/expected outcomes
   a. scoliosis will be diagnosed early
   b. child will recover from therapy without complications
3. Implementation
   a. first treatment usually application of Milwaukee brace or splint
   b. spinal fusion or rod insertion necessary in more severe cases
   c. prepare emotionally and be sensitive to needs of adolescent
   d. if cast in place for several months, teach family care of adolescent and how to meet developmental needs
4. Evaluation
   a. scoliosis diagnosed early
   b. deformity corrected without complications

C. Muscular Dystrophy

Hereditary, progressive degeneration of muscle; inherited as recessive trait

1. Assessment
   a. muscle wasting and weakness
   b. increasing disability, with difficulty in walking, a "waddling gait," and difficulty in standing up
   c. muscle biopsy and electromyography may be done to assist in diagnosis
2. Planning, goals/expected outcomes
   a. diagnosis will be made early
   b. maximal function will be maintained
   c. child/family will cope with altered lifestyle
3. Implementation
   a. prepare for and assist with diagnostic tests
   b. teach child and family to understand disease and accept fact that there is no cure; attempt to maximize child's potential
   c. assist with exercises as ordered to maintain function
   d. teach family to cope with assistive appliances, such as walkers, wheelchairs, crutches, braces, splints
   e. help with developmental testing to monitor child's progression; mild mental retardation frequently occurs
   f. refer to community agencies and support groups
   g. encourage genetic counseling for subsequent pregnancies
4. Evaluation
   a. diagnosis made early
   b. maximal function maintained
   c. child and family coped with altered lifestyle

D. Legg-Calvé-Perthes Disease (Osteochrondritis Deformans Juvenile)

Avascular necrosis of head of femur during rapid growth, followed by slow regeneration

1. Assessment
   a. joint dysfunction with limp and limitation of motion
   b. history of child's complaining of pain; may or may not be preceded by trauma
   c. most common in white males between 4 and 10 years of age
2. Planning, goals/expected outcomes
   a. child will not dislocate femur
   b. child/parents will understand and follow therapeutic regimen
   c. child will recover without complications
3. Implementation
   a. goal of nursing care to keep head of femur within acetabulum
   b. supportive devices, such as abduction brace, bed rest, traction, and casts, must be continued for 2 to 4 years; surgical correction usually permits child to return to normal activities within 3 to 6 months
   c. emotional support crucial to normally active child suddenly immobilized; family support extremely important
   d. activities need to be creatively utilized to maintain development of child; encourage child to begin new hobby or collection that can be done in bed
4. Evaluation
   a. child did not dislocate femur
   b. child/parents complied with therapeutic regimen
   c. child recovered function without complications

Questions

1. An example of a congenital anomaly in a newborn would be the presence of:

① Thrush
② Clubfoot
③ Purpura
④ Vernix

2. Brian, a 10-month-old, has a fractured femur. The most likely type of traction to be used would be:

① Buck's extension
② Bryant's traction
③ Balanced suspension traction
④ Skeletal traction

3. Which of the following best describes Legg-Calvé-Perthes disease?

① Dislocation of the head of the humerus
② Avascular necrosis of the femoral head
③ Evulsion of the tibial tuberosity
④ Pain around the brachial plexus

4. Acute pain is common for the child with Legg-Calvé-Perthes disease. Which of the following provides the most relief?

① Partial weight bearing on the affected side
② Bed rest and analgesics
③ Skeletal traction for 6 months
④ Repeated casting and muscle relaxants

5. Which of the following would be the best way for the PN to screen for scoliosis in school-age children?

① Observe the students in the physical education class touching their toes
② Observe the students in physical education for any students with a waddling gait
③ Advise students with knee pain to see a physician for radiographic follow-up
④ Observe the students in the physical education class for those with prominent buttocks

6. One of the students, Ellie, is found to have scoliosis. She is worried about how long the treatment for this is going to last. You should tell her that the treatment will last:

① For the rest of her life
② Until the curvature is less than 10 degrees
③ Until her body has reached bone maturity
④ About 2 to 3 years

7. It is recommended that Ellie have a Harrington rod insertion and spinal fusion. Which of the following is of greatest concern for the PN?

① Teenagers' need for privacy
② Presence of postoperative pain
③ Tolerance of the diet
④ Number of visitors each day

8. An infant with clubfoot is placed in a Denis Browne splint for discharge. Which of the following would be *inappropriate* in your discharge instructions?

① Prevent Sue from kicking or moving her legs
② Assess her feet regularly for signs of redness
③ Make sure that she always wears socks with her shoes
④ Maintain proper positioning within the splint

9. Harry, age 8 years, fell off his bike and broke his right tibia and fibula, and had a cast applied. Which of the following is a priority nursing intervention in his immediate postoperative care?

① Have him cough and deep breathe every 2 hours
② Elevate the head of his bed 30 degrees
③ Elevate and support his right leg on pillows
④ Wash off any excessive plaster

10. One of the most important assessments for the nurse to make on Harry is neurovascular status. Which of the following findings would provide the least useful information on this?

① Finding that femoral pulses are strong and equal
② Absence of numbness or tingling beneath the cast
③ Presence of positive blanching
④ Complaints of pain and tightness around his right ankle

11. Which of the following best describes Bryant's traction?

① Fractured leg suspended under the knee and held in extension
② Bilateral lower extremities elevated with 90 degrees hip flexion
③ Fractured leg held in extension with a pin through the distal femur
④ Bilateral extension of the lower extremities

12. Alisha, age 14 years, fractured her femur and is placed in skeletal traction. Which of the following is *not* a part of Alisha's care?

① Clean pin sites daily with antibacterial ointment

② Elevate the head of the bed daily

③ Assess neurovascular status below the fracture every shift

④ Turn her from her back to unaffected side every 2 hours

Answers & Rationales

Guide to item identification (see pp. 3–5 for further details about each category)

I, II, III, or IV for the phase of the nursing process
1, 2, 3, or 4 for the category of client needs
A, B, C, D, E, F, or G for the category of human functioning
Specific content category by name; ie, cholecystectomy ·

1. Clubfoot is a congenital anomaly occurring in
② newborns.
I, 4, E. Clubfoot.

2. Bryant's traction is a type of skin traction used
② on young children, usually under 2 years of age, to set fractures.
I, 1, E. Traction.

3. This disease is characterized by avascular ne-
② crosis of the head of the femur. It is not an infection but is related to impairment of the blood supply.
I, 2, E. Legg-Calvé-Perthes Disease.

4. Bed rest and analgesics are used to help relieve
② the pain of this disease. The main goal besides control of pain is the maintenance of function.
III, 1, E. Legg-Calvé-Perthes Disease.

5. When children bend at the waist to touch their
① toes, a child with scoliosis will have unlevel hips. The PN should be able to easily screen for this problem by simply watching the students.
III, 4, E. Scoliosis.

6. Scoliosis treatment must continue until the
③ bones have reached their maximum growth and maturity is reached. As long as the bones are growing, treatment must continue.
III, 2, E. Scoliosis.

7. The presence of pain is an important as-
② sessment because of the extensive nature of the surgery and the need for movement and exercise such as coughing and deep breathing postoperatively. Unless the pain is controlled, other postoperative complications are likely to occur.
I, 1, E. Scoliosis.

8. The Denis Browne splint is designed so that as
① the infant kicks, the feet are automatically moved into alignment. Limiting the child's kicking could delay development.
II, 4, E. Clubfoot.

9. One of the major problems post fracture reduc-
③ tion and casting is edema and impairment of circulation. For this reason it is vital that the affected limb be elevated to decrease the swelling.
III, 2, E. Fracture, Cast.

10. It is important to check the neurovascular status
① distal not proximal to the cast. The other options contain appropriate nursing interventions for the child in a cast.
III, 2, E. Fracture, Cast.

11. Bryant's traction uses the child's body as
② countertraction. Bryant's traction is skin traction.
I, 2, E. Traction.

12. When a child is in skeletal traction, it is impor-
④ tant to maintain the pull of traction without disruption. It is impossible to turn the child without disrupting the skeletal traction.
III, 2, E. Skeletal Traction.

METABOLISM/ELIMINATION

■ Metabolic/Endocrine Disorders

I. CONGENITAL DISORDERS

A. Hypopituitary Dwarfism

Growth retardation due to decreased secretion of growth hormone

1. Assessment
   a. delayed growth and development
   b. history of similar problem in family
   c. treatable if diagnosed early in development, before epiphyses close
2. Planning, goals/expected outcomes
   a. child will be diagnosed early
   b. child will be treated and return to normal growth pattern
3. Implementation
   a. provide emotional support to child and family
   b. administer growth hormone by injections as ordered
   c. teach child and family concerning importance of therapy and expected results
4. Evaluation
   a. child diagnosed early
   b. child returned to normal growth pattern with treatment

B. Congenital Hypothyroidism (Cretinism)

Severe deficiency of thyroid hormone due to some embryonic developmental defect

1. Assessment
   a. large, protruding tongue, dry skin, poor muscle tone, depressed reflexes, hoarse cry, coarse hair, and puffy eyes
   b. difficulty with feeding (slow, frequent choking)
   c. respiratory difficulties, including apnea, noisy respirations, and presence of nasal obstruction
   d. if not treated in infancy, dwarfed stature and mental retardation
   e. symptoms may not appear until 4 to 6 months of age in bottle-fed infants or after weaning in breast-fed infants; check developmental levels at well-child visits
   f. impaired development and mental retardation can be minimized if treated early in infancy

2. Planning, goals/expected outcomes
   a. child will be diagnosed and treatment begun early
   b. parents/child will understand and follow life-long treatment regimen
3. Implementation
   a. prepare for and assist with diagnostic tests, such as thyroid function studies and protein bound iodine
   b. administer thyroid hormone replacement as ordered
   c. teach parent concerning importance of continued, life-long replacement therapy
4. Evaluation
   a. child diagnosed early
   b. child/parent followed life-long therapeutic regimen

C. Phenylketonuria (PKU)

Hereditary metabolic disorder resulting in failure of body to metabolize amino acid phenylalanine

1. Assessment
   a. signs and symptoms of phenylalanine deficiency
      (1) anemia
      (2) anorexia
      (3) diarrhea
      (4) eczema
      (5) occasionally seizures
   b. slow development noted by 3 to 6 months
   c. mental retardation preventable if detected and treated; usually diagnosed in infancy
2. Planning, goals/expected outcomes
   a. child will have condition diagnosed early
   b. child/parents will understand and follow therapeutic dietary modifications
3. Implementation
   a. prepare for and assist with blood test for PKU; mandated by most stated health departments at age 7 days or after feeding but before discharge from hospital after birth
   b. teach parents concerning importance of testing every child to detect this preventable cause of mental retardation
   c. teach parents about strict diet to eliminate phenylalanine from diet until child is 4 to 5 years old
   d. refer to and consult with dietician for reinforcement of diet instruction with parents
   e. recommend genetic counseling for future pregnancies
4. Evaluation
   a. child had condition diagnosed early
   b. child/parents understood and followed therapeutic dietary modifications

II. CHRONIC DISORDERS

A. Celiac Disease

Defect of metabolism characterized by malabsorption of fat

1. Assessment
   a. chronic diarrhea with greasy, bulky, foul-smelling stool
   b. history of anorexia, growth retardation, irritability, distended abdomen
   c. usually diagnosed between 6 and 18 months of age
2. Planning, goals/expected outcomes
   a. child will have disease diagnosed early so complications will be prevented
   b. child/parents will understand and follow therapeutic dietary modifications
3. Implementation
   a. collect stool specimens for determination of fat content; 72-hour stool collection, keep on ice
   b. prepare for and assist with collection of blood specimens for determination of anemia
   c. teach child and family special diet eliminating rye and wheat gluten (starch free and low fat)
   d. provide emotional support to child and family
   e. prevent respiratory tract infections, which may exacerbate celiac crisis (severe vomiting and diarrhea, dehydration, and acidosis)
4. Evaluation
   a. child had diagnosis made early
   b. complications prevented
   c. child/parents complied with therapeutic dietary modifications

B. Diabetes Mellitus

Type I, insulin-dependent diabetes

1. Assessment
   a. inadequate production of insulin by beta cells of pancreas or improper use of insulin results in improper metabolism of nutrients
   b. rapid onset of symptoms in children: polydipsia (excessive thirst), polyphagia (excessive hunger), polyuria (excessive urine output), weight loss, glycosuria (glucose in urine), ketoacidosis
   c. history of diabetes in family
2. Planning, goals/expected outcomes
   a. diabetes will be diagnosed early
   b. child/parents will understand and follow therapeutic regimen
   c. blood glucose will be within normal limits so complications will be minimized
3. Implementation

   a. test blood and urine for glucose; urine for ketones also
   b. assist with glucose tolerance test and other blood glucose tests for positive diagnosis
   c. administer insulin as ordered (Table 7-28)
   d. provide emotional support for child and parents
   e. teach child and parents concerning importance of diet, exercise, urine testing or blood glucose monitoring, skin care, and signs and symptoms of hyperglycemia and hypoglycemia (ketoacidosis and insulin reaction)
4. Evaluation
   a. diabetes diagnosed early
   b. child/parents complied with therapeutic regimen
   c. blood glucose remained within normal limits
   d. child develops with minimal complications

■ Upper Gastrointestinal Disorders

I. CONGENITAL DISORDERS

A. Cleft Lip and Cleft Palate

Split or opening in upper lip that may extend through palate; developmental failure of bone and soft tissues of face to close properly

1. Assessment
   a. lip fissure; palate fissure visible on examination
   b. may choke with feeding; milk may return through nostrils
   c. more common in male infants; repair may be done in stages if defect severe
2. Planning, goals/expected outcomes
   a. parents and infant will be adequately prepared for surgery
   b. infant will recover from surgery without complications
   c. infant will receive adequate nutrition until surgery healed
3. Implementation
   a. provide meticulous mouth care to prevent infection or skin breakdown
   b. feed infant with large, soft nipple; guard against aspiration
   c. provide preoperative teaching for family as appropriate to prepare for closure of lip (as early as 2 to 4 weeks of age) or closure of palate (usually around 18 months of age)
   d. teach family to feed infant and prevent infection pre- and postoperatively
   e. postoperatively: side lying or supine position-

ing with elbow restraints to prevent rubbing on suture line

    f. teach family regarding developmental delays in speech as appropriate

4. Evaluation
    a. parents and child adequately prepared for surgery
    b. child recovered from surgery without complications
    c. adequate nutrition maintained

B. Esophageal Atresia

Developmental defect in which esophagus ends in blind pouch; if esophagus connected to trachea to form fistula, defect called tracheoesophageal fistula

1. Assessment
    a. excessive amounts of saliva and drooling
    b. choking, coughing, and respiratory distress during each feeding; regurgitation of all feedings; weight loss
2. Planning, goals/expected outcomes
    a. infant/parents will be adequately prepared for surgery
    b. nutrition will be maintained until surgery healed
    c. infant will recover from surgery without complications
3. Implementations
    a. prepare for passage of NG tube or catheter to assess patency of esophagus; support infant during diagnostic testing
    b. prepare for radiographic studies; teach family for all diagnostic testing
    c. suction nose and mouth as needed
    d. teach family and provide emotional support concerning surgical repair; not always successful
    e. maintain patent airway
4. Evaluation
    a. infant/parents adequately prepared for surgery
    b. nutrition maintained until surgery healed
    c. infant recovered from surgery without complications

C. Pyloric Stenosis

Congenital hypertrophy of pyloric muscle fibers, resulting in narrowing of pylorus (Fig. 8-5)

1. Assessment
    a. projectile vomiting during or soon after feeding; formula appears undigested or mixed with mucus

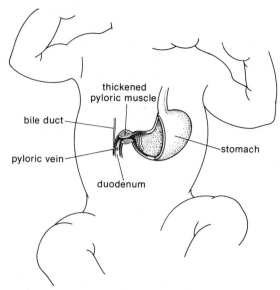

FIGURE 8–5. Pyloric stenosis. Hypertrophy, or thickening, of the pyloric sphincter blocks the stomach contents, causing the infant to regurgitate forcefully. Serious electrolyte imbalances ultimately occur, and surgery is necessary to correct the condition. (From Foster, R.L., Hunsberger, M.M., Anderson, J.J.: Family-Centered Nursing Care of Children. Philadelphia, W.B. Saunders Company, 1989.)

    b. weight loss and dehydration may occur
    c. presence of "olive pit" mass in stomach
    d. more common in male infants
2. Planning, goals/expected outcomes
    a. infant and parents will be adequately prepared for surgery
    b. infant will recover from surgery without complication
    c. infant's nutrition will be maintained until surgical repair heals
3. Implementation
    a. prepare for surgical repair (pyloromyotomy) by Fredet-Ramstedt method
    b. teach family and provide emotional support
    c. maintain hydration: IV fluids with adequate electrolytes
    d. postoperatively: feedings begun slowly with small amounts of glucose water, progressing to formula
4. Evaluation
    a. infant and parents adequately prepared for surgery
    b. infant recovered from surgery without complication
    c. infant's nutrition maintained until surgical repair heals

II. ACUTE DISORDERS

A. Gastroenteritis

Severe vomiting and diarrhea

1. Assessment
   a. may be caused by viral or bacterial infection, allergies to food or drugs, laxatives, or other irritants
   b. frequent emesis or loose, watery stools expelled with force
   c. symptoms of dehydration, including poor skin turgor, sunken fontanels, weight loss
   d. increased peristalsis and visible peristaltic waves
2. Planning, goal/expected outcome: child will recover without complications
3. Implementation
   a. maintain hydration; IV fluids as ordered, clear liquids with progression of diet as symptoms disappear
   b. record accurate intake and output, including diarrhea; daily weights
   c. establish isolation precautions (enteric) as appropriate for organism diagnosed
   d. record character, consistency, and number of emeses and stools
   e. provide meticulous skin care especially to perineum and buttocks; apply medications locally as ordered
   f. provide emotional support to infant, including tender, loving care with cuddling
   g. teach family; encourage parents to participate in infant's care as desired
4. Evaluation: child recovered without complications

III. CHRONIC DISORDERS

A. Anorexia Nervosa and Bulimia

Eating disorders characterized by abnormal weight loss without physical reason caused by self-starvation (anorexia nervosa) or binge eating followed by self-induced purging with vomiting or laxative use (bulimia)

1. Assessment
   a. history of psychologic disturbance concerning incorrect perception of body size, inability to perceive hunger, and poor self-esteem
   b. constipation, dry skin, anemia, weight loss, and amenorrhea
   c. most common in adolescent females
2. Planning, goals/expected outcomes
   a. patient will understand and follow therapeutic regimen
   b. patient will return to normal eating pattern and return to ideal body weight
3. Implementation
   a. provide adequate nutrition and hydration; often challenging to entire health team
   b. cooperate with behavior modification techniques and psychologic counseling
   c. monitor vital signs and daily weight
   d. monitor daily intake of both food and fluids; record number of emesis or stools
4. Evaluation
   a. patient understood and followed therapeutic regimen
   b. patient returned to normal eating pattern and returned to ideal body weight

B. Obesity

Excessive weight over 10% of normal body weight for age, height, and body build

1. Assessment
   a. assess eating habits and pattern
   b. weight 10% above ideal body weight
   c. most common during adolescence
2. Planning, goals/expected outcomes
   a. patient will understand and follow therapeutic dietary modifications
   b. patient will attain and maintain ideal body weight
3. Implementation
   b. provide emotional support and support psychologic counseling to discover cause of overeating
   b. prepare for diagnostic tests to rule out other causes
   c. teach patient and parents concerning proper nutrition and choosing well-balanced meals
4. Evaluation
   a. patient understood and followed therapeutic dietary modifications
   b. patient attained and maintained ideal body weight

■ Lower Intestinal Disorders

I. CONGENITAL DISORDERS

A. Megacolon (Hirschsprung's Disease)

Enlargement of portion of lower colon due to lack of normal innervation

1. Assessment
   a. lack of stools in newborn; progressive constipation as feeding and diet increase

b. abdominal distention, anorexia
2. Planning, goals/expected outcomes
   a. child/parents will be adequately prepared for surgery
   b. parents will understand how to care for colostomy
   c. child/parents will adjust to colostomy
   d. after closure of colostomy, bowel function will return to normal
3. Implementation
   a. prepare for barium enema and rectal biopsy to verify diagnosis
   b. administer daily enemas, irrigations, and stool softeners to evacuate colon
   c. provide emotional support to child and family
   d. maintain adequate nutrition; low residue diet may be ordered
   e. if indicated, surgery done to resect nonfunctional portion of bowel, with colostomy
   f. take temperature using axillary route
4. Evaluation
   a. child/parents adequately prepared for surgery
   b. parents understood how to care for colostomy
   c. child/parents adjusted to colostomy
   d. after closure of colostomy, bowel function returned to normal

B. Imperforate Anus

Developmental abnormality in which anus ends in blind pouch; anal opening may be absent

1. Assessment
   a. no stools within 24 hours of birth
   b. inability to insert rectal thermometer
2. Planning, goal/expected outcome: child will recover from surgery without complications
3. Implementation
   a. prepare for radiographs as ordered
   b. teach family about tests and surgery; provide emotional support
   c. teach parents about diet and postoperative care; anal dilations may continue to be needed
4. Evaluation: child recovered from surgery without complications

C. Omphalocele

Congenital defect of abdominal wall in which abdominal organs protrude into sac; abdomen covered with thin membrane

1. Assessment
   a. presence of sac or membrane in place of abdominal wall

b. outcome of surgery variable, depending on size of defect
2. Planning, goals/expected outcomes
   a. abdominal wall will be closed as soon as possible
   b. child will recover without complications
3. Implementation
   a. maintain sterile environment to prevent infection
   b. cover omphalocele with sterile dressings moistened with sterile normal saline
   c. teach parents about surgical repair; provide emotional support
   d. record passage of any stools
4. Evaluation
   a. abdominal wall closed as soon as possible
   b. child recovered without complications

D. Umbilical Hernia

Protrusion of portion of small intestine through weakness in umbilical ring

1. Assessment
   a. presence of physical defect on examination
   b. more common in blacks
2. Planning, goal/expected outcome: child will recover from surgery to reduce hernia without complication
3. Implementation
   a. teach family to avoid taping or binding hernia to reduce
   b. prepare for surgery; provide emotional support for child and family; surgery may be delayed unless symptoms persist
4. Evaluation: child recovered from surgery without complications

II. ACUTE DISORDERS

A. Intussusception

Telescoping (invagination) of one part of bowel into lower part (Fig. 8-6)

1. Assessment
   a. sudden, severe colicky abdominal pain; infant may draw legs up
   b. vomiting, presence of stools with blood and mucus, "currant-jelly" appearance
   c. signs of shock
   d. emergency situation; most common in male infants between 4 and 10 months of age
2. Planning, goals/expected outcomes
   a. infant/parents will be adequately prepared for surgery

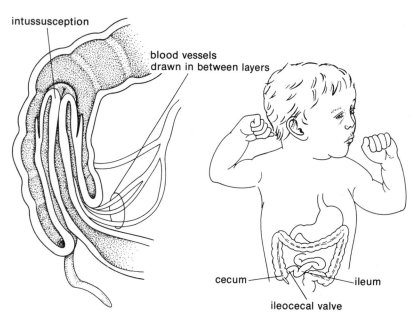

FIGURE 8–6. Intussusception. The most common type begins at or near the ileocecal valve, pushing into the cecum and onto the colon. At first, the obstruction is partial, but as the bowel becomes inflamed and edematous, complete obstruction occurs. (From Foster, R.L., Hunsberger, M.M., Anderson, J.J.: Family-Centered Nursing Care of Children. Philadelphia, W.B. Saunders Company, 1989.)

intussusception

blood vessels drawn in between layers

cecum — ileum

ileocecal valve

  b. infant will recover without complications
3. Implementation
   a. check vital signs frequently; monitor for shock
   b. prepare for barium enema to establish diagnosis; enema may also reduce invagination
   c. maintain hydration with IV fluids; infant usually NPO with NG tube
   d. provide emotional support for infant and family
   e. surgery may be done if not reduced spontaneously or with enema; prepare infant and family
4. Evaluation
   a. infant/parents adequately prepared for surgery
   b. infant recovered without complications

B. Appendicitis

Inflammation of appendix; sometimes follows infection elsewhere in body

1. Assessment
   a. pain in right lower quadrant with rebound tenderness
   b. nausea and vomiting, elevated temperature, leukocytosis
   c. more common in school-age children and adolescents
2. Planning, goals/expected outcomes
   a. diagnosis will be made quickly before complications occur
   b. child will recover from surgery without complications
3. Implementation
   a. provide conservative care prior to definitive diagnosis; NPO, no laxatives or pain medications; monitor vital signs

  b. teach child and parents and provide emotional support in preparation for surgery
   c. administer antibiotics; if appendix ruptured and peritonitis present, massive doses of antibiotics needed to control infection (Table 7-10); maintain NG tube
   d. administer pain medications as needed to keep child comfortable only after diagnosis made
4. Evaluation
   a. diagnosis made quickly before complications occurred
   b. child recovered from surgery without complications

C. Pinworms

Parasitic worms that inhabit intestine

1. Assessment
   a. spread easily by anal–oral contamination on hands, linens, or food
   b. child will scratch around anus in response to itching
   c. eggs or worms in the stool or on the anus seen on examination
   d. history of anorexia
   e. entire family should be treated to prevent infection
2. Planning, goals/expected outcomes
   a. child will be diagnosed early
   b. child/parents will understand and comply with therapeutic regimen
   c. child will recover without complications and reinfection will not occur
3. Implementation

a. collect laboratory specimen for examination with special collection blade or tongue blade covered with cellophane tape, sticky side out; should be collected in early morning before rising

b. practice good hand-washing technique; teach child and family good hand-washing and hygiene habits

c. isolate clothes and linens to prevent reinfection or contamination; wash at high temperature

d. administer vermifuge medications: piperazine (Antepar) and pyrvinium pamoate (Povan) most commonly given

4. Evaluation

a. child diagnosed early

b. child/parents understood and complied with therapeutic regimen

c. child recovered without complications and reinfection did not occur

III. CHRONIC DISORDERS

A. Crohn's Disease

Chronic, recurrent inflammation of the small or large intestine

1. Assessment

a. often affects portion of terminal ileum

b. patchy, skipped inflammatory lesions

c. also called regional enteritis or regional ileitis

d. regional symptoms, such as acute, crampy, low abdominal pain, fever, abdominal distention, and tenderness

e. chronic diarrhea, up to 20 or more stools a day

f. history of weight loss and anemia

g. characteristic radiographic pattern of "skipped lesions"

h. most common in late adolescence and young adulthood; more common in upper- and middle- class individuals

2. Planning, goals/expected outcomes

a. diarrhea will be controlled

b. patient will understand and follow therapeutic regimen

c. disease will remain in remission as long as possible

d. patient will be adequately prepared for surgery

e. patient will recover from surgery without complications

3. Implementation

a. encourage rest and relaxation

b. maintain adequate nutrition and hydration; may need parenteral fluids and nutrition

c. teach dietary modification; usually soft, low fiber diet recommended

d. administer medications as ordered: steroids, to treat inflammation; antidiarrheals, such as Lomotil, to treat diarrhea; and antispasmodics, such as Pro-Banthine, to control intestinal spasms (Tables 7-32 and 7-33)

e. encourage psychologic counseling for support and stress reduction

f. prepare for surgery, both physically and mentally

4. Evaluation

a. diarrhea controlled

b. patient understood and complied with therapeutic regimen

c. disease remained in remission as long as possible

d. patient adequately prepared for surgery

e. patient recovered from surgery without complications

B. Ulcerative Colitis (Granulomatous Colitis)

Chronic, recurrent, inflammatory, and ulcerative disease of colon

1. Assessment

a. differs from Crohn's by presence of patchy granulomas

b. usually starts at rectum and extends upward

c. may lead to perforation; increases risk of colon cancer

d. history of chronic diarrhea, abdominal pain, and distention

e. weight loss and anemia

f. presence of blood and mucus in stools

g. most common in older adolescents and young adults

2. Planning, goals/expected outcomes

a. diarrhea and other symptoms will be controlled

b. patient will understand and follow therapeutic regimen

c. disease will remain in remission as long as possible

d. patient will be adequately prepared for surgery

e. patient will care for and cope with possible permanent colostomy or ileostomy

f. patient will recover from surgery without complications

3. Implementation

a. prepare patient for radiographic and colonoscopic examinations to confirm disease

b. maintain adequate hydration

c. maintain adequate nutrition; soft, bland, low fiber diet may be ordered

d. provide emotional support to patient and family; explain and teach to relieve stress level and help alleviate symptoms

  e. administer steroids to decrease inflammation as ordered

  f. administer antidiarrheals, antibiotics (sulfonamides), and antispasmodics as ordered

  g. teach patient and family to cope with disease or with colostomy or ileostomy

  h. teach care of ileostomy (usual surgery)

    (1) drainage extremely irritating, so avoid getting any drainage on skin; fit pouch well

    (2) empty pouch 3 to 4 times per day

    (3) amount of drainage depends on child's weight

    (4) increased amounts of ileostomy drainage can lead to severe dehydration and electrolyte imbalance; teach parent to report this to physician immediately

4. Evaluation

  a. diarrhea and other symptoms controlled

  b. patient understood and complied with therapeutic regimen

  c. disease remained in remission as long as possible

  d. patient adequately prepared for surgery

  e. patient cared for and coped with possible permanent colostomy or ileostomy

  f. patient recovered from surgery without complications

■ Renal/Urinary Disorders

I. CONGENITAL DISORDERS

A. Epispadias and Hypospadias

Congenital malformation of penis in which urethra opens on dorsal surface of penis (epispadias) or behind glans penis (hypospadias)

1. Assessment

  a. obvious physical defect; defect can be present in varying degrees and, if accompanied by undescended testicles or other anomalies, may leave sex of infant in doubt at birth

  b. may be noted during urination when stream malpositioned

  c. normal return of function depends on degree of defect, how far off glans penis defect occurs

2. Planning, goals/expected outcomes

  a. child/parents will understand and cope with process of surgical repair

  b. child will recover from surgery without complications and with maximal return of function

3. Implementation

  a. surgical correction necessary to improve physi-

cal appearance of penis for psychologic reasons and to improve physical function for urinary and reproductive reasons

  b. teach family concerning surgical correction and expected results

  c. provide emotional support to child and family; if repair done in stages, repeated surgeries and fear of castration and mutilation can lead to psychologic problems

  d. postoperative care to prevent infection and meet psychologic and emotional needs

4. Evaluation

  a. child/parents understood and coped with process of surgical repair

  b. child recovered from surgery without complications and with maximal return of function

B. Cryptorchidism

Failure of one or both testes to descend into scrotum prior to birth

1. Assessment

  a. inability to palpate testes within scrotal sac

  b. testes may descend normally shortly after birth

  c. undescended testes predispose to testicular cancer

2. Planning, goals/expected outcomes

  a. testes will descend normally

  b. child will recover from surgery without complications

3. Implementation

  a. treatment may not be begun in infancy; testes can descend spontaneously during early childhood, but usually treated by age 1–2 years

  b. provide emotional support to family concerning treatment and expected results

  c. administer hormones as ordered to promote descent of testes

  d. prepare child and family for surgery (orchiopexy)

4. Evaluation

  a. testes descended normally

  b. child recovered from surgery without complications

II. ACUTE DISORDERS

A. Wilms' Tumor (Nephroblastoma)

Fast-growing malignant tumor of kidney

1. Assessment

  a. palpation of mass on either side of abdomen or in costovertebral area

b. hematuria, fever, and hypertension
c. prognosis good for early diagnosis and treatment of child under 2 years of age
2. Planning, goals/expected outcomes
   a. diagnosis will be made early
   b. child/parents will understand and comply with treatment regimen
   c. child will recover without complications
3. Implementation
   a. avoid palpation of abdomen and mass to prevent spreading
   b. surgery usually scheduled as soon as possible; chemotherapy and radiation therapy may be used postoperatively; nephrectomy done if remaining kidney functioning normally
   c. teach family and provide emotional support concerning serious nature of tumor, expected treatment, and outcome
4. Evaluation
   a. diagnosis made early
   b. child/parents understood and complied with treatment regimen
   c. child recovered without complications

B. Acute Glomerulonephritis

Inflammation of glomeruli; may occur as antigen–antibody reaction to infection, such as beta-hemolytic streptococcus

1. Assessment
   a. high fever, vomiting, oliguria, hematuria, fatigue, anemia, edema (especially of face)
   b. history of streptococcal infection 1–3 weeks previously
   c. more common in preschool children
2. Planning, goals/expected outcomes
   a. diagnosis will be made early
   b. child will recover without urinary complications
3. Implementations
   a. maintain bed rest throughout fever and active symptoms
   b. administer antibiotics as ordered
   c. administer antihypertensives as ordered (Table 7-3)
   d. monitor vital signs, especially temperature
   e. monitor intake and output and daily weights; observe for edema, especially facial
   f. maintain adequate nutrition; diet may be restricted in salt and fluid as kidney function indicates
   g. test urine for protein and elevated specific gravity
4. Evaluation

a. diagnosis made early
b. child recovered without urinary complications

III. CHRONIC DISORDERS

A. Nephrotic Syndrome (Nephrosis)

Degenerative and noninflammatory disease of glomeruli of kidneys, resulting in edema and large amounts of protein in urine (proteinuria)

1. Assessment
   a. edema of face and generalized edema over whole body
   b. malnutrition, respiratory distress, and irritability
   c. history of frequent infections; increased susceptibility to infections
   d. laboratory tests reveal albuminuria, white blood cells (WBC) in urine, lipids in urine, decreased blood proteins, increased sedimentation rate, increased blood lipids and cholesterol
   e. treatment may continue for 12 to 18 months or longer
   f. more common in preschool children
2. Planning, goals/expected outcomes
   a. infections will be prevented
   b. child will remain in remission as long as possible
   c. child/parents will understand and follow therapeutic regimen
3. Implementation
   a. prevent infections
   b. provide meticulous skin care and position changes to avoid skin breakdown
   c. monitor intake and output, daily weights
   d. test urine for protein and albumin
   e. administer diuretics as ordered (Table 7-3)
   f. administer steroids as ordered to control inflammation (Table 7-17)
   g. observe for drug side effects and toxicities
   h. maintain adequate nutrition; diet modifications may include high protein and low salt (Tables 5-3 and 5-10)
   i. because this is a chronic disease, teach child and parents home care, medication administration, and prevention of infections; crucial to success of therapy
   j. provide emotional support to child and parents to accept conditions and to follow through in treatment regimen
4. Evaluation
   a. infections prevented
   b. child remained in remission as long as possible
   c. child/parents understood and complied with therapeutic regimen

Questions

Jeremy, 4 1/2 years old, has been admitted to the hospital with the diagnosis of nephrosis.

1. The prime presenting symptom of the child with nephrosis is:

① Hematuria
② Edema
③ Petechial rash
④ Dehydration

2. A urinalysis would reveal:

① Gross albuminuria
② Gross hematuria
③ Glycosuria
④ No significant abnormalities

3. The diet ordered for a child with nephrosis would be most likely to contain:

① Decreased amounts of protein and possibly sodium
② Decreased amounts of sodium and limited fluids
③ Increase in fiber and vitamin content with increased fluid
④ Increased amounts of protein and possibly decreased amount of sodium

4. Andy, age 2 years, suffers from nephrosis and is on steroids. As a result of the steroid therapy, he would be unlikely to suffer from:

① Cushing's syndrome
② Depression
③ Delayed wound healing
④ Increased growth spurts

5. A severe emergency that may occur when a portion of the intestine becomes trapped in a passageway and the blood supply is impaired is known as a:

① Hernia
② Reducible hernia
③ Strangulated hernia
④ Irreducible hernia

6. Phenylketonuria (PKU) is caused by:

① Faulty metabolism of phenylalanine
② Excessive ketone bodies in the urine
③ Faulty metabolism of trypsin, amylase, and lipase
④ Embryonic defect

7. A child is admitted with acute appendicitis. The most comfortable position for this child would be:

① Left lateral Sims'
② Prone
③ Supine
④ Semi-Fowler's

8. Pinworms may be transmitted by:

① Droplet infection
② Stepping in the worms or eggs
③ Improper hand washing after bowel movements
④ Using the same comb or brush

Adam is the third child born to Mr. and Mrs. Lewis, their first son, and weighed 8 lb at birth. They were shocked to learn that he had a complete cleft lip and palate. Mrs. Lewis was quite alarmed by the appearance of her baby and for some time she was unable to look at him without crying. Adam's lip will be repaired in 3 weeks, his palate later.

9. Preoperatively, which of the following are necessary for Adam?

① Feed him in a flat position for ease of swallowing
② Feed him with a cup, spoon, or straw
③ Offer small, frequent feedings so as not to tire him
④ Burp him frequently during feeding

10. In the recovery room, Adam suddenly becomes cyanotic. Which of the following would you do first?

① Call for assistance
② Administer oxygen
③ Check for obstruction in the mouth
④ Insert an oral airway

11. The *best* position for Adam while in the recovery room is:

① Prone with the head turned to one side
② Left lateral Sims'
③ Supine with the head turned to the side
④ Flat on his back

12. Postoperatively, the nurse should feed Adam slowly by using a:

① Premature-type nipple
② Rubber-tipped Asepto syringe
③ Newborn nipple
④ Nasogastric tube

13. It is very important to prevent crying postoperatively because:

① Cyanosis is common postoperatively
② Adam could feel rejected if he is allowed to cry
③ He could injure a fresh suture line
④ Crying will interfere with his feedings

14. Adam will be discharged before the sutures have been removed. You should teach his mother to:

① Avoid contact with the suture line
② Carefully remove crusts that have formed on the suture line with soap and water
③ Apply zinc oxide ointment on the suture line before feeding
④ Gently cleanse the suture line with peroxide on a cotton swab

Carl, age 10 years, has a history of a strep throat 2 weeks ago. Now he has edema around his eyes, decreased urine output, and complains of headache. He is admitted to the hospital with a diagnosis of acute poststreptococcal glomerulonephritis.

15. The nurse would expect Carl's urine to:

① Be cloudy yellow
② Test +4 for protein
③ Have specific gravity of 1.005 or less
④ Be increased in quantity

16. The diet allowed Carl should:

① Contain extra protein
② Consist of favorite foods
③ Be severely salt restricted
④ Provide a maximum of 120 mL of fluid

17. Carl's parents are concerned about his prognosis. The best response by the nurse is:

① Most children recover with no renal damage
② He may require medicine to control his blood pressure
③ There's a chance the disease could recur at any time
④ Permanent renal damage cannot be evaluated for a year

18. Preoperative care for the child suspected of having a Wilms' tumor includes:

① Every shift takes abdominal circumferences
② Avoidance of palpating abdomen
③ Monitoring for intestinal obstruction
④ Assessing for signs of infection

19. Which of the following is *not* a classic sign of insulin dependent diabetes?

① Polyuria
② Weight gain
③ Polydipsia
④ Polyphagia

Answers & Rationales

Guide to item identification (see pp. 3–5 for further details about each category)

I, II, III, or IV for the phase of the nursing process
1, 2, 3, or 4 for the category of client needs
A, B, C, D, E, F, or G for the category of human functioning
Specific content category by name; ie, cholecystectomy

1. ② Edema is the prime clinical symptom of nephrosis. It may become so severe that the child may gain to twice his normal weight.
I, 2, F. Peds Nephrosis.

2. ① Laboratory tests show "marked proteinuria," with blood not usually present.
IV, 1, F. Peds Nephrosis.

3. ④ Increase in dietary proteins, though contrary to dietary treatment of most kidney disorders, is needed for replacement of urinary protein loss and for maintaining correct blood albumin levels.
III & IV, 4, F. Peds Nephrosis.

4. ④ Growth is retarded in children on steroid therapy.
IV, 2, F. Peds Nephrosis.

5. ③ A hernia that is not reducible and has a compromised blood supply is called a strangulated hernia. If it is not treated immediately, it can result in gangrene of that portion of the bowel.
I, 2, F. Hernia.

6. ① Improper metabolism of phenylalanine leads to a build-up of PKU.
IV, 4, F. PKU.

7. ① Side lying with the right leg drawn up is the most comfortable position.
III, 2, C. Appendicitis.

8. ③ Pinworms are transmitted through the rectal to hands to oral route. Good hand washing after bowel movements decreases their transmission.
I, 2, A, G–H. Pinworms.

9. ④ Frequent burping is necessary because he tends to swallow large amounts of air. He must be fed upright to make swallowing easier and decrease the chance of aspiration. Straws are not to be used, because he is not to form a vacuum seal that may injure his mouth.
III, 1, F. Cleft Lip and Palate.

10. ③ Making sure that the airway is free of mechanical obstruction is the priority.
III, 2, F. Cleft Lip and Palate.

11. ③ This is the best position for safety. The foot of the bed may also be elevated to further prevent aspiration of drainage.
III, 2, F. Cleft Lip and Palate.

12. ② To prevent regurgitation through the nose and sucking during the postoperative period, use a rubber-tipped Asepto syringe (Brech feeder).
III, 2, F. Cleft Lip and Palate.

13. ③ Prevent crying to minimize undue stress to the suture line. Cuddling, holding, and other comfort methods are effective.
III, 2, F. Cleft Lip and Palate.

14. ④ The best way to remove crusts is with peroxide. Arm/elbow restraints are used to prevent the infant from rubbing the suture line. If ordered, use A and D Ointment or mineral oil to keep the area lubricated, because zinc oxide would dry the area.
III, 2, F. Cleft Lip and Palate.

15. ② The urine is cola-colored, contains albumin, output is low, and specific gravity is high.
I, 2, E. Glomerulonephritis.

16. ② The diet should be as unrestricted as possible, because these children are anorexic.
III, 2, E. Glomerulonephritis.

17. ① Children with poststreptococcal glomerulonephritis usually recover without any residual effects.
III, 2, E. Glomerulonephritis.

18. ② Because the tumor tends to be fragile and can rupture and disseminate when palpated, the nurse should never palpate the abdomen.
III, 2, E. Wilms' Tumor.

19. ② Classic signs of diabetes include weight loss despite polyphagia.
I, 1, E. Diabetes.

BIBLIOGRAPHY

Bates, B. (1990). *A Guide to Physical Examination and History Taking, 5th ed.* J.B. Lippincott Co., Philadelphia.

Behrman, R.E., & Vaughan, V.C. (1987). *Nelson Textbook of Pediatrics, 13th ed.* W.B. Saunders Co., Philadelphia.

Brunner, L.S. & Suddarth, D.S. (1986). *The Lippincott Manual of Nursing Practice, 4th ed.* J.B. Lippincott Co., Philadelphia.

Foster, R.L., Hunsberger, M.M., & Anderson, J.J. (1989). *Family-Centered Nursing Care of Children.* W.B. Saunders Co., Philadelphia.

Govoni, L.E., & Hayes, J.E. (1988). *Drugs and Nursing Implications, 6th ed.* Appleton and Lange, E. Norwalk, Connecticut.

Guyton, A.C. (1991). *Textbook of Medical Physiology, 8th ed.* W.B. Saunders Co., Philadelphia.

Ingalls, A.J., & Salerno, M.C. (1991). *Maternal and Child Nursing, 7th ed.* C.V. Mosby Co., St. Louis.

Keane, C.B. (1986). *Essentials of Medical-Surgical Nursing, 2nd ed.* W.B. Saunders Co., Philadelphia.

Luckmann, J., & Sorensen, K.C. (1987). *Medical-Surgical Nursing: A Psychophysiologic Approach, 3rd ed.* W.B. Saunders Co., Philadelphia.

Marlow, D.R., & Redding, B.A. (1988). *Textbook of Pediatric Nursing, 6th ed.* W.B. Saunders Co., Philadelphia.

Murray, R.B., & Zentner, J.P. (1989). *Nursing Assessment and Health Promotion Through the Lifespan, 4th ed.* Prentice-Hall, Englewood Cliffs, NJ.

Thompson, E.D. (1987). *Pediatric Nursing: An Introductory Text, 5th ed.* W.B. Saunders Co., Philadelphia.

Whaley, L.F., & Wong, D.L. (1991). *Nursing Care of Infants and Children, 3rd ed.* C.V. Mosby Co., St. Louis.

The Childbearing Family

YOUNG ADULT DEVELOPMENT

I. PHYSIOLOGIC DEVELOPMENT

A. Females

1. Reproductive system
   a. maturation process begins during puberty
   b. influenced by hormones
   c. responsible for development of secondary sexual characteristics
2. Estrogen: secreted by maturing ovarian follicle and responsible for
   a. growth and development of ovaries, uterus, and vagina
   b. enlargement of breasts
   c. development of secondary sex characteristics
   d. aiding in growth of skeleton, resulting in cessation of bone growth
3. Progesterone: secreted by corpus luteum or, if pregnancy occurs, secreted by placenta
   a. prepares lining of uterus for implantation of embryo
   b. decreases rapidly with estrogen if fertilization does not occur
4. Menstrual cycle (Fig. 9–1)
   a. begins at puberty (menarche), ends at menopause
   b. usually on 28-day cycle
   c. consists of four phases
      (1) menstruation phase
         (a) lasts 4 to 6 days, shedding of endometrial lining
         (b) luteinizing hormone (LH), estrogen, and progesterone at lowest level
         (c) follicle-stimulating hormone rises, which enables graafian follicle to begin to mature
      (2) proliferative phase
         (a) uterine lining grows and thickens, leveling off at ovulation
         (b) estrogen level increases
         (c) lasts about 9 days
      (3) secretory or luteal phase
         (a) initiated by ovulation in response to surge of LH
         (b) corpus luteum produces large quantities of progesterone and estrogen
         (c) uterine lining prepared to receive and nourish fertilized ovum
         (d) implantation occurs 7 to 10 days after ovulation
         (e) fertilized ovum produces human chorionic gonadotropin (HCG), which stimulates continued estrogen and progesterone production
      (4) premenstrual or ischemic phase
         (a) occurs only if fertilization does not occur
         (b) progesterone and estrogen decrease as corpus luteum degenerates
         (c) arteries in endometrium constrict, causing uterine lining to shrink and die
         (d) lasts 3 to 5 days

B. Males

1. Reproductive system
   a. maturation begins at puberty
   b. influenced by hormones
   c. responsible for development of secondary sexual characteristics
2. Testosterone: produced by interstitial cells in testes and responsible for
   a. producing sex drive and potency
   b. enlargement of scrotum and elongation of penis
   c. causing seminiferous tubules of testes to produce sperm
   d. developing secondary sexual characteristics
      (1) affects height
      (2) increases size and number of muscles
      (3) promotes cessation of bone growth

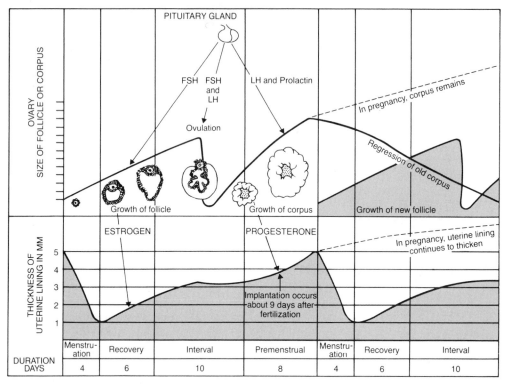

FIGURE 9–1. Average 28-day menstrual cycle. The cycle begins when hormones from the pituitary gland stimulate the development of an egg in a follicle inside one of the ovaries. About the 14th day, ovulation occurs: the follicle bursts, and the egg is discharged from the ovary. If the egg is not fertilized, the cycle ends in menstruation on the 28th day. If the egg is fertilized, pregnancy begins. (From Miller, B.F., Keane, C.B.: Encyclopedia and Dictionary of Medicine, Nursing, and Allied Health. 4th ed. Philadelphia, W.B. Saunders Company, 1987.)

3. Sperm development
   a. develop in testes
   b. mature and remain in epididymis 2 to 10 days
   c. move into vas deferens after maturing
4. Reproduction
   a. sperm mixes with seminal fluid to form semen
   b. semen may be secreted during intercourse before ejaculation
   c. ejaculation helps propel sperm toward uterus

II. PSYCHOLOGIC DEVELOPMENT

A. Females and Males

1. Similar for both sexes
2. Major developmental tasks: Erikson's stage of intimacy vs. isolation
   a. achieve relative independence from parental figures and develop sense of responsibility for own life
   b. increased self-development and achievement of appropriate roles and positions in society
   c. begin to develop personal lifestyle away from home; begin work life
   d. adjust to marital relationships and intimacy with another person

   e. develop parenting behaviors for offspring or for society if childless
   f. integrate personal values with career development and socioeconomic constraints

PSYCHOLOGIC AND PHYSICAL CHANGES DURING PREGNANCY

I. DEVELOPMENTAL TASKS OF PREGNANCY

A. Tasks

1. Pregnancy validation: first trimester
   a. often shock and denial first
   b. introversion begins and lasts 7 to 8 months: encouraged by weight gain and other outward signs of pregnancy
2. Fetal embodiment: second trimester
   a. attempts to incorporate fetus into her body image as integral part of self
   b. readjusts to life roles
   c. develops feeling of inner strength
   d. appears to be time of maturation
3. Fetal distinction

a. encouraged by quickening
b. fetus becomes distinct and apart from herself
c. daydreams about baby and herself as mother; dreams are often unrealistic
4. Role transition: third trimester
a. separates fetus from herself and makes concrete plans
b. becomes more irritable and wants pregnancy to end

II. EFFECTS ON BODILY SYSTEMS

A. Effects

1. Reproductive system
   a. amenorrhea occurs, ovulation inhibited by increased progesterone and estrogen levels
   b. softening of cervix (Goodell's sign) due to increased blood supply
   c. softening of lower segment of uterus (Hegar's sign)
   d. purplish hue to vaginal mucosa (Chadwick's sign)
   e. uterus enlarges
   f. secretions of vaginal cells increase: leukorrhea, acts as body's first line of defense against infection
2. Endocrine system
   a. fatigue result of increased hormonal levels, causing sodium and water retention and smooth muscle relaxation
   b. HCG produced by 14th day
      (1) secreted by trophoblastic tissue of conceptus
      (2) critical to corpus luteum
      (3) measured as part of pregnancy test
   c. melanocyte-stimulating hormone (MSH) causes increased pigmentation in localized areas
   d. estrogen produced by corpus luteum first 5 weeks then placenta with levels rising throughout pregnancy; main functions of estrogen:
      (1) growth of uterine muscles and ability of uterine muscles to contract
      (2) aids in development of breast ducts and secretory system to prepare for lactation
   e. progesterone produced by corpus luteum for first 5 weeks, then by placenta; functions of progesterone include:
      (1) acting as regulatory mechanism to handle increased needs of woman and fetus
      (2) causing slight increase in basal metabolic rate
      (3) causing smooth muscle of uterus to relax
      (4) sustaining pregnancy
      (5) relaxing uterine muscle

f. aldosterone increases
3. Cardiovascular system
   a. main functions to:
      (1) deliver blood to uterine vessels at pressures adequate to fulfill requirements of placental circulation
      (2) effect physical, chemical, and cellular changes in blood to provide adequate oxygen exchange between mother and fetus
   b. major changes include:
      (1) cardiac enlargement
      (2) cardiac output increased by 30% to 50%
      (3) cardiac rate and stroke volume increase
      (4) blood volume increased 30% to 50%
      (5) increased potential for varicose veins
      (6) pseudo anemia due to increased fluid volume
4. Respiratory system
   a. increased volume of air per minute
   b. increased alveolar ventilation
   c. improved exchange of CO_2 and O_2 at cellular level
   d. increased estrogen leads to nasal swelling and stuffiness
   e. enlarging uterus puts pressure on diaphragm, decreasing respiratory movement
5. Urinary system
   a. increased renal blood flow
   b. increased renal plasma flow
   c. increased glomerular filtration rate, increasing efficiency of clearance, resulting in polyuria
   d. increased susceptibility to infection from dilation of ureters and renal pelvis
   e. pressure from uterus and loss of bladder tone lead to urinary frequency
6. Gastrointestinal system
   a. increased appetite and thirst
   b. increased food requirements
   c. gastric acids and pepsin levels decreased
   d. heartburn, caused by esophageal reflux
   e. increased time of contents in bowel leads to increased absorption of water, and to constipation
   f. delayed gastric emptying time, resulting in better absorption of nutrients, especially glucose and iron

III. SIGNS OF PREGNANCY

A. Presumptive, Probable and Positive Signs

1. Presumptive signs: more subjective signs; cannot be used to diagnose pregnancy
   a. amenorrhea
      (1) other causes may be strenuous exercise,

changes in nutrition, and endocrine problems

    (2) menses may not cease immediately with pregnancy

  b. nausea and vomiting

    (1) present in half of all pregnancies

    (2) referred to as "morning sickness," but can occur at any time

    (3) common food or odor distaste early problem

    (4) HCG secretion major cause

  c. Breast changes

    (1) result of progesterone secretion

    (2) increase in size, tenderness, and darkening of the areola

  d. urinary frequency

    (1) enlarging uterus puts extra pressure on bladder

    (2) blood supply to pelvis increases

    (3) frequency and urgency common in first trimester until uterus enlarges enough during second trimester to rise into abdomen

  e. fatigue

    (1) exact cause unknown

    (2) may be most common early sign of pregnancy in healthy young women

  f. quickening

    (1) faint abdominal fluttering felt by mother at 18–20 weeks

    (2) may be used as reference point in determining gestational age

2. Probable signs: objective signs determined during physical examination; result of vascular congestion in pelvis

  a. uterine enlargement

    (1) occurs irregularly at beginning

    (2) uterus above pubic symphysis by 12th week

    (3) reaches umbilicus by 20–22 weeks

  b. Hegar's sign

    (1) softening of lower uterine segment

    (2) occurs in 2nd and 3rd months of pregnancy

  c. Goodell's sign

    (1) softening of cervix and vagina

    (2) caused by vascular congestion of pelvis

  d. Chadwick's sign

    (1) bluish or purplish discoloration of cervix, vagina, and vulva

    (2) caused by vascular congestion of pelvis

  e. ballottement: rebounding of fetus against examiner's fingers on palpation

  f. Braxton-Hicks contractions: irregular, painless contractions throughout pregnancy

  g. abdominal enlargement

    (1) gradual process

    (2) more rapid after 12th week when uterus rises into abdominal cavity

  h. Abdominal striae

    (1) stretch marks

    (2) occur when elastic tissue stretched beyond its capacity

    (3) found on breasts, abdomen, thighs, and buttocks

  i. skin pigmentation changes

    (1) results from hormonal changes

    (2) nipples may darken

    (3) linea nigra: brown or pink line from umbilicus to pubic symphysis

    (4) chloasma gravidarum: mask of pregnancy

  j. positive pregnancy test

    (1) measures HCG

    (2) 90% to 98% reliable

3. Positive signs: absolute indicators of pregnancy

  a. fetal heart sounds

    (1) may be heard at 10 to 12 weeks by Doppler

    (2) may be heard through regular fetoscope by 18 to 20 weeks

    (3) normal rate 120 to 160 beats/minute

  b. fetal movements: felt by second trimester

  c. ultrasound of fetus

    (1) at 6 to 8 weeks, fetal identification positive

    (2) earliest positive method of diagnosing pregnancy

PREGNANCY

I. PRENATAL DEVELOPMENT

A. Conception

1. Fertilization of egg by sperm

  a. human body cells normally contain 46 chromosomes; of these, two are sex chromosomes

  b. sperm and ovum each contain 22 chromosomes and 1 sex chromosome

  c. the sex chromosome is either X or a Y chromosome

  d. a female develops if the sex chromosomes are X and X

  e. a male develops if the sex chromosomes are X and Y

  f. the sex chromosome of the sperm determines the sex of the fetus

2. Fertilized egg normally implants into upper portion of uterine wall 7 to 10 days after conception

3. Known as zygote until 3rd week

B. Embryonic Stage: 3rd to 8th Week

1. Embryo

  a. differentiates into three distinct layers

    (1) ectoderm

(2) mesoderm

(3) endoderm

b. critical period of organ development, disruption can cause abnormal development

c. size approximately:
  (1) 2 mm at 3 weeks
  (2) 5 mm at 4 weeks
  (3) 12 mm at 6 weeks
  (4) 3 cm at 8 weeks and weighs 2 g

d. fingers, toes, eyes, mouth, nose, and ears formed

e. differentiation of sexes occurs

f. heart function and fetal circulation established

2. Placenta
  a. developed by the first month of pregnancy
  b. provides fetal oxygenation, nutrition, and elimination
  c. produces progesterone, estrogen, HCG, and human placental lactogen (HPL)

3. Umbilical cord
  a. develops at same time as placenta
  b. connects fetal circulation to placenta
  c. consists of two arteries and one vein
  d. attached at center of placenta in normal development
  e. about 55 cm long and 2 cm in diameter

4. Amniotic sac
  a. surrounds the fetus and fetal side of placenta
  b. made up of two membranes, chorion and amnion
  c. contains amniotic fluid
    (1) between 500–1000 mL by end of pregnancy
    (2) protects the embryo
    (3) allows fetal movement
    (4) provides a constant temperature
    (5) swallowed by the fetus
    (6) primarily water, but contains small amount of protein, glucose, fetal hair, fetal urine, and vernix caseosa

C. Fetal Period

Lasts from start of third month to delivery

1. General development
  a. by 12 weeks
    (1) eyes, ears, mouth, nose, heart and circulatory system, limbs, tail, spinal cord, and bones present
    (2) bile secreted into stomach
    (3) fetus weighs 45 g, moves body parts, and swallows
  b. refinement and completion of all systems occurs
  c. by 20 weeks
    (1) hair grows, skeleton hardens, sex visible, and fetal heart audible

(2) able to suck and swallow

(3) weight about 450 g

d. by 28 weeks
  (1) eyelids open
  (2) skin red and wrinkled, with vernix caseosa
  (3) surfactant production begins
  (4) some nervous system regulation begins
  (5) testes descend into scrotum
  (6) weight about 1250 g

e. by 36 weeks
  (1) increased fat deposits, nervous and breathing systems, and blood developed enough to support extrauterine life
  (2) lanugo decreases, with vernix caseosa
  (3) weight 2600 to 2750 g

f. major development of brain and nervous system during last 3 months

2. Fetal circulation (Fig. 9-2)
  a. placenta supplies oxygen and nutrients and removes wastes; responsible for:
    (1) metabolism, fetal digestive tract
    (2) transfer, fetal lungs and kidneys
    (3) endocrine secretions, major endocrine gland
  b. umbilical cord contains two arteries and one vein
    (1) vein brings oxygen to fetus
    (2) arteries remove wastes from fetus
  c. major bypasses in fetal circulation
    (1) foramen ovale, opening between right and left atria of heart, bypassing lungs
    (2) ductus arteriosus, connects pulmonary artery to aorta, bypassing the lungs
    (3) ductus venosus, connecting umbilical vein and ascending vena cava, bypassing fetal liver

II. PRENATAL PERIOD

A. Prenatal Care

1. Initial assessment
  a. complete history and physical
  b. assess tolerance to pregnancy
    (1) past pregnancies
    (2) family situation
  c. presence of any health problems
  d. estimated date of deliver, Nägele's rule (take first day of last menstrual period, subtract 3 months and add 7 days)
  e. pelvic measurements
  f. vital signs, weight, and lab tests
  g. fetal heart rate and presentation

2. Nutritional status
  a. gain 25 to 30 lb, if weight normal before conception

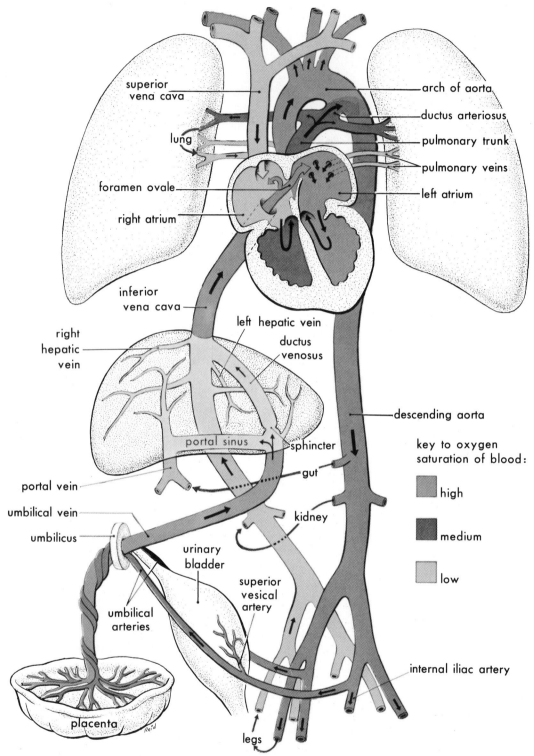

FIGURE 9–2. Fetal circulation. (From Moore, K.L.: Before We Are Born. 3rd ed. Philadelphia, W.B. Saunders Company, 1989.)

(1) women who are underweight should be encouraged to gain to normal weight plus 25 to 30 lb

(2) women who are overweight must watch weight carefully

b. increased calories needed to meet requirements for mother and baby (see Chapter 5)

c. increased protein, vitamins, and minerals, especially calcium and iron

d. sodium not restricted unless specifically ordered

e. diet based on four basic food groups

3. Prenatal visits
   a. initial visit for pregnancy test
   b. monthly visits for the first 7 months if pregnancy without problems
   c. during 8th month, visits usually every 2 weeks, and then weekly during last month until delivery

B. Environmental Risks to Pregnancy

1. German measles
   a. can cause major defects in fetus between second to sixth week after conception
   b. measles titer should be done before pregnancy to determine risks
2. Sexually transmitted diseases
   a. syphilis
      (1) passed to fetus; usually leads to spontaneous abortions
      (2) treated with penicillin up to last trimester; important to prevent congenital syphilis
      (3) increased incidence of mental subnormality and physical deformities
   b. herpes
      (1) contamination of fetus after membranes rupture or with vaginal delivery
      (2) generalized herpes results in 100% mortality
      (3) cesarean section indicated if labor occurs during an episode
3. Drugs/alcohol/tobacco
   a. drugs cross placenta
      (1) no drugs unless prescribed by doctor
      (2) no over-the-counter medications
      (3) no illegal drugs
   b. alcohol during pregnancies may lead to fetal alcohol syndrome, physical abnormalities, congenital anomalies, growth deficits, or jitteriness
   c. cigarette smoking
      (1) leads to low birth weights and higher incidence of birth defects and stillbirths
      (2) research indicates that even second-hand smoke is harmful
4. Radiation exposure
   a. no level of radiation safe; women should always be asked about possibility of pregnancy before radiographs are taken
   b. increased risk of spontaneous abortion
   c. increased risk of physical deformities
5. Other risk factors
   a. stress causes increased activity in fetus in response to increased epinephrine

b. women over age 35 years have greater risk of genetic abnormalities

c. girls under age 15 years have greater risk of stillbirths, spontaneous abortions, and premature births

C. Diagnostic Tests During Pregnancy

1. Pregnancy test
   a. measures HCG in urine
   b. accurate early in pregnancy
2. Ultrasound
   a. identifies fetal and maternal structures
   b. PN responsibilities
      (1) explain test to patient
      (2) have patient drink six to eight glasses of water, without voiding, before test
3. Amniocentesis: determines genetic disorders, sex, and fetal lung maturity (L : S ratio)
4. Oxytocin challenge test or stress test: determines fetal well-being and fetus's ability to withstand stress of labor
5. Nonstress test: evaluates fetal heart rate in response to fetal movement
6. Maternal estriol levels: provides information about stability of fetal-placental/maternal unit

D. Discomforts of Pregnancy

1. First trimester
   a. nausea and vomiting due to elevated HCG levels and changes in carbohydrate metabolism
      (1) small frequent meals
      (2) dry crackers often help
      (3) drink liquids between meals
   b. fatigue
      (1) get plenty of rest
      (2) usually disappears, then returns during late third trimester
   c. urinary urgency and frequency due to pressure of fundus on bladder
      (1) do not limit fluid intake
      (2) burning and disagreeable odor abnormal
      (3) decreases in second trimester
   d. breast tenderness from increased levels of estrogen and progesterone
   e. increased vaginal discharge from hyperplasia of mucosa and increased mucus production
      (1) take shower daily
      (2) do not use commercial vaginal cleansing products
   f. nasal stuffiness and epistaxis from elevated estrogen levels
2. Second and third trimester

a. heartburn: from esophageal reflux
   (1) avoid caffeine and spicy foods
   (2) sit up after meals
b. ankle edema: from venous stasis
   (1) elevate legs when sitting and do not cross legs
   (2) avoid prolonged standing
   (3) wear support stockings
c. varicose veins: from weakening walls of veins or faulty valves
   (1) elevate legs when sitting and do not cross legs
   (2) avoid prolonged standing
   (3) wear support stockings
d. hemorrhoids: from increased venous pressure or constipation
   (1) avoid constipation
   (2) increase bulk and fluid in diet
e. constipation: from sluggish bowel from progesterone and steroid metabolism, displaced intestines, and iron supplements
   (1) increase fluid and bulk in diet
   (2) maintain regular exercise regimen
f. backache from exaggerated lumbosacral curve from enlarged uterus
   (1) maintain good body mechanics and posture
   (2) wear low-heeled shoes
   (3) sit in chairs with proper back support
g. leg cramps: from pressure on nerves
   (1) stretch and exercise legs
   (2) maintain good posture and body mechanics
h. faintness: due to orthostatic changes
   (1) change position slowly
   (2) sit up for several minutes before rising
i. shortness of breath: from pressure on diaphragm
   (1) rest with head elevated
   (2) sleep in reclining position rather than flat

E. Complications of Pregnancy

1. Pregnancy-induced hypertension (PIH)
  a. also known as toxemia
  b. leading cause of maternal mortality
  c. incidence
    (1) common in teenage pregnancies and low income mothers
    (2) women with previous history of hypertension
    (3) multiple pregnancy; ie, twins
  d. cause unknown; predisposing factors include:
    (1) diabetes mellitus
    (2) hypertension
    (3) kidney disease
    (4) obesity
    (5) protein malnutrition

    (6) previous hydatidiform mole
    (7) excessive amniotic fluid (hydramnios)
    (8) family history of PIH
  e. symptoms
    (1) hypertension
    (2) proteinuria
    (3) generalized edema
  f. classified as preeclampsia and eclampsia
    (1) mild preeclampsia
      (a) edema minimal
      (b) blood pressure only about 30 mm Hg higher systolic and 15 mm Hg higher diastolic
      (c) proteinuria of +1 or +2
    (2) severe preeclampsia
      (a) sudden, severe edema with rapid weight gain
      (b) systolic blood pressure 40 mm Hg or more higher and diastolic 20 mm Hg or more higher
      (c) proteinuria +3 or +4 with oliguria
      (d) blurred vision and headaches
      (e) hyperreflexia
      (f) epigastric pain from engorgement of liver, usually precedes convulsions
    (3) eclampsia
      (a) fever
      (b) convulsions
      (c) severe hypertension
  g. treatment
    (1) mild
      (a) close monitoring of blood pressure
      (b) high protein, moderate sodium diet
      (c) bed rest in left lateral recumbent position
    (2) severe
      (a) hospitalization
      (b) monitor vital signs, fetal heart tones, urine output, and maternal daily weights
      (c) maintain high protein moderate sodium diet
      (d) monitor closely for convulsions
      (e) maintain quiet, nonstressful environment
      (f) if continues and hypertension severe, magnesium sulfate administered very carefully IV (Table 9-1)
  h. only real cure, termination of pregnancy
  i. attempt to control hypertension long enough to deliver viable fetus
2. Hyperemesis gravidarum: persistent nausea/vomiting, after first trimester, causing dehydration and starvation
  a. cause unknown but related to psychologic factors
  b. treatment

TABLE 9–1. Drugs Affecting Reproduction

UTERINE SMOOTH MUSCLE STIMULANTS

Description: Drugs that stimulate uterine smooth muscle, especially the gravid uterus; sensitivity of uterus increases during gestation and increases sharply before parturition

Uses: For initiation and improvement of uterine contractions for term or preterm delivery in maternal or fetal distress situations; postpartum to control postpartum bleeding or hemorrhage; nasal oxytocin indicated for initial letdown of milk

Side Effects: Fetal bradycardia; anaphylaxis; hemorrhage; nausea, vomiting; uterine hypertonicity; rupture of uterus; water intoxication

Nursing Implications: Obtain good obstetric history; do not administer IV without physician available; have magnesium sulfate (MgSO$_4$) on hand to treat tetany; use infusion pump with IV; monitor mother and fetus continually during administration; monitor for postpartum bleeding; monitor uterine contractions

Example: oxytocin (Pitocin)

BETA-RECEPTOR ANTAGONIST

Description: Drugs that have antagonistic effect on B$_2$-adrenergic receptors, such as those in uterine smooth muscle

Uses: Management of preterm labor in suitable patients; safe and effective under 20 weeks gestation

Side Effects: Dose-related alterations in maternal and fetal heart rates and maternal blood pressure; palpitations; tremors; nausea, vomiting; headache; erythema; malaise

Nursing Implications: Check maternal vital signs and monitor fetus; monitor uterine contractions; run as IV piggyback; use IV infusion pump; teach patient use of oral form; keep in left lateral position during IV administration

Example: ritodrine hydrochloride (Yutopar).

ANTICONVULSANT

Description: Acts as anticonvulsant for seizures associated with toxemia of pregnancy, partly by acting as central nervous system depressant and by reducing neuromuscular transmissions

Uses: Control convulsions associated with epilepsy, toxemia of pregnancy, and convulsions associated with low magnesium levels

Side Effects: Flushing; hypotension; cardiac depression; sedation; depressed reflexes; respiratory depression; circulatory collapse

Nursng Implications: Keep IV calcium gluconate on hand as antidote; check reflexes closely for early signs of toxicity; monitor vital signs, especially blood pressure and pulse; do not administer without close supervision

Example: MgSO$_4$

---

    (1) correct electrolyte imbalance and dehydration
    (2) carefully monitor intake and output
    (3) provide good oral care before meals
    (4) try small meals, not highly seasoned or odorous
    (5) have someone other than pregnant women prepare food
    (6) provide emotional support
3. Hemorrhagic disorders
  a. abortion: termination of pregnancy before fetus is viable, 20 weeks or weight of 500 G
    (1) types
      (a) spontaneous: natural causes; sometimes termed miscarriage or complete abortion
      (b) induced: therapeutic or elective reasons
      (c) threatened: bleeding, cramping, and backache but cervix remains closed
      (d) imminent or inevitable: persistent cramping and bleeding with dilation of cervix and rupture of membranes
      (e) incomplete: portion of products of conception expelled, usually fetus, but placenta remains
      (f) missed: fetus dies in utero without being expelled; may expel after about 6 weeks or may need dilatation and curettage (D&C)
      (g) habitual: loss of three or more consecutive pregnancies, preterm
    (2) nursing interventions
      (a) maintain bed rest
      (b) monitor vital signs
      (c) monitor amount of bleeding and loss of tissue
      (d) provide emotional support to parents
  b. ectopic pregnancy: implantation of fertilized ovum in site other than endometrial lining of uterus
    (1) usually occurs in fallopian tubes
    (2) causes
      (a) pelvic inflammatory disease (PID)
      (b) tubal adhesions
      (c) endometriosis
    (3) rupture of tube when fetal size increases, with severe pain and bleeding
      (a) often requires blood transfusions/fluid replacement
      (b) untreated may lead to shock and death
    (4) surgical removal
      (a) if diagnosed before rupture, tube may be left intact
      (b) if after rupture, fetus and affected tube removed
  c. hydatidiform mole: rare condition of abnormal change of placental villi into grape-like cysts filled with viscid material (Fig. 9-3)
    (1) signs and symptoms
      (a) larger than expected for gestational age uterus
      (b) higher than normal level of HCG
      (c) prolonged, severe nausea/vomiting
      (d) ultrasound shows no sign of fetus
      (e) signs of PIH
    (2) embryo dies and mole grows rapidly
    (3) often brown vaginal discharge
    (4) treated by D&C; avoid pregnancy for 1 year
    (5) increases incidence of choriocarcinoma
  d. placenta previa: improperly implanted placenta in lower uterine segment or over internal os (Fig. 9-4)
    (1) types
      (a) low or marginal: placenta attached close to internal cervical os

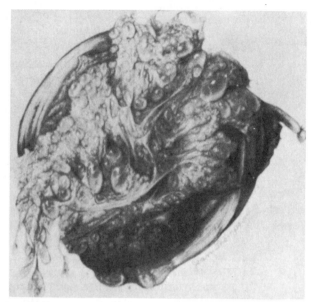

FIGURE 9–3. Drawing of a uterus containing a hydatidiform mole. (From Villee, C.A., Villee, D.B.: Human Reproduction. 3rd ed. Philadelphia, W.B. Saunders Company, 1981.)

     (b) partial: small part of placenta over internal cervical os
     (c) complete: placenta completely over internal cervical os
   (2) as lower uterine segment dilates and effaces, placental villi torn from uterine wall
   (3) classic symptom painless vaginal bleeding after 7 months

     (4) treatment for incomplete placenta previa is attempt to continue pregnancy until fetus viable
     (5) may require cesarean section for delivery
  e. abruptio placenta: premature separation of placenta from uterine wall (Fig. 9-5)
   (1) medical emergency
   (2) classic symptom painful vaginal bleeding
   (3) abdomen is board-like and symptoms of shock
   (4) hasten labor if bleeding not severe
   (5) cesarean section for severe bleeding
4. Infectious diseases
  a. cystitis
   (1) causative organism is usually *Escherichia coli*
   (2) antibiotics usually control
   (3) tetracycline contraindicated because of effect on fetus
   (4) instruct woman on proper perineal cleansing
  b. pyelonephritis
   (1) IV antibiotics required
   (2) increase fluid intake to help wash out bacteria
   (3) maintain acid urine with fluids like cranberry juice
  c. *TO*xoplasmosis, *R*ubella, *C*ytomegalovirus, *H*erpes (*TORCH*)
   (1) toxoplasmosis
     (a) organism transmitted through feces of infected animals
     (b) avoid changing cat litter box

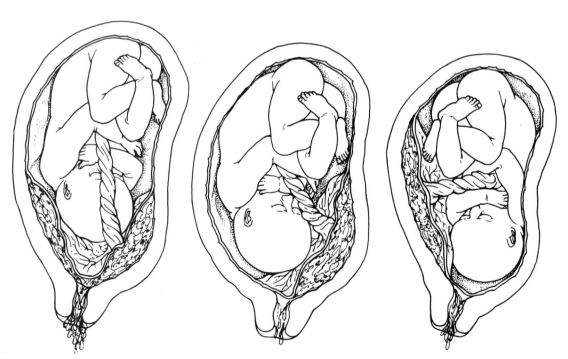

FIGURE 9–4. Three types of placenta previa. (From Thompson, E.D.: Introduction to Maternity and Pediatric Nursing. Philadelphia, W.B. Saunders Company, 1990.)

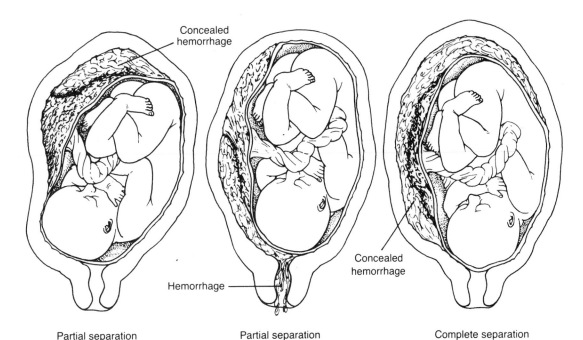

Concealed
hemorrhage

Concealed
hemorrhage

Hemorrhage

Partial separation   Partial separation   Complete separation

FIGURE 9–5. Three types of abruptio placentae. (From Thompson, E.D.: Introduction to Maternity and Pediatric Nursing. Philadelphia, W.B. Saunders Company, 1990.)

(c) although mother recovers, fetus affected

(d) fetal damage greatest if infection first 20 weeks

(2) rubella or German measles

  (a) causes chronic infection in fetus

  (b) exposure in first trimester often results in fetal death

  (c) in second trimester leads to hearing loss and other abnormalities, including growth retardation

  (d) draw rubella titer in all women at first prenatal visit; if low, then must avoid exposure

  (e) vaccinate, if possible, at least 3 months before pregnancy occurs, if women's titer low

(3) cytomegalovirus (CMV)

  (a) herpes virus

  (b) may be present in adults without symptoms

  (c) presence of antibodies means mother has virus

  (d) no treatment currently

  (e) may cause severe damage to fetus, or even fetal death

(4) herpesvirus, type 2 (HVH), herpes simplex

  (a) symptoms of herpes simplex in mother

  (b) may cause spontaneous abortion in first trimester

  (c) fetus may be infected during vaginal delivery, cesarean section indicated

  (d) if infected during vaginal delivery, high incidence of fetal death

5. Noninfectious diseases

a. diabetes mellitus: inherited metabolic disorder caused by insulin deficiency

  (1) gestational diabetes: diabetes that is first diagnosed during pregnancy

  (2) pregnancy increases mother's insulin need

  (3) fetus compensates by oversecreting insulin, resulting in excessively large fetus

  (4) increased incidence of stillbirth, congenital abnormalities, fetal, maternal, and neonatal complications

b. cardiac disease

  (1) unable to cope with added volume and increased cardiac output

  (2) symptoms of fatigue and shortness of breath, palpitations, tachycardia, murmurs, rales, and hemoptysis

  (3) classified and treated based on the severity of symptoms

c. Rh incompatibility

  (1) Rh-negative mother and Rh-positive fetus

  (2) mother produces antibodies against Rh antigens

  (3) first pregnancy fetus not usually affected, because this occurs near time of delivery, but subsequent fetuses affected

  (4) Rh_o (D) immune globulin, RhoGAM, given to destroy antibodies in mother's bloodstream; given at 28 weeks gestation and within 72 hours after termination of pregnancy

  (5) once sensitized, effect is permanent and no treatment available

Questions

1. In which of the following situations is the fetus at highest risk if born to an Rh-negative mother?

   ① First pregnancy, Rh-positive fetus
   ② First pregnancy, Rh-negative fetus
   ③ Second pregnancy, Rh-positive fetus, mother received RhoGAM right after first delivery
   ④ Second pregnancy, Rh-positive fetus, mother received RhoGAM before second pregnancy

2. Which of the following statements is *not* true concerning a hydatidiform mole?

   ① It is a malignant neoplasm
   ② Bleeding is associated with its presence
   ③ The uterus enlarges out of proportion to gestational age
   ④ Transparent vesicles resembling grapes develop from the chorion

Judy is a 16-year-old single primigravida whose membranes ruptured spontaneously. She has a slight bloody show and contractions 10–12 minutes apart that last about 20 seconds. Her chart indicates that she was seen by a physician for the first time 2 weeks ago.

3. Judy is considered a high-risk pregnancy because of:

   ① Lack of prenatal care
   ② Her age
   ③ Her marital status
   ④ All of the above

4. You plan to do as much teaching as possible to assist Judy. The best time to do this would be:

   ① During the latent phase of labor, giving simple, short instructions
   ② During the active phase of labor, so Judy will know what you are talking about
   ③ During transition, because now Judy knows that delivery is near
   ④ After delivery, when Judy is less anxious and more comfortable

5. While taking Judy's vital signs, you discover that her blood pressure is 148/98, her face is edematous, and her urine shows 2+ protein. These are signs of:

   ① Normal progression of labor
   ② Preeclampsia
   ③ Gestational diabetes
   ④ Impending delivery

6. The physician examines Judy and orders an infusion of $MgSO_4$ (magnesium sulfate). This drug is administered to:

   ① Stimulate labor
   ② Relieve discomfort
   ③ Prevent hemorrhage
   ④ Prevent convulsions

7. Which of the following occurs first in fetal development?

   ① Appearance of vernix caseosa
   ② Muscle contraction
   ③ Increased subcutaneous fat deposits
   ④ Secretion of urine by the kidneys

8. The fetus receives oxygen and excretes its wastes through:

   ① The amniotic fluid
   ② Two umbilical arteries and one umbilical vein
   ③ One umbilical artery and two umbilical veins
   ④ The lungs and kidneys

9. The first movements of the fetus in utero are referred to as:

   ① Lightening
   ② Quickening
   ③ Involution
   ④ Expulsion

10. The first movements of the fetus in utero are usually felt:

    ① 2 weeks prior to delivery
    ② At about 8 weeks
    ③ Within the first week after conception
    ④ Between 16 to 20 weeks of gestation

11. Normal changes that occur during pregnancy include:

    ① Increased vaginal discharge
    ② Persistent vomiting
    ③ Headaches and dizziness
    ④ Swelling of fingers and ankles on rising

12. The hemoglobin and hematocrit change during pregnancy. The normal changes experienced include:

① A decrease in both due to the increased blood volume
② An increase in both due to the decreased blood volume
③ An increase in the hemoglobin and a decrease in the hematocrit
④ Neither actually changes significantly during pregnancy

13. Symptoms of placenta previa include:

① Bleeding in the early months of pregnancy
② Painless bleeding in the last months of pregnancy
③ Sharp pains with the absence of bleeding
④ Separation of a normally implanted placenta

14. Your patient is admitted with hyperemesis gravidarum. Your nursing interventions should include:

① Placing a padded tongue blade at the head of the bed
② Accurately measuring intake and output
③ Identification of foods especially nauseating to her
④ Limiting visitors

15. Your patient is admitted with preeclampsia in week 32 of pregnancy. Her blood pressure is 160/110, she has 3+ albumin in her urine and she is complaining of severe headaches. Which of the following should be included in your nursing care of this patient?

① Complete bed rest
② Rest on the right side
③ Blood pressure measurement every shift
④ Limit fluids

16. Your patient begins to experience convulsions. Your priority nursing intervention would be to:

① Run for help immediately
② Put on the call light and ask for help
③ Yell for help
④ Ask her roommate to get help

17. Which of the following nursing interventions would be appropriate for the pregnant patient during a convulsion?

① Place a padded tongue blade between her teeth
② Put a blanket over the side rails to protect her
③ Monitor the fetal heart tones
④ Restrain her movements

18. The expectant mother at the greatest risk for developing toxemia would be a:

① 22-year-old Rh-negative multigravida
② 17-year-old primigravida with a positive roll-over test
③ 25-year-old anemic primigravida
④ 28-year-old slightly obese primigravida

19. Which of the following is *not* a cause of ectopic pregnancies

① Adhesions of the fallopian tubes
② Congenital abnormalities of the fallopian tubes
③ Tumors outside the fallopian tubes, pressing on it
④ Complete obstruction of the fallopian tubes

Answers & Rationales

Guide to item identification (see pp. 3–5 for further details about each category)

I, II, III, or IV for the phase of the nursing process
1, 2, 3, or 4 for the category of client needs
A, B, C, D, E, F, or G for the category of human functioning
Specific content category by name; ie, cholecystectomy

1. ④ RhoGAM must be given within 72 hours after delivery in Rh incompatible births so that the mother does not form antibodies.
I & IV, 4, A. Complications of Pregnancy.

2. ① A hydatidiform mole is considered a benign tumor, but follow-up for a malignancy is always recommended.
I & IV, 2, A. Complications of Pregnancy.

3. ④ All of these factors increase the risk of pregnancy.
I, 4, A. Prenatal Care.

4. ① During the latent phase of labor, the patient is fairly comfortable, and instructions regarding what to expect as labor progresses relieve anxiety and promote cooperation. A person under stress has limited ability to concentrate; thus instructions should be short and simple.
III, 4, A. Prenatal Care.

5. ② Classic signs of preeclampsia are elevated blood pressure, proteinuria, and edema.
I, 4, B and C. Prenatal Care.

6. ④ Magnesium sulfate decreases nerve impulses from the brain to the muscles.
IV, 4, C. Prenatal Care.

7. ④ The kidneys begin to secrete urine as early as week 12 after conception.
IV, 4, A. Fetal Development.

8. ② The normal umbilical cord contains two arteries and one vein.
I, 4, A. Fetal Development.

9. ② The first fetal movement is quickening.
IV, 4, A. Fetal Development.

10. ④ Quickening usually occurs between weeks 16 and 20.
I, 4, A. Fetal Development.

11. ① Increased vaginal discharge is normal and quite common. All others require that the doctor be notified.
I, 4, A. Prenatal Care.

12. ① As the blood volume increases, the relative levels of the hemoglobin and hematocrit are lowered.
I, 4, A and B. Prenatal Care.

13. ② Because the placenta is located on or near the cervical os, as the cervix prepares for birth, painless bleeding occurs.
I, 4, A. Prenatal Care.

14. ② Measurement of intake and output is very important to make sure that the patient is not developing a severe imbalance. Food should not be discussed, as it often increases the nausea.
III, 4, A and F. Prenatal/Hyperemesis.

15. ① Complete bed rest promotes diuresis. Patient should rest on left side. Blood pressure is monitored frequently, fluids are not limited.
III, 4, B and C. Preeclampsia.

16. ② The nurse must remain with the patient experiencing convulsions, protecting her from injury. Yelling may needlessly upset many other patients and family, and the call light should be answered immediately.
III, 1 & 4, C. Preeclampsia.

17. ② During the convulsion, the mother's protection must be the priority. The fetal heart tone can be monitored as soon as the convulsion is over. Padded tongue blades are rarely used. Do not restrain.
III, 1 & 4, C. Preeclampsia.

18. ② Younger patients are always at higher risk and the roll-over test is usually accurate in detecting women at risk for toxemia.
IV, 4, A and C. Preeclampsia.

19. ④ If the tubes are completely obstructed, fertilization cannot occur anywhere.
IV, 4, A. Ectopic Pregnancy.

LABOR AND DELIVERY

I. NORMAL LABOR AND DELIVERY

A. Normal Labor Process

1. Onset: exact cause unknown
   a. contributing factors
      (1) enlarged uterus
      (2) aging placenta
      (3) hormonal changes
          (a) increased oxytocin
          (b) decreased estrogen
   b. lightening: fetal head settles into pelvis
   c. show: discharge of blood-tinged mucus from cervical canal
   d. cervical changes
      (1) cervix "ripens": becomes soft
      (2) effacement: thinning and shortening of cervix to 100%
      (3) dilation: opening of cervical os to 10 cm (complete dilation)
2. Spontaneous rupture of membranes (SROM)
   a. verified by Nitrazine paper (pH), gives alkaline reaction
   b. microscopic examination of fluid shows ferning pattern
   c. risk of infection increases in direct proportion to length of time membranes are ruptured prior to delivery
   d. risk of prolapsed cord
   e. if labor does not begin, may require induction
      (1) Pitocin IV (Table 9-1)
      (2) physician must be present
      (3) mother and fetus must be closely and continually monitored
   f. record time, color, and amount of fluid, presence of unusual odor, and fetal heart rate (FHR)
   g. note presence of meconium-stained fluid if fetus is in vertex position; may indicate fetal distress
   h. observe for cord prolapse
3. Presentation and positions of fetus
   a. lie: relationship of long axis of fetus to long axis of mother
      (1) longitudinal
      (2) transverse
   b. attitude: degree of flexion of fetal head
   c. presentation: part of fetus coming through pelvis first
      (1) cephalic: head first
          (a) vertex: head well flexed onto chest
          (b) face: head hyperextended
      (2) breech: fetal buttocks or lower limbs first
      (3) shoulder: transverse lie with shoulder first

   d. position: relationship of presenting part to quadrants of maternal pelvis (Table 9-2)
4. Normal progression
   a. station: relationship of presenting part to ischial spine in maternal pelvis (Fig. 9-6)
      (1) presenting part above ischial spines measured as −1 cm, −2 cm, −3 cm, ballottable, or floating
      (2) presenting part even with ischial spines: 0 station
      (3) presenting part below ischial spine progressing towards perineum, +1 cm, +2 cm, +3 cm, crowning
      (4) crowning: fetal head or presenting part seen on perineum during contraction
   b. cardinal movements: mechanisms of labor
      (1) descent, enlargement, flexion: may occur concurrently and continue during labor
      (2) internal rotation: fetal head reaches perineum
      (3) extension: head emerges from vaginal opening
      (4) external rotation (restitution): head realigns with shoulders
      (5) expulsion: delivery of fetus
   c. contractions: rhythmic, involuntary tightening of uterine muscles
      (1) frequency: time from beginning of one contraction to beginning of next
      (2) duration: time from beginning to end of one contraction
      (3) intensity
          (a) strength of contraction determined by palpation

TABLE 9-2. Fetal Presentations

VERTEX	
ROA	Right occiput anterior
LOA	Left occiput anterior
ROP	Right occiput posterior
LOP	Left occiput posterior
ROT	Right occiput transverse
LOT	Left occiput transverse
FACE	
RMA	Right mentoanterior
LMA	Left mentoanterior
RMP	Right mentoposterior
LMP	Left mentoposterior
RMT	Right mentotransverse
LMT	Left mentotransverse
BREECH	
RSA	Right sacroanterior
LSA	Left sacroanterior
RSP	Right sacroposterior
LSP	Left sacroposterior
RST	Right sacrotransverse
LST	Left sacrotransverse
SHOULDER	
RADA	Right acromiodorsoanterior
LADA	Left acromiodorsoanterior
RADP	Right acromiodorsoposterior
LADP	Left acromiodorsoposterior

FIGURE 9–6. Stations of the presenting part. (From Burroughs, A.: Bleier's Maternity Nursing. 5th ed. Philadelphia, W.B. Saunders Company, 1986.)

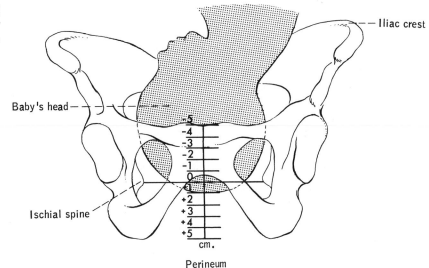

(b) described as mild, moderate, or strong
(c) also can be measured by internal uterine monitor, which measures pressure of amniotic fluid
(4) record and report to physician
  (a) change in pattern of contractions
  (b) tetanic contractions: those lasting more than 2 minutes
  (c) decreased relaxation between contractions
  (d) cessation of contractions
  (e) abrupt increase in pain
5. Factors influencing course of labor
  a. parity
    (1) primigravida: usual length of labor, 10–12 hours
    (2) multigravida: usual length of labor, 6–8 hours
  b. contractions
    (1) quality
    (2) frequency
  c. position, presentation, attitude, and lie of fetus
  d. maternal pelvic to fetal proportions
  e. maternal characteristics
    (1) physical status of mother
    (2) psychologic status of mother
    (3) prenatal education
    (4) attitude
    (5) support system
    (6) ability to relax and to cooperate with labor process

B. Assessment of Patient in Labor

1. Impending labor
  a. nesting instinct
    (1) sudden burst of energy
    (2) want to clean house, rearrange furniture
    (3) make sure mother avoids overexertion
  b. weight loss
    (1) fluid loss
    (2) related to changes in estrogen and progesterone levels
  c. lightening
    (1) fetus moves into pelvic inlet
    (2) mother notices decreased pressure on diaphragm and urinary frequency
  d. increasing backache
    (1) hormone relaxin causes relaxation of pelvis
    (2) fetus moves lower into pelvis
  e. other
    (1) indigestion, nausea, and vomiting from changing hormone levels
    (2) increased pressure on bladder as fetus settles into pelvis
2. Active labor
  a. admission criteria
    (1) membranes leaking or ruptured
    (2) vaginal bleeding present
      (a) do not do rectal examination
      (b) do not do vaginal examination
      (c) do not give enema
    (3) contractions regular and effective with cervical changes
    (4) premature dilation and effacement present
    (5) abnormally high blood pressure, proteinuria, and edema present or known PIH
    (6) fetal heart rate (FHR) and rhythm abnormal
    (7) mother in labor with history of multiparity with short labor
    (8) severe abdominal pain, not associated with contraction, present
  b. Leopold's maneuver
    (1) systematic palpation of abdomen

(2) done to determine fetal position prior to delivery

c. sterile vaginal examination (SVE)
   (1) done to determine station, dilation, effacement, and presentation
   (2) **never do examination if active bleeding present**
d. maternal vital signs
   (1) on admission, establish baseline; also check prenatal record for baseline assessments
   (2) temperature: elevation may indicate dehydration or infection
   (3) pulse: elevation may indicate anxiety, bleeding, or maternal distress
   (4) blood pressure
       (a) hypotension: may indicate bleeding
       (b) hypertension: may indicate anxiety or preeclampsia (PIH)
e. rupture of membranes (ROM)
   (1) spontaneous rupture of membranes (SROM)
       (a) record and report time of rupture, color, amount, or unusual odor of fluid
       (b) assess FHR and for prolapsed cord
   (2) artificial rupture of membranes (AROM): amniotomy performed by physician
       (a) allows placement of fetal electrode
       (b) allows placement of internal uterine monitor
       (c) stimulates labor
       (d) induces labor
       (e) performed between contractions and not until fetal head engaged
       (f) record time of procedure, color, amount, and unusual odor of fluid
       (g) assess FHR and for prolapsed cord
   (3) premature rupture of membrane (PROM) and more than 12 hours elapsed
       (a) if labor not started, intervention needed
       (b) temperature should be taken every hour due to increased risk of infection
f. fetal assessment: cardiac activity
   (1) normal FHR, 120–160 beats per minute (bpm)
   (2) bradycardia: less than 120 bpm
   (3) tachycardia: greater than 160 bpm
   (4) classification of fetal decelerations
       (a) Type I: early decelerations
           (i) start at onset of contraction
           (ii) most often due to head compression of infant
           (iii) pattern benign and requires no intervention
       (b) Type II: late decelerations
           (i) slow down of fetal cardiac activity, beginning after peak of contraction with slow return to baseline

(ii) indicates uteroplacental insufficiency
(iii) associated with high-risk pregnancies, uterine hyperactivity, and maternal hypotension
(iv) requires intervention to decrease or eliminate fetal distress
    (a) decrease in uterine activity (stop oxytocin if applicable)
    (b) change maternal position to correct maternal hypotension
    (c) administer oxygen at 6 to 12 L/minute via mask
    (d) prepare for delivery
       (c) Type III: variable deceleration
           (i) periodic and unpredictable
           (ii) most often due to cord compression
           (iii) most common pattern associated with fetal distress
           (iv) often alleviated by changing maternal position
           (v) if persistent and increasing, other intervention required
               (a) check for prolapsed cord
               (b) turn patient or place in Trendelenburg position
               (c) administer oxygen at 6 to 12 L/minute via mask
               (d) prepare for delivery
   (5) fetal accelerations
       (a) usually benign and initiated by fetal activity
       (b) may precede late decelerations when associated with contractions
   (6) other signs of fetal distress
       (a) meconium-stained amniotic fluid with baby in cephalic position
       (b) sudden, exaggerated fetal movement

C. Stages of Labor

1. First stage: period of time that elapses from beginning of regular contractions until cervix completely dilated and effaced
   a. latent phase
      (1) dilation of cervix from 1 to 4 cm
      (2) contractions
          (a) may be mild to moderate
          (b) occur every 4 to 5 minutes
          (c) last 30 to 40 seconds
      (3) mother:
          (a) may complain of backache; provide backrub, position on left side, and provide pillow for back
          (b) does not want to be left alone; stay with

mother, encourage significant other to stay with mother

b. active phase
- (1) dilation from 4 to 8 cm
- (2) contractions
  - (a) may be moderate to strong
  - (b) occur every 2 to 4 minutes
  - (c) last 45 to 60 seconds
- (3) mother:
  - (a) may be more apprehensive; reassure her, provide support, and inform her of progress of labor and what to expect
  - (b) does not want to be left alone; stay with mother, or have significant other stay with her
  - (c) may be uncertain if she can cope with contractions; encourage her, and use relaxation and breathing techniques

c. transition phase
- (1) dilation from 8 to 10 cm
- (2) contractions
  - (a) may be moderate to moderately strong
  - (b) occur every 2 to 4 minutes
  - (c) last 45 to 90 seconds
- (3) mother may:
  - (a) have increased bloody show; give frequent perineal care, change Chux frequently, and assure mother this is normal
  - (b) feel rectal pressure; encourage her not to push at this point and to use deep-breathing exercises
  - (c) show marked restlessness; continue relaxation exercises and encourage mother
  - (d) become nauseated; encourage deep breaths, provide frequent mouth care, and clean if vomiting occurs and prevent aspiration
  - (e) experience shaking of legs; provide blankets and gently massage legs
  - (f) have perspiration on upper lids and forehead; change bed linens and gown as needed, and apply cold cloth to forehead
  - (g) display irritability and unwillingness to be touched; speak slowly and clearly, help mother focus attention on task, and be understanding
  - (h) show frustration and inability to cope with contractions if left alone; do not leave mother alone, and encourage mother and focus on progress
  - (i) be eager to be "put to sleep"; provide encouragement, advise mother of progress, and provide noninvasive pain relief through breathing and massage
  - (j) be bewildered by intensity of contractions; tell her what to expect and encourage her about her progress

2. Second stage: lasts from time of complete dilation of cervix through delivery of baby
   a. contractions
   - (1) may be moderate to moderately strong
   - (2) occur every 1 to 2 minutes
   - (3) last 60 to 90 seconds
   b. mother may:
   - (1) experience desire to move bowels
     - (a) reassure her that she will not have bowel movement
     - (b) use pushing only when necessary
   - (2) panic when head reaches perineum
     - (a) reassure mother
     - (b) use breathing and relaxation techniques
   - (3) feel splitting sensation due to extreme vaginal stretching
     - (a) assist with local anesthesia
     - (b) assist with episiotomy
   - (4) be vague in communication
     - (a) speak slowly and clearly to mother
     - (b) avoid unnecessary distractions
   - (5) be amnesic between contractions
     - (a) avoid unnecessary distractions
     - (b) avoid explanations at this time
   - (6) Have tremendous satisfaction or great pain with each push: praise progress

3. Third stage: lasts from after birth of baby until placenta expelled
   a. physical characteristics include:
   - (1) rise of fundus
   - (2) uterus assumes globular shape
   - (3) visible descent of cord, lengthening
   - (4) trickle or gush of blood
   b. mother should be:
   - (1) alert
   - (2) proud and happy
   - (3) anxious to see baby
   - (4) relieved
   c. nursing interventions
   - (1) assess mother's vital signs
   - (2) monitor for excessive bleeding
   - (3) assist with episiotomy repair
   - (4) lower mother's legs slowly and simultaneously
   - (5) take mother to recovery room

4. Fourth stage: from after delivery of placenta to postpartum stabilization
   a. time, 2 to 4 hours
   b. assessments
   - (1) fundus firm; in midline, at, or below umbilicus
   - (2) lochia scant to moderate
   - (3) mother may be very excited or exhausted; response individualized

c. nursing interventions
  (1) palpate fundus every 15 minutes for first hour and massage fundus if boggy
  (2) check for bladder distention; offer bedpan
  (3) monitor vital signs for signs of shock
  (4) check vaginal drainage and report any fresh, heavy bleeding, especially if uterus is boggy
  (5) monitor mother on IV Pitocin to treat boggy uterus and hemorrhage
  (6) check perineum for signs of trauma
    (a) watch for swelling and hematoma formation
    (b) apply ice to perineum to treat pain and swelling

D. Anesthesia and Analgesia During Labor and Delivery

1. Analgesia: alters pain perception
  a. nonpharmacologic: relief of fear, tension, or pain syndrome
    (1) encourage mother and significant other to use Lamaze if prepared
    (2) relaxation
      (a) allows release of endorphins
      (b) good for tension and anxiety
      (c) can treat real physical pain
    (3) education: information and understanding
    (4) cognitive control: use of dissociation, imagery, and focusing
  b. pharmacologic
    (1) timing of depressant drug administration
      (a) respiratory depression of fetus may occur if given within 2 hours of delivery
      (b) progress of labor may be impeded if given during latent phase
      (c) should be administered during active phase of labor
    (2) classifications
      (a) sedatives/barbiturates: allow rest and sleep; can depress fetal respirations and heart rate
      (b) tranquilizers: promote relaxation and potentiate action of barbiturates and narcotics
      (c) narcotics: alter perception of pain
      (d) narcotic antagonist, naloxone (Narcan): administered to infant to reverse respiratory depression effects of narcotics; *note:* does not reverse effects of sedatives or tranquilizers
2. Anesthesia
  a. general
    (1) rarely used—emergency cesarean section only

    (2) produces unconsciousness
    (3) may cause severe respiratory depression of fetus/infant
  b. regional
    (1) subarachnoid block (saddle block)
      (a) dilation must be complete
      (b) may cause maternal hypotension, which causes fetal bradycardia
      (c) bearing-down reflex lost
    (2) epidural
      (a) given during first or second stage of labor
      (b) may prolong latent phase if given too early
      (c) loss of bearing-down reflex
    (3) pudendal block
      (a) infiltration of pudendal nerve
      (b) produces pain relief and relaxation of perineum
      (c) no fetal side effects if given properly
    (4) paracervical block
      (a) infiltration of tissues around cervix
      (b) given during first stage of labor
      (c) lasts 1 to 2 hours
      (d) rapid placental transmission, causing fetal bradycardia lasting up to 10 minutes; position mother on left side, increase fluid intake, monitor closely for maternal hypotension, and administer oxygen at 6 to 12 L/minute if maternal hypotension occurs
    (5) local
      (a) infiltration of perineal tissues
      (b) purpose: episiotomy
      (c) no fetal side effects

II. DEVIATIONS IN NORMAL LABOR PROCESS

A. Preterm Labor

1. Occurs: before end of week 37 of gestation
2. Causes
  a. spontaneous rupture of membranes
  b. cervical incompetence
  c. uterine anomalies
  d. fetal anomalies
  e. multiple fetuses
  f. chronic maternal disease, such as diabetes or hypertension
3. Treatment
  a. bed rest
  b. medications to decrease or stop contractions (ritodrine, Brethine, Vasodilan, MgSO$_4$) (Table 9-1)
  c. delivery, if fetus is viable

4. Contraindications for halting preterm labor
   a. rupture of membranes
   b. gross vaginal bleeding
   c. gross fetal anomalies
   d. severe maternal hypertension, eclampsia
   e. fetal demise

B. Precipitate Labor

1. Definition: labor lasting less than 3 hours
2. Nursing intervention: never attempt to hold back infant's head to slow or prevent delivery

C. Dystocia (Difficult Labor)

1. Hypotonic contractions
   a. contractions ineffective and irregular
   b. treatment: Pitocin augmentation, if no complications present
   c. cesarean section for cephalopelvic disproportion (CPD), fetal distress, or maternal distress
   d. nursing interventions
      (1) provide rest for mother
      (2) offer emotional reassurance
      (3) monitor Pitocin infusion for effects on contractions and maternal response
2. Hypertonic contractions
   a. decrease in resting tone between contractions, with uncoordinated activity between upper and lower uterine segments
   b. contractions painful but ineffective in producing cervical dilation
   c. treatment
      (1) sedation and analgesia
      (2) cesarean section for fetal distress
   d. nursing interventions
      (1) provide rest
      (2) offer emotional support
      (3) monitor for maternal exhaustion
      (4) administer medications as ordered
      (5) monitor fetal status
3. Rupture of uterus: may be partial or complete
   a. causes
      (1) prolonged labor with CPD
      (2) poorly managed induction of labor
      (3) unsupervised labor after previous cesarean section
   b. treatment: immediate laparotomy
   c. nursing interventions
      (1) report changes in contraction pattern, especially tetanic contraction with sudden cessation of contraction
      (2) monitor for signs of shock
      (3) be calm and supportive to mother
4. Prolapsed cord (Fig. 9-7)

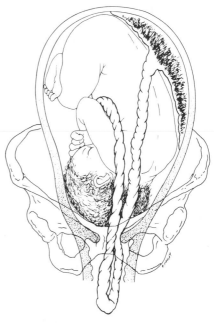

FIGURE 9–7. Prolapsed umbilical cord. (From Burroughs, A.: Bleier's Maternity Nursing. 5th ed. Philadelphia, W.B. Saunders Company, 1986.)

   a. caused by rupture of membranes when presenting part not engaged in pelvis
   b. nursing interventions
      (1) relieve pressure on cord by placing mother in Trendelenburg or knee chest position
      (2) notify physician immediately
      (3) do **not** attempt to replace cord into uterus
      (4) if cord protrudes outside vagina, cover with saline-moistened sterile towel
      (5) monitor FHR closely
      (6) prepare for delivery by cesarean section

D. Complications with Amniotic Fluid

1. Hydramnios
   a. excessive amounts of amniotic fluid; over 2000 mL
   b. etiology unknown: associated with:
      (1) maternal diabetes mellitus
      (2) Rh sensitivities
      (3) fetal malformations of esophagus or neural tube anencephaly
   c. problems associated with increased fluid amount
      (1) 2000 to 3000 mL causes some discomfort but no real problems
      (2) greater than 3000 mL
         (a) severe respiratory discomfort from pressure on diaphragm
         (b) lower extremity edema from pressure on pelvic vessels

(c) abruptio placenta with ROM due to rapid change in uterine size

(d) postpartum hemorrhage from overdistended uterine muscles

(e) increased fetal mortality and increased risk of prolapsed cord with ROM

d. treatment

(1) identification of problem during prenatal period

(2) amniocentesis if maternal problems great

2. Oligohydramnios

a. amniotic fluid less than 100 mL

b. associated with:

(1) postmaturity

(2) intrauterine growth retardation

(3) fetal renal system abnormalities

c. labor may be dysfunctional

d. fetal hypoxia may occur from cord compression during labor

III. OPERATIVE PROCEDURES

A. Episiotomy

Surgical incision into perineum

1. Rationale

a. facilitate delivery

b. prevent lacerations

(1) first-degree laceration: tear in mucous membrane and skin only

(2) second-degree laceration: includes above plus tear into perineal muscle

(3) third-degree laceration: both of above plus tear into rectal sphincter

(4) fourth-degree laceration: all of above plus tear into rectal mucosa

2. May be midline or mediolateral

B. Forceps

May be used to facilitate delivery

1. High forceps: above 0 station—never recommended

2. Mid forceps: 0 station—only occasionally used

3. Low forceps (outlet forceps): baby's head on perineum—most common

C. Cesarean Delivery (Section)

Delivery of fetus through abdominal incision

1. Elective

a. repeat of previous section

b. prediagnosed placenta previa, herpes, or abnormal presentation

2. Emergency

a. abruptio placenta: premature separation of placenta

b. placenta previa: abnormal implantation of placenta, in which placenta partially or completely covers cervical os

c. CPD

d. abnormal presentation

e. prolapsed cord

f. fetal distress

g. uterine dystocia

3. Types

a. classic

(1) midline section

(2) performed when speed is important

b. transverse incision in lower uterus

c. extra-peritoneal

4. Nursing interventions

a. remain calm

b. insert Foley catheter

c. be sure operative permit signed before administering any medications

d. notify nursery

5. Postoperative care

a. same as for every abdominal surgery patient

b. remember to monitor uterus as after any delivery

c. attention to postpartum needs

d. psychosocial support to facilitate mother–infant bonding

IV. SPECIAL CONCERNS

A. HIV-Positive Mother During and After Delivery

1. Assessment

a. knowledge of condition

b. plans for discharge care of self and infant

c. self-concept

d. mother's knowledge of own prognosis and infant's prognosis

(1) mother HIV-positive or with active AIDS

(2) one-third of infants born to HIV-positive mothers will be HIV-positive

(3) most of HIV-positive infants die within first 2 years

2. Implementation

a. use universal precaution guidelines from Centers for Disease Control (CDC) (Table 9-3)

b. provide routine postpartum care and support

c. teach self-care

TABLE 9–3. Universal Precautions Guidelines from the Centers for Disease Control

1. Precautions should be used in care of ALL patients
2. Barrier precautions to prevent skin and mucous membranes exposed
   a. Gloves for contact with blood and body fluids of mother and infant
   b. Masks, protective eye wear, and gowns for procedure that might involve droplet or splash exposure
3. Handwashing
   a. Immediately after exposure
   b. After removing gloves
4. Precautions to prevent needle-stick injuries
5. Health care workers with skin lesions should avoid direct patient contact until condition resolves

     (1) usual postpartum information
     (2) information needed to treat own disease
  d. teach infant care

     (1) HIV-positive infant, special needs
     (2) mother may be unable to care for infant
  e. encourage consultation with social services
3. Evaluation
  a. mother demonstrates feelings of self-worth
  b. mother verbalizes understanding of precaution
     (1) hand-washing
     (2) breast-feeding discouraged; HIV can be transmitted in breast milk
     (3) interactions with family and friends
     (4) disposal of soiled materials from self and infant (if infant HIV-positive)
  c. mother verbalizes knowledge of support systems
  d. mother verbalizes knowledge of disease process and prognosis for self and infant (if infant HIV-positive)

Questions

At 8 AM Susan Smith, a 24-year-old gravida 3 para 1, arrives at the labor and delivery unit. She states that her "water broke" about 7:30 this morning and she has been having contractions 6–7 minutes apart lasting 30 seconds since that time.

1. During the admission procedures, the LPN obtains Susan's temperature, pulse, and respiration (TPR), blood pressure (BP), and fetal heart rate (FHR). Vital signs are taken upon admission primarily because:

① It is hospital policy
② A baseline is necessary for further assessment
③ It is part of the admission record
④ The nursing care plan is based on this information

2. Before taking the FHR, the nurse palpates Susan's abdomen to determine fetal position. This procedure is known as:

① Ritgen's maneuver
② Homans' sign
③ Leopold's maneuver
④ Chadwick's sign

3. Rupture of the membranes (ROM) may be verified by testing:

① Fluid in the vagina with pH paper and obtaining an acid reaction
② Fluid in the vagina with pH paper and obtaining an alkaline reaction
③ Fluid in the vagina for glucose
④ Fluid in the vagina for meconium

4. Sterile vaginal examination (SVE) reveals that Susan's cervix is dilated 2–3 cm and 50% effaced and the presenting part is at 0 station. Complete dilation of the cervix is considered to be:

① 10 cm
② 8 cm
③ 20 cm
④ 5 cm

5. Effacement refers to:

① The amount of show
② The size of the pelvis
③ The position of the infant's head
④ Thinning and shortening of the cervix

6. Station refers to:

① Position of the baby's head in relation to the ischial spines
② Degree of flexion of the baby's head
③ Relationship of the presenting part to the four quadrants of the maternal pelvis
④ Ballottement

7. Susan is placed in bed, and the external fetal–maternal monitor is applied. The phono-transducer indicates an FHR of 140 bpm. The normal FHR is:

① 60–90 bpm
② 90–120 bpm
③ 120–160 bpm
④ 160–190 bpm

8. To time the frequency of Susan's contractions, the nurse counts the time from:

① The beginning of one contraction to the beginning of the next contraction
② The end of one contraction to the beginning of the next contraction
③ The beginning of the contraction to the end of the contraction
④ The peak of one contraction to the peak of the next contraction

9. Susan's contractions are 2–3 minutes apart and lasting 60 seconds. She is 5–6 cm dilated and is using good breathing techniques. Susan requests some medication for discomfort. The nurse's best reply would be:

① "Sure, I'll get you something right away."
② "No, you're in transition, and if we give you anything, it will make your baby sleepy."
③ "You are in the active phase of labor now. I will check with doctor to see if you can have something."
④ "I thought you wanted to have natural childbirth."

10. The doctor orders Demerol, 50 mg IM, to be given now. The nurse knows that:

① This is an incorrect dose
② Demerol can be given only by mouth
③ Demerol is a narcotic analgesic
④ The infant will require Narcan

11. Susan is taken to the delivery room. The doctor does an episiotomy to facilitate the birth of the baby. An episiotomy is an incision into:

① The peritoneum
② The abdomen
③ The perineum
④ The cervix

12. As soon as possible after delivery, the baby is placed next to Susan and her husband is encouraged to stroke and talk to the baby. This helps to promote:

① Involution
② Bonding and attachment
③ Separation of the placenta
④ Breast-feeding

13. The placenta separates and is expelled during the:

① First stage of labor
② Second stage of labor
③ Third stage of labor
④ Fourth stage of labor

Doris is a primigravida at term who was scheduled for a cesarean section but was admitted in active labor with a breech presentation. Her membranes are intact, and she is 4 cm dilated and at −1 station.

14. If her membranes rupture, she would be at risk for:

① A prolapsed cord
② A nuchal cord
③ Hemorrhage
④ Precipitate delivery

15. The LPN knows that a breech presentation means that the baby is in:

① A transverse position
② A vertex position
③ A buttocks presentation
④ Distress

16. The doctor decides to do an immediate cesarean section and orders a Foley catheter inserted. The purpose of the catheter is to:

① Prevent rupture of the membranes
② Slow down labor
③ Prevent incontinence postoperatively
④ Prevent trauma to the bladder during surgery

17. To provide the best outcome for both the mother and the baby, the anesthesia of choice would be a (an):

① Epidural
② General
③ Pudendal
④ Bier's block

18. Doris asks if she will be able to breast-feed her baby after a cesarean section. The nurse's best reply would be:

① "You will probably have a lot of pain, so perhaps you should consider bottle feeding."
② "Yes, and one of us will help you."
③ "You will have to ask the doctor."
④ "Don't think about that now—you can decide later."

Karen is admitted to the labor floor in active labor. A diagnosis of pregnancy-induced hypertension is made. An infusion of MgSO$_4$ is begun.

19. While Karen is receiving the MgSO$_4$, you observe that her respirations are 8 and her patellar reflexes have decreased. This should be:

① Brought to the attention of the charge nurse immediately
② Considered to be the desired result
③ Recorded and monitored to see if it continues
④ Considered as an indication that a higher dose of medication is needed

20. As you care for Karen, you watch the fetal monitor for signs of fetal distress. Fetal distress may be indicated by:

① An increase in the frequency and duration of contractions
② Meconium stained amniotic fluid when the baby is in a breech position
③ Decelerations in the fetal heart rate (FHR)
④ Increased bloody show as Karen nears the end of transition

21. The most common type of fetal deceleration is:

① Early
② Late
③ Variable
④ Periodic

22. Early decelerations are most often due to:

① Cord compression
② Fetal head compression
③ Uteroplacental insufficiency
④ Prolapsed cord

23. When oxygen is administered via mask to relieve fetal distress, the correct rate is:

① 2–3 L/min
② 4–6 L/min

③ 8–10 L/min
④ 15–20 L/min

24. Labor progresses, and Karen delivers a healthy baby boy and is taken to the recovery room. The chart indicates a blood loss of approximately 350 mL. This is:

① Considered to be postpartum hemorrhage
② Normal
③ A sign of retained placenta
④ An indication that a transfusion will be needed

Answers & Rationales

Guide to item identification (see pp. 3–5 for further details about each category)

I, II, III, or IV for the phase of the nursing process
1, 2, 3, or 4 for the category of client needs
A, B, C, D, E, F, or G for the category of human functioning
Specific content category by name; ie, cholecystectomy

1. While the other answers may be correct, it is
② most important to establishment a baseline so that changes may be assessed.
I, 4, A. Labor & Delivery.

2. Ritgen's maneuver assists in delivery of the fe-
③ tal head. Homans' sign assesses for thrombophlebitis. Chadwick's sign is a bluish coloration of the vagina found early in pregnancy.
III, 4, A. Labor & Delivery.

3. The pH of amniotic fluid is 7.5, or alkaline. The
② pH of vaginal fluid is 5–6.5, or acid.
III, 2 & 4, A. Labor & Delivery.

4. Complete dilation of the cervix is 10 cm.
① I, 1 & 4, A. Labor & Delivery.

5. Effacement is a thinning and shortening of the
④ cervix that occurs prior to or concurrent with dilation of the cervix.
I, 4, A. Labor & Delivery.

6. As the baby descends toward the perineum,
① progress is measured by the relationship of the presenting part to the ischial spines of the maternal pelvis.
I, 4, A. Labor & Delivery.

7. A fetal heart rate of less than 120 bpm is con-
③ sidered bradycardia, and an increase above 160 bpm is tachycardia. A 30 bpm deviation from the baseline may also be used to determine these conditions.
I, 4, A & B. Labor & Delivery.

8. Frequency is always timed from the beginning
① of one contraction to the beginning of the next contraction. Duration is the time period from the beginning of a contraction to the end of that contraction.
III, 4, A. Labor & Delivery.

9. During the active phase of labor is the optimum
③ time for the patient to receive medication. However, an order must always be obtained from the physician after complete assessment of the patient's progress. Answer 2 is not a correct assessment of the patient's progress, and answer 4 is judgmental.
III, 1 & 4, A & G. Labor & Delivery.

10. The dosage is within acceptable limits. The oral
③ route is the slowest acting. The infant will probably not require Narcan (naloxone) if the Demerol (meperidine) is given during the active phase of labor.
III, 1 & 4, A. Labor & Delivery.

11. An incision is made into the perineum to facili-
③ tate the delivery of the infant and to prevent lacerations.
I, 4, A. Labor & Delivery.

12. Early contact with the infant promotes a close
② relationship with both parents.
IV, 4, A & G. Labor & Delivery.

13. The first stage of labor is from the beginning of
③ contractions to complete dilation of the cervix. The second stage of labor is from complete dilation of the cervix through the delivery of the infant. The fourth stage of labor is the time from the delivery of the placenta to postpartum stability, about 2 hours.
I, 4, A. Labor & Delivery.

14. Rupture of the membranes when there is other
① than a cephalic presentation or when the presenting part is not engaged predisposes to a prolapsed cord. A nuchal cord is found around the back of the infant's neck. Precipitate delivery is a rapid delivery often without benefit of sterile preparations.
I, 4, A. Labor & Delivery.

15. In a transverse lie, the long axis of the infant is
③ crosswise to the long axis of the mother. A vertex is a head, or cephalic, presentation.
I, 4, A. Labor & Delivery.

16. During a cesarean section the bladder must re-
④ main empty to avoid trauma during surgery.
III, 4, A & D. C-section.

17. General anesthesia predisposes the infant
① to respiratory depression. A pudendal and a Bier's block are regional anesthetics that would have no effect on the abdomen.
IV, 4, A & D. C-section.

18. A cesarean section is not a contraindication to
② breast feeding. Encouragement and assistance
from the nursing staff will decrease anxiety and
promote successful breast-feeding.
III, 1 & 4, A & G. C-section.

19. Respirations less than 14, absent patellar re-
① flexes and urinary output of less than 24 mL/
hour are signs of magnesium toxicity, and the
physician should be notified immediately.
I & III, 1, 2, & 4, A, B & C. Labor & Delivery.

20. Decelerations in the FHR indicate an attempt by
③ the fetus to compensate for stress.
I, 1, 2, & 4, A & B. Labor & Delivery.

21. Variable decelerations are the most common
③ type and are associated with cord compression
and are often relieved by a change in maternal
position.
I, 4, A & B. Labor & Delivery.

22. Early decelerations are most often due to fetal
② head compression as the head progresses
through the maternal pelvis. Late decelerations
are considered ominous and are related to placental insufficiency.
I, 4, A & B. Labor & Delivery.

23. The rate of oxygen administration must be great
③ enough to cross the placenta and reach the
fetus.
III, 4, A & B. Labor & Delivery.

24. Normal blood loss during delivery is 300–
② 450 mL. A blood loss of more than 450–500 mL
is considered postpartum hemorrhage.
I, 2 & 4, A & B. Labor & Delivery.

POSTPARTUM PERIOD

Involution: Process occurring in time period from delivery until reproductive organs return to prepregnant state (usually about 6 weeks)

I. NORMAL POSTPARTUM PERIOD

A. Assessment

1. Fundus
   a. should be firm, 1–2 cm below umbilicus, in midline, and not palpable after day 10
   b. cramping sensation felt by mother as uterus contracts, called "afterpain"
      (1) more pronounced in multiparous patients
      (2) stimulated by breast-feeding
      (3) relieved by mild analgesic (Tylenol, Motrin)
      (4) ergovine may be prescribed to hasten process
2. Lochia
   a. rubra: bright red; lasts 1 to 2 days
   b. serosa: pinkish to brown; lasts 2 to 10 days
   c. alba: whitish; usually appears after day 10
   d. amount: should be scant
   e. report: any foul odor or increase in bright red blood
3. Perineum and rectum
   a. check episiotomy suture line for intactness, bruising, edema, or hematoma
   b. check for hemorrhoids
   c. apply ice packs or anesthetic sprays as ordered
   d. teach mother perineal care and proper application of perineal pads
   e. monitor for first bowel movement
      (1) usually within 3 days postpartum
      (2) administer stool softener (Colace) as ordered
4. Vital signs
   a. temperature
      (1) elevation 2 to 3 days postpartum and lasting less than 12 hours may be due to breast engorgement
      (2) elevation immediately after delivery may mean dehydration or beginning of infection
      (3) elevation greater than 100.2°F lasting or recurring for 24 hours or more may indicate endometritis, urinary tract infection, or other systemic infection
      (4) elevation accompanied by positive Homan's sign may indicate thrombophlebitis
   b. pulse
      (1) bradycardia (50–60 bpm) normal and may last 5 to 10 days
      (2) tachycardia may indicate pain, infection, anxiety, or excessive blood loss
   c. blood pressure
      (1) hypotension: blood loss
      (2) hypertension: ongoing disorder related to pregnancy, such as preeclampsia, PIH
5. Elimination
   a. urination
      (1) diuresis common first 24 hours and may last up to 5 days
      (2) be alert for signs of urinary tract infection
   b. defecation
      (1) stool softeners, such as Colace, usually ordered
      (2) monitor closely those patients with third- or fourth-degree lacerations
   c. diaphoresis (excessive sweating) is common as body adjusts to eliminate excess fluid
6. Weight loss
   a. 10–12 lb lost immediately after delivery from fetus, placenta, and fluid
   b. 5 lb lost in early postpartum period through diuresis and diaphoresis
   c. loss may be hastened by exercise and balanced diet
7. Lactation
   a. controlled by secretion of hormones prolactin and oxytocin
   b. stimulated by sucking of infant
   c. may be suppressed by drugs (TACE, Deludemone)
   d. breast-feeding requires high protein diet, with 500 additional calories
   e. initial milk called colostrum
8. Other
   a. Rh-negative mothers with Rh-positive fetus
      (1) mother develops antibodies
      (2) must be given RhoGAM within 72 hours after delivery
   b. mother who had low or no rubella titer
      (1) rubella vaccine given
      (2) may cause fever and symptoms of mild case of measles
      (3) mother should be told of dangers of becoming pregnant within 3 months after vaccination
9. Bonding and attachment
   a. relationship formed between parents and infant that has lifelong effects
   b. infants separated from parents at birth at risk for difficulties in bonding
   c. monitor for signs of bonding progression
   d. create atmosphere on nursing unit to enhance bonding

II. COMPLICATIONS OF POSTPARTUM PERIOD

A. Postpartum Hemorrhage

Blood loss greater than 500 mL

1. Causes
    a. uterine atony
    b. retained placenta
    c. lacerations of reproductive tract
2. Control and correction of hemorrhage
    a. massage fundus
    b. additional Pitocin given
    c. if bleeding continues and fundus boggy, patient may need to return to delivery room for sterile examination to look for retained placenta fragments or other problem
    d. blood loss may need to be replaced by transfusions

B. Puerperal Infections

1. Endometritis
    a. predisposing factors
        (1) prolonged labor
        (2) postpartum hemorrhage
        (3) premature rupture of membranes
        (4) intrauterine manipulation
        (5) anemia
        (6) retention of placental fragments
    b. assessment
        (1) sustained fever 100.4°F or higher
        (2) uterine tenderness
        (3) profuse, foul-smelling lochia, sometimes frothy
    c. treatments and nursing interventions
        (1) antibiotic therapy, usually IV
        (2) Tylenol for temperature above 101°F
        (3) sitz bath
        (4) position to promote excretion of lochia
2. Mastitis (inflammation of breasts)
    a. cause: usually due to *Staphylococcus aureus* derived from:
        (1) infant's nose or mouth
        (2) mother herself because of poor hand washing
        (3) hospital personnel because of poor hand washing
    b. assessment
        (1) usually appears third or fourth week of puerperium
        (2) marked by breast engorgement
        (3) chills
        (4) elevated temperature
        (5) increased pulse rate
        (6) hardness and redness of breasts
        (7) pain in breast
    c. treatment and nursing interventions
        (1) antibiotic therapy
        (2) administer pain medication as needed
        (3) teach and maintain good hygiene
        (4) breast-feeding may or may not be discontinued

C. Thrombophlebitis

1. Etiology
    a. injury (bruise) to vein
    b. extension of infection from tissues surrounding vessel
    c. pregnancy, when women must be in bed for prolonged time
    d. unusual activity in person who has been sedentary
2. Assessment
    a. soreness or stiffness in calf
    b. edema of leg
    c. redness over area affected
    d. pain in upper posterior calf on dorsiflexion of foot (Homan's sign)
    e. assumption of "frog-like" position (leg externally rotated, knee flexed)
    f. muscle ache, may be falsely assumed to result from wearing flat bedroom slippers postoperatively
    g. signs of circulatory obstruction (thrombus)
        (1) swelling
        (2) vasospasm followed by cyanosis
        (3) increasing coolness of area
        (4) loss of pulses distal to obstruction
    h. signs of pulmonary embolus
        (1) restlessness
        (2) severe shortness of breath
        (3) unrelieved chest pain
        (4) frothy blood-tinged sputum
        (5) respiratory arrest
3. Preventative measures
    a. initiate early ambulation as soon as possible in postpartum or postoperative period
    b. avoid keeping extremities in one position for long period of time
    c. avoid using knee gatch on bed
    d. do not sit with legs crossed
    e. use elastic stockings before thrombophlebitis occurs
4. Treatment and nursing interventions
    a. institute all preventative measures appropriate for this patient
    b. avoid massaging or rubbing calf because of danger of breaking clot loose

c. apply heat in form of warm, moist packs to area to promote circulation and provide comfort
d. administer anticoagulants as ordered
  (1) IV heparin first
  (2) oral Coumadin next, and after discharge
e. bed rest with affected leg elevated, without pressure behind knee
f. apply support hose to unaffected leg only
g. instruct patient for discharge
  (1) wear support stockings (remove several times daily for short periods)
  (2) avoid prolonged sitting or standing
  (3) elevate extremity as much as possible
  (4) take precautions against injury to area
  (5) exercise extremity for 5 minutes every hour
  (6) take Coumadin as ordered
    (a) return per physician's orders for blood tests
    (b) do not stop taking Coumadin until told by physician
    (c) instruct on bleeding precautions

D. Urinary Tract Infections

1. Predisposing factors
  a. urinary stasis
  b. indwelling catheters
  c. renal disease
  d. lowered body resistance
2. Assessment
  a. some patients completely asymptomatic (diagnosis made by presence of bacteria in urine culture in more than 100,000 microorganisms/mL)
  b. dysuria
  c. urgency
  d. frequency
  e. burning sensation on voiding
  f. fever
  g. flank pain; costovertebral angle (CVA) tenderness
3. Treatment and nursing interventions
  a. antibiotics for 10 to 14 days
  b. encourage fluids, especially acid–ash fluids, such as cranberry juice

c. follow-up cultures should be done after antibiotic therapy (disappearance of symptoms does not mean patient has been adequately treated)

E. Wound Separations

1. Predisposing factors
  a. sutures giving way
  b. obesity
  c. infections
  d. marked distention
  e. heavy coughing without splinting incision
  f. pulmonary or cardiovascular disease
  g. diabetes mellitus
  h. steroid therapy
2. Types of wound separations
  a. dehiscence: separation of wound edges down to peritoneum, without exposure of viscera
  b. evisceration: separation of wound edges, with protrusion of viscera through open incision
3. Assessment
  a. patient complains feeling that something suddenly gave way in wound
  b. edges of wound separated, intestines may be exposed and gradually pushing out (observe for drainage of peritoneal fluid on dressing)
  c. pain, anxiety, and vomiting
4. Treatment and nursing interventions
  a. return patient to bed in semi-Fowler's position with knees flexed to relieve tension on abdominal muscles
  b. notify surgeon immediately
  c. if intestines are exposed, cover with sterile dressing, wet with normal saline
  d. reassure patient, keep patient quiet and relaxed
  e. for eviscerations, prepare patient for surgery and wound repair
  f. for smaller dehiscence, irrigations with saline or hydrogen peroxide may be ordered; wound eventually heals, by granulation, leaving wider scar

Questions

1. Following a normal vaginal delivery, the patient's vital signs, fundus, and lochia are checked every 15 minutes until stable. The fundus should be:

   ① Firm, below the umbilicus and in the midline
   ② Soft, below the umbilicus and in the midline
   ③ Firm, dextroverted and above the umbilicus
   ④ Soft, above the umbilicus and in the midline

2. A postpartum patient is receiving an infusion of dextrose 5% in lactated Ringer's solution with Pitocin, 20 U, while in the recovery room. The purpose of the Pitocin is to:

   ① Decrease discomfort
   ② Prevent uterine tetany
   ③ Remove retained placental fragments
   ④ Prevent uterine atony

3. A nursing mother often does not menstruate for several months after delivery or until she discontinues breast-feeding. She should be taught that:

   ① Ovulation is suppressed and pregnancy is impossible while she is breast-feeding
   ② Ovulation is not suppressed and pregnancy is possible even though she is breast-feeding
   ③ The uterus will not return to a normal size while she is breast-feeding
   ④ If she does not begin to menstruate in 3 months, she should stop breast-feeding

4. The nurse notes that the lochia has a foul smell. The most appropriate nursing intervention is:

   ① Report immediately that the patient may have an infection
   ② Nothing, as this is normal during the first few days after delivery
   ③ Begin vaginal irrigations to decrease the odor and increase patient comfort
   ④ Stop the use of perineal pads for the next few days

5. When administering an enema to a postpartum patient, it is important that the nurse:

   ① Use a small caliber tube
   ② Administer no more than 100 mL of solution
   ③ Be careful not to irritate the perineum while inserting the rectal tube
   ④ Encourage the patient to administer her own so she will learn how for home care

6. The incidence of postpartum thrombophlebitis has been decreased owing to which of the following nursing interventions?

   ① Early ambulation
   ② Immobilization and elevation of the lower extremities
   ③ Administration of anticoagulants routinely after the birth
   ④ Breast-feeding the newborn

Mary is a single 17 year old who delivers a healthy baby girl.

7. Two hours after Mary's delivery, you notice that Mary's fundus is firm, rising and displaced to the right. This indicates:

   ① Postpartum bleeding
   ② A normal position
   ③ Retained placental fragments
   ④ A full bladder

8. Mary had a laceration into the vaginal mucosa and the perineal muscle. This is a:

   ① First-degree laceration
   ② Second-degree laceration
   ③ Third-degree laceration
   ④ Fourth-degree laceration

9. Mary plans to bottle-feed her infant, and the doctor orders medication to suppress lactation. Which of the following drugs is used for this purpose?

   ① TACE
   ② Motrin
   ③ Pitocin
   ④ Colace

10. Even though Mary's family has been supportive, she expresses concern about how she will support herself and her baby. Your best response would be:

   ① "You should have thought of that before you got pregnant."

   ② "Getting on welfare is probably your best bet."

   ③ "The baby's father has a responsibility to help you out."

   ④ "Tell me some of the things you have considered, and we can find out more about them."

11. Because of Mary's educational level, socioeconomic status, and age:

   ① She has special need for information about maternal and infant nutrition

   ② Her baby is at risk for neglect and abuse

   ③ She is at risk for postpartum complications

   ④ All of the above

Answers & Rationales

Guide to item identification (see pp. 3–5 for further details about each category)

I, II, III, or IV for the phase of the nursing process
1, 2, 3, or 4 for the category of client needs
A, B, C, D, E, F, or G for the category of human functioning
Specific content category by name; ie, cholecystectomy

1. ① A soft, boggy uterus is associated with postpartum bleeding. If the fundus is firm, rising and displaced to the right or left side, the patient probably has a full bladder.
IV, 4, A. Postpartum.

2. ④ Pitocin (oxytocin) promotes contraction of the uterus.
IV, 4, A & D. Postpartum/Medications.

3. ② Although menstruation usually does not occur, ovulation may occur, so lactation is not a method of contraception.
III, 4, A. Postpartum.

4. ① Foul odor may indicate the presence of an infection and should be reported to the doctor so antibiotics can be started.
III, 4, A & D. Postpartum.

5. ③ It is important to be gentle, because the area around the episiotomy is easily irritated and hemorrhoids are quite common.
III, 4, A & F. Postpartum.

6. ① Early ambulation is the most effective and safe way to prevent thrombophlebitis.
III, 4, A, B, & E. Postpartum.

7. ④ The fundus should be firm, below the umbilicus and in the midline. A firm, rising fundus often displaced to the right is an indication of a full bladder.
I & IV, 4, A & F. Postpartum.

8. ② Second-degree lacerations include the skin, mucous membrane and the muscles of the perineal block.
I & IV, 4, A & D. Postpartum.

9. ① TACE is a lactation inhibitor.
I & III, 4, A & D. Postpartum.

10. ④ It is important to discover what plans and ideas the person has and explore those possibilities. Giving advice is judgmental, serves no useful purpose and only increases the person's feelings of insecurity and any guilt feeling they may have.
III, 4, A & G. Postpartum.

11. ④ A single teenage mother usually has limited resources and coping mechanisms. Support systems can assist the mother in gaining maturity and in learning parenting skills. Her health status may also be lowered.
II & IV, 4, A & G. Postpartum.

NEONATE

First 4 weeks of life

I. NORMAL PHYSICAL DEVELOPMENT

A. Appearance

1. Head often misshapen; one-fourth total body size
   a. caput succedaneum
   b. molding
2. Skin discolored and puffy
3. Protruding umbilical stump for first 3 weeks
4. Soft fontanels
   a. posterior closes in about 2 to 3 months
   b. anterior closes about 8 to 18 months

B. Head Circumference

1. Measurement taken over eyebrows, just above eyes, across posterior occipital protuberance
2. Normal size about 14 inches (or 35 cm)
3. Head may be molded from birthing process

C. Cardiovascular System

1. Foramen ovale functionally closes after 1 minute; anatomically after 2 weeks
2. Ductus arteriosus functionally closes after 15 hours; anatomically closes in 3 weeks
3. Unstable temperature regulation system
   a. dependent on ambient (room) temperature and amount of covering
   b. observe facial color to gauge warmth
      (1) flushed face, too warm
      (2) pale or bluish face, too cold

D. Skin

1. Lanugo: downy hair, lost after few months
2. Vernix caseosa: cheesy skin covering that rubs off in several days
3. Milia: small collections of sebaceous secretions that disappear within several weeks
4. Hemangiomas: pink spots that may or may not be permanent
5. Mongolian spots: slate colored areas found in Blacks, Asians, or Mediterraneans, which normally fade; usually over sacrum and gluteal areas
6. Jaundice: yellowish discoloration of skin
   a. physiologic: normal by about day 3 or 4 and disappears in 1 week
   b. abnormal: occurs in first 24 hours, usually due to Rh incompatibility
7. Acrocyanosis: normal blueness of hands and feet
8. Desquamation: peeling of skin; normal for about 2 to 4 weeks after birth
9. Umbilical cord
   a. dries and shrinks rapidly dropping off in 6 to 14 days
   b. area should be cleaned daily with alcohol and watched for presence of infection

E. Weight/Length

1. Weight at birth is about 7 to 8 lb
2. Normal loss of 10% of birth weight right after birth
3. Steady weight gain begins at 1 to 2 weeks
4. Average length about 19 to 21 inches

F. Vital Signs

1. Unstable in newborn
2. Respirations vary from 50 to 80 right after birth to 35 to 50 soon thereafter
3. Temperature ranges from 97°F to 100°F, with body heat lost very rapidly
4. Heart rate at birth is 120 to 150 bpm and varies from 170 to 180 bpm when crying to 90 bpm when asleep, dropping throughout first years of life
5. Blood pressure is 40 to 70 systolic, reaching 80/40 by end of first month of life

G. Elimination

1. Gastrointestinal (GI)
   a. Meconium: first fecal material passed 8 to 24 hours after birth
      (1) mix of amniotic fluid and intestinal glandular secretions
      (2) dark green, thick, sticky stool
   b. transition stools with mucus for first week
   c. 2 to 4 stools/day normal at first, decreasing to 1 to 2 stools/day
   d. breast-fed baby: stools soft, yellow, and pasty; more frequent than bottle-fed baby
   e. bottle-fed baby: stools more solid and yellow to brown
   f. stools are darker if infant is receiving iron
   g. stools are greener if infant is under bilirubin lamp
2. Genitourinary (GU)
   a. decreased ability to concentrate urine
      (1) more prone to dehydration
      (2) limited ability to reabsorb important substances

b. voids soon after birth
c. voids frequently during early life

H. Reflex Activities

1. Consummatory: survival, such as rooting and sucking
2. Avoidant: elicited by potentially harmful stimuli, such as Moro's reflex and blinking
3. Postural: tonic neck reflex seen when baby asleep
4. Exploratory: when awake and upright
5. Social: such as smiling
6. Attentional: orienting and attending
7. Born with reflexes, such as gag, sneeze, blink, suck, and grasp
8. Absence of any reflexes should be noted

II. SENSORY DEVELOPMENT

1. Vision
   a. can see at birth
   b. able to fixate points of contrast
   c. shows preference for human face
   d. can follow moving objects
   e. likes bright or contrasting colors
2. Hearing
   a. responsive to verbal stimuli
   b. avoid auditory overload
   c. attends to auditory toys
3. Sleep
   a. usually sleeps 15 to 20 hours/day at first
   b. may begin sleeping through night after 4 to 6 weeks

III. CARE OF NEONATE

A. Immediate Assessment

1. Airway
   a. first concern after delivery, clearing airway
   b. use soft rubber bulb syringe to aspirate mouth gently and then the nose
   c. spontaneous breathing usually occurs soon after birth
   d. if breathing does not occur
      (1) immediate resuscitation
      (2) tactile stimulation
      (3) ventilation
      (4) use of naloxone (Narcan) to reverse narcotics given to mother
2. Apgar: system of immediate assessment of newborn to evaluate physical status
   a. assess
      (1) heart rate
      (2) respiratory effort: frequency and regularity
      (3) muscle tone
      (4) reflex irritability
      (5) color
   b. each scored as 0, 1, or 2, then added together, with 10 being highest score
      (1) 7–10: condition good
      (2) 4–6: condition fair
      (3) 0–3: poor condition and need for further evaluation and care
   c. first assessment at 1 minute after delivery
   d. second assessment at 5 minutes
3. Assess for gestational age
   a. Dubowitz evaluation
      (1) done within 24 hours after birth
      (2) scoring system including evaluation of physical characteristics and neuromuscular tone
   b. also figured by counting weeks fetal development from first day of mother's last normal period until delivery
4. Meconium aspiration
   a. suggestive of fetal distress in utero
   b. common if fetus is a cephalic presentation, with meconium-stained amniotic fluid
   c. neonate needs immediate suctioning
   d. may exhibit respiratory distress
      (1) mild, usually disappears in 48 hours
      (2) severe, may lead to aspiration pneumonia and require intensive care

B. Immediate Nursing Care

1. Prevention of infection
   a. sterile technique for cutting cord
   b. use of 1% silver nitrate solution or erythromycin opthalmic ointment in eyes to prevent ophthalmia neonatorum (blindness from maternal gonococcal infection)
2. Provision of warmth
   a. use of preheated tables, warming lamps, and warm blankets
   b. dry neonate well
   c. can be placed on mother's chest, with direct contact providing body warmth
   d. cap on neonate to prevent heat loss
3. Vitamin K given IM to aid in clotting and preventing bleeding
4. Neonate footprinted and identification bracelets applied to mother and neonate before removing neonate from delivery room

C. Continuing Care of Neonate

1. Bonding: psychosocial attachment of neonate to mother and father
   a. both parents allowed to hold and touch neonate

b. need to assure themselves of neonate's sex and wholeness
c. parents encouraged to point out family resemblances
d. way to begin to establish parental role and love neonate
2. Screening tests
   a. phenylketonuria (PKU)
      (1) screening for inability to metabolize phenylalanine
      (2) done after neonate feeds for first time
   b. hypothyroidism
   c. galactosemia
   d. hypoglycemia
3. Teaching infant care
   a. mother needs to learn to care for infant
      (1) bathing
      (2) diapering
      (3) safety
      (4) care of umbilical cord
      (5) need for sleep
   b. feeding
      (1) bottle
      (2) breast-feeding

Questions

1. The jaundice associated with erythroblastosis fetalis is generally seen:

   ① During the first 24 hours after birth
   ② 72–96 hours after birth
   ③ 96–120 hours after birth
   ④ 1 week after birth

2. Baby Boy Harris, 6 lb 1 oz, was just delivered after a long labor. His initial Apgar is 3. Which of the following is the priority nursing intervention for this baby?

   ① Suction him
   ② Dry him with a warm towel
   ③ Ventilate him with 100% oxygen at 40 to 60 breaths/minute
   ④ Place baby under warmer to maintain body temperature

3. Baby Boy Harris is in the newborn nursery. In assessing his eyes and vision, which of the following would be an abnormal finding?

   ① Crossed eyes
   ② Absent blink reflex
   ③ Positive red reflex
   ④ Edema of the eyelids

4. Which of the following would be an abnormality in the newborn's cardiovascular system?

   ① Heart rate of 154
   ② Irregular heart beats
   ③ Acrocyanosis of the extremities
   ④ Circumoral cyanosis

5. Baby Boy Harris is breathing with 10- to 15-second periods of apnea. The PN knows that this is a sign of:

   ① Normal newborn breathing
   ② Impending respiratory distress
   ③ Prenatal asthma
   ④ Impending respiratory infection

6. When you assess the newborn's renal system, which of the following would be considered abnormal?

   ① Urine specific gravity of 1.008
   ② First void after the first 24 hours
   ③ Voiding up to 20 times a day
   ④ "Brick dust" colored urine with the first void

7. Which of the following is *not* part of the care of a newborn with hyperbilirubinemia?

   ① Withhold fluids during treatment
   ② Maintain neutral temperature
   ③ Administer phototherapy
   ④ Assist with exchange transfusions if needed

8. Baby Fran, 6 lb 8 oz, was born today. She is in the newborn nursery and you are caring for her. Which of the following is appropriate when caring for the umbilical cord?

   ① Apply a petrolatum gauze dressing over the site
   ② Apply a simple dry dressing over the site
   ③ Clean the site daily vigorously with soap and water
   ④ Apply topical triple dye or bacitracin ointment initially and apply alcohol daily

9. Gastric emptying time in the newborn is about:

   ① 1–1 1/2 hours
   ② 2 1/2 –3 hours
   ③ 1 1/2–2 hours
   ④ 3–3 1/2 hours

10. About how many calories/day does the average newborn need?

    ① 50 cal/kg/day
    ② 75 cal/kg/day
    ③ 120 cal/kg/day
    ④ 150 cal/kg/day

11. The newborn infant exhibits a number of reflexes at birth. Which reflex is *not* present at birth?

    ① Parachute reflex
    ② Moro's reflex
    ③ Sucking reflex
    ④ Extrusion reflex

12. Which of the following is not a risk factor for respiratory distress syndrome?

    ① Prematurity
    ② Maternal diabetes
    ③ Birth trauma
    ④ Post-term birth

Answers & Rationales

Guide to item identification (see pp. 3–5 for further details about each category)

I, II, III, or IV for the phase of the nursing process
1, 2, 3, or 4 for the category of client needs
A, B, C, D, E, F, or G for the category of human functioning
Specific content category by name; ie, cholecystectomy

1. ① Pathologic jaundice appears within the first 24 hours after birth.
I, 4, A & E. Newborn.

2. ③ An Apgar score of 3 indicates a very depressed infant. He will be intubated and ventilated at a rate of 40 to 60 breaths/minute with 100% oxygen.
III, 4, A & B. Newborn.

3. ② The blink reflex is a protective reflex that is present at birth; absence is abnormal.
III, 2, A & C. Newborn.

4. ④ Circumoral cyanosis is an ominous sign of severe hypoxia and is not a normal finding.
III, 1, A & B. Newborn.

5. ① Short periods of apnea are normal in the newborn and no action is needed.
III, 1, A & B. Newborn.

6. ② It is normal for the first voiding to be within the first 24 hours, not after it.
III, 1, A & F. Newborn.

7. ① It is important that the newborn be adequately hydrated to help prevent further complications from hyperbilirubinemia.
III, 4, A & F. Newborn.

8. ④ The cord needs to dry and should be open to the air. An antibiotic ointment is applied initially and the cord cleaned daily with alcohol. The baby should receive sponge baths until the cord drops off.
III, 4, A. Newborn.

9. ② Normal gastric emptying in the newborn is about $2\frac{1}{2}$ to 3 hours.
III, 1, A & F. Newborn.

10. ③ The normal newborn needs about 120 cal/kg/day to grow normally.
III, 1 & 4, A & E. Newborn.

11. ① The parachute reflex appears at about 7 to 9 months and remains indefinitely.
III, 1, A & C. Newborn.

12. ④ The post-term infant is not at special risk for RDS. The other options listed are risk factors for RDS.
III, 1, A & B. Newborn.

BIBLIOGRAPHY

Bobak, I.M., Jensen, M., and Zalar, M. (1989). *Maternity and Gynecological Care, The Nurse and the Family.* 4th ed. C.V. Mosby Co., St. Louis.

Burroughs, A. (1986). *Bleier's Maternity Nursing.* 5th ed. W.B. Saunders Co., Philadelphia.

Freiberg, K.L. (1987). *Human Development—A Life Span Approach.* 3rd ed. Jones and Bartlett Publishers, Boston.

Friedman, H.S., and DiMatteo, M.R. (1989). *Health Psychology.* Prentice Hall, Englewood, NJ.

Hamilton, P.M. (1989). *Basic Maternity Nursing.* 6th ed. C.V. Mosby Co., St. Louis.

Ingalls, A.J., and Salerno, M.C. (1987). *Maternal and Child Health Nursing.* 6th ed. C.V. Mosby Co., St. Louis.

Lewis, A. (1988). *Nursing Care of the Person with AIDS/ARC.* Aspen Publishers, Rockville, MD.

Thompson, E.D. (1990). *Introduction to Maternity and Pediatric Nursing.* W.B. Saunders Co., Philadelphia.

The Mental Health Patient

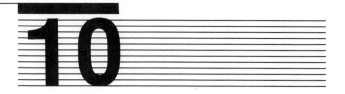

COMMUNICATION, INTERACTION, AND BEHAVIOR

Involves exchange of attitudes, feelings, and ideas; done through:

1. **Active listening:** allowing individual to own problem, using techniques of reflection and clarification
2. **"I" messages:** clear and honest statements of fact about individual, rather than "you" messages, which put receiver on defensive

■ Communication Process

I. PROCESS

A. Assessment

1. Assess patient's level of functioning, ability to process information
2. Observe what is happening to patient at present time
3. Assess overall behavior and appearance of patient
4. Identify environmental conditions that may affect communication process
5. Assess relationship between persons communicating
   a. sender's purpose
   b. content of message
   c. nonverbal manner in which message is conveyed
   d. effect of message on receiver
6. Verbal versus nonverbal communication
   a. verbal refers to what is actually said
   b. nonverbal refers to message conveyed by means other than speaking
      (1) body language
      (2) facial expressions
      (3) gestures
      (4) distancing
      (5) often "implied" message
      (6) patient may be unaware of these messages
   c. verbal and nonverbal messages may or may not be same

d. nonverbal communication easily misunderstood

B. Planning, Goals/Expected Outcomes

1. Patient will know purpose of interaction
2. Patient will be able to understand messages being sent
3. Patient will be able to convey needs, feelings, and thoughts
4. Patient will develop agreement between verbal and nonverbal communication
5. Patient will maintain control over own life

C. Implementation

1. Identify situations to be discussed with patient
   a. define purpose of relationship
   b. identify expectations
   c. provide safe, comfortable, and protective environment
2. Use active listening techniques to encourage patient to describe what is happening
   a. ask patient to clarify message received
   b. use "I" messages rather than "you" messages, such as "I do not like what you are doing," not "you shouldn't do that"
   c. avoid selective listening
   d. avoid insensitive listening
3. Assist patient to identify own thoughts and feelings
   a. tune into verbal and nonverbal cues from patient
   b. maintain accepting, nonjudgmental attitude
4. Focus on patient's verbal and nonverbal communication
   a. assist patient to recognize inconsistencies between verbal and nonverbal communication
   b. give honest, nonbiased feedback to patient
5. Allow patient to problem solve
   a. assist patient to use problem-solving process
   b. help patient to identify goals, to meet individual needs
   c. focus on positive aspects of patient's attempt to communicate effectively

D. Evaluation

1. Communication, patient centered
2. Patient's ability to understand messages received is increased
3. Patient's ability to communicate needs, feelings, and thoughts improved
4. Patient's verbal and nonverbal communications consistent with one another
5. Patient's coping mechanisms improved

■ Interpersonal Relationships

I. INTERACTIONS

Between two or more persons over period of time

II. THERAPEUTIC INTERPERSONAL RELATIONSHIPS

Characterized by

1. Acceptance
2. Honesty
3. Understanding
4. Empathy

A. Phases

1. Initial, introductory, or orientation phase
   a. guidelines for relationship established
   b. problems and expectations identified
2. Working, problem solving, or working through phase
   a. problem-solving techniques developed for identified problems
   b. methods of working through problems implemented and evaluated
   c. focus on increasing patient's independence
3. Terminating phase
   a. closing of relationship planned for early in development of relationship
   b. problems of termination anticipated and discussed openly

B. Assessment

1. Self-assessment questions for PN
   a. do you honestly want to help?
   b. are you able to experience positive attitudes toward others: caring, warmth, acceptance, interest, and respect?
   c. can you give, or must you always be on receiving end?
   d. can you enter into patient's world and view what's happening from patient's perspective?
   e. can you allow patient to grow by encountering his/her independence and, eventually, separation?
2. Patient assessment
   a. determine purpose of relationship with patient
   b. observe what is happening with patient in here and now and how patient perceives your assistance
   c. identify developmental level of patient so that realistic expectations of relationship are developed
   d. assess verbal and nonverbal communication patterns of patient
   e. examine expectations of patient and self in terms of outcome of relationship

C. Planning, Goals/Expected Outcomes

1. Patient will develop sense of trust
2. Patient will be able to verbalize thoughts and feelings clearly
3. Patient will be able to set goals for self within relationship
4. Patient will use problem-solving process with ineffective behaviors
5. Patient will become as independent as possible and be able to terminate relationship in positive way

D. Implementation

1. Help identify times that trust occurs in patient's behavior; for example, when patient makes positive decision about own life, respond by saying, "That was a positive choice you made. See, you can trust your decisions."
   a. accept patient as is currently
   b. be open, honest, and consistent in relationship with patient
   c. demonstrate to patient that you can be trusted; only make promises you can keep
2. Encourage patient to verbalize thoughts and feelings in clear way
   a. tune into verbal cues to increase expression
   b. use nonverbal techniques
   c. use open-ended statements
   d. clarify misinterpretations or misconceptions of feelings by patient
3. Define expectations of relationship: assist patient in developing realistic and attainable goals
4. Help patient define problem
   a. explore alternative solutions to problem with patient

b. encourage patient to test out one of solutions in safe and supportive environment

c. reinforce patient's growth-producing behaviors

5. At start of relationship, plan, with patient, for termination of relationship
   a. encourage expression of feelings during this time
   b. help patient work through any negative reactions

E. Evaluation

1. Patient able to initiate contact on own
2. Patient interacted and expressed self more clearly
3. Patient took active part in goal setting
4. Patient explored alternative solutions to problems
5. Patient demonstrated greater self-confidence by functioning more independently

■ Patterns of Behavior

I. WITHDRAWAL PATTERN OF BEHAVIOR

A. Assessment

1. Definition: disintegrative behavior pattern characterized by thinking disorder, withdrawal from reality, bizarre, regressive behavior, poor communication, and impaired interpersonal relationships; this pattern of behavior seen in persons suffering from schizophrenic disorders

B. Classifications of Schizophrenia

1. Catatonic
   a. stuporous state: mute, immobile, waxy flexibility, urinary and fecal retention
   b. excited state: assaultive, aggressive, hyperactive, agitated
2. Disorganized: incoherent, foolish, regressive
3. Paranoid: delusions of persecution and grandeur
4. Undifferentiated: variety of symptoms found in other classifications

C. Incidence

1. Onset of active disease before age 45 years
2. Mainly affects adolescents and young adults
3. Occurs in about 1% of population; most prevalent of major psychoses
4. Increased incidence in lower socioeconomic classes
5. Occupy 50% of psychiatric hospital beds

D. Prognosis

1. 25% recover completely
2. 50%–60% retain some residual symptoms
3. 10% never improve

E. Signs and Symptoms

1. Associative looseness, flattened affect, ambivalence, autism
2. Disrupted thought process
3. Inability to express appropriate emotions
4. Hallucinations
5. Unable to relate to others in meaningful way
6. Delusions

F. Planning, Goals/ Expected Outcomes

1. Patient will take prescribed medications
2. Patient will maintain contact with reality
3. Patient will initiate a social contact independently
4. Patient will take care of own physical needs and function more independently

G. Implementation

1. Establish trusting relationship; open, honest communication
2. Alleviate patient's anxiety
3. Maintain patient's biologic integrity
4. Give antipsychotic medications as ordered (Table 10-1)
5. Distract patient from preoccupation by approaching patient in warm, friendly way to take walk
6. Design reality-oriented activities that will make external environment more satisfying to patient
7. Approach patient for short intervals at patient's level of functioning
8. Accept patient where he or she is and realize that, at this time, it is best patient can do
9. Provide consistent, honest interaction with patient to develop trust
10. Gradually increase social contacts from one-to-one to include other people in environment
11. Initially, supervise and assist patient, as needed, in caring for physical needs
12. Gradually encourage patient to make decisions and assume responsibility for personal care
13. Praise patient when patient does things for self and let patient know that he or she can trust self to make choices

TABLE 10–1. Antipsychotic Agents (Major Tranquilizers)

Classification

Antipsychotic agents (major tranquilizers)

Action

Target symptoms most likely to decrease include: hyperactivity, combativeness, agitation, hostility, hallucinations, irritability, negativism, acute delusions, insomnia, poor self-care, anorexia

Use

Psychotic disorders, such as schizophrenic disorders, paranoid disorders, affective disorders, and organic mental disorders

Common Side Effects

Sedation, extrapyramidal side effects (EPS), anticholinergic effects, allergic side effects

Nursing Implications/Teaching

Additive effect when combined with other central nervous system (CNS) depressants; check tongue regularly for vermiform movements (early sign of tardive dyskinesia); relieve dry mouth by rinsing—sips of water, chewing sugarless gum or "Quench," a saliva-stimulating gum; use paste adhesive for dentures; add chewing time with extra fluid between bites of food; fluids running out of mouth may signal dysphagia; dangle, especially after injections; check for urinary retention and constipation; extra tears for contact lens or may not be able to wear contacts because of dryness; red, hot, dry skin is sign of anhydrosis—cool immediately; sunscreen factor is for photosensitivity; dilute liquid medication

Examples

Haldol (haloperidol), Mellaril (thioridazine), Prolixin (fluphenazine), Loxitane (loxapine), Navane (thiothixene), Thorazine (chlorpromazine)

H. Evaluation

1. Patient complied with medication regimen
2. Patient realized when he or she distorted reality and verbalized more realistic perception of self
3. Patient related to others in more effective ways
4. Patient assumed more self-care responsibility

II. OVERLY SUSPICIOUS PATTERN OF BEHAVIOR

A. Assessment

1. Definition: disruptive lifestyle characterized by extreme suspiciousness, lack of trust, anger, delusions of persecution or jealousy, tendency to blame others, rigidity, and feelings of being mistreated or misjudged; this pattern seen in people suffering from paranoid disorders
2. Signs and symptoms
   a. suspicious of others' behavior
   b. secretiveness
   c. overconcerned with hidden motives and special meanings
   d. feeling of constant persecution
   e. tense, rigid, insecure
   f. clear, elaborate, and lasting delusions
   g. distorted religious beliefs
   h. alienation (basic mistrust of all others)
   i. may be hostile and possibly violent

B. Planning, Goals/ Expected Outcomes

1. Patient will take prescribed medications
2. Patient will learn to trust self and others
3. Patient will have needs met in more realistic way
4. Patient will use constructive outlets to deal with anger

C. Implementation

1. Give antipsychotic medications as ordered (Table 10-1)
2. Approach patient slowly, one-to-one, allow plenty of personal space
3. Help patient learn to trust self by identifying times that trust occurs in behavior; for example, when patient makes positive decision about own life, respond by saying, "That was a good choice that you made; see, you can trust yourself to make decisions about your life."
4. Listen to patient without agreeing or disagreeing
5. Communicate understanding to patient, but explain that what patient is presenting is not reality, always in calm and matter of fact way
6. Give honest, specific praise for patient's accomplishments
7. Provide noncompetitive, solitary tasks, such as puzzles, ceramics, punching bag, or running, as outlets for anger and aggressive drives
8. Move patient into group activities after patient develops trust in self and environment

D. Evaluation

1. Patient complied with medication regimen
2. Overly suspicious behavior decreased through establishment of trusting relationship
3. Patient's delusional system subsided as needs met in more realistic way
4. Patient has found safe outlets for aggressive drives

III. PATTERNS OF BEHAVIOR INVOLVING MOOD AND AFFECT

A. Assessment

1. Definition: variety of states that include extremes of mood and affect
   a. depression: sense of loss that overwhelms patient

b. mania: denial of loss with temporary improvement in self-esteem; reaction formation to depression; elation

c. bipolar (manic-depressive disorders): alternating mania and depression

B. Incidence

1. Depression
   a. any age, both sexes, but women and people over age 65 years more common
   b. 1.5 million patients diagnosed per year
   c. almost half recover without treatment
   d. most common emotional illness
2. Mania
   a. more common in women
   b. occurs much more commonly in siblings or family of sufferers
   c. highest occurrence in Northern Europeans and descendants
3. Bipolar: occurs before age 30 years

C. Signs and Symptoms

1. Depression
   a. sense of worthlessness, hopelessness, and helplessness
   b. frequent crying
   c. withdrawal from others
   d. sleep disturbance
   e. changes in appetite and weight
   f. lack of energy
   g. flat affect, look of sadness
   h. decreased mental activities
   i. potential for suicide
2. Mania
   a. sense of euphoria, excitement, and talkativeness
   b. hyperactive, talks continuously
   c. aggressive behavior
   d. flight of ideas and delusions
   e. increased energy with infrequent eating or sleeping
   f. increased productivity
3. Bipolar: shift from depression to mania and back

D. Planning, Goals/ Expected Outcomes

1. Depression
   a. patient will take prescribed medications
   b. patient will become more involved in simple activities
   c. patient will talk about things outside of self
   d. patient will care for personal needs, eat regular meals, and sleep through night
   e. patient will not harm self
2. Mania
   a. patient will take antimanic medications as ordered
   b. patient will channel energy into constructive outlets
   c. patient will be able to get involved in social interactions without losing control
   d. patient will receive adequate nutrition and rest and be able to care for own personal needs

E. Implementation

1. Depression
   a. administer antidepressant medications (Tables 10-2 and 10-3) as ordered; monitor closely for side effects
   b. assist with electroconvulsive therapy (ECT) as ordered
   c. design simple routine, including activities and tasks that patient can accomplish that do not require deep concentration
   d. express appreciation to patient for contribution
   e. focus patient on own strengths
   f. sit with patient; avoid overcheerfulness; let patient know when you are leaving and when you will return
   g. assist patient with exploring alternative ways of handling feelings, such as anger or guilt
   h. assist patient with personal hygiene; offer positive reinforcement for what patient accomplishes
   i. encourage eating by offering small, attractive portions; use supplemental feedings as needed

TABLE 10–2. Antidepressive Agents (Tricyclic)

Classification
Antidepressive agents (tricyclic)
Action
Mood elevator
Use
Tricyclic antidepressants first line of treatment for depression
Common Side Effects
Anticholinergic effects, orthostatic hypotension, sedation
Nursing Implications/Teaching
Take 1–4 weeks for onset of effect; side effects tend to show up rapidly; client experiences depression plus side effects; body adjusts to side effects in a week or two (ways of relieving side effects included on medication write-up for antipsychotic medications); overdose can be lethal; often ordered as a single dose at bedtime (exception, Vivactil)—sedating effect promotes sleep; danger early in therapy is suicide; client is able to channel energy to formulate and implement a plan before depression significantly improves; not given with monoamine oxidase inhibitor (MAOI) antidepressants
Examples
Tofranil (imipramine), Elavil (amitriptyline), Vivactil (protriptyline), Desyrel (trazodone)

TABLE 10–3. Antidepressive Agents (MAOIs)

Classification
Antidepressive agents (MAOIs)

Action
MAOIs inhibit the oxidase enzyme that breaks down monoamine transmitters at many places in the body, including the intestine; results in greater availability of these transmitters for improved message transmission in the brain

Use
Reserved for symptomatic relief of depression in clients who have failed to respond to other antidepressant therapy

Common Side Effects
Similar to those of tricyclic antidepressants

Toxic Side Effects
Hypertensive crisis resulting in a cerebrovascular accident if foods or medication containing tyramine, a monoamine, is ingested

Nursing Implications/Teaching
Antidepressant effect experienced in 48 hours to 3 weeks
1. Instruct client about foods to avoid
2. Tell client what medications to avoid
3. Warn client how to recognize danger signs of impending hypertensive crisis
4. Monitor blood pressure regularly at onset of medication therapy

Examples
Marplan (isocarboxazid), Nardil (phenelzine), Parnate (tranylcypromine)

TABLE 10–4. Antimanic Agents

Classification
Antimanic agents

Action
Decrease hyperactivity, verbalism, agitation, irritability, insomnia, anorexia

Use
Drug of choice for clients with mania and for long-term maintenance to prevent both depressive and manic episodes in bipolar disorder

Common Side Effects
Nausea and fatigue early in therapy; tremor, thirst, edema, and weight gain throughout therapy

Toxic Side Effects
Confusion (often missed), ataxia, impaired coordination, dizziness, headaches, blurred vision, muscle weakness, gastrointestinal symptoms; if untreated, can lead to coma and *death*

Nursing Implications/Teaching
Serum lithium level monitored; 12-hour sample; blood drawn (usually) 12 hours after last dose of medication
1. 1.2–1.6 mEq/L: therapeutic for most clients
2. 2 mEq/L: risk of toxicity
3. 0.8–1.2 mEq/L: maintenance
Takes 2–3 weeks for therapeutic effect; patient receives temporary treatment with antipsychotic medication until therapeutic blood level of lithium obtained; impaired renal function, decreased sodium intake and diuretic therapy provide risk of toxicity; teach client relationship of sodium and lithium; as long as sodium intake and output is stable, lithium absorption and excretion will be stable; client needs help to adjust to new feeling state

Examples
Eskalith, Lithane, Lithonate (lithium carbonate)

---

    j. establish sleep routine; warm milk and relaxation techniques helpful in inducing sleep; avoid use of sleeping pills, which are depressants

2. Mania
    a. give patient prescribed antimanic medications (Table 10-4) and monitor closely for side effects
    b. provide quiet, nonstimulating environment
    c. set limits on behavior harmful to self or others, as well as on behavior interfering with others' rights
    d. use patient's poor attention span and easy distractibility to avoid difficult situations
    e. provide constructive outlets for patient's excess energy: jogging, swimming, walking, or noncompetitive sports
    f. maintain calm, matter-of-fact, nonjudgmental attitude when patient is sarcastic or critical; do not take patient's remarks personally
    g. protect patient from humiliating self in front of others when grandiose
    h. laugh with, not at, patient; set limits on patient's playful, joking behavior
    i. encourage patient to express negative feelings that may underlie overactivity
    j. provide high carbohydrate, high protein diet with vitamin supplements; use finger foods and high calorie liquids if patient cannot sit still
    k. provide extra rest periods, soothing warm baths, quiet music, and nonstimulating environment
    l. encourage acceptable hygiene and clothing
    m. monitor elimination; may be too busy to go to bathroom

F. Evaluation

1. Depression
    a. patient complied with medication regimen
    b. patient became more involved in simple activities
    c. patient talked about things outside of self
    d. patient cared for personal needs, ate regular meals, and slept through night
    e. patient did not harm self
2. Mania
    a. patient took antimanic medications as ordered
    b. patient channeled energy into constructive outlets
    c. patient able to get involved in social interactions without losing control
    d. patient received adequate nutrition and rest and became able to care for own personal needs

IV. SUICIDAL PATTERN OF BEHAVIOR

A. Assessment

1. Definition: deliberate action to end one's life
2. Predisposing factors
   a. pathologic depression most common factor
   b. alcoholism next most common factor
   c. inability to deal with unexpected outcomes, so that individual feels overwhelmed
   d. need to control significant others
   e. inability to deal with intolerable emotional pain

B. Signs and Symptoms

1. Previous suicide attempts, suicide threats, or extreme depression
2. Giving away prized possessions, especially in young
3. Putting affairs in order after depression
4. Asking questions, such as "How many pills would it take to kill someone?"
5. Cries easily
6. Hears voices telling person to kill self
7. Talks about seeing again people who have died
8. Talks about plan for suicide
9. Sudden euphoria after severe depression

C. Planning, Goals/ Expected Outcomes

1. Patient will use positive ways of solving problems instead of attempting suicide
2. Patient will form relationship with significant other(s) for support during difficult times
3. Patient's physical status will return to pre-illness pattern
4. Patient will focus on more positive aspects of living
5. Patient will not commit suicide

D. Implementation

1. Maintain safe and unchallenging environment; if needed, provide constant supervision during suicide crisis
2. Monitor patient's medication usage closely
3. Take every complaint and feeling individual expresses seriously
4. Talk openly about patient's ideas of suicide
5. Build on patient's strengths; previous positive coping mechanisms might be used
6. Be affirmative, but supportive
7. Provide emotional strength by communicating that you know what you are doing and that everything possible will be done for patient
8. Contact persons in patient's life who are significant and can be supportive, such as ministers, relatives, and friends
9. Pay attention to more subtle and hidden clues that patient is self-destructive, such as not eating or caring for personal needs
10. Supervise patient when eating and performing hygienic measures
11. Give reassurance that patient's feelings of despair and pain are temporary and will pass
12. Mention that as long as life exists, there is a chance for help; death is final
13. Encourage change of pace, such as exercise or relaxation techniques
14. Remove objects that could be used in a suicide attempt

E. Evaluation

1. Patient used positive ways of solving problems instead of attempting suicide
2. Patient formed relationship with significant other(s) for support during difficult times
3. Patient's physical status returned to pre-illness pattern
4. Patient focused on more positive aspects of living
5. Patient did not commit suicide

V. BEHAVIOR PATTERNS OF YOUNG, CHRONICALLY MENTALLY ILL

A. Assessment

1. Definition: population of previously institutionalized patients, who experience repeated hospitalizations; little or no improvement
2. Behaviors include
   a. developmental disorders
   b. disruptive behavior disorders
   c. anxiety disorders of childhood
   d. eating disorders
   e. gender-identity disorders

B. Signs and Symptoms

1. Denial of need for treatment
2. Refusal to take prescribed antipsychotic medications
3. Use of street drugs

4. May exhibit violent behavior toward self or others
5. Ability to perform activities of daily living may be impaired

C. Planning, Goals/ Expected Outcomes

1. Patient will admit that mental illness exists
2. Patient will participate in developing *realistic, short-term* goals for self
3. Patient will use *rationalization* to explain why not ready to take on too large a task (failure would further deflate ego and evoke guilt about having failed you after all you did for patient)
4. Patient will work with more than one therapist on scheduled basis

D. Implementation

1. Involve patient in interests outside self; projects, people, and structured activities
2. Discuss possibility of sheltered employment
3. Encourage involvement with support system
   a. stable one-to-one relationship
   b. ongoing group therapy
   c. follow-up home visits
4. Support use of coping/mental mechanism, rationalization, when patient plans tasks that would lead to failure
5. Introduce patient to co-therapist relationship during hospitalization to prevent patient from feeling abandoned when one therapist is not available
6. Respond to age-related needs; attitude important
7. Administer antipsychotic medications (Table 10-1) as ordered

E. Evaluation

1. Patient involved in structured activity, project, or relationship that can be continued after hospitalization
2. Patient consented to testing for sheltered employment
3. Patient exhibited beginning trust in self and others
   a. took medications from staff
   b. participated marginally in group therapy
   c. indicated willingness to talk to follow-up home visit staff
4. Patient offered rationalization for why patient cannot pursue goal at this time, such as go to college
5. Patient agreed to see two separate therapists

VI. ANXIOUS PATTERNS OF BEHAVIOR

A. Anxiety

1. Assessment
   a. Definition: normal function; diffuse feeling of dread; apprehension or unexplained discomfort; subjectively painful warning of impending danger
   b. Characteristics
      (1) subjective feeling
      (2) mild
         (a) normal
         (b) motivates person to action
      (3) severe
         (a) disabling
         (b) requires outside intervention
      (4) unrelated to specific object
   c. incidence
      (1) all people experience mild to moderate anxiety
      (2) severe anxiety to panic state affects about 5% of population
2. Signs and symptoms
   a. mild
      (1) increased perception and alertness
      (2) observations clearer
   b. moderate
      (1) decreased perception
      (2) increased alertness
      (3) concentration centered; irrelevant tasks ignored
   c. severe
      (1) decreased and narrowed perception
      (2) poor communication
   d. generalized
      (1) muscle tension, hyperactivity
      (2) vigilant behavior
   e. panic state
      (1) sudden, intense periods of extreme fear
      (2) accompanied by physical symptoms of palpitations, dyspnea, chest pain, sensation of choking, dizziness, hot and cold flashes, sweating, trembling
      (3) fear of impending doom
      (4) nonpurposeful behavior
      (5) unable to fight or take flight
3. Planning, goals/expected outcomes
   a. patient will learn constructive ways of dealing with anxiety
   b. patient will recognize symptoms of onset of anxiety and intervene before reaching panic state
   c. patient will care for personal needs, such as bathing, oral hygiene, nutrition, and sleep

4. Implementation
   a. assist patient to recognize feelings of anxiety when they arise and to connect these feelings to relief behaviors, such as use of relaxation, imagery, humor, and other coping behaviors
   b. try to interest patient in things outside of self, such as simple concrete task or game, walking, physical activity, sweeping, clearing table, and washing dishes
   c. remind patient to care for own physical needs
   d. monitor patient's weight
   e. administer antianxiety medications (Table 10-5) as ordered
   f. provide calm, quiet, safe environment
   g. reinforce effective and constructive coping behaviors
   h. reassure patient of safety and security
5. Evaluation
   a. patient learned constructive ways of dealing with anxiety
   b. patient recognized symptoms of onset of anxiety and intervened before reaching panic state
   c. patient cared for personal needs, such as bathing, oral hygiene, nutrition, and sleep

B. Phobias

1. Assessment
   a. definition: intense irrational fear of object or situation; may interfere with normal function of patient

   b. types
      (1) xenophobia: fear of strangers
      (2) agoraphobia: fear of open or public places from which escape is difficult
      (3) claustrophobia: fear of enclosed or small places
      (4) acrophobia: fear of heights
2. Signs and symptoms
   a. panic attack when exposed to phobic object or situation
   b. refusal to leave home or face exposure to phobic situation or object
   c. apprehension, diffuse anxiety
   d. uses avoidance coping style
   e. fight or flight behaviors when exposed to phobia
3. Planning, goals/expected outcomes
   a. patient will become desensitized to phobic object or situation and no longer experience phobic response
   b. patient will acknowledge and discuss fear
   c. patient will accept and participate in treatment program aimed at reducing phobic response
4. Implementation
   a. assist in desensitization
   b. administer antidepressant drugs (Table 10-2), antianxiety drugs, and tranquilizers (Tables 10-1 and 10-5)
   c. help patient understand that facing phobia can lead to adaptive coping behaviors
   d. identify and reinforce positive coping by patient
   e. encourage patient to identify life situations that generate anxiety and conflict
   f. offer hope that treatment will reduce phobic response
5. Evaluation
   a. patient became desensitized to phobic object or situation and no longer experienced phobic response
   b. patient acknowledged and discussed fear
   c. patient accepted and participated in treatment program aimed at reducing phobic response

C. Obsessive-Compulsive Behaviors

1. Assessment
   a. definition: involuntary, recurring thoughts or images that cannot be ignored or treated logically; recurring impulses to perform seemingly purposeless activities
   b. signs and symptoms
      (1) excessive conformity and conscientiousness
      (2) perfectionist, overly meticulous
      (3) rigidity, difficulty making decisions
      (4) selective inattention to new ideas

TABLE 10–5. Antianxiety Agents (Minor Tranquilizers)

Classification
Antianxiety agents (minor tranquilizers)

Action
Relieve anxiety and muscle tension, anticonvulsant (*no* antipsychotic activity)

Use
Relieve uncomfortable anxiety and muscular tension; leave client with sufficient anxiety to motivate client to seek solution to actual problem; have anticonvulsive action; useful during alcohol detoxification in preventing or decreasing intensity of end-stage withdrawal symptoms (anxiety disorders, somatoform disorders, alcohol detoxification)

Common Side Effects
Additive effect with other CNS depressants; drowsiness, fatigue, ataxia most common, confusion especially in the elderly; drug dependence with chronic use; withdrawal symptoms if abruptly withdrawn

Nursing Implications/Teaching
Have client set treatment goals; avoid use with other CNS depressants (alcohol, barbiturates); use only as prescribed to avoid psychic or physical dependence; withdrawal symptoms of long-acting drugs such as Valium may be delayed for days and then may be confused with anxiety

Examples
Ativan (lorazepam), Valium (diazepam), Librium (chlordiazepoxide)

    (5) concentration on insignificant details
    (6) lack of personal convictions
    (7) when severe, worry borders on delusion
    (8) when anxious, performs repetitive behavior to relieve stress

2. Planning, goals/expected outcomes
  a. patient will cope effectively with activities of daily living without resorting to obsessive-compulsive behaviors
  b. patient will accept limits on repetitive behaviors and participate in alternative adaptive activities

3. Implementation
  a. develop affirming, dependable relationship
  b. determine situations that precipitate repetitive behavior
  c. show acceptance of person without showing disapproval of behavior
  d. provide structure and time so that rituals can be completed without increased anxiety
  e. provide environment so patient can decrease rituals and increase other activities
  f. positively reinforce nonritualistic behaviors
  g. teach patient to recognize and anticipate situations that might precipitate rituals
  h. teach techniques to allow patient to stop thoughts that precipitate rituals, such as relaxation techniques, constructive activity, and exercise
  i. assist patient with dependency conflict
  j. help patient find initial source of anxiety

4. Evaluation
  a. patient coped effectively with activities of daily living without resorting to obsessive-compulsive behaviors
  b. patient accepted limits on repetitive behaviors and participated in alternative adaptive activities

VII. BEHAVIOR PATTERN RELATED TO ORGANIC MENTAL DISORDERS

A. Assessment

1. Description: pattern of behavior characterized by changes in organic functioning due to injury or disease, substance abuse, aging, or medication; can produce either temporary or permanent brain damage
2. Types
  a. delirium: usually stable or self-limiting
  b. dementia: progressive, static, or remitting
  c. primary, degenerative dementia of Alzheimer type most common dementia
3. Signs and symptoms
  a. memory impairment
  b. impairment of abstract thinking

  c. impaired judgment and impulse control
  d. loss of other higher cortical functions
  e. personality changes
  f. altered state of consciousness
  g. perceptual disturbances
  h. altered sleep–wakefulness cycle
  i. decreased psychomotor activity
  j. emotional disturbances

B. Planning, Goals/ Expected Outcomes

1. Patient will do as much as possible for self in caring for own physical needs
2. Patient will maintain sense of self-control by doing for self within modified environment
3. Patient will maintain human dignity through interaction with staff, other patients, and significant others

C. Implementations

1. Establish structured, consistent, daily routine
  a. supervise health habits, including eating, personal hygiene, exercise, and toileting
  b. have patient assist with personal care as much as possible
2. Patiently answer questions in short, simple sentences; repeat answers when needed
  a. demonstrate nonverbally and concretely what you are trying to convey to patient
  b. try to help patient, whenever necessary, to become oriented through use of clocks, calendars, signs, and written and verbal reminders
  c. modify environment for safety according to individual needs
3. Tell patient when you do not understand what he or she is talking about
  a. use patient's past memory to bring patient to present through reminiscing during one-to-one encounters and reminiscing group
  b. assist family members in their contact with patient
4. Administer antipsychotic medications (Table 10-1) as ordered

D. Evaluation

1. Patient did as much as possible for self in caring for own physical needs
2. Patient maintained sense of self-control by doing for self within modified environment
3. Patient maintained human dignity through interaction with staff, other patients, and significant others

Questions

May Witherspoon, age 23 years, was brought to the mental health center by her parents. They are concerned because she does not want to come out of her room, makes up words, and spends hours "decoding" messages that she hears being transmitted to her through television. When you arrive on the unit, you find her sitting in her room, her face expressionless. She does not raise her head or answer when you call her by name.

1. What is May's major pattern of behavior?

① Overly suspicious
② Withdrawal
③ Depressive
④ Manic

2. May is exhibiting which of the following behaviors?

① Schizophrenia
② Reactive depression
③ Paranoid state
④ Borderline personality

3. What is a core problem for this behavioral pattern?

① Inability to deal with hostile feelings
② Inability to adjust to personal confrontation
③ Inability to develop relationships outside of self
④ Inability to accept decreasing intelligence

4. What is the major defense mechanism used by May?

① Denial
② Reaction formation
③ Projection
④ Regression

5. How do you respond if May asks if you believe that she hears secret messages through TV?

① "It's probably the Russians; ignore them!"
② "No, but I know the 'so-called voices' are real to you."
③ "Why do you think you hear messages over the TV?"
④ "What do you think? Do you think I hear them?"

6. Which of these reflects a positive improvement for May?

① Rejects you after spending time with her
② Is no longer verbally explosive when approached
③ No longer believes that she is terminally ill
④ Eats and sleeps regularly without special arrangements

Del Peery was brought to the hospital by the police. Neighbors became concerned because they saw him looking out his window with a shotgun in his hand. When people walked by, he shouted, "You can't take my property away! Get away or I will shoot!" Upon admission, Mr. Peery tells you of his neighbors' plot to take his property away.

7. What is his major pattern of behavior?

① Compulsive
② Overly suspicious
③ Withdrawal
④ Anxious

8. What does Mr. Peery's behavior pattern tell you about him?

① His compulsive behavior relieves tension
② He needs group interaction and stimulation
③ He uses sublimation to deal with anxiety
④ He has not learned to trust himself

9. What is an idea not supported by logic called?

① Hallucination
② Illusion
③ Delusion
④ Blocking

10. Why would you address this client as "Mr. Peery" during your contact with him?

① Casualness may lead him to think you are incompetent
② All clients need to be addressed formally
③ His use of introjection lowers his self-esteem
④ It supports his use of symptoms for now

11. What will you do if Mr. Peery refuses to eat because of his fear of being poisoned?

① Have his family bring him food
② Remind him that this is crazy behavior
③ Tell him that no one poisoned his food
④ Offer to let him serve himself and taste his food for him

12. How would you advise someone regarding use of touch with this client?

① Touch is comforting to him
② A backrub will help him sleep
③ He may misinterpret someone's touching him
④ Touch is a way to reorient him

13. What is a desired response if you are alone and a physically assaultive client tells you to open the door?

① Open the door without resistance
② Block the door with your body
③ Use body language; roll your eyes
④ Attempt to flirt with the client

14. What is meant by "Images go directly to the nervous system"?

① Images can cause damage to the central nervous system (CNS)
② You become what you imagine you will become
③ Fantasizing is considered unhealthy
④ Imaging is done under supervision

Dee Dee Droop, a nurse, has been calling in sick to the unit where she works. She is always tired, complains of not sleeping well and has lost 10 lb within the last 2 weeks owing to loss of appetite. Three months ago, administration announced that some staff may expect a "layoff" within the next 6 months. Yesterday, she called her mother to say goodbye: "I couldn't take this any longer." When you meet her, you note a deeply sad expression.

15. What is her major pattern of behavior?

① Depression
② Overly suspicious
③ Antisocial personality
④ Withdrawal

16. Which of the following will help you in planning her care?

① Your cheerfulness will help elevate her mood
② Sharing your problems will help her focus on others
③ Depression often lifts slightly in the late afternoon
④ Telling her that she is angry increases insight

17. What is her major coping/mental mechanism?

① Symbolism
② Projection
③ Denial
④ Introjection

18. What would you suggest as a way of dealing with her suicidal feelings?

① Encourage her to talk about her suicidal feelings
② Maintain detailed notes concerning her actions
③ Tell her you will keep her from killing herself
④ Remind her that other employees are facing the same problem

19. What approach will you use to get this client involved in her care?

① "Do you want to take a bath now?"
② "Stop feeling sorry for yourself."
③ "It's time for us to have our breakfast."
④ "I want you to brush your teeth now."

20. Why might this client experience constipation?

① An expression of anger toward you
② A way of manipulating you
③ Emotional needs expressed physically
④ A lack of activity and intake

21. What will you stress as a nursing intervention for a client who is receiving monoamine oxidase inhibitors (MAOIs)?

① Set treatment goals
② Avoid tyramine-rich foods
③ Plan for drug holidays
④ Avoid CNS depressants

Freddie Fast, age 50 years, was admitted this afternoon. He was previously hospitalized with a similar episode 10 years ago. During the past 2 weeks, he has become increasingly agitated and excitable. Both verbalization and physical activity have increased. His wife notes that he "goes from topic to topic and has hardly slept at all." Two days ago, he went on a buying spree and gave all his purchases away.

22. What diagnosis best describes this behavior?

① Panic attack
② Schizophreniform
③ Manic episode
④ Paranoid state

23. Which of the following is a helpful nursing intervention when the client is agitated?

   ① Include him in a card game with other clients
   ② Set firm, fixed limits on his behaviors
   ③ Separate him from others in a quiet area
   ④ Encourage him to organize a baseball game

24. What is the core problem for this behavior?

   ① Attempt to increase self-esteem
   ② Inability to develop relationships
   ③ Overwhelming desire to be liked
   ④ Exaggeration of basic personality traits

25. How will you respond if the client calls you a "fat, gum-chewing, dumb nurse"?

   ① Ask him for clarification of his statement
   ② Be nondefensive and avoid arousing guilt
   ③ Tell him he is inappropriate; send him to his room
   ④ Join Weight Watchers, throw out your gum, and go back to school

26. What is Freddie's major coping/mental mechanism?

   ① Regression
   ② Projection
   ③ Sublimation
   ④ Conversion

27. Which of the following is an example of an assertive response?

   ① "Yes, I'd be willing to go along with your second idea but not with the first one."
   ② "You make me so angry! You always act like you know all the answers."
   ③ "Well, if you really think I should, I'll go along with the suggestion."
   ④ "You are so critical! Why don't you evaluate your own behavior?"

28. Which of the following statements is an example of assuming responsibility for content of personal conversation?

   ① "We decided that we want to continue with group meetings."
   ② "You know that the group meetings benefit all of us together."
   ③ "Most guys, me included, feel that it's a good idea to continue."
   ④ "I feel that it's important for me to continue with the group."

Jan Brainard, age 22 years, has experienced repeated hospitalizations because of chronic mental illness (CMI). Although she has been stabilized on medication repeated times, she discontinues the medications on her own shortly after she leaves the hospital.

29. What is a major consideration in developing Jan's care plan?

   ① Natural rebelliousness of this age group
   ② The staffing pattern on the unit at night
   ③ Age range of the present unit staff
   ④ Age of the parents

30. What coping/mental mechanism may be helpful in dealing with unrealized expectations?

   ① Denial
   ② Projection
   ③ Repression
   ④ Rationalization

Lilly Fidget, age 36 years, was admitted to the center last night because her repetitive hand washing has increased to the point where she is no longer able to complete her work on the job and at home.

31. What is Lilly's major pattern of behavior?

   ① Depression
   ② Aggression
   ③ Suspiciousness
   ④ Compulsion

32. What is the major coping/mental mechanism?

   ① Repression
   ② Projection
   ③ Introjection
   ④ Reaction formation

33. What is the reason Lilly washes her hands repeatedly?

   ① To be clean
   ② To get attention from others
   ③ For temporary relief of anxiety
   ④ To sublimate her aggressiveness

34. Why is it important for staff to deal with personal feelings evoked by Lilly's behavior?

   ① Prevent support of negative coping methods
   ② Interpret meaning of Lilly's ritual to her
   ③ Clearly tell her how to stop hand washing
   ④ Share personal solution to problems with Lilly

35. What classification of medications will the doctor order for relief of symptoms?

① Antipsychotic
② Antianxiety
③ Antidepressant
④ Antimanic

36. Which of the following statements is true about use of relaxation techniques?

① Everyone benefits from practicing relaxation.
② Relaxation techniques are desirable for psychotic clients.
③ Relaxation has no known effect on medication.
④ A small percent of the population experience an opposite effect.

37. How can you direct Lilly to use humor to deal with a present situation?

① Help her see the humor in other clients' behavior.
② Have her draw a cartoon that exaggerates the situation.
③ Point out what is funny about her problem.
④ Tease Lilly when she gets "too serious."

38. What is empathy?

① Respectful, detached concern
② Experiencing the patient's emotion
③ Identifying with the patient
④ Focusing on patient's condition

39. Electroconvulsive therapy is used as a treatment for which of the following conditions?

① Primary dementia
② Schizophrenia
③ Paranoid disorder
④ Severe depression

Answers & Rationales

Guide to item identification (see pp. 3–5 for further details about each category)

I, II, III, or IV for the phase of the nursing process
1, 2, 3, or 4 for the category of client needs
A, B, C, D, E, F, or G for the category of human functioning
Specific content category by name; ie, cholecystectomy

1. "The withdrawal pattern of behavior is usu-
② ally seen in those people who are suffering from schizophrenic disorders." (Bauer & Hill, 1986:57)
I, 3, G. Schizophrenia.

2. Same as above.
①

3. "One of the most pronounced difficulties these
③ persons have is the inability to relate in a meaningful way to other people. To avoid further rejection, they set up barriers that make it difficult for persons to establish contact." (Bauer & Hill, 1986:57)
I, 3, G. Schizophrenia.

4. "Clients with withdrawal patterns of behavior
④ may have been exposed to a great deal of conflict and turmoil during their early developmental periods. As a result of these early experiences they never fully develop a basic sense of trust. They continue throughout life to search for acceptance and approval. After numerous rejections, they eventually give up, and, utilizing the coping/mental mechanism of *regression*, retreat to a simpler form of existence in a world of their own. In this world, they turn their attention to themselves and relate to their imaginary environment as if it were real." (Bauer & Hill, 1986:57)
I, 3, G. Defense Mechanisms.

5. "Discuss real events with client; focus on
② reality. Refer to voices as 'so-called voices.' Do not act attentive to discussion regarding hallucinations. This will decrease importance of hallucinations." (Bauer & Hill, 1986:46)
III, 3, G. Schizophrenia.

6. "A rejection from such a client is often a clue
① that he has not allowed the health provider to enter his world. . . . The health provider should not view this as a permanent rejection by the client. Instead, he should move more slowly." (Bauer & Hill, 1986:58)
IV, 3, G. Schizophrenia.

7. "The overly suspicious pattern of behavior is
② usually seen in people suffering from a paranoid disorder." (Bauer & Hill, 1986:59)
I, 3, G. Overly Suspicious Behavior.

8. "These clients have usually had a childhood
④ in which distrust, hate, and poor interpersonal relationships developed." (Bauer & Hill, 1986:59)
I, 3, G. Overly Suspicious Behavior.

9. "Delusion—belief or idea that is not supported
③ by logic." (Bauer & Hill, 1986:194)
I, 3, G. Overly Suspicious Behavior.

10. "The health provider must be professional at all
① times with this client to decrease use of the mechanism of projection. He denies his shortcomings to himself and uses the coping/mental mechanism of projection to attribute his feelings to objects and people outside himself. In doing so, the client feels more comfortable with himself and superior to others. He is a lonely person, frightened of being exposed as inadequate." (Bauer & Hill, 1986:59, 60)
III, 3, G. Overly Suspicious Behavior.

11. ". . . if the client thinks his food is poisoned, it
④ may be necessary to serve food in closed containers and to allow the client to open the containers. Sometimes the client may want you to taste his food before he will eat it." (Bauer & Hill, 1986:60)
III, 3, G. Overly Suspicious Behavior.

12. ". . . the behavior pattern may influence the
③ client's response to touch." (Bauer & Hill, 1986:165)
III, 3, G. Overly Suspicious Behavior.

13. "Don't try to be a hero. Get out of the way and
① get help, if possible." (Bauer & Hill, 1986:176)
III, 3, G. Overly Suspicious Behavior.

14. "Feelings and thoughts are pulled toward one's
② mental images, and the client, most often, becomes what he imagines he can become." (Bauer & Hill, 1986:160)
I, 3, G. Coping Behaviors.

15. "Deeply sad and hopeless expression, loss of
① energy, fatigability or tiredness, sleeping difficulty, recurrent thoughts of death or suicide or
any suicidal behavior, including thoughts of
wishing to be dead, poor appetite or weight
loss, are common characteristics of depression." (Bauer & Hill, 1986:28, 61)
I, 3, G. Depression.

16. "Usually there is a period in early evening
③ when the depression lifts slightly. Use this time
to reach the client and share simple activities
with him." (Bauer & Hill, 1986:62)
II, 3, G. Depression.

17. "The client who is clinically depressed can deal
④ with his anger through the coping technique
of *introjection*. By turning his anger in on himself—intra-aggression—it no longer poses an
external threat to him as an individual." (Bauer
& Hill, 1986:61)
I, 3, G. Depression.

18. "Do not be afraid to ask directly if the individ
① ual has suicidal thoughts. Talking about it
frankly can help prevent an individual from
carrying out his idea. He usually welcomes the
opportunity to open up and discuss it." (Bauer
& Hill, 1986:66)
III, 3, G. Depression.

19. "If a client's illness limits his problem-solving
④ abilities, then the provider must communicate
in simple, clear 'I' statements." (Bauer & Hill,
1986:101–102)
III & IV, 3, A & C. Depression.

20. "All internal body functions are slowed down,
④ so elimination can become a problem." (Bauer
& Hill, 1986:62)
IV, 3, F & G. Depression.

21. "Clients who are receiving MAOIs need to
② be cautioned about ingesting products that
would cause a significant additional supply of
monoamines. Some foods contain significant
amounts of tyramine, a monoamine that affects
blood pressure. Large amounts of tyramine can
lead to a hypertensive crisis (an extreme elevation in blood pressure), leading to rupture of
blood vessels that results in a cerebrovascular
accident (stroke)." (Bauer & Hill, 1986:133)
III, 3, F & G. Antipsychotic Medications.

22. "During *manic* episodes, all processes speed
③ up." (Bauer & Hill, 1986:28)
I, 3, G. Mania.

23. "The client needs protection from overstim
③ ulation. A quiet area removed from the center
of activity is often helpful." (Bauer & Hill,
1986:64)
III, 3, G. Mania.

24. "His frantic activity is an attempt to increase his
① self-esteem." (Bauer & Hill, 1986:63)
I, 3, G. Mania.

25. "The client needs a nonchallenging atmo
② sphere and health providers who can accept his
verbal abuse calmly and matter-of-factly."
(Bauer & Hill, 1986:64)
III, 3, G. Mania.

26. "The client with overactive behavior uses the
② technique of projection to turn his anger outward toward objects and people in his environment." (Bauer & Hill, 1986:63)
IV, 3, G. Mania.

27. "Make your feelings known by being direct and
① by beginning your statements with 'I'." (Bauer
& Hill, 1986:102)
IV, 1 & 3, G. Therapeutic Communication.

28. "The underlying theme in communication is to
④ allow individuals to own their problems."
(Bauer & Hill, 1986:101)
IV, 1 & 3, G. Therapeutic Communication.

29. "Two important factors seem to be involved:
① (1) the client views the admission of mental
illness as being equal with failure, and (2) the
natural rebelliousness of this age group."
(Bauer & Hill, 1986:68)
II, 3, G. Chronic Mental Illness.

30. "Help the client develop *rationalization* for why
④ he may not be ready to take on too large a task,
such as a difficult job or a demanding collegiate
program. Failure would further deflate his ego
and evoke guilt about having failed you after all
you did for him." (Bauer & Hill, 1986: 69)
I, 3, G. Chronic Mental Illness.

31. "In order to cope with the overwhelming anxi
④ ety, the individual may separate (dissociate) the
anxiety from the rest of his personality. The
resulting symptoms give clues (symbolism) to
the underlying problem, of which he is not consciously aware." (Bauer & Hill, 1986: 28–29)
Compulsive behavior helps to decrease anxiety.
I, 3, G. Compulsive Behavior.

32. "Through *repression*, they attempt to keep the threatening experiences and thoughts hidden." (Bauer & Hill, 1986: 72)
① I, 3, G. Compulsive Behavior.

33. "An example of a common compulsion is handwashing. When the person attempts not to give in to the compulsion, the mounting tension is overwhelming and can be immediately relieved by giving in to the act." (Bauer & Hill, 1986: 29)
③ IV, 3, G. Compulsive Behavior.

34. ". . . client problems and behaviors can unleash unresolved personal problems that the health provider has not come to terms with." (Bauer & Hill, 1986: 119)
① II & IV, 3, G. Compulsive Behavior.

35. "Antianxiety agents, previously known as minor tranquilizers, primarily relieve anxiety and muscle tension." (Bauer & Hill, 1986: 132)
② III, 3, G. Compulsive Behavior.

36. Approximately 3% of clients respond to relaxation training by actually increasing arousal (eg, increasing blood pressure instead of decreasing)
④ IV, 3, G. Compulsive Behavior.

37. Have the client draw or visualize the present situation as a cartoon, exaggerating it so it is ridiculous. By injecting some humor into the situation, the client may be able to deal with it more effectively.
② III, 3, G. Compulsive Behavior.

38. "Empathy is a respectful, detached concern; the provider understands what the client is experiencing but does not experience the emotion with him." (Bauer & Hill, 1986: 119)
① IV, 3, G. Mental Health.

39. "It is most effective with clients who are severely depressed and/or compulsively suicidal." (Bauer & Hill, 1986: 135)
④ IV, 3, G. Depression.

EMOTIONS, BEHAVIOR, AND MENTAL HEALTH

The way people deal with emotions (feelings, such as ambivalence, love, hate, and so on) has a significant relationship to how mentally healthy they are; Mental Health is a state of being defined as:

1. Feeling comfortable about yourself
2. Feeling right about others
3. Meeting demands of life
4. Coping and adjusting to recurrent stresses of everyday living

■ Coping/Mental Mechanisms

I. DEFENSE MECHANISMS

A. Assessment

1. Definition: unconscious, automatic ways of dealing with discomfort
2. May develop in childhood when individual is placed in difficult situations person cannot handle
3. Can have healthy or unhealthy effect on individual; depends on degree of use
4. Use of mechanism continues throughout person's life, even when original stress no longer exists

B. Types*

1. Compensation
   a. definition: covering for real or imagined inadequacy by developing or exaggerating desirable trait
   b. example: undersized boy develops intellectual ability instead of participating in sports
2. Conversion
   a. definition: channeling of anxiety into physical symptoms
   b. example: Mrs. Smith develops headache on evening she is scheduled to present paper at convention and is unable to make presentation because of illness
3. Denial
   a. definition: rejection of things, events, or feelings as they actually exist, thus eliminating need for anxiety
   b. example: alcoholic denies alcoholism; "I am a social drinker and can quit anytime"
4. Displacement
   a. definition: occurs when feelings toward object

are distorted and transferred to less threatening object
   b. example: boy, angry at weather, which he cannot control, kicks cat
5. Dissociation
   a. definition: occurs when painful ideas, situations, or feelings are separated from awareness
   b. example: Carol has forgotten details of accident in which loved one was killed
6. Fantasy
   a. Definition: using imagination to solve problems; on conscious level, fantasy used to reduce stress through relaxation; on unconscious level, fantasy used as retreat from threatening environment
   b. example: children work through situations they will encounter in adult life by assuming parental roles in play and using pets or dolls as their children
7. Identification
   a. definition: occurs when persons take on characteristics and values of someone they admire, recognizing that they are not that person
   b. example: teenager dresses like favorite "rock" star
8. Introjection
   a. definition: incorporating or internalizing of conflicting values, standards, persons, objects, or attitudes so that they are no longer external threats
   b. example: political candidate professes to represent every interest group so that none attack platform
9. Projection
   a. definition: attributing to other people or objects motives and emotions that are unacceptable to oneself
   b. example: overweight woman blames her 2-year-old son for her condition, saying that he makes her nervous
10. Rationalization
   a. definition: logical-sounding excuses that conceal real reason for actions, thoughts, or feelings
   b. example: young boy explains why he left for school without feeding dog—"I did it because Johnny came over and told me we had to leave right away"
11. Reaction formation
   a. definition: sometimes viewed as an overcompensation, means of disguising from self an unacceptable desire or drive by developing its exact opposite to an exaggerated degree
   b. example: wife angry at husband for attention he gives dog but reacts by being overly sweet
12. Regression

---

* Bauer & Hill (1986), pp 15–21.

a. definition: retreat to an earlier, less stressful time of development

b. example: adult is faced with stress that cannot be tolerated and throws a tantrum

13. Repression
    a. definition: unconscious withholding of unpleasant thoughts, feelings, or experiences
    b. example: Ginger unable to remember name of demanding neighbor when she meets neighbor at market

14. Sublimation
    a. definition: substituting socially acceptable behavior for unacceptable or unattainable desire
    b. example: person channels his or her paternal/maternal feelings into caring and loving interest in plants or animals

15. Symbolization
    a. definition: representation of an internal feeling, wish, attitude, or idea through external object or quality (eg, color)
    b. example: diamond ring and its presentation symbolizes love and commitment

16. Undoing
    a. definition: attempt to conceal negative action by other positive action
    b. example: father offers his son an allowance after punishing him

■ Crisis Intervention

Short-term therapy that focuses on solving immediate problem

I. DEALING WITH LOSS (GRIEF AND GRIEVING)

A. Loss

Includes both physical and biologic loss; involves total human experiencing grieving process

B. Stages of Grief

1. Shock and disbelief
2. Development of awareness
3. Restitution
4. Resolution of loss

C. Grieving Process

1. Assessment
   a. assess for presence of psychologic symptoms, such as anger, guilt, depression
   b. assess for presence of physiologic symptoms, such as insomnia, exhaustion, digestive disturbances
   c. determine stage of grief process that patient is experiencing
   d. observe for abnormal reactions to loss, such as absence of grieving, or illness

2. Planning, goals/expected outcomes
   a. patient will be able to express feelings of loss openly
   b. patient will move through stages of grieving process at own pace

3. Implementation
   a. encourage patient to talk about loss
   b. explore what loss means to patient
   c. find out how patient feels about loss
   d. be aware of own feelings of sadness so that they do not get mixed up with patient's feelings
   e. assist and support patient through grief process

4. Evaluation
   a. patient verbalized feelings about loss
   b. patient accepted loss and found healing process helpful experience

II. PERSON ABUSE (TRAUMA)

A. Spouse Abuse

Deliberate and repeated physical or verbal assault on mate

1. Assessment
   a. beginning of violent behaviors
   b. types of violence and frequency
   c. coping techniques that spouse used to deal with violence
   d. resources available in community
   e. effects of violence on family
   f. assess background of abusive mate
   g. assess physical condition of abused mate

2. Planning, goals/expected outcomes
   a. patient will seek professional help when violence occurs
   b. patient will explore alternative situations available that will alter cycle of abuse
   c. patient will increase independent functioning, focusing on strengths and other roles available

3. Implementation
   a. provide safety for patient and treat any existing physical injuries
   b. encourage patient to get out of dangerous situations
   c. assist patient with problem solving, allowing patient to make own decisions
      (1) provide needed information on available resources

408 THE MENTAL HEALTH PATIENT

(2) assist patient, as needed, in initial contacts with resource agencies

d. assist patient in identifying personal strengths, resources, goals

(1) support use of assertive skills

(2) encourage patient to join support group of persons who have had similar experiences

4. Evaluation

a. patient used professional resources when abused

b. patient demonstrated decision-making skills and developed plan of action that will break abuse cycle

c. patient secured employment and pursued additional vocational training to develop skills further

d. patient joined support group, if available

B. Child Abuse

Physical, mental, or sexual assault on child; often occurs within family

1. Assessment

a. physical condition of child: burns; bruises; abrasions; multiple, old, poorly healed fractures

b. need for child to be removed from harmful situation

c. assess behavior of child

(1) relationship to parents; often seem closest to abusive parent

(2) functioning at school

(a) truancy

(b) fatigue at school

(3) somatic complaints

(4) acting out types of behavior: running away, promiscuity, hurting other children, destructive behaviors

d. assess behavior of parents

(1) anger or contradictions in discussing child's injury

(2) deny involvement in child's injury

(3) elaborate stories about child's "clumsiness" and how child hurt self

(4) parents who were abused as children are more likely to abuse their own children

2. Planning, goals/expected outcomes

a. child will be protected from further harm; if necessary, will be removed from home

b. child's physical condition will be stabilized, as evidenced by relief of discomfort

c. child's parents will become involved in ongoing treatment program

d. child's family will use effective problem-solving techniques, providing safe environment for child

3. Implementation

a. provide protection for child; follow procedure for reporting suspicions of child abuse to proper authorities

b. provide care for child's injury

c. inform child's parents of resources available, such as Parents Anonymous and parenting classes

d. support child's family in their use of effective problem-solving techniques to deal with their feelings; use positive reinforcement

4. Evaluation

a. abused child now in safe environment as determined by legal authorities and demonstrated by more positive behaviors

b. abused child's physical condition stabilized

c. child's parents participated in treatment groups and applied positive parenting skills

d. child's family demonstrated use of effective problem-solving skills in dealing with their anger and frustrations

C. Sexual Abuse

Involves sex acts without consent of victim, except for child who may be too young to give consent or understand actions

1. Assessment

a. assess emotional status of patient: fear, shame, anger, suspiciousness, panic

b. assess patients who come in with vague problems; be suspicious of abuse

c. with children, assess for suspicious signs, such as rectal pain, itching, or bleeding; unexplained bruises; bladder infections; edema around rectum or genitalia

2. Planning, goals/expected outcomes

a. patient will be able to give accurate and complete information about sexual assault

b. patient's physical condition will be stabilized

c. patient's emotional state will be improved, as evidenced by decrease of fear, panic, anger, and shame

d. patient will participate in support groups, counseling, and legal proceedings, if necessary

e. child will be removed from abusive situation

3. Implementation

a. note date and time of assault and what measures patient took prior to examination

b. assist with physical examination of patient

c. label all specimens and chart clearly; may be part of legal proceeding

d. identify resources that patient has for support

e. encourage patient to use services, such as Rape Crisis Centers, emergency shelters, and so on

f. care of physical injuries and follow through with laboratory tests ordered

g. communicate caring and concerned attitude; encourage client to talk about sexual assault and feelings associated with it

h. contact social services for abused children who may need to be removed from dangerous situation

4. Evaluation

a. patient gave accurate and complete information about sexual assault

b. patient recovered from any physical injuries related to sexual assault

c. patient verbalized feelings associated with sexual assault

d. patient participated in support groups and other follow-up treatment, if necessary

e. child removed from abusive situation

D. Elder Abuse

Includes acts of physical, mental, sexual, material (including financial) abuse, and violation of rights of older person, usually age 65 years or older

1. Assessment

a. assess needs of patient being abused: physical, emotional, or material

b. determine if patient is aware of alternatives to remaining in abusive situation

c. assess if patient is fearful of abusive situation or is unaware of being abused

d. note physical or emotional disability of patient

2. Planning, goals/expected outcomes

a. patient will be protected from physical, emotional, or material abuse

b. patient will be aware of support systems for dealing with abusive situations

c. patient will verbalize fears of being harmed and will talk about abusive situation

d. patient will increase independent functioning within physical and emotional capabilities

3. Implementation

a. care for physical injuries, if present

b. provide for alternate living arrangements for patient to avoid fear of abuse

c. discuss abusive situation(s) with patient and encourage patient to express fears

d. encourage patient to use strengths to explore activities to provide interest outside self

4. Evaluation

a. abuse of patient ceased

b. patient identified available options other than remaining in abusive situation

c. patient verbalized feelings about abusive situation

d. patient made decisions about life according to ability, so that patient's rights were respected

■ Substance Abuse and Dependence

I. ABUSE AND DEPENDENCE

A. Definitions

1. Substance abuse: pathologic use of substance, although individual aware of harm to self

a. category includes substances that alter mood or depress or stimulate central nervous system (CNS) and those abused or causing dependence

b. repeated use results in problems with interpersonal relationships, job functioning, poor judgment and impulse control, changes in behavior, and for some, involvement in criminal activity

c. abusing individual deteriorates in both physical and psychologic functioning

2. Substance dependence: user experiences physiologic and often psychologic dependence, evidenced by tolerance or withdrawal

a. tolerance: increasing amounts of drugs needed to achieve desired effect

b. withdrawal: syndrome experienced by user when amount of drug decreased or discontinued; course of withdrawal varies depending on drug

B. Classes of Substances Associated with Both Abuse and Dependence

1. Alcohol: abrupt withdrawal can result in death

2. Barbiturates (plus antianxiety agents and sedative hypnotic drugs, all CNS depressants)

a. Withdrawal or overdose: medical emergency

b. Abrupt withdrawal without detoxification can result in death

3. Opiates (including opium, morphine, codeine, heroin, Dilaudid, Percodan, and Demerol)

a. risks for IV addicts include hepatitis, overdose, acquired immune deficiency syndrome (AIDS), and infection

b. overdose: medical emergency, often fatal

4. Amphetamines (includes dexedrine, benzedrine, and biphetamine, CNS stimulants)

a. risk of amphetamine psychosis (mimics paranoid schizophrenia)

b. medical complaints: cardiac arrhythmias, hyperthermia, hypertension, and malnutrition

c. withdrawal: depression, fatigue, disturbed sleep, and potential suicide risk

5. Cannabis (includes marijuana, hashish, hash oil)
   a. intoxication can lead to bizarre, aggressive behavior
   b. harmful changes in respiratory, reproductive, and nervous systems

C. Classes of Substances Associated with Abuse Only

1. Cocaine
   a. total preoccupation with drug
   b. reluctant to give it up
   c. stimulant
   d. usually no physical withdrawal symptoms, but produces psychologic dependence
2. PCP (phencyclidine)
   a. hallucinogenic and CNS depressant effect
   b. CNS depression in high-dose intoxication; can lead to coma and death
   c. violent outbursts and psychosis
3. Hallucinogens (peyote, psilocybin, psilocin, LSD)
   a. sensory illusions
   b. hallucinations and delusions rare

D. Class of Substance Associated with Dependence Only: Tobacco

1. Nicotine: an alkaloid found in tobacco
   a. rapidly absorbed by the lungs
   b. mild central stimulatory effect
   c. decreased skeletal muscle tone, reduced appetite, occasional nausea, vomiting, dizziness and irritability
   d. withdrawal: nausea, diarrhea, increased appetite, headache, drowsiness, insomnia, irritability, and poor concentration
2. Risk factors associated with cigarette smoking: bronchogenic carcinoma, coronary artery disease, emphysema, and chronic pulmonary disease
3. Abrupt withdrawal more effective

E. Behavior Patterns Related to Other Substance Abuse or Dependence

1. As with alcohol abuse, all assessment, planning, goals/expected outcomes, implementation, and evaluation relate to:
   a. pattern of pathologic use, how much, and how often
   b. problems in social or occupational functioning due to drug abuse
   c. length of time pathologic use of drug has cre-
ated problems with social or occupational functioning
   d. history of withdrawal symptoms (limited to drugs that cause physical dependence)
   e. history of drug-related medical complications
2. All abused substances require patient to go through stages similar to those with alcohol (detoxification, rehabilitation, and follow-up)

II. CESSATION OF USE

A. Behavior Pattern Related to Use of Alcohol (Detoxification)

1. Assessment
   a. symptoms of alcohol withdrawal: coarse tremors of hands, tongue, and eyelids; nausea and vomiting; malaise; tachycardia; diaphoresis; hypertension; anxiety; depressed mood; irritability; orthostatic hypotension; grand mal seizures may occur
   b. alcohol withdrawal delirium (delirium tremens [DTs]): symptoms of delirium plus tachycardia, diaphoresis, and hypertension; also, delusions, vivid visual hallucinations, and agitated behavior
   c. hydration
   d. nutritional intake
   e. signs of physical illness
   f. liver function
2. Planning, goals/expected outcomes
   a. patient will improve physically and be able to care for self in 1 to 3 days
   b. patient will not suffer injury during withdrawal
3. Implementation
   a. close observation of symptoms for 1 to 3 days
   b. position on side to prevent aspiration from possible vomiting; reposition frequently
   c. visual check of patient every 15 minutes, especially restrained patient; monitor for signs of impending DTs
   d. monitor and record vital signs every 2 hours for first 12 hours, then four times per day for next 3 days (unless abnormal), and every day for next 4 days
   e. administer medications as ordered for one or more of following symptoms:
      (1) elevated blood pressure (ie, above 140/90)
      (2) elevated pulse (ie, above 90)
      (3) diaphoresis
      (4) hallucinations
      (5) seizures or history of seizures during withdrawal
      (6) agitation
   f. administer IVs with B vitamins as ordered

g. Check vital signs every 2 hours after each dose of medication given

h. Contact physician for further direction if vital signs do not stabilize after usual dose of medication

i. Reorient patient as needed

j. Offer cup of juice every hour

4. Evaluation

a. patient moved through detoxification without developing symptoms of end-stage alcohol withdrawal delirium (DTs): convulsions, coma and death

b. patient able to care for self in 1 to 3 days after withdrawal

B. Behavior Pattern Related to Use of Alcohol (Rehabilitation)

1. Assessment

a. use of denial as coping/mental mechanism

b. willingness to participate in developing personal goal

c. willingness to participate in structured daily activities

d. willingness to participate in planned therapeutic activities

2. Planning, goals/expected outcomes

a. patient will move through denial phase

b. patient will learn alternate ways of dealing with stress other than alcohol, ways that will produce "natural highs," such as running, meditation, and swimming

3. Implementation

a. involve patient in developing own plan of care so that patient assumes responsibility and accountability for own care

b. structure daily living and leisure activities; provide consistency

(1) set and maintain limits; minimize manipulative behavior

(2) provide various group experiences: alcohol education, Alcoholics Anonymous (AA) lessons and meetings, work opportunities, social interactions, family sessions, gripe sessions, values clarification sessions, relaxation techniques, nutritional groups, leisure counseling, job interviews, and community living skills

4. Evaluation

a. patient admitted inability to control own drinking

b. patient involves self in ways of dealing with stress other than alcohol

C. Behavior Pattern Related to Use of Alcohol (Follow-up Care)

1. Assessment: support systems needed by patient to maintain sobriety

2. Planning, goals/expected outcomes: patient will maintain sobriety in home and work setting on continuing basis with help of support systems

3. Implementation

a. attend weekly community AA meetings with other patients and staff prior to discharge

b. attend closed AA meetings after discharge, starting with day of discharge

c. continue weekly counseling sessions with family members

d. encourage continuation of hobbies and recreational activities that patient participated in during inpatient stay

e. practice relaxation techniques daily to lower anxiety level

f. administer tranquilizers (Table 10-5) as ordered

(1) chemical taken daily to discourage patient from drinking

(2) Antabuse plus alcohol results in violent physical reaction

4. Evaluation: after discharge, patient maintained sobriety in home and work settings on continuing basis with help from support systems

Questions

1. What is the coping/mental mechanism used by someone who experiences many aggressive fantasies and channels these feelings into playing football?

   ① Identification
   ② Sublimation
   ③ Reaction formation
   ④ Projection

Gene Frealoe, age 38 years, is experiencing his fourth admission to the chemical dependency unit. He has signed himself out before completing the treatment program during each of his other admissions. He has insisted that it is his wife who causes him to drink because of her behavior. This time she has threatened to follow through with a divorce if he does not complete the program; she is tired of being abused by him. On this admission, Gene is actively involved in treatment, which is based on the Alcoholics Anonymous format.

2. What is Gene's major coping/mental mechanism?

   ① Regression
   ② Denial
   ③ Reaction formation
   ④ Undoing

3. Why are fluids increased during detoxification?

   ① They wash the alcohol from the body
   ② Alcohol has a diuretic effect
   ③ They counteract the constipating effect
   ④ It is a way of preventing cirrhosis

4. What are signs of alcohol withdrawal delirium (DTs)?

   ① Elevated temperature, catatonia, convulsions, tremors
   ② Decreased vital signs, increased agitation, hallucinations
   ③ Hypertension, diaphoresis, tachycardia, delusions
   ④ Hypotension, psychomotor retardation, visual hallucinations

5. Which classification of medication is useful in controlling alcohol withdrawal delirium symptoms?

   ① Antipsychotic
   ② Antianxiety
   ③ Antidepressant
   ④ Antimanic

6. What problem will you anticipate when working with Gene?

   ① Orienting him
   ② Controlling depression
   ③ Managing guilt
   ④ Setting limits

7. What disease directly related to alcohol consumption can be treated by thiamine?

   ① Wernicke's
   ② Alzheimer's
   ③ Pick's
   ④ Subdural hematoma

8. Why is work therapy a part of psychiatric care?

   ① Helps pay for hospitalization fees
   ② Provides a setting for adjusting medications
   ③ Provides for a sense of self-worth
   ④ Keeps the client from focusing on own problems

9. Which of the following is appropriate occupational therapy (OT) for the client with alcoholism?

   ① Noncompetitive, solitary, meaningful tasks
   ② Group activities that use his talents
   ③ Simple, concrete, repetitive tasks
   ④ Activities that take concentration

10. What option is available to Mrs. Frealoe to deal with feelings about being abused?

   ① Focus on Gene; he needs her, and it is her duty to stand by her man.
   ② Focus on the children; Gene is her only means of support for the children.
   ③ Focus on herself; getting help for herself will influence Gene's behavior
   ④ Focus on their marriage; he really loves her, because he is so considerate when sober.

11. Which of the following is an essential tool to teach the patient in doing crisis intervention?

   ① Giving advice
   ② Interpreting behavior
   ③ Problem solving
   ④ Anticipatory grieving

12. Abrupt withdrawal from which of the following drugs can lead to death?

① Heroin
② Cocaine
③ Barbiturates
④ Morphine

13. Developing trust and cooperation results from:

① Alleviating fears by joking about patient's concerns
② Selecting the diet for the patient, to eliminate unnecessary decisions
③ Giving involved nursing care until discharge
④ Involving the patients in meeting their own needs

Answers & Rationales

Guide to item identification (see pp. 3–5 for further details about each category)

I, II, III, or IV for the phase of the nursing process
1, 2, 3, or 4 for the category of client needs
A, B, C, D, E, F, or G for the category of human functioning
Specific content category by name; ie, cholecystectomy

1. "Sublimation is substituting socially acceptable behavior for an unacceptable and/or unattainable desire." (Bauer & Hill, 1986:20)
② IV, 3, G. Coping.

2. "The alcoholic's use of denial perpetuates a continuous cycle of low self-concept, guilt over behavior connected with drinking, and drinking again to deal with guilty feelings." (Bauer & Hill, 1986: 87)
② IV, 3, G. Alcoholism.

3. "Because of the diuretic effect of alcohol, adequate hydration is important when dealing with the alcoholic client." (Bauer & Hill, 1986: 173)
② III, 3, F & G. Alcoholism.

4. "Major symptoms are those of delirium, plus tachycardia, diaphoresis, and hypertension. Other symptoms that usually occur include delusions; vivid, visual hallucinations; and agitated behavior." (Bauer & Hill, 1986: 87)
③ I, 3, G. Alcoholism.

5. "These medications also have an anticonvulsive action, and they are useful during alcohol detoxification in preventing or decreasing the intensity of end-stage withdrawal symptoms." (Bauer & Hill, 1986: 132)
② I & III, 3, G. Alcoholism.

6. "Set and maintain limits to minimize manipulative behavior." (Bauer & Hill, 1986: 88)
④ III, 3, G. Alcoholism.

7. "Wernicke's disease is a neurologic disease manifested by confusion, ataxia, eye movement abnormalities, and other neurologic symptoms. If Wernicke's disease is treated early with large doses of thiamine, alcohol amnestic disorder may not develop." (Bauer & Hill, 1986: 172–173)
① IV, 3, C & G. Alcoholism.

8. "Work results in productivity and productivity conveys a sense of self-worth and self-dignity." (Bauer & Hill, 1986: 153)
③ III, 3, G. Alcoholism.

9. "Group activities in which client uses his talents and assets. For example, involve client in planning social activities; encourage interaction with others." (Bauer & Hill, 1986: 156)
② III, 3, G. Alcoholism.

10. There is a need to get in touch with personal feelings and to understand the reaction to those feelings and how they influence others' behavior.
③ II, 3, G. Alcoholism.

11. "The problem-solving process is a conscious growth-producing method of dealing with stressful situations. By confronting the felt anxiety, the individual is able to move through the stressful situation." (Bauer & Hill, 1986: 21)
③ III, 3, G. Crisis Intervention.

12. In severe cases, coma and death occur.
③ IV, 3, G. Addictive Behaviors.

13. Encouraging the patient to take responsibility for as many aspects of his or her own care as possible will prove genuine interest on the part of the nurse and will result in trust and cooperation from the patient.
④ III, 1, G. Mental Health

BIBLIOGRAPHY

Bauer, B. & Hill, S. (1986). *Essentials of Mental Health Care: Planning and Interventions.* W.B. Saunders Co., Philadelphia.

Griest, J. & Jefferson, J. (1984). *Depression and Its Treatment: Help for the Nation's #1 Mental Problem.* American Psychiatric Association Press, Washington, D.C.

Irving, S. (1983). *Basic Psychiatric Nursing, 3rd ed.* W.B. Saunders Co., Philadelphia.

Kolb, L. & Brodie, K. (1982). *Modern Clinical Psychiatry, 3rd ed.* W.B. Saunders Co., Philadelphia.

Perko, J. & Kreigh, H. (1983). *Psychiatric and Mental Health Nursing: A Commitment to Care and Concern, 2nd ed.* Reston Publishing Co., Inc., Reston, VA.

Purtilo, R. (1984). *Health Professional/Patient Interaction, 3rd ed.* W.B. Saunders Co., Philadelphia.

Robinson, L. (1983). *Psychiatric Nursing as a Human Experience.* W.B. Saunders Co., Philadelphia.

Practice Test

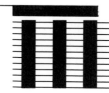

Questions

1. According to the American Heart Association, the first step in performing CPR is to:
   ① Establish an airway
   ② Establish unresponsiveness
   ③ Check the pulse
   ④ Check for respirations

2. The most common airway obstruction in sudden death is caused by the:
   ① Absence of nerve stimuli to the brain
   ② Inability to swallow secretions
   ③ Swelling of the epiglottis
   ④ Tongue falling backwards

3. The ratio of compressions to breaths by one rescuer on an adult is:
   ① 2 breaths to 15 compressions
   ② 4 breaths to 12 compressions
   ③ 1 breath to 5 compressions
   ④ 1 breath to 15 compressions

4. Which of the following would be an appropriate reason to discontinue CPR?
   ① Resuscitation efforts have been unsuccessful after 15 minutes
   ② You are too tired to continue
   ③ The pupils are dilated
   ④ The victim has vomited

5. The primary goal in shock management is to:
   ① Raise the systolic blood pressure to 90 mm Hg or above
   ② Restore and maintain tissue oxygenation
   ③ Maintain heart rate between 70 and 90
   ④ Increase urine output

6. The emergency management of a hemorrhagic shock victim requires that an airway is established, blood loss stopped, and then:
   ① An intravenous infusion is established
   ② An indwelling catheter is inserted
   ③ Blood is drawn for arterial blood gases
   ④ An ECG is done

7. When assessing the patient in hypovolemic shock, which of the following findings would be evident?

   ① Warm, dry skin and tachycardia
   ② Pale skin and a slow pulse
   ③ Decreasing level of consciousness and increased urine output
   ④ Cold, clammy skin, and hypotension

8. Mrs. Potts is admitted to the ER in anaphylactic shock following an insect bite. Initially, nursing care should focus on:

   ① Assessing level of consciousness
   ② Maintaining an open airway
   ③ Providing fluid replacement
   ④ Maintaining body temperature

Jill Cohen, a 64-year-old factory worker, is admitted through the emergency department. She is diaphoretic, nauseated, and complains of severe chest pain. Ms. Cohen weighs 180 lb and is 64 inches tall. She is an insulin-dependent diabetic with a history of hypertension. Her vital signs are BP, 80/60; T, 97°F; P, 120; and R, 36. Her diagnosis is myocardial infarction.

9. Which of the following interventions should *first* be performed by the nurse?

   ① Call the lab to draw blood for baseline cardiac enzymes
   ② Call respiratory therapy to draw blood gases
   ③ Begin cardiac monitoring and take vital signs
   ④ Place the crash cart in the patient's room

10. Morphine sulfate, IV, is given for chest pain. During the administration of this medication, the nurse must observe carefully for:

    ① Respiratory depression
    ② Wheezing
    ③ Anxiety and restlessness
    ④ Hypertension

11. Nursing care during the acute phase following an MI includes:

    ① Recording vital signs every 4 hours
    ② Positioning the patient in Trendelenburg position
    ③ Range of motion exercises
    ④ Administration of oxygen

12. Which of the following is *not* a cardiac enzyme?

① Creatine kinase (CPK)
② Alanine aminotransferase (SGPT or ALT)
③ Lactic acid dehydrogenase (LDH)
④ Aspartate aminotransferase (SGOT or AST)

13. What usual immediate complication of a myocardial infarction do Ms. Cohen's symptoms indicate?

① Pulmonary edema
② Angina pectoris
③ Congestive heart failure
④ Cardiogenic shock

14. Ms. Cohen finds breathing more difficult unless she is in high Fowler position. She has also begun to have a cough with blood tinged, frothy sputum. You assessment leads you to believe she has developed:

① Atrial fibrillation
② Right-sided heart failure
③ Left-sided heart failure
④ Mitral valve prolapse

15. Her respiratory status will be recorded as:

① Stertorous
② Apneic
③ Orthopneic
④ Cheyne-Stokes

16. Propranolol (Inderal), has been orderd for an atrial arrhythmia. A note should be made on the nursing care plan to assess patient frequently for:

① Increased blood pressure
② Restlessness and anxiety
③ Bradycardia
④ Decreased level of consciousness

17. Ms. Cohen is also placed on heparin sodium IV. Considering the side effects of this drug, nursing care should including monitoring the patient for:

① Diarrhea
② Hematuria
③ Increased white blood count
④ Shortness of breath

18. The heparin has been changed to subcutaneous injections instead of IV. Injections should be:

① Massaged to promote absorption
② Limited to upper arms and anterior thigh
③ Given in the lower abdomen
④ Rotated between the arms, thighs, gluteal area, and abdomen

19. Ms. Cohen becomes very depressed 2 days after admission. The nurse should:

① Remind her that she is fortunate to be alive after her heart attack
② Show her a tape of what happens during an MI
③ Encourage her to get more exercise to take her mind off her problems
④ Encourage her to express her fears and answer her questions

---

Lucy, a widow age 85 years, is admitted to the hospital and scheduled for extraction of a cataract of her left eye and insertion of an intraocular lens. Her right eye also has a cataract, but has better vision. Her general health is good. She lives alone in a small apartment, but her daughter and son-in-law live nearby and check on her daily.

20. Admission procedures have been completed and the patient has been oriented to her surroundings. In contributing to her care plan, the nurse added the diagnosis of potential for injury related to impaired vision. An important intervention to include in her plan is to:

① Maintain all four side rails at all times
② Restrain her with a vest restraint when in bed to assure that she does not climb out
③ Maintain the location of items at her bedside, furnishings and other items in her immediate environment
④ Encourage a family member to stay with her at all times

21. When Lucy returns to her room after surgery, the nurse should observe for:

① Sudden or severe pain in the eye
② Diplopia
③ Equality of carotid pulses
④ Equality of pupil reactions to light and accommodation

22. A postoperative nursing diagnosis for Lucy is potential for injury related to hemorrhage. An important nursing intervention is to:

① Maintain Lucy on complete bed rest for 24 hours

② Remind Lucy not to cough or sneeze
③ Reinforce loose dressing to maintain pressure
④ Maintain Lucy on her operative side

Abigail Mullen, age 17 years, is admitted to the emergency room with suspected drug abuse. It has not as yet been determined what drug or drugs Abigail has been using.

23. If Abigail has been using heroin, the nurse would expect her pupils to appear:

① Dilated
② Constricted
③ Fixed
④ Unequal

24. If Abigail has been using amphetamines, she may be suffering from malnutrition. This is because amphetamines:

① Cause vitamins to be excreted
② Decrease the appetite
③ Cause malabsorption syndrome
④ Inhibit protein synthesis

25. If Abigail has been using cocaine, the nurse should assess for:

① Necrosis of nasal septum
② Parkinson's syndrome
③ Toxic shock
④ Dehydration

26. Abigail is tested for marijuana use. The nurse knows Abigail's parents understand the test when they explain that the chemical ingredient in marijuana:

① Is water soluble and leaves the body in less than 12 hrs
② Is fat soluble and may be stored by the body for up to 1 month
③ Is water soluble and may remain in the blood stream for up to 1 week
④ Is fat soluble and cannot pass the blood–brain barrier

27. In addition to marijuana use, Abigail has been drinking excessively on weekends. Because of the weekend pattern her parents do not believe she is an alcoholic. The nurse's response to the parents should indicate that Abigail:

① Is not yet an alcoholic, but may become one

② May be an alcoholic and have physical dependency
③ Is only psychologically dependent on alcohol
④ Is not an alcoholic but is responding to peer pressure

28. Abigail's parents feel that her problem is not addiction. After teaching, the nurse evaluates Abigail's parents' knowledge of alcohol metabolism by an alcoholic when they explain that it (is):

① Same as for a nonalcoholic
② Slower than for a nonalcoholic
③ Toxin producing
④ Produces a heroin-like substance

29. Abigail's physician orders a pregnancy test. Her mother has expressed confusion about the need for this test. To explain the rationale for the test to Abigail's mother, the nurse must know alcohol use during pregnancy is dangerous because it:

① Lowers the blood pressure
② Causes menstruation in the first trimester
③ Causes birth defects
④ Decreases blood supply to the placenta

Ms. Duncan is 36 weeks pregnant and admitted with a diagnosis of preeclampsia.

30. Which of the following assessments are a priority in Ms. Duncan's case?

① Glucosuria, hypotension, dependent edema, and depressed reflexes
② Bacteriuria, flank pain, malaise, and low-grade fever
③ Hypertension, proteinuria, and generalized edema
④ Uterine contractions, concentrated urine, and low-grade fever

31. Planning for Ms. Duncan's care should include:

① Rest on her left side in a quiet room with restricted visitors
② Force fluids, continuous uterine monitoring and a bright sunny room
③ Activity as desired by low carbohydrate diet and frequent monitoring of her blood sugar
④ Keep her in the labor room and administer tocolytic drugs

32. The physician orders an infusion of MgSO₄ (magnesium sulfate). This drug is administered to:

① Promote labor
② Promote relaxation
③ Prevent convulsions
④ Lower blood sugar

33. While Ms. Duncan is receiving the MgSO₄, you observe that her urinary output is decreasing, her respirations are 10, and her knee reflexes are diminished. You should:

① Notify the charge nurse immediately
② Realize that this is the desired result
③ Continue to observe her for further changes
④ Expect that the dosage will be increased

34. When Ms. Duncan goes into labor she will be monitored for fetal distress. Which of the following indicates fetal distress?

① Presence of meconium-stained fluid when the fetus is in the breech position
② Increase in maternal blood pressure
③ Decelerations in the fetal heart rate
④ Increase in the frequency and duration of uterine contractions

Mary is seen in the clinic with a diagnosis of urinary tract infection.

35. Mary reports the following symptoms. Which one is unrelated to her primary diagnosis?

① Elevated BUN
② Frequency of urination
③ Nocturia
④ Burning on urination

36. How would the PN report painful voiding, using medical terminology?

① Enuresis
② Anuresis
③ Dysuria
④ Urinary colic

37. Cranberry juice is frequently recommended for patients with urinary tract infections because cranberry juice tends to:

① Promote diuresis
② Increase acidity of urine
③ Decrease urinary tract spasms
④ Relax the bladder

38. Mary is discharged on Gantrisin. Discharge instructions should include:

① Take your temperature twice a day
② Limit food with high salt content
③ Set alarm in order to take fluids hourly
④ Take fluids hourly while awake

A young woman comes to the clinic because she thinks she may have a venereal disease.

39. The appropriate action for the PN to take initially is to:

① Determine if she is promiscuous
② Ask her for a list of all sexual partners
③ Explore the reasons she thinks she has a venereal disease
④ Determine if she is a minor

40. She says that her boyfriend has VD, that about a month ago she had a painless sore on her genitals that disappeared, and that she is afraid. Given her description, which of the following venereal diseases may be the likely diagnosis?

① Syphilis
② Gonorrhea
③ Chancre
④ Herpes

41. The routine test for syphilis involves a:

① Urine test
② Blood test
③ Vaginal smear
④ Wound culture

42. The MD orders probenecid and penicillin for the patient. The rationale for administering probenecid with penicillin is that it:

① Inhibits renal secretion of penicillin
② Prevents allergic reactions
③ Decreases side effects of penicillin
④ Prevents hepatic damage

Mr. John Smith has been hospitalized with a myocardial infarction. He is being transferred from the ICU to a cardiac step-down unit. He no longer has chest pain but still requires oxygen prn.

43. Shortly after Mr. Smith is transferred, he complains of shortness of breath. The first action that the PN should take is to:

① Call the doctor

② Document the complaint in the nurse's notes
③ Connect Mr. Smith to oxygen
④ Offer to stay with Mr. Smith until the symptoms disappear

44. Oxygen is connected to Mr. Smith via nasal cannula. The flow rate for oxygen delivered by nasal cannula should not exceed:

① 6 L
② 10 L
③ 12 L
④ 20 L

45. Which of the following observations would indicate that the oxygen is relieving the complaint.

① The pulse rate is increasing
② Mr. Smith is sitting in a chair playing cards with his grandson
③ Mr. Smith is leaning over his bedside table
④ The respiratory rate is 36

Mrs. Smith has stopped by the nurse's desk on her way out after visiting hours. She states, "Keep an eye on my husband, will you? He doesn't seem himself tonight." Because of her worried expression you decide to check on Mr. Smith immediately and find him *slumped over the side rails.* He does not respond when you shake his shoulder or loudly call his name.

46. Your first reaction should be to:

① Call for help
② Place the client on a hard surface
③ Give two sharp thumps to the left chest
④ Administer two quick breaths

47. You position Mr. Smith horizontally and hyperextend his neck. Your next action should be to:

① Call for help
② Check for a pulse
③ Give two sharp thumps to the left chest
④ Ventilate twice

48. The rate of ventilation to cardiac compression with two nurses is:

① 1:5
② 2:15
③ 1:10
④ 4:15

Mr. Smith is successfully resuscitated and has an uneventful stay in the ICU. He is experiencing episodes of angina following meals.

49. Angina pectoris that occurs after eating may be due to:

① Increased abdominal distention
② Esophageal reflux
③ Blood being shunted to the gut
④ Decreased oxygen intake while eating

50. Mr. Smith is given nitroglycerin. Which of the following information concerning the medication should you include in your teaching?

① Take the medicine every 6 hours
② You may experience flushing
③ Take your pulse prior to taking the medication
④ The medication should not be taken if burning under the tongue is noted

Olivia, 4 months old, is brought to the hospital by her mother. The mother reports that Olivia has been ill for several days with a cold and that today she awakened with a cough and problems breathing.

51. Which of the assessment findings would indicate that Olivia is in acute respiratory distress?

① Respiratory rate of 35 at rest
② Flaring of the nares
③ Bronchial breath sounds
④ Experiencing diaphragmatic respirations

The RN charge nurse reports that Olivia's diagnosis is viral bronchiolitis and that she is to be placed in a mist tent.

52. In which of the following positions would you expect Olivia to be most comfortable?

① Left side
② Abdomen
③ Semi-Fowler's
④ High Fowler's

53. Which of the following actions would it be most important for the nurse to implement while Olivia is in the mist tent?

① To maintain hydration, feed Olivia every 3 hours
② To keep her dry, change her clothing frequently
③ Observe for cyanosis by turning off the mist frequently
④ Take her out of the mist tent hourly for cuddling

54. How should the PN plan to take Olivia's temperature?

① Orally
② Axillary
③ Rectally
④ Skin-heat sensor

55. Which urine specific gravity would indicate that Olivia is in good fluid balance?

① 1.002
② 1.015
③ 1.030
④ 1.035

56. Which of the following would be correct information to be given to Olivia's mother?

① A vaccine will prevent future attacks
② She should be placed on prophylactic antibiotics
③ Repeated attacks may be associated with asthmatic allergic reactions
④ She will most likely be placed on bronchodilators

Olivia has also been diagnosed as having bilateral otitis media. Her physician has ordered ear drops and an IM antibiotic.

57. When administering the ear drops to Olivia, the PN should pull her ear:

① Up and back
② Down and back
③ Straight up
④ Straight down

58. Which of the following injection sites should be used for the injection of the antibiotic?

① Ventrogluteal
② Deltoid
③ Dorsogluteal
④ Laterofemoral

59. In observing Olivia for pain, which of the following would be an unexpected physiologic response to pain?

① Flushing
② Restlessness
③ Constriction of pupils
④ Increase in pulse rate

60. Olivia's mother tells you that she is due for her immunization. The PN should know that:

① This should be her first immunization
② She is out of sequence for the normal immunization series
③ She should be due her second DPT
④ Olivia should have completed her DPT immunizations

Jason is 5 years old. He has had several hospitalizations for recurrent ear infections and myringotomy. He is being admitted to the hospital for a tonsillectomy and adenoidectomy.

61. In preparing Jason for his admission, the PN should initially:

① Meet Jason and his parents at their home
② Supply him with a book about going to the hospital
③ Due to his past experience, nothing is necessary
④ Explore Jason's concept of hospitalization

62. Considering Jason's age, his dominant fear during hospitalization will be that of:

① Body mutilation
② Abandonment
③ Death
④ Stranger anxiety

63. Jason is to receive an injection preoperatively. He is most concerned and asks you, the PN, "Will it hurt?" Your best reply is:

① "Yes, it will hurt a little, but not for long."
② "Big boys are not afraid."
③ "I can't believe that you are afraid."
④ "You may watch TV as soon as this is over."

Jason's preoperative orders are: Demerol 35 mg and Vistaril 12.5 mg.

64. The Demerol available is 50 mg per 1 mL. Which of the following is the appropriate amount of Demerol that Jason should receive?

① 1.7 mL
② 0.7 mL
③ 0.8 mL
④ 0.5 mL

65. The Vistaril available is 100 mg per 2 mL. Which of the following is the appropriate amount of Vistaril that Jason should receive?

① 1 mL
② 0.5 mL
③ 0.25 mL
④ 0.1 mL

66. The PN is unsure if the Demerol and Vistaril are compatible when mixed in the same syringe. Which of the following options would be best for her to choose?

① Mix the medications but discard if clouding occurs
② Assume that they are not compatible and give the medications in two syringes
③ Ask another nurse
④ Check the compatibility chart in the medication room

67. As you come into the room to give Jason his injection, he starts to cry and scream "I hate you. Get out of my room." Which of the following actions would be most appropriate for the nurse to take?

① Ask another nurse to give Jason his shot because he does not like you
② Explain to Jason in a calm voice what you are going to do and then do it
③ Ask Jason's parents to leave the room as you will then be able to calm him
④ Tell Jason that he acting like a baby and that big boys do not act like that

68. Which of the following would be an appropriate liquid to give Jason postoperatively?

① Orange juice
② Tepid water
③ Hot tea
④ Milk

69. Jason's parents ask you why Jason is susceptible to hemorrhage in about 5 days? The most likely reason for this is:

① Decreased platelet count
② Sloughing of the membrane from the throat
③ An anticoagulative effect of aspirin
④ Eating rough foods

Ann is a 3-year-old who has a tentative diagnosis of pinworm infestation.

70. Ann's physician has ordered a cellophane tape test to be performed at home. The PN should explain to Ann's mother that the most effective time to perform this test is:

① At bedtime before bathing
② Following a bowel movement
③ Immediately after lunch
④ Early morning before arising

71. Which of the following should the nurse included in the teaching plan for Ann and her family?

① Good hand-washing technique
② Proper food preparation
③ Proper isolation techniques
④ Sterilization techniques

Provan has been ordered for Ann.

72. It is important to note on Ann's care plan that a side effect of Provan is that it makes the stool:

① Black
② Green
③ Red
④ Blue

Terri, age 3 years, is admitted to the pediatric unit with a diagnosis of Wilms' tumor.

73. The PN should be aware that the most important aspect of Terri's care preoperatively is to:

① Avoid palpating the abdomen
② Maintain a high protein and low salt diet
③ Obtain daily weights
④ Enforce strict bed rest

74. When it is time for Terri's parents to leave, the nurse should encourage the parents to:

① Wait until the child is asleep to leave
② Tell Terri truthfully that they are leaving
③ Wait until Terri is distracted in play
④ Tell the child that the nurse said that they must go

75. Which type of behavior would you expect from Terri the first time that her parents leave?

① Wave bye to them
② Cry
③ Hide under the bed
④ Ask to go to the playroom

Terri has surgery.

76. When taking Terri's blood pressure, the blood pressure cuff:

① Will produce a higher reading if too wide
② Should cover about two-thirds of the upper arm
③ Should only be applied to the thigh
④ Will produce a low reading if too narrow

77. In assessing Terri for pain, the PN should know that the *first* observable behavioral change is usually:

① Irritability
② Lethargy
③ Loss of appetite
④ Disturbed sleep patterns

Nine-year-old Paul has been admitted to the pediatric unit with the diagnosis of Legg-Calvé-Perthes disease.

78. In completing your nursing assessment of Paul, you should expect Paul to complain of pain in which of the following areas?

① Hip
② Calf
③ Lower abdomen
④ Lumbar spine

79. Treatment for Paul is aimed at:

① Preventing deformity of the femur
② Preventing degeneration of the knee joint
③ Reducing muscle spasms of the back
④ Preventing pressure on the head of the femur

80. In dealing with Paul, one of the most difficult aspects of his care is expected to be the:

① Compliance with the prescribed diet
② Overwhelming feeling of fatigue
③ Overconcern for missing school
④ Necessity of prolonged immobility

81. Paul is being discharged with braces. His teaching for home care of the braces should include which of the following instructions?

① Apply alcohol to bony prominences
② Check skin weekly for signs of irritation
④ Clean plastic molds weekly with soap and water
④ Use crutches if braces need repair

82. Which of the following activities might Paul be able to participate in following discharge?

① Swimming
② Tennis
③ Football
④ Horseback riding

83. Paul should be mastering Erikson's stage of:

① Industry versus inferiority
② Intimacy versus isolation
③ Trust versus mistrust
④ Autonomy versus shame

Shannon, a 17 year old, has been admitted to the hospital with infectious mononucleosis. Her symptoms are fever, sore throat, muscle soreness, and general malaise.

84. The PN should expect to find which of the following during her initial nursing assessment?

① Abdominal distention
② Productive cough
③ Lesions of the lips
④ Enlarged lymph nodes

85. The PN should plan to prevent the spread of the disease by following which of the following precautions?

① Good hand-washing
② Respiratory isolation
③ Enteric isolation
④ Complete isolation

86. The diagnosis of infectious mononucleosis is confirmed by which of the following?

① Chest radiograph
② Urinalysis
③ Blood test
④ Skin test

87. In planning to meet the dietary needs of Shannon, which of the following items should be excluded?

① Orange juice
② Puddings
③ Milk shakes
④ Warm tea

88. Which of the following is a potential complication that occur with Shannon's diagnosis?

① Cystitis
② Diarrhea
③ Weight gain
④ Hepatomegaly

89. Which of the following statements indicates that Shannon understands the teaching regarding her convalescence?

① "I must have complete bed rest to prevent relapse."
② "Bed rest is not necessary, but I can only have quiet activities."
③ "Additional rest periods will be necessary, but I must avoid only strenuous activities."
④ "Activity limitations are not necessary, but I must avoid crowds."

90. In caring for Shannon while she is hospitalized, it is most important to recall that adolescents are most likely to be fearful of:

① Separation from family and school
② Falling behind in academic studies
③ Loss of body integrity
④ Loss of self-control in front of others

91. In response to Shannon's parents' questions regarding the spread of her disease, it is correct to tell them that mononucleosis is spread by:

① Contact with oral secretions
② Contact with the stools
③ The respiratory system
④ Contact with blood

Yolanda, age 3 years, has developed a pink rash and is diagnosed as having rubella.

92. Identify the correct statement regarding Yolanda's condition.

① Yolanda should have Koplik spots in her mouth
② She should not be visited by her aunt, who is 2 months pregnant
③ Yolanda's treatment should consist of antibiotics

④ Encephalitis is a frequent complication of this condition

The PN hears in report that Mike in room 400 has Koplik spots.

93. Koplik spots are considered diagnostic of:

① Rubella
② Roseola
③ Rubeola
④ Chickenpox

94. Which of the following statements regarding rubeola is *false*?

① The duration of symptoms is about 3 days
② The disease is highly contagious
③ The incubation period is 10 to 14 days
④ Photophobia is a frequent symptom

Tony, age 3 years, has been admitted to the pediatric unit with the admitting diagnosis of nephrotic syndrome.

95. Which assessment finding would the PN most likely find, given Tony's diagnosis?

① Edema
② Hypernatremia
③ Hematuria
④ Increased urinary output

96. In response to Tony's parents questions about the cause of Tony's disease, the PN could reply that the etiology is:

① Unknown
② Hyperimmune response
③ Acute glomerulonephritis
④ An allergic response

97. Tony is placed on steroid therapy. The aim of this therapy is to prevent:

① Diuresis
② Hematuria
③ Proteinuria
④ Potassium loss

98. The diet for Tony during the acute stage will most likely be:

① Normal for age
② High protein, low sodium
③ Low protein, low sodium
④ High protein, high sodium

99. Which of the following nursing actions will help to insure an accurate urinalysis?

① Force fluids to 1000 mL prior to collection
② Take the urine to the lab as soon as it is obtained
③ Collect all of the urine
④ Cleanse the container with betadine prior to collecting the specimen

Cathy is admitted to the hospital with acute glomerulonephritis.

100. Many infections commonly precede glomerulonephritis. Which of the following is *not* known to precede the disease?

① Tonsillitis
② Mononucleosis
③ Scarlet fever
④ Impetigo

101. The PN should expect that Cathy's urinalysis would reflect the presence of:

① A specific gravity of 1.045
② Blood
③ Glucose
④ Bacteria

Carl, age 6 years, fell from his bike, resulting in a fracture to his lower leg. He has been admitted to the hospital for casting.

102. When obtaining the admission history, the PN should first:

① Assess Carl's reaction to the hospital
② Inquire about health insurance
③ Review Carl's development with his mother
④ Establish a rapport with Carl and his parents

103. The nurse should use the palms of her hands when handling the wet cast to:

① Assess dryness of the cast
② Facilitate easy turning
③ Keep the limbs balanced
④ Prevent indenting the cast

104. Which of the following assessment findings would cause the PN to suspect that an infection has developed under the cast?

① Complaint of numbness
② Cold toes

③ Increased respirations
④ Foul smell

105. In planning for Carl's discharge, which intervention may be used to relieve itching?

① Blow cool air under the cast with a fan
② Squeeze lotion beneath the cast
③ Use a straightened coat hanger to scratch the area
④ Sprinkle powder beneath the cast

Your neighbor, Mrs. Smith, tells you that her baby has impetigo. She has many questions.

106. Which of the following statements regarding impetigo is false?

① Impetigo is caused by a bacterium
② Scarring rarely occurs
③ Impetigo commonly occurs on the face
④ It is usually not contagious

107. Which of the following is a potentially dangerous complication of impetigo?

① Reye's syndrome
② Erythema multiforme
③ Pyelonephritis
④ Glomerulonephritis

During a rotation on the pediatric unit, the PN should review what she knows about child abuse.

108. In which of the following situations would a PN be most likely to suspect the incidence of child abuse?

① A child who cries during the physical examination
② A broken arm in a 6-year-old child
③ Bruises on a child's forehead and knees
④ A 4-year-old with a broken nose

109. Which would be inappropriate in the case of suspected child abuse?

① Document all bruises and cuts
② Chart interactions between the child and parent
③ Document staff perceptions of the family relationships
④ Report to the state child welfare agency or law enforcement agency

Herm is brought to the hospital with a sickle cell crisis. His father also has the disease.

110. Because the father has sickle cell disease and the mother has not had it, the mother:

① Must have the disease too
② Must have the trait
③ Is disease-free
④ May or may not have the trait

111. An increased fluid intake is most important in treating sickle cell crisis because:

① A child may refuse to drink due to discomfort
② Hydration will increase blood volume and decrease blood viscosity
③ It will increase the excretion of toxins
④ It will prevent heart failure

112. Herm is on intake and output. In recording the fluid content of a popsicle (2½ oz), you should record:

① 25 mL
② 75 mL
③ 120 mL
④ 240 mL

113. Herm is from a culture different from the PN's. Ignoring Herm's cultural values and beliefs may cause:

① Indifference
② Confusion
③ Alienation
④ No effect

As a PN, you are assigned to work in the immunization clinic.

114. Immunizations should be started when a child is:

① 6 months
② 2 months
③ 12 months
④ 2 weeks

115. There is no active immunization for:

① Measles
② Smallpox
③ Chickenpox
④ Mumps

116. DPT is used to immunize children against:

① Diphtheria, polio, and tetanus
② Diphtheria, polio, and typhoid
③ Diphtheria, pertussis, and tetanus
④ Diphtheria, pertussis, and typhoid

117. Mrs. Jones is admitted to your unit with a diagnosis of anxiety. She is able to concentrate on a particular problem and is very alert. Which of the following stages of anxiety is she experiencing?

① Mild
② Moderate
③ Severe
④ Panic

118. Which of the following would *not* be a common cause of anxiety?

① Nonspecific threats to self
② When one's defenses are not working well
③ Aggressive behavior
④ Threat to the biologic integrity

119. When administering a major tranquilizer such as a phenothiazine, which of the following symptoms should be reported to the physician immediately?

① Dry mouth
② Drowsiness
③ Orthostatic hypotension
④ Abnormal facial grimaces

120. If your patient is placed on diazepam (Valium) to treat anxiety, which of the following should be included in your patient teaching?

① Take the drug with milk or food to decrease nausea
② If you are drowsy, stop taking the drug
③ Do not drink alcohol while on the drug
④ Food and drink with caffeine should be eliminated

Answers & Rationales

Guide to item identifications (see pp. 3–5 for further details about each category)

I, II, III, or IV for the phase of the nursing process
1, 2, 3, or 4 for the category of client needs
A, B, C, D, E, F, or G for the category of human functioning
Specific content category by name; ie, cholecystectomy

1. ② The first step in the CPR procedure, according to the American Heart Association, is to establish whether or not the patient is responsive. Next, establish the airway, restore breathing, and then circulation.
III, 1, B. CPR.

2. ④ The tongue falls back into the throat when the patient loses consciousness. This can obstruct the airway and cause death.
I, 2, B. CPR.

3. ① One rescuer should ventilate/compress at the rate of 2 breaths for every 15 compressions. If there are 2 rescuers, the ratio is 1 breath to every 5 compressions.
III, 1, B. CPR.

4. ② CPR should be carried out until: (a) the person regains a satisfactory intrinsic pulse, (b) the person is pronounced dead, or (c) the rescuer is exhausted and unable to continue, and no one else is available to perform CPR. Pupils could be dilated for other reasons.
III, 1, B. CPR.

5. ② The primary goal in treating shock is to restore effective tissue perfusion. Oxygenation is the overall objective.
II, 2, B. Shock.

6. ① The third priority is in treating shock is establishing an IV line so that fluids, medications, and blood can be given immediately. Following this blood gases are drawn, an ECG monitor is attached, and a catheter is inserted.
III, 1, B. Shock.

7. ④ When the patient suffers from shock, vasoconstriction is one of the first compensatory mechanisms associated with shock. The vasoconstriction causes the cold clammy skin and if the shock continues, hypotension occurs. Urine output is decreased to conserve fluids and the heart rate increases.
I, 2, B. Shock.

8. ② Anaphylactic shock is the result of a severe antibody–antigen reaction. This reaction causes damage to the cells of the respiratory epithelium resulting in edema.
I, 2, B. Shock.

9. ③ When a patient is admitted with a suspected MI, it is important to immediately assess the status of the heart. The other actions would be done, but not first.
III, 2, B. MI.

10. ① A major side effect of morphine, a narcotic analgesic, is respiratory depression.
III, 2, B. Medications.

11. ④ Oxygen is administered during the acute phase to relieve respiratory distress associated with MI.
III, 2, B. MI.

12. ② Alanine aminotransferase (SGPT or ALT) is not a cardiac enzyme. The other options are all cardiac enzymes.
IV, 2, B. MI.

13. ④ Cardiogenic shock is characterized by the more acute symptoms the patient is exhibiting. Although CHF and pulmonary edema are possible complications, they are not indicated by the symptoms.
I, 2, B. MI.

14. ③ Left-sided heart failure is characterized by a back up of pressure and fluid in the lungs. Her symptoms indicate that this has occurred. Right-sided failure would produce back up in the periphery, the venous system.
III & IV, 2, B. MI.

15. ③ Orthopnea refers to the need to assume an upright position to breathe.
III & IV, 2, B. MI.

16. ③ Inderal will lower the blood pressure and pulse rate, not raise it. It does sometimes cause depression in older patients.
III & IV, 2, B. MI/Medication.

17. Heparin can cause bleeding from mucous membranes if the level is too high. It is important to evaluate the urine for the presence of blood.
② I & IV, 2, B. MI/Medication.

18. Subcutaneous heparin should be given in the fat of the abdomen. This area is less prone to trauma and bleeding. Do not massage the area since this will increase bruising.
③ III, 2, B. MI/Medication.

19. Depression is common following a myocardial infarction. It is important for patients to be able to express what is concerning them and have their questions answered fully.
④ III, 3, G. MI

20. Items in environment should not be moved after the patient is oriented to her location to prevent her from tripping, falling, or walking into items. Thus, safety and patient dignity are preserved.
③ III, 1, C. Cataract/Surgery.

21. Sudden or severe pain in the eye could indicate increased intraocular pressure or hemorrhage.
① I, 1 & 2, C. Cataract/Surgery.

22. Any actions which increase intraocular pressure should be avoided, especially coughing or sneezing. The eye patch, if in place, is to collect drainage and should not be applying pressure to the eye. Turning to the operative side might increase intraocular pressure, so is an inappropriate nursing action. Complete bed rest is unnecessary.
② II, 1 & 2, C. Cataract/Surgery.

23. Heroin causes the pupils to become pinpoint in size or miotic. #1, #3, and #4 are not commonly associated with heroin use.
② I, 2, G. Adolescent Drug Abuse.

24. Amphetamines cause a lack of appetite and can be used therapeutically for this purpose. #1, #3, and #4 are not associated with amphetamine use.
② I, 2, G. Adolescent Drug Abuse.

25. Cocaine use, in its various forms, can lead to destruction of the nasal septum, myocardial infarction, and stroke. #2 and #3 are not associated with cocaine use and #4 is incorrect.
① I, 2, G. Adolescent Drug Abuse.

26. THC, the chemical in marijuana, may be detected for up to 1 month because it is stored in the body's fat. #1, #3, and #4 are incorrect.
② III, 2, G. Adolescent Drug Abuse.

27. Even though a person can abstain for moderate lengths of time, they may still experience withdrawal symptoms. #1 and #3 cannot yet be stated by the nurse. "Drunk" is not a medical term and has no meaning here.
② I, 2, G. Adolescent Drug Abuse.

28. Many alcoholics metabolize alcohol into a substance related to heroin and sharing much of its addictive qualities. #1, #2, and #3 are incorrect.
④ II, 2, G. Adolescent Drug Abuse.

29. Alcohol is to be withheld during pregnancy due to the possibilities of birth defects. #1, #2, and #4 are incorrect.
③ III, 2, G. Adolescent Drug Abuse.

30. These are the classic symptoms of preeclampsia. The other answers contain unrelated symptoms.
③ I, 4, A & B. Prenatal.

31. Bed rest on the left side is usually helpful in increasing placental blood flow and lowering blood pressure. A quiet room is advised to decrease stimulation. Continuous uterine monitoring and dietary restrictions are usually not recommended.
① II, 4, B. Prenatal.

32. Eclampsia can precipitate convulsions. $MgSO_4$ reduces the transmission of nerve impulses from the brain to the muscles and is used, in this case, as an anticonvulsant.
③ IV, 4, C. Prenatal.

33. These symptoms are typical of magnesium toxicity and should be reported to the charge nurse and the physician immediately.
① III, 4, C. Prenatal.

34. Signs of fetal distress include meconium-stained fluid if the fetus is in a vertex position and decelerations in the fetal heart rate.
③ I, 4, B. Labor and Delivery.

35. Signs of urinary tract infections include #2, #3, and #4. An elevated BUN would not occur as a result of a UTI.
① I, 2, F. Urinary Tract Infection.

36. Dysuria is the medical term for painful void-
③ ing. The usage of correct medical terminology
is desirable when reporting information.
II, 1, F. Urinary Tract Infection.

37. Cranberry juice is offered to clients with uri-
② nary tract infections because it increases the
acidity of the urine. Acidic urine decreases the
rate of bacterial multiplication. The other options are not known actions of cranberry juice.
II, 1, F. Urinary Tract Infection.

38. Gantrisin is a sulfa derivative that can cause
④ crystal and stone formation in the urine. Patients on Gantrisin should increase their fluid
intake. It is not necessary to interrupt her
sleep.
III, 1, D & F. Urinary Tract Infection.

39. The first step should be to find out why she
③ believes that she has the disease. This information will determine the second step. It is
not within the role of the nurse to make judg-
ments about her sexual activities. #2 would
not be done initially. #4 is incorrect in that
most states provide for the treatment of sexually transmitted diseases without parental
consent.
III, 4, D. Syphilis.

40. Syphilis is a sexually transmitted disease that
① occurs in stages. In the primary stage the lesion, chancre, which is painless, appears then
disappears in 2 to 6 weeks. Primary syphilis
can be cured with large doses of penicillin.
Symptoms of primary herpes are dysuria,
vaginal discharge, and a very painful lesion.
Gonorrhea is characterized by vaginal discharge, pelvic pain, and dysuria.
I, 4, D. Syphilis.

41. While #1 and #3 could be correct in some
② cases, they are not routinely done. Cultures
take 24 to 48 hours to grow and would be
impractical in many cases.
I, 4, D. Syphilis.

42. Large doses of penicillin are administered for
① the treatment of syphilis. Penicillin is lost in
the urine. Probenecid inhibits the excretion of
penicillin. The PN should be able to explain
the action of drugs that are administered.
II, 1, D. Syphilis/Medications.

43. Mr. Smith has an order to cover this type of
③ complaint. The doctor may wish to be notified

but he would expect you to follow his orders
prior to calling. Also if the situation warrants
a call to the doctor, the charge nurse should be
notified. You should document his complaint, but this should be done at a later time.
You might offer to stay with Mr. Smith, but
this action alone would probably not relieve
his symptom.
III, 1, B. MI.

44. Nasal oxygen, in excess of 6 L, can result in air
① swallowing and irritation of the nasal and
pharyngeal mucosa.
III, 1, B. MI.

45. This observation would indicate comfort. An
② increasing pulse rate could be indicative of
hypoxia. #3 describes a posture seen commonly in patients with hypoxia. A respiratory
rate of 36 is abnormal for an adult.
IV, 1, B. MI.

46. It is important to call for help first, so that
① needed personnel and equipment can be
brought to the room.
III, 1, B. MI.

47. Once an airway is established, two ventila-
④ tions are given. A precordial thump is no
longer given. A pulse is determined after the
quick breaths.
III, 1, B. CPR.

48. The American Heart Association has estab-
① lished that the correct rate of ventilation to
cardiac compression with two-person rescue
is 1:5.
III, 1, B. MI/CPR.

49. Following a meal, an increased amount of
③ blood is shunted to the small intestine. This
increase in blood for digestion will result in
less blood being available for the heart and
may precipitate angina.
I, 1, B. Angina Pectoris.

50. Flushing is an expected reaction to ni-
② troglycerin. The medication should be taken
as needed. There is no reason to take the
pulse prior to taking nitroglycerin. Nitroglycerin usually causes burning under the
tongue.
III, 4, B. Angina Pectoris/Medication.

51. The other choices are all normal findings in a 4
② month old.
I, 2, B. Bronchiolitis.

52. The Semi-Fowler position allows for expansion of the lungs by lowering the contents of the abdominal cavity. High Fowler's is poorly tolerated by infants.
③ II, 2, B. Bronchiolitis.

53. Children in mist tents require frequent change of clothing to keep dry. The child can be observed inside the tent and parents may get into the tent for cuddling. She should spend as much time as possible in the mist tent. She should not be disturbed for feeding every 3 hours.
② III, 1, B. Broncholitis.

54. Olivia's temperature should be taken rectally. She is too young for oral temperatures. The cool mist tent would result in lower skin temperature.
③ II, 1, D. Basic Skills.

55. Specific gravity measurement is ordered to determine the concentration of urine. #1 indicates the urine is very dilute. #3 and #4 indicate the urine is highly concentrated.
② IV, 2, B & F. Fluid Balance.

56. This is the only option that is factually correct. It has been noted that children with a history of bronchiolitis frequently develop asthmatic allergic reactions. #1, #2, and #4 are false statements.
③ III, 4, B. Bronchiolitis.

57. The correct method to administer ear drops to an infant is to pull the ear down and back. This action is necessary to straighten the eustachian tube.
② III, 2, C. Medication Administration.

58. Thigh muscles are the best site for IM injections for infants. Other muscles are small and poorly developed.
④ III, 2, A & D. Medication Administration.

59. In response to pain, the pupils dilate. Pupil constriction may be observed following the administration of pain medication. #1, #2, and #4 are other responses to pain.
③ I, 2 & 3, C. Bronchiolitis.

60. The normal schedule for DPT immunizations for an infant is 2, 4, and 6 months.
③ II, 1, A & D. Immunizations.

61. Jason's previous experience with hospitaliza-
④ tion will have resulted in certain preconceptions.
II, 3, G. Tonsillectomy.

62. Fear of body mutilation is a dominant fear of the preschool child.
① II, 3, G. Growth & Development.

63. It reflects honesty. #2 and #3 indicates that the nurse is critical of Jason's fear. #4 ignores the question.
① III, 3, G. Perioperative Care.

64. By using ratio and proportion, the correct response is #2. 50:1::35:X.
② III, 2, D. Medication Administration.

65. By using ratio and proportion, the only correct answer is #3. 100:2::12.5:X.
③ III, 2, D. Medication Administration.

66. The compatibility chart is the correct source of information. #1 and #2 are incorrect practices. #3 is a poor choice as the other nurse may not know the correct answer either.
④ III, 1, D. Medication Administration.

67. Jason must have the injection. In response #1, Jason's reaction is to the situation not the nurse. Jason's parents should be allowed to stay as their presence may be a comfort.
② III, 3, G. Medication Administration.

68. Of the listed choices, tepid water is the best option. Fluids that are too hot or too cold should be avoided. Orange juice is acidic and may cause burning. Milk causes coating and thickened secretions.
② III, 2, F. Tonsillectomy.

69. This is the best response because post-tonsillectomy children are prone to hemorrhage as the membrane in the throat is sloughed. This occurs in about 5 days. There is nothing to indicate that Jason has #1 or #3. The eating of rough foods would more likely result in bleeding earlier.
② III, 2 & 4, B. Tonsillectomy.

70. The best time to schedule the procedure is early morning. The parasites emerge at night. The parasites adhere to the sticky surface of the tape. A commercially prepared swab is also available.
④ III, 1, F. Pinworms.

71. Good hand-washing helps prevent spread of the pinworm eggs from the hands to the mouth.
① II, 1, D & F. Pinworms.

72. Everyone caring for the child should be made aware that the stools may be red. This information will help to avoid any misunderstanding of the finding.
③ III, 2, F. Pinworms.

73. It is imperative that nurses avoid palpating the tumor as this could result in rupture of the tumor capsule. #2 & #3 are not components of care for a child with Wilms' tumor. The child would most likely not be on complete bed rest.
① II, 1, F. Wilms' Tumor.

74. Parents should be honest with their children. #1 & #3 might result in the child not wanting to go to sleep or to play. #4 might result in poor, nontrusting relationship between the child and the nurse.
② III, 3, A & G. Growth and Development.

75. It is normal for the toddler to cry when she is left by her parents. #1 & #4 would reflect a poor parent/child relationship. Hiding under the bed is not a behavior to anticipate in this situation.
② I, 3, A. Growth & Development.

76. #1 is incorrect in that a large cuff will result in a lower pressure reading. #4 would result in a higher reading. The thigh would be the second choice.
② I, 2, B. Basic Skills.

77. This is the first observable behavioral sign. All may be correct, but not first.
① I, 2, C. Pain.

78. Children with Legg-Calvé-Perthes disease frequently complain of hip and knee pain. The other symptoms would most likely be due to other causes.
① I, 4, E. Legg-Calvé-Perthes.

79. The aim of conservative treatment is to prevent pressure on the femoral head.
④ II, 1, E. Legg-Calvé-Perthes.

80. Prolonged immobility is difficult for school-aged children. There is usually no diet restriction. The disease does not cause fa-
④ tigue. The child may return to school with braces.
IV, 3, E. Legg-Calvé-Perthes.

81. Alcohol will help to toughen the skin. #2 & #3 should be performed daily. The child should be placed on bed rest until the braces are repaired.
① III, 4, E. Legg-Calvé-Perthes.

82. This is the only safe activity of those listed. The other activities could result in slippage of the head of the femur.
① I, 2, E. Legg-Calvé-Perthes.

83. The school-age child is placed in the stage of industry versus inferiority. He should have mastered trust and autonomy. He is too young to be mastering intimacy.
① I, 3, A. Growth & Development.

84. Enlarged lymph nodes are a typical finding of clients with infectious mononucleosis. The other symptoms might indicate a secondary diagnosis. Lesions of the gums are more common than lip lesions.
④ I, 2, A. Infectious Mononucleosis.

85. Infectious mononucleosis is slightly contagious. The other types of isolation are inappropriate in this situation.
① III, 1, B & D. Infectious Mononucleosis.

86. Knowledge of diagnostic tests aids the PN in patient education. #1, #2, & #4 would not confirm the diagnosis.
③ I, 4, B & D. Infectious Mononucleosis.

87. Orange juice, which is acidic, would not be given to Shannon as an extremely sore throat is a frequent complaint. Bland liquids and puddings are better tolerated. The remainder of the options are appropriate choices.
① III, 2, B & F. Infectious Mononucleosis.

88. Hepatomegaly occurs in about 10% of the cases. It usually resolves within 3 months. The other symptoms are not known complications of mononucleosis.
④ II, 4, B & D. Infectious Mononucleosis.

89. This reflects the best understanding of follow-up convalescence. She would not have to be on complete bed rest. She should slowly resume her normal activities with additional rest periods. Avoiding crowds would be appropriate only in the early stages of the disease.
③ IV, 4, B & D. Infectious Mononucleosis.

90. The major stress for hospitalized adolescents is fear of loss of control in front of others. While the other options may be true of a particular client, #4 is considered the best of the options.
④ I, 3, A. Growth and Development.

91. Infectious mononucleosis is spread by contact with oral secretions. This knowledge aids the PN in preventing spread of the disease.
① III, 1, B & D. Infectious Mononucleosis.

92. Rubella (German measles) can cause serious congenital malformations if contracted by a pregnant woman, particularly during the first trimester.
② III, 1, D. Rubella.

93. Koplik spots are bluish white pinpoint spots that appear in the mouth on about the second or third day of the disease. They usually appear prior to the skin rash.
③ I, 2, D. Rubeola.

94. The duration of the rubeola is about 7 days. Sometimes rubeola is referred to as the 7 day measles.
① II, 2, D. Rubeola.

95. Nephrotic syndrome is characterized by proteinuria, hypoproteinemia, oliguria, and generalized edema. This excess extra fluid volume should be a nursing priority in care plan development.
① I, 2, F. Nephrotic Syndrome.

96. The etiology of nephrotic syndrome remains unknown. Parents frequently feel guilty and anxious when their child is ill and every member of the health team should give consistent information.
① I, 4, F. Nephrotic Syndrome.

97. The aim of steroid therapy is to prevent the loss of protein in the urine by decreasing inflammation of the glomeruli. The benefits outweigh the numerous side effects in this situation.
③ II, 2, F. Nephrotic Syndrome.

98. The child will lose massive amounts of protein in the urine. Lowering the salt content may aid in reducing edema.
② III, 1, F. Nephrotic Syndrome.

99. Stored urine can result in false-positive results, thus urine should either be stored in a
② refrigerator or transported immediately to the laboratory. Forcing fluids will result in dilute urine. The specimen collected should be mid stream. Betadine will affect the results.
III, 1, F. Basic Skills.

100. Mononucleosis does not precede glomerulonephritis: Glomerulonephritis is usually preceded by a Group A beta-hemolytic streptococcal infection. The other three options may be caused by a streptococcal infection.
② IV, 2, F. Glomerulonephritis.

101. Urinalysis findings with glomerulonephritis include specific gravity less than 1.030, positive blood and protein and white blood cells. Glucose and bacteria in the urine are not clinical findings with the disease.
② I, 1, F. Glomerulonephritis.

102. The PN should recognize that in order to complete her assessment, she must first establish a rapport. Insurance information should be obtained by the financial department.
④ I, 3, E. Cast.

103. Wet casts are easily indented. The other options are incorrect.
④ III, 1, E. Cast.

104. Complaints #1 and #2 indicate decreased circulation. Increased respirations have many causes.
④ I, 2, E. Cast.

105. This can be accomplished by using a fan. Nothing should ever be put inside the cast.
① III, 1, E. Cast.

106. Impetigo is a skin infection usually caused by a staphylococcus or a streptococcus. It usually occurs on the face and hands. Impetigo is contagious and steps should be taken to prevent the spread. The disease usually leaves no scars.
④ III, 2, D. Impetigo.

107. Impetigo that is caused by the streptococcus can result in glomerulonephritis. Reye's syndrome is associated with viral infections and the use of aspirin.
④ I, 1, D. Impetigo.

108. Normally, central facial injuries are unusual because children protect this area. Children often cry during examinations. Bruises on the forehead and knees can be accidental. A bro-
④

ken arm in a child of 6 years is not as questionable as one in a child under 2 years.
I, 1, A. Child Abuse.

109. ③ Documentation is extremely important. Care should be taken to chart and report what you observe, but perceptions should never be charted. It is the law that suspected child abuse be reported.
III, 1, G. Child Abuse.

110. ② Sickle cell anemia is an autosomal recessive disease. In order for it to occur both parents must be carriers.
I, 4, B. Sickle Cell Anemia.

111. ② It is important for the child with sickle cell anemia to be well hydrated to prevent sickling and to delay the stasis-thrombosis-ischemia cycle during crisis.
I, 2, B. Sickle Cell Anemia.

112. ② To solve this problem, the PN must recall that there are 30 mL in 1 oz.
III, 1, B. Sickle Cell Anemia.

113. ③ Cultural beliefs and values should be taken into consideration when planning nursing care. Failure to do so will frequently result in alienation.
II, 3, G. Growth & Development.

114. ② Healthy children should start immunizations at 2 months.
I, 4, D. Immunizations.

115. ③ At present there is no immunization available for chickenpox.
I, 4, D. Immunizations.

116. ③ DPT stands for diphtheria, pertussis, and tetanus. DPTs are given to healthy children in a series of 3 at 2, 4, and 6 months. Boosters are given at 18 months and 4 to 6 years. Thereafter, diphtheria and tetanus are given every 10 years.
I, 4, D. Immunizations.

117. ② With moderate anxiety, the individual's alertness increases but her perceptual field narrows to allow the person to focus more. Mild anxiety exhibits lesser symptoms and the other two options have much more severe symptoms.
IV, 3, G. Anxiety.

118. ③ Aggressive behavior is not a cause of anxiety. The other options refer to common causes of anxiety.
I, 3, G. Anxiety.

119. ④ One of the major side effects are the development of extrapyramidal symptoms. The most common of these is tardive dyskinesia, which is a ruminating-like effect characterized by facial grimaces and involuntary movements of the lips, tongue, and jaw. If this develops, the physician should be notified because nonphenothiazine tranquilizers could be substituted. The other options are common side effects which do not require physician interventions.
III, 3, G. Medications/Anxiety.

120. ③ When the patient is on a drug such as Valium, the use of any other CNS depressant is contraindicated. There is no need to take the drug with food or milk. The drug typically causes drowsiness and the patient should be warned of this, but it does not require the drug to be stopped. Caffeine can inhibit the drug's effects.
III, 3, G. Medications/Anxiety.

Practice Test IV

Questions

121. The chest pain of angina pectoris is caused by:
1. Excessive action of the myocardium
2. A blockage in the conductive system of the heart
3. Reduced blood supply to the myocardium
4. Vasodilation of the coronary arteries

122. The pain associated with angina is best described as:
1. Similar to indigestion
2. Severe, substernal, radiating to left arm and neck
3. Crushing pain, beginning in shoulders and radiating to center of chest
4. A dull ache in the entire chest and neck

Ray Cox, age 64 years, was admitted to the medical unit with a diagnosis of unstable angina pectoris. Mr. Cox is retired and enjoys playing tennis each morning with friends, an activity he's done for 30 years.

123. Mr. Cox should be instructed that to prevent acute attacks of angina he should:
1. Not continue playing tennis
2. Avoid crowds
3. Sleep at least 10 hours a night
4. Avoid exposure to severe cold

124. The physician may best distinguish between the chest pain of angina from other forms of illness by doing a:
1. BUN and creatinine
2. Echocardiogram
3. Exercise stress test
4. Ultrasound of the heart

125. A vasodilator that is specific for relief of acute anginal pain during an acute attack is:
1. Nitroglycerin
2. Isosorbide dinitrate (Isordil SR)
3. Dypyridamole (Persantin)
4. Isoxsuprine hydrochloride (Vasodilan)

126. Because Mr. Cox is of normal weight for his height, the nurse should include in his dietary instructions:
1. That no dietary restrictions are needed
2. To eat large meals each day and avoid snacking
3. Avoid all high sodium foods
4. To reduce fat intake to reduce his cholesterol

127. Mr. Cox is taught that the nitroglycerin is used for anginal pain because it:
1. Has a long-acting effect and prevents heart attacks
2. Works quickly to dilate coronary arteries
3. Increases the heart rate to improve blood flow to the myocardium
4. Slows and strengthens heart action

128. The nurse evaluates Mr. Cox's knowledge of nitroglycerin when he correctly states that a common side effect is:
1. Vertigo
2. Headache
3. Glycosuria
4. Increased blood pressure

John works in a factory using an electric saw. He was not wearing his protective goggles and a small wood-shaving flew into his eye. The company nurse examined his eye and irrigated it, but noted that the shaving was embedded in the sclera. She patches both eyes and has John transported to the local emergency room.

129. The rationale for covering both eyes, when only one has been injured, is that:
1. The patient is more relaxed in complete darkness
2. It is easier to cover both eyes with a wrap encircling the head
3. One-sided vision is blurred
4. The use of one eye causes movement of the other eye

While working in the laboratory, Sue accidentally splashed an irritating chemical into her eye.

130. The first action for chemical splashes to the eye should be *immediate*:

① Rinsing with a small amount of sterile normal saline
② Covering with a sterile patch and rushing the patient to the hospital
③ Copious flushing with water
④ Applying a neutralizing agent to the eye

131. Sue's co-workers assisted her to the emergency room. After assessment and eye irrigation, the doctor prescribed an ophthalmic antibiotic ointment. The nurse explained the reason for the prescription was to:

① Prevent an abscess
② Destroy bacteria in the chemical
③ Prevent scarring to the cornea
④ Prevent chemical conjunctivitis

Mrs. Kelly is at term, comes to the hospital, and tells you that she is having bright red vaginal bleeding and no pain.

132. In performing the initial assessment the nurse would **not**:

① Apply the external fetal monitor
② Monitor uterine contractions
③ Perform a vaginal or rectal examination
④ Perform a routine admission as the patient is not in labor

133. Bright red, painless bleeding is a classical sign of:

① Preeclampsia
② Placenta previa
③ Abruptio placenta
④ Ruptured uterus

134. The physician decides to perform a cesarean section. The anesthesia that would provide the best outcome for the mother and infant is:

① A general
② A local
③ An epidural
④ A pudendal block

135. The baby is delivered with an Apgar score of 8 and 9. Apgar scoring assesses:

① Brain damage and respiratory distress
② Heart rate, reflex irritability, muscle tone, respirations, and color
③ Cyanosis, vision, and hearing
④ Heart rate, blood pressure, respiratory rate, and response to light

136. Following a cesarean section the nurse palpates the fundus and expects to find the fundus:

① Difficult to palpate because of dressings
② Firm and in the midline
③ Soft and immediately above the pubis
④ Firm and displaced to the side of the incision

137. Mrs. Kelly asks if she will be able to breast-feed her infant. Your best response would be:

① "No, because your baby suffered a lot of stress at birth."
② "No, because you will have a lot of pain and require medication."
③ "Yes, as soon as you are able to be up and around."
④ "Yes, and we will help you to be comfortable."

138. On her fourth postpartum day, you enter the room and find Mrs. Kelly crying. An appropriate nursing intervention is:

① Tell her not to worry, everyone gets the "postpartum blues"
② Quietly leave the room without speaking so you will not embarrass her
③ Sit with her and ask if she feels like talking
④ Tell her that if she would like to talk you will come back later when she has everything under control

Your recovery room patient is HIV positive.

139. In keeping with the guidelines set up by the Centers for Disease Control, the nurse caring for postpartum patients should wear:

① Gloves when handling soiled materials
② Gloves and a mask
③ Gloves, mask, and a special gown
④ No special precautions are necessary after delivery

140. A postpartum patient who is HIV positive should:

① Not handle her infant
② Room in if possible
③ Be in complete isolation
④ Wear gloves and a mask when handling her infant

141. The single most important precaution in preventing infection is:

① Wearing gloves at all times
② Wearing a gown and mask
③ Hand-washing
④ Wearing scrub uniforms

142. The nurse caring for the HIV-positive mother understands:

① Breast-feeding is not allowed
② The infant is always infected
③ The mother is an IV drug user
④ The mother should breast-feed and care for her infant as usual

143. Which of the following actions indicates successful postpartum teaching for the HIV-positive mother?

① Patient washes her hands after handling the infant
② Patient wears gloves when holding the infant
③ Patient demonstrates appropriate care and feeding of infant
④ Verbalizes understanding as to why she should not care for the infant

144. The progressive increase in function and the acquisition of new functions *best* describes:

① Maturation
② Development
③ Growth
④ Learning

145. Based on the principles of cephalocaudal development, which of the following would the child gain control of last?

① Neck
② Arms
③ Feet
④ Back

146. The type of play most characteristic of toddlers is:

① Cooperative
② Solitary
③ Competitive
④ Parallel

147. By what age should infants double their birth weight?

① 4 months
② 6 months

③ 8 months
④ 12 months

148. The feeling of guilt that the child "caused" his disability is especially critical in which of the following age groups?

① Toddler
② Preschooler
③ School-age
④ Adolescent

149. At what period do children have the most difficulty coping with death, particularly if it is their own?

① Toddlers
② Preschooler
③ School-age
④ Adolescence

150. Which age group is most likely to personify death as a devil or monster?

① Toddler
② Preschooler
③ School-age
④ Adolescence

151. A social smile can be elicited from most infants by:

① 2 weeks
② 1 month
③ 2 months
④ 4 months

152. According to Erikson, if a mother is inconsistent and careless in the care of her infant, the infant can develop:

① A sense of shame and doubt
② A feeling of inferiority
③ A sense of mistrust
④ Identity confusion

153. The age at which stranger anxiety appears is:

① Birth to 2 months
② 2 to 4 months
③ 6 to 9 months
④ After 12 months

154. According to Erikson, the developmental task of adolescence is the acquisition of a sense of:

① Autonomy
② Industry
③ Initiative
④ Identity

155. Which of the following would be an unusual characteristic in an adolescent?

① Predictability
② Tendency toward idealism
③ Rebellion
④ Moodiness

156. A mother of a 24-month-old child asks the PN to recommend an appropriate toy for her child. Which of the following items would be most appropriate for a child of this age?

① Clay
② Sewing cards
③ Toy soldiers
④ Matching picture games

157. Mrs. Johnson tells the PN that she is upset because her 12-month-old son is not yet walking. Which of the following is the most appropriate reply?

① "Have you talked this over with your pediatrician?"
② "This is normal development for his age."
③ "You should encourage him to walk by holding his hands."
④ "I understand your concern, because most children walk by 12 months of age."

158. At what age level is castration anxiety at its height?

① Toddler
② Preschooler
③ School-age
④ Adolescence

159. Rhymes, riddles, and jokes are most characteristic of:

① Toddlers
② Preschoolers
③ School-agers
④ Adolescents

160. Mrs. Kent tells the PN that her 3 year old refuses to share his toys with other children. On which of the following statements should the PN base her response?

① A toddler of this age is seldom able to share toys
② By this age a child should be able to share his toys
③ A child of age 3 should be firmly encouraged to share
④ Inability to share at this age indicates abnormal egocentric behavior

161. By the age of 8 months, an infant should have mastered the ability to:

① Drink from a cup, independently
② Walk holding on to an adult's hand
③ Feed himself with a spoon
④ Eat finger foods, independently

162. Which of the following is an unexpected finding in a 3-month-old child?

① Smiling in response to the mother's face
② Holding a rattle
③ Holding the head erect
④ Reaching and grabbing objects

163. Which of the following is an expected assessment in a 7-month-old child?

① Walking unassisted
② Creeping up and down several steps
③ Sitting up alone for short periods
④ Beginning to hold the head up

164. Which of the following is expected in a normal 15-month-old child?

① Has an imaginary friend
② Has 20 teeth
③ Dresses without assistance
④ Appears to be bowlegged

165. Which of the following observations indicates that a child is ready for school?

① The demonstrated ability to wait his or her turn
② Dresses self on a consistent basis
③ Is creative in play activities
④ Enjoys educational programs on TV

166. An 11-year-old boy tells the school nurse that he hates being short and that even girls are taller than he. Which of the following responses would be appropriate in this situation?

① "Not everyone gets to be tall."
② "How tall are your parents?"
③ "It's normal for you to want to be tall."
④ "I know it's hard now but in a few years you will experience a growth spurt."

167. Which of the following contributes to egocentrism in early adolescence?

① Preoccupation with bodily development
② Need for peer recognition
③ Desire for independence
④ Increased sexual drive

168. A child's teeth usually emerge at age:

① 4 months
② 6 months
③ 10 months
④ 1 year

169. Which of the following is **not** a risk factor for uterine cancer?

① Postmenopausal bleeding
② History of genital herpes
③ Obesity
④ History of infertility

170. The major diagnostic test to confirm the presence of uterine cancer is a:

① Pap smear
② Colposcopic examination
③ Fractional D&C
④ Ultrasonography

171. The leading cause of death in adults in the United States is:

① Diabetes mellitus
② Cancer
③ Chronic obstructive pulmonary disease (COPD)
④ Cardiovascular disease

172. The physician orders nitroglycerin sublingually to relieve chest pain. When Mr. Jones asks how this drug affects his heart, the nurse tells him that it:

① Relieves the muscle spasms
② Increases the blood flow through the chambers
③ Increases the diameter of the coronary arteries
④ Has a sedative effect that relieves the chest pain

173. Which of the following side effects is common with coronary vasodilators and should be explained to Mr. Jones?

① Loss of appetite
② Increased urine output
③ Headache
④ Increased blood pressure

174. Oxygen is taken to the myocardial cells by the:

① Pulmonary arteries
② Subclavian arteries
③ Aorta
④ Coronary arteries

175. Which of the following is not classified as coronary artery disease (CAD)?

① Congestive heart failure
② Myocardial infarction
③ Coronary occlusion
④ Angina pectoris

176. The nurse explains to Mr. Jones that isoenzyme blood levels are checked to determine:

① If there is myocardial damage
② If he has an arrhythmia
③ The strength of his myocardium
④ If the heart valves are effective

177. Mr. Jones is to have a Holter monitor. He is instructed that he will be required to:

① Wear the monitor 24 hours, keeping a log of activity
② Have special ECG while walking on a treadmill
③ Be on bed rest during this period
④ Not take any medication during this test

178. Mr. Jones is on a 2-g sodium, low fat diet. He should be instructed:

① To use salt substitutes as desired
② That cheese may be substituted freely for meat
③ That canned soups are low in sodium
④ To use alternative condiments for salt

179. Mr. Jones is to have an arteriogram; immediately following this procedure the nurse should assess for bleeding at the insertion site and the:

① Pulses below the dressing
② Urinary output
③ Level of consciousness
④ Ability to move the affected limb

Mr. Bynum is admitted to the health clinic with a diagnosis of peripheral vascular disease.

180. Teaching for Mr. Bynum should include:

① Massaging feet and legs briskly twice a day to promote circulation
② Wearing open-toed sandals only
③ Cutting his nails at least weekly
④ Inspecting feet daily for any injuries

181. Mr. Bynum has intermittent claudication. This is:

① Burning and tingling of the extremities
② Periodic severe pain not associated with activity
③ Cramping pain brought on by exercise and relieved by rest
④ Dull aching calf pain brought on by activity and not relieved by rest

Mr. Burns has a stasis ulcer on his left ankle.

182. This ulcer will probably:

① Heal very slowly with periods of exacerbation
② Require debridement often to promote healing
③ Not heal without surgery such as sympathectomy
④ Heal quickly if protected from injury

183. Thrombophlebitis is most accurately described as:

① Venostasis
② A blood clot occurring in the legs or pelvis
③ Inflammation of a vein associated with clot formation
④ Infection resulting from injury to a superficial blood vessel

184. Assessment of the patient with thrombophlebitis would reveal:

① A positive Homan's sign in the affected leg
② Cold, pale extremities
③ Vasoconstriction of the surrounding veins
④ Cyanosis of the entire affected limb

185. Patients with deep vein thrombosis should be instructed to:

① Elevate legs when sitting
② Check peripheral pulses often
③ Perform Berger-Allen exercises daily
④ Keep knees flexed with a pillow when in bed

186. The most serious complication of deep vein thrombosis is a:

① Stasis ulcer
② Pulmonary embolus
③ Phlebitis
④ Varicose veins

Mrs. Jan Smith has bilateral varicose veins.

187. Which of the following would *not* be discussed with the patient prior to discharge?

① Putting support stockings on before getting out of bed
② Maintaining proper weight
③ Avoiding exercises such as walking or jogging
④ Elevating the foot of the bed for sleeping

188. Mrs. Smith is to have a ligation and stripping of the saphenous vein. An appropriate priority in postoperative nursing care will include:

① Maintaining knee level pressure bandages on both legs
② Assessing for pain related to inadequate circulation
③ Encouraging dangling of legs for 5 to 10 minutes before getting up to ambulate
④ Keeping legs flat and providing sand bags to prevent external rotation

189. Symptoms of carditis include:

① Cardiac murmurs and a pericardial rub
② Bradycardia
③ ECG changes showing ST segment elevation
④ Slow, regular, bounding apical pulse

190. The nurse should observe the patient with pericarditis for signs of:

① Mitral stenosis
② Atelectasis
③ Renal insufficiency
④ Congestive heart failure

George Ellis is admitted to the hospital with a diagnosis of pulmonary tuberculosis (TB).

191. The persons most susceptible to tuberculosis are:

① Middle-aged, white females
② People who work in high pollution conditions
③ Elderly, nonwhite males
④ Obese, multiparous females

192. The most accurate diagnostic test for TB is a:

① MRI
② PPD skin test
③ Chest radiograph
④ Sputum for acid-fast bacillus

193. Mr. Ellis asks how long he will need to continue his antitubercular medicines. He is instructed that treatment is usually:

① 3 months
② 6 months
③ 1 to 2 years
④ 4 to 5 years

194. Mr. Ellis's wife was given a Tine test; she is instructed to return to have it read in:

① 24 hours
② 72 hours
③ 1 week
④ 2 weeks

195. Mrs. Ellis's skin test was positive. This means that she:

① Has inactive TB
② Has active TB
③ Is immune to TB
④ Has antibodies against TB

196. Prophylactic treatment for Mrs. Ellis will probably last for:

① 6 weeks
② 6 months
③ 1 year
④ 2 years

197. Characteristics of mycobacterium tuberculosis is that it:

① Only affects the lungs
② Is an acid-fast bacillus
③ Is an anaerobic organism
④ Multiplies rapidly

Charles Brown, age 55 years, is admitted to the oncology ward. Mr. Brown has a history of weight loss, a persistent cough which has increased, and has had blood-tinged sputum for 2 weeks. He has smoked up to 2 packs of cigarettes for 20 years. He is an accountant and has delayed seeking medical attention until his work load was lighter. His chest radiograph revealed a mass in the right lung. He is being admitted for further evaluation and treatment.

198. An early sign/symptom of lung cancer seen in Mr. Brown's history is:

① Persistent cough
② Hemoptysis
③ Weight loss
④ Dyspnea

199. An MRI is scheduled. You prepare Mr. Brown for this study by telling him that:

① He will have to take laxatives prior to the study
② A dye will be injected into his veins just before the test
③ No physical preparation is needed before the test
④ A nuclear medication is administered by the radiology department 24 hours before the test

200. Mr. Brown is scheduled for a bronchoscopy to biopsy the lesion. Mr. Brown's preoperative teaching will include an explanation that following the biopsy he will:

① Be unable to talk for several days
② Have nothing by mouth until his gag reflex returns
③ Will be unable to swallow for 12 hours
④ Experience no soreness of the throat

201. Which of the following would *not* be a common method of obtaining a specimen to diagnose lung cancer?

① Thoracentesis
② Needle biopsy
③ Mediastinoscopy
④ Wedge resection

202. The risk factor for lung cancer demonstrated by Mr. Brown is:

① A sedentary occupation
② Stress
③ Cigarette smoking
④ Weight loss

203. To assist Mr. Brown and his family to cope with his diagnosis, the nurse should:

① Explain procedures and their purposes before they are carried out
② Tell him the physician will have to tell him about the tests
③ Limit the number of visitors for a few days
④ Provide extensive teaching regarding his illness

204. Following his thoracotomy, the nurse positions the patient:

① Only on the affected side
② On his back or affected side
③ On his back or unaffected side
④ On either side or his back

205. Which of the following surgical procedures would not require the insertion of chest tubes?

① Pneumonectomy
② Lobectomy
③ Wedge resection
④ Open biopsy

206. The main purpose of a chest tube is to:

① Remove drainage from the alveoli
② Remove air and fluid from the pleural space
③ Supply oxygen to the lung
④ Provide an easy access for chemotherapy

207. The PN is caring for a patient with a chest tube connected to a three-bottle drainage system connected to suction. Which of the following observations concerning the drainage system should be reported to the physician immediately?

① Fluctuation of fluid in the water-seal tube during ventilatory movements
② Intermittent bubbling in the water-seal bottle
③ Bubbling in the suction control bottle
④ Continuous bubbling in the water-seal bottle

208. If the chest tube becomes disconnected from the drainage system the nurse should first:

① Reconnect and tape the tube
② Remove the tube and apply a dressing
③ Clamp the tube close to the disconnected area
④ Clamp the tube near the chest wall

Caroline Maynard, a 16-year-old primigravida, is a single high school student. She and her boyfriend have moved into a low-income housing area and subsist on his unemployment benefits. At 24 weeks gestation, she visits the prenatal clinic for the first time. She complains to the nurse that her appetite has been poor for several weeks, but she is discouraged to see that her weight has increased by 3 lb the last week and her rings are even tight on her fingers.

209. The priority nursing intervention for Caroline is assessing:

① Blood pressure
② Fetal heart rate
③ Pedal pulses
④ Nutritional state

210. On examination, Caroline's BP is 120/88. Her lab report reveals albuminuria. The nurse interprets the lab report to mean:

① Normal kidney functioning
② There is excessive pressure on the ureters from an enlarging uterus
③ An increased glomerular filtration rate
④ A kidney malfunction related to her diagnosis

211. The nursing goal in caring for Caroline is Patient will not develop:

① Eclampsia
② Kidney shutdown
③ Epilepsy
④ Chorea gravidarum

212. Caroline returns home with instructions from the nurse. Which of the following would be an *inappropriate* statement for the nurse to make to Caroline?

① "Be sure to eat lots of foods on the high protein diet list."
② "You will likely have a headache, but don't worry, it is expected."
③ "Call the clinic immediately if you begin to see spots before your eyes."
④ "You must remain in bed most of the day resting on your left side."

213. The following week at her next clinic visit, Caroline's blood pressure is 124/90 and she has gained 2½ lb more. The physician admits her to the hospital antepartum unit. Which of the nursing actions should be included on Caroline's care plan?

① Encourage resting on the right side
② Limit fluid intake
③ Encourage low protein, low salt diet
④ Maintain quiet, dark room; limit visitation

214. Caroline's condition improves and she is discharged. At 37 weeks gestation she is admitted to the hospital's labor and delivery suite with rising blood pressure and worsening albuminuria. The physician orders magnesium sulfate by intravenous drip. The practical nurse on duty knows this medication has a:

① Stimulating effect on the central nervous system
② Side effect of hyperreflexia
③ Depressant effect on the central nervous system

④ Stimulating effect on the uterine musculature

215. The practical nurse will assist the labor room RN to monitor Caroline closely. The practical nurse would most likely be asked to:

① Insert a Foley catheter
② Administer IM sedation frequently
③ Ambulate the patient to stimulate labor contractions
④ Maintain the patient in a supine position

216. The practical nurse checks the supply of emergency medications. She is aware that the antidote for magnesium sulfate toxicity is:

① Calcium gluconate
② Calcium chloride
③ Sodium bicarbonate
④ Narcan

217. Caroline eventually delivered a 5-lb, 6-oz female infant in satisfactory condition. After the 1-hour recovery period, it would be most appropriate for the practical nurse to:

① Transfer Caroline to the postpartum unit
② Continue to assist the RN to monitor Caroline's condition
③ Assist Caroline to the bathroom and instruct her in routine peri-care
④ Encourage Caroline's visitors to keep her company at this time

218. Which of the following patients, scheduled for surgery, would be most prone to develop dehydration postoperatively?

① Adolescent patients
② Patients with history of cancer
③ Patients with history of gout
④ Elderly patients

219. Preoperative medications ordered for your patient were Demerol 100 mg and atropine 0.3 mg. Dosages available were Demerol 50 mg/mL and atropine 0.4 mg/mL. You should prepare:

① Demerol 0.75 mL; atropine 1.2 mL
② Demerol 1.5 mL; atropine 0.5 mL
③ Demerol 2 mL; atropine 1 mL
④ Demerol 2 mL; atropine 0.75 mL

220. Atropine is given to the patient preoperatively to:

① Provide general muscle relaxation
② Cause a decrease in pulse and respiration

③ Produce a decrease in oral and respiratory secretions
④ Enhance the effectiveness of Demerol

221. Which of the following interventions is appropriate in the recovery room for the patient who had spinal anesthesia?

① Monitor for the possibility of hypotension
② Maintain semi-Fowler's position
③ Never give medication if the patient is unable to move his/her legs
④ High Fowler's position is best for these clients

222. An early sign/symptom of a transfusion reaction is:

① Hypertension
② Flank pain
③ Cyanosis
④ Bradycardia

223. Which of the following findings would be considered abnormal for the first postoperative day after upper abdominal surgery?

① Nausea
② Pain over the incision site when coughing
③ Drainage on dressing the size of a half dollar
④ Frequently voiding in small amounts

224. Your surgical patient is NPO after midnight the night before surgery. The rationale for this is to prevent:

① Fluid overload postoperatively
② Urinary incontinence during surgery
③ Vomiting and aspiration during surgery
④ Pneumonia postoperatively

225. Which of the following laboratory data would be necessary to report to the surgeon prior to any patient undergoing major surgery?

① Serum potassium of 2.5 mEq/L
② Hematocrit of 42 mL/100 mL
③ Platelet count of 300,000 mm^3
④ Total serum protein of 8 g/100 mL

226. IV fluids are given after major surgery. If the order reads "1000 cc D$_5$/Water to infuse over 8 hours" and the drip factor is 15, the correct rate of the infusion would be:

① 22 gtt/min
② 51 gtt/min
③ 42 gtt/min
④ 31 gtt/min

227. When a patient initially enters the recovery room, the nurse should first:

① Remove the oropharyngeal airway
② Increase the IV fluid rate
③ Assess the level of consciousness and vital signs
④ Assess the wound and any drainage

228. Which of the following positions is most appropriate for a semiconscious patient recovering from anesthesia in the recovery room?

① Supine
② Low Fowler's
③ Semi-Fowler's
④ Lateral Sims

229. Which of the following assessments made by the practical nurse would indicate an oxygenation problem postoperatively?

① Bradycardia
② Incisional pain when coughing
③ A nonproductive cough
④ Restlessness

Mrs. Arnold has surgery for an abdominal perineal resection and a colostomy as a result of rectal cancer.

230. Your immediate postoperative nursing care includes:

① Checking for incisional infection
② Teaching the client colostomy care
③ Placing the permanent colostomy appliance
④ Checking for color, size, and patency of stoma

231. Within the first week after surgery, you would expect Mrs. Arnold to experience:

① A change in body image
② A change in social role
③ Guilt feelings due to cancer
④ Regression

232. A patient with leukopenia is most susceptible to:

① Infection
② Bleeding
③ Hyperuricemia
④ Hypercalcemia

233. Which of the following assessments would be *unlikely* to occur if your patient is hypocalcemic?

① Laryngeal spasms
② Difficulty talking
③ Carpopedal spasms
④ Hyperpnea

234. Local care of irritated skin resulting from radiation treatments should include:

① Applying oil-based cream three times a day
② Washing the area with water only
③ Exposing the area to sunlight at least 1 hour/day
④ Keeping the area covered with a clean dry dressing

235. The PN is caring for a patient receiving radiation therapy. Which of the following should be reported immediately to the physician?

① Platelet count of 50,000
② Increasing fatigue
③ Nausea and vomiting
④ WBC count of 2000

236. Which of the following would predispose a person to immunosuppression?

① Diabetes mellitus
② Obesity
③ Hormone imbalances
④ Maladaptive behavior

237. An optimal preventive measure against acquired immunodeficiency syndrome is:

① Protective isolation
② Meticulous skin care
③ Respiratory isolation
④ Blood and body fluid precaution

238. Which of the following would *not* be a characteristic of a phobia?

① Anxiety attributed to an external source
② Displacement keeps the source of anxiety out of the consciousness
③ Can be helped by insight-oriented therapy
④ Secondary gains may be very important to patient

239. Mr. Applegate is afraid of heights. A term used to describe this type of phobia is:

① Agoraphobia
② Acrophobia
③ Claustrophobia
④ Xenophobia

240. Which of the following nursing interventions would be useful in helping a patient overcome a phobia?

① Place patient in phobic situations to desensitize the patient

② Point out adaptive coping mechanisms and reinforce them

③ Help patient avoid anxiety-producing situations

④ Never administer tranquilizers

Answers & Rationales

Guide to item identifications (see pp. 3–5 for further details about each category)

I, II, III, or IV for the phase of the nursing process
1, 2, 3, or 4 for the category of client needs
A, B, C, D, E, F, or G for the category of human functioning
Specific content category by name; ie, cholecystectomy

121. ③ The cause of angina is myocardial ischemia. When there is not enough oxygen going to these tissues, pain results.
IV, 2, B. Angina.

122. ② The pain of angina takes on the characteristic of being severe and substernal. It typically radiates to the left arm and possibly the neck. Crushing pain is more characteristic of an MI.
III & IV, 2, B. Angina.

123. ④ Cold is one of the common precipitating factors for angina. The tennis should not cause pain, because it is an exercise he is used to. As his disease progresses, he may find that tennis also precipitates it.
I, 2, B. Angina.

124. ③ The exercise stress test is designed to trigger the angina if it is present. None of the other tests would provide any information about the heart and its circulation.
IV, 2, B. Angina.

125. ① All of the drugs are vasodilators, but only the nitroglycerin acts on coronary arteries immediately. Isordil and Persantin may be used for prophylactic or long-term use. Vasodilan is more for peripheral vasodilation.
III, 2, B. Angina.

126. ④ If he is of normal weight, the only restriction he needs to follow is to keep his cholesterol level low.
III, 4, B. Angina.

127. ② Nitroglycerin is the fastest drug for dilating coronary arteries. Given sublingually or IV it works immediately.
III, 2, B. Angina/Medication.

128. ② As a vasodilator, nitroglycerin also dilates cerebral vessels causing a headache. This is a common side effect of the drug. If dizziness occurs at all, it is secondary to the drop in blood pressure.
IV, 2, B. Angina/Medication.

129. ④ Eye movement may cause increased pain and may further the damage by embedding the foreign body more deeply. Eye muscles work in coordination; therefore, movement of one eye causes movement of the other. #1 is incorrect as it probably increases anxiety; #2 and #3 are not appropriate rationale; safety for the patient is the primary concern.
II, 1 & 2, C & D. Trauma/Foreign Body.

130. ③ Irritating substances should immediately be diluted and rinsed out of the eye with large amounts of solution to minimize damage to the eye. Because water is usually readily available, it should be used rather than wasting valuable minutes searching for a sterile solution while allowing the chemical to further the damage to the eye. #1, #2, & #4 all allow further damage to the eye.
III, 1 & 2, C & D. Trauma/Conjunctivitis.

131. ④ Irritation and inflammation from chemicals and other substances predispose the eye to bacterial invasion; therefore, antibiotics are used prophylactically. The situation gives no indication for #1 or #2. An antibiotic ointment cannot prevent scarring.
II & III, 1 & 2, C & D. Trauma/Conjunctivitis.

132. ③ The mother should **never** be examined, either vaginally or rectally, when she is bleeding. Either rectal or vaginal examinations may worsen the bleeding.
I, 4, A & B. Labor and Delivery.

133. ② Placenta previa refers to a placenta that is implanted either partially or completely over the cervical os. As the cervix begins to dilate, the placenta pulls away and bleeding occurs. Placenta abruptio refers to premature separation of the placenta from the uterine wall which can cause pain as well as bleeding.
I, 4, A & B. Labor and Delivery.

134. ③ Spinal anesthesia is considered safer to both mother and infant than general anesthesia. It offers the advantage that the mother may see the infant at birth. A pudendal block and local anesthesia are used to simply anesthetize the perineum mainly for the episiotomy.
IV, 4, A & D. Labor and Delivery.

135. Apgar scoring is a method to evaluate the neonate's physical status at birth. A score of 7 to 10 at 1 and 5 minutes is considered to indicate a vigorous neonate.
② I, 1 and 4, B. The Neonate.

136. The fundus should be assessed gently and with care after a cesarean section. It should be firm and in the midline as with any normal delivery.
② III, 4, A & D. Postpartum.

137. A cesarean section is not a contraindication for breast-feeding. Assistance from the staff is necessary to maintain comfort and to provide comfort for the postoperative patient.
④ III, 4, A. Postpartum.

138. Postpartum "blues" is a transitory, mild depression that occurs frequently after childbirth. Many times, the mother does not even know why she is having these feelings. Sitting down with her implies interest and caring.
III, 3 and 4, A & G. Postpartum.

139. Mask and gown are only necessary if there is a possibility of splash or droplet exposure. Gloves should be worn when handling any material exposed to blood or other body fluids.
① III, 4, D. Postpartum.

140. The HIV-positive mother may need additional support in caring for her infant and in establishing bonding with the newborn. Rooming-in is not contraindicated for the mother or newborn.
② III, 4, D & G. Postpartum.

141. Hand-washing is absolutely mandatory before and after all procedures with *all* patients. It is the most basic and important action in infection control.
③ III, 4, D. Postpartum.

142. The HIV virus has been isolated in breast milk and breast-feeding is discouraged. Approximately 40% of the infants born to HIV-positive mothers test seropositive themselves. If the newborn is negative, breast-feeding could pass the virus to it.
① III, 4, D. Postpartum.

143. The mother should care for the infant using appropriate techniques. It is not necessary to
③

wear gloves for contact with unsoiled articles or intact skin.
III, 4, D. Postpartum.

144. Maturation (#1) refers to maturing and #3, Growth, refers to increase in size. Assessment of development should be a part of the admission process, which aids in all steps of the nursing process.
② I, 4, A. Growth and Development.

145. The term cephalocaudal refers to head to tail or top to bottom. This knowledge should be used in assessment and in planning for patient safety.
③ I, 2 & 4, A. Growth and Development.

146. Toddlers are not cooperative or competitive in their play. While they play alone for short periods, the type of play that is most characteristic of this age group is #2.
④ I, 4, A. Growth and Development.

147. The only correct answer is #2. This information is important for the PN to know as a first step in nursing assessment of the infant.
② I, 4, A. Growth and Development.

148. It is typical for preschoolers to view hospitalization as punishment for real or imagined misdeeds. The response to such thinking is frequently a feeling of guilt.
② IV, 4, A & G. Growth and Development.

149. Adolescents have the most difficulty in coping with death, especially their own. Their concern is the present. They frequently feel alone.
④ I, 4, A & G. Growth and Development.

150. Due to an increased ability to comprehend, school-age children experience fear in regards to death and dying. They frequently personify death as a devil, monster, or a bogey man.
③ IV, 4, A & G. Growth and Development.

151. At 2 months, the infant develops a social smile in response to various stimuli. Infants prefer people to objects.
③ I, 4, A. Growth and Development.

152. Erikson's first phase, from birth to one year, involves acquiring a basic sense of trust while overcoming a sense of mistrust. The crucial element of trust development is the consistent quality of care given to the infant by the
③

mother. If this child/mother trust does not develop, mistrust is the outcome.
IV, 4, A & G. Growth and Development.

153. ③ Stranger anxiety, where the infant begins to fear strangers, appears between the age of 6 and 9 months. The friendly infant begins to cling to mother and become fretful when he can not see his mother. The PN should assure parents that this is normal.
I, 4, A. Growth and Development.

154. ④ Erikson's theory holds that the developmental crisis of adolescence leads to the formation of a sense of identity. The adolescent first identifies with a group and then develops a sense of personal identity.
l, 4, A. Growth and Development.

155. ① Adolescence is generally a time of turmoil. They demonstrate turbulent, rebellious, and unpredictable behavior. They experience frequent mood swings. They are idealistic and rather judgmental.
I, 4, A. Growth and Development.

156. ① A 24-month-old child can manipulate clay. The other toys are more appropriate for the preschool child who has more developed motor skills and the ability for more imaginative play.
I, 4, A. Growth and Development.

157. ② 90% of all children will be able to walk well by 14 months. Because the age varies for onset of walking, this age may be a more useful guideline for assessment of gross motor skills development.
III, 4, A. Growth and Development.

158. ② Castration anxiety is at its height during the preschool years. The concept of body integrity is poorly developed. Concerns of mutilation are paramount at this age.
I, 4, A. Growth and Development.

159. ③ School-age children enjoy sharing secrets and private jokes with same-sex peers. They like to solve riddles and make rhymes. Their increasing intellectual skills allow for this type of activity.
IV, 4, A. Growth and Development.

160. ① Before age 4 to 5 years, a child is seldom able to share toys. Parents should not force a toddler to share.
II, 4, A. Growth and Development.

161. ④ By 8 months, an infant has developed the ability to use his index finger and thumb as a pincer. This facilitates finger feeding. The other skills will develop at a later stage.
I, 4, A. Growth and Development.

162. ④ It is unexpected for a 3-month-old child to reach and grab objects. All other findings are within normal limits.
I, 4, A. Growth and Development.

163. ③ A 7-month-old child should be sitting up alone.
I, 4, A. Growth and Development.

164. ④ Young toddlers appear bowlegged. This sometimes causes parental concern. The PN should assure them that this a normal finding in this age group.
I, 4, A. Growth and Development.

165. ① The only option that indicates a readiness for school is #1. A child must have the ability to wait his or her turn if the child is to be successful in school.
II, 4, A. Growth and Development.

166. ④ Female growth spurts usually precede male growth spurts by about 2 years. This sometimes creates social problems for both sexes.
II, 4, A. Growth and Development.

167. ① Physical changes during early and middle adolescence causes the young person to focus on his or her bodily development. This contributes to egocentrism or self-centeredness.
I, 4, A. Growth and Development.

168. ② Teething begins at about 6 months with eruption of two lower central incisors.
I, 4, A. Growth and Development.

169. ② History of genital herpes is a risk factor for cervical cancer. The other options are all risk factors for uterine cancer.
III, 1, A & D. Uterine Cancer.

170. ③ Uterine cancer can only be diagnosed through obtaining endometrial tissue. A fractional D&C provides this tissue. A Pap smear is positive only about 50% of the time in the presence of uterine cancer. A colposcopic examination is done to locate cervical lesions. Ultasonography may be used in assessing for ovarian cancer.
III, 2, A & D. Uterine Cancer.

171.
④ Heart disease is the leading cause of death in adults in the United States. Cancer is the second leading cause of death among adults in this country.
I, 4, B. Heart Disease.

172.
③ Nitroglycerin dilates coronary arteries causing increased blood flow to the coronary muscle.
I, 1, B. CAD.

173.
③ Coronary vasodilators also dilate other arteries causing side effects, such as headache, orthostatic hypotension, and fainting.
III, 2, B. CAD.

174.
④ The coronary arteries provide blood to the myocardium. If these arteries are occluded, then the patient may suffer a heart attack.
I, 2, B. CAD.

175.
① Coronary artery disease includes any disease that affects the blood supply to the myocardium.
I, 1, B. CAD.

176.
① When the muscle of the myocardium infarcts, isoenzymes are released. These can be measured and they give an indication of how much damage has been done to the myocardium.
III, 2, B. CAD.

177.
① The Holter monitor is a type of continuous ECG worn during normal activity so that any changes can be observed. The patient is asked to keep a log during this time so that if any changes are noted on the ECG, the activity that caused them can be identified.
III, 1, B. CAD.

178.
④ Salt substitutes may be high in potassium and are not necessary on a 2-g restriction. Substituting condiments such as lemon juice can provide the seasoning usually provided by salt.
III, 4, B & F. CAD.

179.
① It is important to assess for both bleeding and thrombus formation after an arteriogram. The pulses below the site should be taken before the arteriogram so that baseline can be established. Any changes should be reported to the physician immediately.
III, 1, B. CAD.

180.
④ It is important to not only protect the feet, but to inspect them closely at regular intervals for injury. It is important to catch injuries early while treatment is more likely to be effective.
III, 1, B. PVD.

181.
③ Intermittent claudication is defined as the pain caused by ischemia during exercise. When the pain occurs without activity, it is termed as "rest pain."
IV, 1, B. PVD.

182.
① Stasis ulcers are venous ulcers and heal very slowly because of the venous congestion associated with the vascular disease. The surgery that might be done to treat vascular ulcers is a skin graft to cover the ulcer once it is clean.
IV, 1, B. PVD.

183.
③ Thrombophlebitis is an inflammation of the vein associated with a blood clot within the vein. A thrombus is simply a clot and phlebitis is inflammation of a vessel.
IV, 1, B. PVD.

184.
① Homan's sign is diagnostic of thrombophlebitis in the calf. When the calf muscle is contracted with a clot in the vessel, sharp pain is felt in the calf. The other symptoms might be associated with an arterial occlusion.
I, 1, B. PVD.

185.
① Elevating the leg with a clot is important to improve venous return. Peripheral pulses are checked with arterial disease and the Berger-Allen exercises improve arterial flow. A pillow should never be used behind the knee in any patient.
III, 1, B. PVD.

186.
② If a thrombosis becomes dislodged, it becomes an embolus. Clots dislodged from the lower extremities travel to the lungs becoming pulmonary emboli. This is a life-threatening complication of thrombophlebitis.
II & IV, 1, B. PVD.

187.
③ Walking and exercise are important to exercise the muscles and to help venous return which is slowed from the incompetent veins. The other options are appropriate to treat varicose veins.
III, 1, B. PVD.

188.
② Excessive swelling postoperatively would be demonstrated by pain under the Ace wraps

that are put on the legs after the stripping. Swelling may indicate bleeding postoperatively. The legs are elevated and never dangled.
III, 1, B. PVD.

189. ① Carditis is an inflammation of the pericardium causing rubbing within the pericardium.
I, 2, B. Inflammation.

190. ④ Pericarditis can cause damage of the heart muscle leading to congestive heart failure.
IV, 2, B. Inflammation.

191. ③ TB is increasing in poor, elderly, and non-whites, especially Native Americans. The lower a person's resistance, the more malnutrition present, and the lower their immunity, the more likely they are to develop TB.
IV, 1, B. TB.

192. ④ The tuberculin bacillus is an acid-fast bacillus. Obtaining a culture of this bacillus is diagnostic of TB. The skin test tells you only that the patient has been exposed to TB and has formed antibodies. The chest radiograph cannot differentiate between active or encapsulated TB.
IV, 1, B. TB.

193. ③ The tuberculin bacillus is very difficult to control. Treatment can never cure or eradicate the bacillus. The bacteria become encapsulated only after 1 to 2 years of treatment with the antibiotics.
III & IV, 1, B. TB.

194. ② A tuberculin skin test is simply an antigen–antibody response. It takes about 72 hours for the full reaction to be seen.
III & IV, 1, B. TB.

195. ④ A positive skin test indicates only the person has antibodies against TB. It does not mean the person has active or inactive TB.
IV, 2, B. TB.

196. ③ Prophylactic treatment for a person who has been exposed to TB but has not developed it lasts at least 1 year.
III & IV, 1, B. TB.

197. ② Tuberculosis is an acid-fast bacillus. It can affect almost any organ such as the kidneys.
I, 2, B. TB.

198. ① Unfortunately, the only early symptom of lung cancer is a persistent cough. Many smokers, the largest group of people developing lung cancer, have a chronic cough anyway. Many do not notice the cough until they begin to cough up blood.
I, 2, B & D. Lung Cancer.

199. ③ An MRI does not require any preparation. The MRI is not a radiographic examine, but instead uses magnetically stimulated images.
III, 2, B & D. Lung Cancer.

200. ② When a patient has a bronchoscopy, local anesthesia is used in the back of the throat to deaden the gag reflex. Nothing can be taken by mouth until the gag reflex returns so that the patient will not choke. It usually takes several hours for this reflex to return.
III, 1, B & D. Bronchoscopy/Lung Cancer.

201. ④ Specimens can be obtained without the surgery. Chest tubes are required if a wedge resection is done. This procedure would be performed if a small tumor had already been diagnosed and needed to be resected.
IV, 2, B & D. Lung Cancer.

202. ③ The highest risk factor for lung cancer is cigarette smoking. It is also the most modifiable cause of disease.
I, 2, B & D. Lung Cancer.

203. ① It is important for the patient and family to be well informed of tests and procedures to be done. Fear of the unknown is one of the most anxiety-producing problems for the ill patient. Visitors can provide a great deal of support to the patient. The patient should not be bombarded with a great deal of information at this time.
III, 3, B & D & G. Lung Cancer.

204. ③ After a thoracotomy, it is important for the patient to be positioned so that the affected lung can best re-expand. Lying on the affected side could slow or interfere with this re-expansion.
III, 1, B & D. Lung Cancer.

205. ① Chest tubes are inserted to re-expand the lung. A pneumonectomy means that the entire lung is removed so there is nothing to be re-expanded. The other procedure would require chest tubes for re-expansion.
IV, 2, B. Lung Cancer.

206. The chest tube drains fluid and removes air
② from the pleural space after the integrity of
this space has been violated. It could be used
for access of chemotherapy, but this is a minor
use.
IV, 2, B. Lung Cancer.

207. Continuous bubbling during ventilation indi-
④ cates that air is leaking into the drainage system or pleural cavity. The other observations
are normal with the three-bottle system.
III, 1, B & D. Lung Cancer.

208. The tube is clamped if it becomes dislodged
④ since if it is left open to the air, the lung will
collapse. It should be clamped close to the
chest wall so that no further leakage can occur. The tubing should then be repaired and
reattached properly to water-seal drainage so
that it can be unclamped as soon as possible.
III, 1, B. Lung Cancer.

209. Symptoms of pregnancy induced hyperten-
① sion are increased weight gain and fluid retention with edema.
I, 2, B. Complications of Pregnancy/PIH.

210. Albumin in the urine indicates kidney mal-
④ function related to pregnancy induced hypertension. Increased glomerular filtration rate is
normal for pregnancy. Pressure on the ureters
should not cause this symptom.
I, 2, B. Complications of Pregnancy/PIH.

211. Eclampsia is the worst stage of pregnancy in-
① duced hypertension.
II, 2, B. Complications of Pregnancy/PIH.

212. Headache is indicative of increasing blood
② pressure. Other instructions are appropriate.
III, 2, B. Complications of Pregnancy/PIH.

213. The patient should rest in a quiet environ-
④ ment. Lying on the left side promotes maximum blood flow to vital organs. Fluid intake
should be increased. Protein intake should be
adequate.
II & III, 2, B. Complications of Pregnancy/
PIH.

214. Magnesium sulfate has a CNS depressant af-
③ fect, and a depressant affect on reflexes and
uterine contractions.
I, 2, B & C. Medication/PIH.

215. A catheter will be used to monitor urine out-
① put. The patient will likely not be given heavy

sedation, but will remain on bed rest on the
left side.
III, 2, B. PIH.

216. Calcium gluconate is the antidote for
① magesium sulfate.
II, 2, B & C. Medications/PIH.

217. Patients on magnesium sulfate stay on bed
② rest under close observation in the labor suite
with minimal disturbance until their condition stabilizes.
III, 2, B & C. Complications of Labor and Delivery.

218. The elderly are often dehydrated preopera-
④ tively and have difficulty maintaining homeostasis. None of the other patients are at particular risk.
I, 1, B & D. Surgical Intervention.

219. Demerol 50 mg/1 mL = 100 mg/X mL,
④ 50X = 100, X = 2. Atropine 0.4 mg/1
mL = 0.3 mg/X ml, 0.4X = 0.3, X = 0.75.
III, 2, D. Medication Administration.

220. Atropine acts to reduce tracheobronchial se-
③ cretions and dries the mucous membranes. It
increases the pulse, is not a muscle relaxant
and does not affect Demerol.
IV, 2, B & D. Medications.

221. Hypotension is the major complication of
① spinal anesthesia since it causes peripheral
vasodilation. None of the other answers is
correct.
III, 1, B & D. Surgical Intervention.

222. A early clinical manifestation of a transfusion
② reaction is flank pain and low back pain because of the renal involvement.
I, 1 and 2, D & F. Surgical Intervention.

223. Frequent voiding of small amounts of urine
④ could be a sign of bladder distention. Nausea
can occur after surgery but should be reported
if it persists. Pain at the incision site and
drainage are to be expected.
IV, 1, D & F. Surgical Intervention.

224. Keeping the patient NPO prevents aspiration
③ of gastric contents during or after the surgery.
IV, 1, D & F. Surgical Intervention.

225. The normal serum potassium is 3.5–
① 5.0 mEq/L. A low level can lead to cardiac

abnormalities and death. The other values are within normal limits.
III and IV, 1 and 2, B & D. Surgical Intervention.

226. ④ 1000/480 × 15 = gtt/min,   100/48 × 15 = 1500/48 = 31 gtt/min.
III, 2, D. Medication Administration.

227. ③ In the immediate postoperative period, the priority is to assess for respiratory distress. Always compare your assessments with the patient's preoperative normals.
III, 1 & 2, B & D. Surgical Intervention.

228. ④ The best position for a patient recovering from the effects of general anesthesia is the lateral Sims' position with the head to the side and the chin extended forward to prevent airway obstruction.
III, 1, B & D. Surgical Intervention.

229. ④ Restlessness is the earliest sign of cerebral anoxia.
I, 1 and 2, C & D. Surgical Intervention.

230. ④ Immediate postoperative care of the colostomy patient must include close observation of the stoma for possible circulatory impairment. This is the most significant observation.
I, 2, B & F. Colostomies.

231. ① Change in body image is a reality within the first week after a colostomy is performed. Change in social role and regression are not expected, and guilt feelings about cancer are only a conjecture.
I, 3, F & G. Colostomies.

232. ① Patients with leukopenia are most susceptible to infections. Bleeding may occur due to thrombocytopenia or due to chemical toxicity on fragile blood vessels, whereas hyperuricemia may occur due to massive cell destruction due to cancer or due to effects of chemotherapeutic drugs or radiation therapy. Hypercalcemia may result from cancer, not leukopenia.
IV, 1 & 2, A. Chemotherapy.

233. ④ Hypocalcemic tetany is manifested by laryngeal spasms, difficulty talking, and carpopedal spasms.
I, 2, A & F. Chemotherapy.

234. ② Irradiated skin is fragile and susceptible to injury. Protection from the sun and other irritants is necessary. Care of the skin includes washing gently with warm water, patting gently dry and using lanolin or A&D ointment to dry areas with physician's orders. A dressing is not necessary.
III, 1, A & C. Radiation Therapy.

235. ① A platelet count of less than 100,000 should be reported, because bleeding can result. Nausea, vomiting, and fatigue do occur with radiation therapy. WBC counts less than 1,000 should be reported.
III, 1, F & H. Radiation Therapy.

236. ① Immunosuppression may be linked to diabetes mellitus but not to obesity, maladaptive behaviors, or hormone imbalances.
I, 1, A & G. Immune Suppression.

237. ④ Preventing direct contact with body fluids and secretions is the best safeguard against acquired immune deficiency syndrome. The other options are required for other infectious conditions.
III, 1 & 2, D. AIDS.

238. ③ A phobia cannot be treated by insight-oriented therapy. Desensitization is the most common form of therapy. The others are common characteristics associated with phobias.
I, 3, G. Phobias.

239. ② Xenophobia is fear of strangers, agoraphobia fear of outdoors, acrophobia fear of heights, and claustrophobia is fear of close spaces.
I, 3, G. Phobias.

240. ② When attempting to help the patient overcome a phobia, the nurse should help the patient recognize and strengthen any adaptive coping mechanisms the patient develops. The patient cannot be placed directly into situations that confront the phobia but they must be helped to gradually face anxiety-producing situations. Tranquilizers are commonly used to help control the anxiety the patient is feeling.
III, 3, G. Phobias.

Analysis of Questions in Practice
Tests III and IV

PHASES OF THE NURSING PROCESS

Assessment

2, 7, 8, 13, 17, 21,
23, 24, 25, 27, 30,
34, 35, 36, 37, 40,
41, 49, 51, 59, 71,
75, 76, 77, 78, 82,
83, 84, 86, 90, 93,
95, 96, 101, 102,
104, 107, 108, 110,
111, 114, 115, 116,
118, 123, 132, 133,
135, 144, 145, 146,
147, 149, 151, 153,
154, 155, 156, 157,
158, 161, 162, 163,
164, 167, 168, 171,
172, 174, 175, 184,
189, 197, 198, 202,
209, 210, 214, 218,
222, 229, 230, 231,
233, 236, 238, 239.

Planning

5, 19, 22, 28, 31,
42, 52, 54, 60, 61,
62, 70, 73, 79, 88,
94, 97, 113, 129,
131, 160, 165, 166,
186, 213, 216.

Implementation

1, 3, 4, 6, 9, 10, 11,
14, 15, 16, 18, 20,
26, 29, 33, 38, 39,
43, 44, 46, 47, 48,
50, 53, 56, 57, 58,
63, 64, 65, 66, 67,
68, 69, 72, 74, 81,
85, 87, 91, 92, 98,
99, 103, 105, 106,
109, 112, 119, 120,
122, 125, 126, 127,
130, 131, 136, 137,
138, 139, 140, 141,
142, 143, 169, 170,
173, 176, 177, 178,
179, 180, 185, 187,
188, 193, 194, 196,
199, 200, 203, 204,
207, 208, 212, 213,
215, 217, 219, 221,
225, 226, 227, 228,
234, 235, 237, 240.

Evaluation

12, 14, 15, 16, 17,
19, 32, 45, 55, 80,
89, 100, 117, 121,
122, 124, 128, 134,
148, 150, 152, 159,
181, 182, 183, 186,
190, 191, 192, 193,
194, 195, 196, 201,
205, 206, 220, 223,
224, 225, 232.

CATEGORIES OF CLIENT NEEDS

Safe, Effective Care Environment

1, 3, 4, 6, 20, 21,
22, 36, 37, 38, 42,
43, 44, 45, 46, 47,
48, 49, 53, 54, 60,
66, 70, 71, 73, 79,
85, 91, 92, 98, 99,
101, 103, 105, 107,
108, 109, 112, 129,
130, 131, 135, 169,
172, 175, 177, 179,
180, 181, 182, 183,
184, 185, 186, 187,
188, 191, 192, 193,
194, 196, 200, 204,
207, 208, 218, 221,
222, 223, 224, 225,
227, 228, 229, 232,
234, 235, 236, 237.

Physiologic Integrity

2, 5, 7, 8, 9, 10, 11,
12, 13, 14, 15, 16,
17, 18, 21, 22, 23,
24, 25, 26, 27, 28,
29, 35, 51, 52, 55,
57, 58, 59, 64, 65,
68, 69, 72, 76, 77,
82, 84, 87, 93, 94,
95, 97, 100, 104,
106, 111, 121, 122,
123, 124, 125, 127,
128, 129, 130, 131,
145, 170, 173, 174,
176, 189, 190, 195,
197, 198, 199, 201,
202, 205, 206, 209,
210, 211, 212, 213,
214, 215, 216, 217,
219, 220, 222, 225,
226, 227, 229, 230,
232, 233, 237.

Psychosocial Integrity

19, 59, 61, 62, 63,
67, 74, 75, 80, 83,
90, 103, 113, 117,
118, 119, 120, 138,
203, 231, 238, 239,
240.

Health Promotion and Maintenance

30, 31, 32, 33, 34,
39, 40, 41, 50, 56,
69, 78, 81, 86, 88,
89, 96, 110, 114,
115, 116, 126, 132,
133, 134, 135, 136,
137, 138, 139, 140,
141, 142, 143, 144,
145, 146, 147, 148,
149, 150, 151, 152,
153, 154, 155, 156,
157, 158, 159, 160,
161, 162, 163, 164,
165, 166, 167, 168,
171, 178.

Appendix I

Administration of Examination Committee
Testing Dates

NCLEX for *Practical Nurse* Licensure
1992: April 15 and October 21
1993: April 14 and October 13
1994: April 13 and October 12
1995: April 12 and October 24
1996: April 17 and October 16
1997: April 16 and October 9

Appendix II

State and Territorial Boards of Nursing and Practical Nursing

NATIONAL COUNCIL OF STATE BOARDS OF NURSING, INC.

ALABAMA
Executive Director
Alabama Board of Nursing
RSA Plaza, Suite 250
770 Washington Avenue
Montgomery, Alabama 36130
Tel: (205) 242-4060

ALASKA
Executive Secretary
Alaska Board of Nursing
Department of Commerce and Economic
Development
Div. of Occupational Licensing
3601 C Street, Suite 722
Anchorage, Alaska 99503
Tel: (907) 561-2878

AMERICAN SAMOA
Executive Secretary
American Samoa Health Service Regulatory Board
LBJ Tropical Medical Center
Pago Pago, American Samoa 96799
Tel: (684) 633-1222, ext. 206
Telex No.: #782-573-LBJ TMC

ARIZONA
Executive Director
Arizona State Board of Nursing
2001 W. Camelback Road, Suite 350
Phoenix, Arizona 85015
Tel: (602) 255-5092

ARKANSAS
Executive Director
Arkansas State Board of Nursing
1123 South University
Little Rock, Arkansas 72204
Tel: (501) 371-2751

CALIFORNIA
Executive Officer
California Board of Vocational Nurse and
Psychiatric Technician Examiners
1414 K Street, Suite 103
Sacramento, California 95814
Tel: (916) 445-0793

COLORADO
Program Administrator
Colorado Board of Nursing
1560 Broadway, Suite 670
Denver, Colorado 80202
Tel: (303) 894-2430

CONNECTICUT
Executive Officer
Connecticut Board of Examiners for Nursing
150 Washington Street
Hartford, Connecticut 06106
Tel: (203) 566-1041

DELAWARE
Executive Director
Delaware Board of Nursing
Margaret O'Neill Building
P.O. Box 1401
Dover, Delaware 19903
Tel: (302) 739-4522

DISTRICT OF COLUMBIA
District of Columbia Board of Nursing
614 H Street, N.W.
Washington, D.C. 20001
Tel: (202) 727-7468

FLORIDA
Executive Director
Florida Board of Nursing
111 Coastline Drive, East, Suite 516
Jacksonville, Florida 32202
Tel: (904) 359-6331

For Exam Information:
Florida Department of Professional Regulation
1940 N. Monroe Street
Tallahassee, Florida 32399-0750

GEORGIA
Executive Director
Georgia Board of Nursing
166 Pryor Street, S.W.
Atlanta, Georgia 30303
Tel: (404) 656-3943

Executive Director
Georgia State Board of Licensed Practical Nurses
166 Pryor Street, S.W.
Atlanta, Georgia 30303
Tel: (404) 656-3921

GUAM
Nurse Examiner Administrator
Guam Board of Nurse Examiners
P.O. Box 2816
Agana, Guam 96910
Tel: (671) 734-7304

HAWAII
Executive Secretary
Hawaii Board of Nursing
P.O. Box 3469
Honolulu, Hawaii 96801
Tel: (808) 586-2695

IDAHO
Executive Director
Idaho Board of Nursing
280 North 8th Street
Suite 210
Boise, Idaho 83720
Tel: (208) 334-3110

ILLINOIS
Nursing Education Coordinator
Illinois Department of Professional Regulation
320 West Washington Street
3rd Floor
Springfield, Illinois 62786
Tel: (217) 782-0800
    (217) 782-0458 (Application requests)

INDIANA
Executive Director
Indiana State Board of Nursing
Health Professions Bureau
402 West Washington Street
Room #041
Suite 1020, Box 82067
Indianapolis, Indiana 46282-0004
Tel: (317) 232-2960

IOWA
Executive Director
Iowa Board of Nursing
Executive Hills East
1223 East Court Avenue
Des Moines, Iowa 50319
Tel: (515) 281-3256

KANSAS
Executive Administrator
Kansas Board of Nursing
Landon State Office Building
900 SW Jackson, Suite 551 S
Topeka, Kansas 66612-4929
Tel: (913) 296-4929
    (913) 296-4068

KENTUCKY
Executive Director
Kentucky Board of Nursing
4010 Dupont Circle, Suite 430
Louisville, Kentucky 40207
Tel: (502) 897-5143

LOUISIANA
Executive Director
Louisiana State Board of Practical Nurse Examiners
Tidewater Place
1440 Canal Street, Suite 2010
New Orleans, Louisiana 70112
Tel: (504) 568-6480

Executive Director
Louisiana State Board of Nursing
907 Pere Marquette Building
150 Baronne Street
New Orleans, Louisiana 70112
Tel: (504) 568-5464

MAINE
Executive Director
Maine State Board of Nursing
State House Station #158
Augusta, Maine 04333-0158
Tel: (207) 289-5324

MARYLAND
Executive Director
Maryland Board of Examiners of Nurses
4201 Patterson Ave.
Baltimore, Maryland 21215
Tel: (301) 764-4741

MASSACHUSETTS
Executive Secretary
Massachusetts Board of Registration in Nursing
Leverett Saltonstall Building

100 Cambridge Street
Room 1519
Boston, Massachusetts 02202
Tel: (617) 727-7393
    (617) 727-9962

MICHIGAN
Licensing Administrator
Michigan Board of Nursing
Dept. of Licensing & Regulation
Ottawa Towers North
611 West Ottawa
P.O. Box 30018
Lansing, Michigan 48909
Tel: (517) 373-1600

MINNESOTA
Executive Director
Minnesota Board of Nursing
2700 University Ave. West, #108
St. Paul, Minnesota 55114
Tel: (612) 642-0567

MISSISSIPPI
Executive Director
Mississippi Board of Nursing
239 N. Lamar Street, Suite 401
Jackson, Mississippi 39206-1311
Tel: (601) 359-6170

MISSOURI
Executive Director
Missouri State Board of Nursing
P.O. Box 656
3524A North Ten Mile Drive
Jefferson City, Missouri 65102
Tel: (314) 751-0681

MONTANA
Executive Secretary
Montana State Board of Nursing
Department of Commerce
Division of Business and Professional Licensing
111 N. Jackson
Lower Level, Arcade Building
Helena, Montana 59620-0407
Tel: (406) 444-4279

NEBRASKA
Associate Director
Bureau of Examining Boards
Nebraska Department of Health
P.O. Box 95007
Lincoln, Nebraska 68509
Tel: (402) 471-2115

NEVADA
Executive Director
Nevada State Board of Nursing
1281 Terminal Way, Suite 116
Reno, Nevada 89502
Tel: (702) 786-2778

NEW HAMPSHIRE
Executive Director
New Hampshire Board of Nursing
Health & Welfare Building
6 Hazen Drive
Concord, New Hampshire 03301
Tel: (693) 271-2323

NEW JERSEY
Executive Director
New Jersey Board of Nursing
1100 Raymond Blvd., Room 508
Newark, New Jersey 07102
Tel: (201) 648-2570

NEW MEXICO
Executive Director
New Mexico Board of Nursing
4253 Montgomery Blvd., Suite 130
Albuquerque, New Mexico 87109
Tel: (505) 841-8340

NEW YORK
Executive Secretary
New York State Board for Nursing
State Education Department
Cultural Education Center
Room 9B30
Albany, New York 12230
Tel: (518) 474-6591

NORTH CAROLINA
Executive Director
North Carolina Board of Nursing
P.O. Box 2129
Raleigh, North Carolina 27602
Tel: (919) 782-3211

NORTH DAKOTA
Executive Director
North Dakota Board of Nursing
919 South 7th Street
Suite 504
Bismarck, North Dakota 58504
Tel: (701) 224-2974

NORTHERN MARIANA ISLANDS
Chairperson
Commonwealth Board of Nurse Examiners
Public Health Center

P.O. Box 1458
Saipan, MP 96950
Tel: (0-11-670) 234-8950
Ask for Public Health Center
Extension: 2018 or 2019
Telex No.: 783-744
Answer back code: PNESPN744

OHIO
Executive Director
Ohio Board of Nursing Education and Nurse
  Registration
77 South High Street
17th Floor
Columbus, Ohio 43266-0316
Tel: (614) 466-3947

OKLAHOMA
Executive Director
Oklahoma Board of Nurse Registration & Nursing
  Education
2915 North Classen Boulevard
Suite 524
Oklahoma City, Oklahoma 73106
Tel: (405) 525-2076

OREGON
Executive Director
Oregon State Board of Nursing
10445 S.W. Canyon Road, Suite 200
Beaverton, Oregon 97005
Tel: (503) 664-2767

PENNSYLVANIA
Executive Secretary
Pennsylvania Board of Nursing
Department of State
P.O. Box 2649
Harrisburg, Pennsylvania 17105
Tel: (717) 783-7142

RHODE ISLAND
Executive Secretary
Rhode Island Board of Nurse Registration &
  Nursing Education
Cannon Health Building
Three Capital Hill, Room 104
Providence, Rhode Island 02908-2488
Tel: (401) 277-2827

SOUTH CAROLINA
Executive Director
South Carolina State Board of Nursing
220 Executive Center Drive, Suite 220
Columbia, South Carolina 29210
Tel: (803) 731-1648

SOUTH DAKOTA
Executive Secretary
South Dakota Board of Nursing
3307 South Lincoln Avenue
Suite 205
Sioux Falls, South Dakota 57105-5224
Tel: (605) 335-4973

TENNESSEE
Executive Director
Tennessee State Board of Nursing
283 Plus Park Boulevard
Nashville, Tennessee 37247
Tel: (615) 367-6232

TEXAS
Executive Director
Texas Board of Vocational Nurse Examiners
9101 Burnet Road, Suite 105
Austin, Texas 78758
Tel: (512) 835-2071

Executive Secretary
Texas Board of Nurse Examiners (RN)
P.O. Box 140466
Austin, Texas 78714
Tel: (512) 835-8650

UTAH
Executive Secretary
Utah State Board of Nursing
Division of Occupational and Professional Licensing
P.O. Box 45805
Salt Lake City, Utah 84145-0805
Tel: (801) 530-6628

VERMONT
Executive Director
Vermont State Board of Nursing
Redstone Building
26 Terrace Street
Montpelier, Vermont 05602
Tel: (802) 828-2396

VIRGIN ISLANDS
Chairperson
Virgin Islands Board of Nursing
P.O. Box 4247
Charlotte Amalie
St. Thomas, Virgin Islands 00803
Tel: (809) 776-7397

VIRGINIA
Executive Director
Virginia State Board of Nursing
1601 Rolling Hills Drive

Richmond, Virginia 23229-5005
Tel: (804) 662-9909

WASHINGTON
Executive Secretary
Washington State Board of Practical Nursing
1300 Quince Street S.E., EY-28
Olympia, Washington 98504
Tel: (206) 753-2807

Executive Secretary
Washington State Board of Nursing (RN)
Department of Licensing
1300 Quince Street SE, MS:EY-28
Olympia, Washington 98504
Tel: (206) 753-2206

WEST VIRGINA
Executive Secretary
West Virginia State Board of Examiners for Practical
   Nurses
922 Quarrier Street
Embleton Building, Suite 506
Charleston, West Virginia 25301
Tel: (304) 348-3572

Executive Secretary
West Virginia Board of Examiners for Registered
   Nurses
922 Quarrier Street
Embleton Building, Suite 309
Charleston, West Virginia 25301
Tel: (304) 348-3596

WISCONSIN
Director
Wisconsin Bureau of Health Professions
1400 East Washington Ave.
P.O. Box 8935
Madison, Wisconsin 53708-8935
Tel: (608) 266-0257

WYOMING
Executive Director
Wyoming State Board of Nursing
Barrett Building, 4th Floor
2301 Central Avenue
Cheyenne, Wyoming 82002
Tel: (307) 777-7601

Canadian Nursing Assistant Jurisdictions

01 - MANITOBA
Executive Director
Manitoba Association of Licensed Practical Nurses
P.O. Box 249, Transcana
615 Kemaghan Avenue
Winnipeg, Manitoba
R2C 2Z4
(204) 222-6743

02 - ONTARIO
Director, Registration
College of Nurses of Ontario
101 Davenport Road
Toronto, Ontario
M5R 3P1
(416) 928-0900

03 - NEWFOUNDLAND
Registrar
Council for Nursing Assistants
LeMarchant Medical Centre
195 LeMarchant Road
St. John's, Newfoundland
A1C 2H5
(709) 579-3843

04 - SASKATCHEWAN
Executive Director
Saskatchewan Association of Certified Nursing
   Assistants
2310 Smith Street
Regina, Saskatchewan
S4P 2P6
(306) 525-1436

05 - NOVA SCOTIA
Executive Director
Board of Registration of Nursing Assistants
   of Nova Scotia
2021 Brunswick Street
Suite 404
Halifax, Nova Scotia
B3K 2Y5
(902) 423-8517

06 - ALBERTA
Executive Director/Registrar
Professional Council of Registered Nursing
   Assistants
10604 - 170th Street

Edmonton, Alberta
T5S 1P3
(403) 484-8886

07 - NEW BRUNSWICK

Registrar
Association of New Brunswick Registered Nursing
  Assistants
384 Smythe Street
Fredericton, New Brunswick
E3B 3E4
(506) 453-0747

08 - BRITISH COLUMBIA

Registrar
British Columbia Council of Licensed Practical
  Nurses
3405 Willingdon Avenue
Room B-118
Burnaby, British Columbia
V5G 3H4
(604) 660-5750

10 - PRINCE EDWARD ISLAND

Registrar
Prince Edward Island Nursing Assistants'
  Registration Board
P.O. Box 3235

Charlottetown, Prince Edward Island
C1A 7N9
(902) 566-1512

11 - NORTHWEST TERRITORIES

Registrar
Certification & Student Assistance Division
Department of Education
Government of the Northwest Territories
Yellowknife, Northwest Territories
X1A 2L9
(403) 873-7669

12 - YUKON

Registrar of Nursing Assistants
Justice Service Division
Consumer Services
P.O. Box 2703
Whitehorse, Yukon
Y1A 2C6
(403) 667-5811

Executive Director
Yukon Nurses Society
P.O. Box 5371
Whitehorse, Yukon
Y1A 4Z2
(403) 667-4062

Index